The ADA Practical Guide to Patients with Medical Conditions

Companion website

This book is accompanied by a companion website:

www.wiley.com/go/patton

The website includes:
- Webliography
- Powerpoints of all figures and tables from the book for downloading

The ADA Practical Guide to Patients with Medical Conditions

Edited by

Lauren L. Patton, DDS

WILEY-BLACKWELL
A John Wiley & Sons, Inc., Publication

ADA American Dental Association®
America's leading advocate for oral health

This edition first published 2012 © 2012 by American Dental Association

Wiley-Blackwell is an imprint of John Wiley & Sons, formed by the merger of Wiley's global Scientific, Technical and Medical business with Blackwell Publishing.

Editorial offices: 2121 State Avenue, Ames, Iowa 50014-8300, USA
The Atrium, Southern Gate, Chichester, West Sussex, PO19 8SQ, UK
9600 Garsington Road, Oxford, OX4 2DQ, UK

For details of our global editorial offices, for customer services and for information about how to apply for permission to reuse the copyright material in this book please see our website at www.wiley.com/wiley-blackwell.

Authorization to photocopy items for internal or personal use, or the internal or personal use of specific clients, is granted by Blackwell Publishing, provided that the base fee is paid directly to the Copyright Clearance Center, 222 Rosewood Drive, Danvers, MA 01923. For those organizations that have been granted a photocopy license by CCC, a separate system of payments has been arranged. The fee codes for users of the Transactional Reporting Service are ISBN-13: 978-1-1182-4530-9/2012.

Designations used by companies to distinguish their products are often claimed as trademarks. All brand names and product names used in this book are trade names, service marks, trademarks or registered trademarks of their respective owners. The publisher is not associated with any product or vendor mentioned in this book. This publication is designed to provide accurate and authoritative information in regard to the subject matter covered. It is sold on the understanding that the publisher is not engaged in rendering professional services. If professional advice or other expert assistance is required, the services of a competent professional should be sought.

Library of Congress Cataloging-in-Publication Data

The ADA practical guide to patients with medical conditions / edited by Lauren L. Patton.
    p. ; cm.
Practical guide to patients with medical conditions
Includes bibliographical references and index.
ISBN 978-1-118-24530-9 (pbk. : alk. paper)
I. Patton, Lauren L. II. American Dental Association. III. Title: Practical guide to patients with medical conditions.
[DNLM: 1. Dental Care. 2. Dental Care for Chronically Ill. 3. Medical History Taking.
4. Oral Manifestations. 5. Patient Care Planning. 6. Risk Assessment. WU 29]
617.6–dc23
                        2012009291

A catalogue record for this book is available from the British Library.

Wiley also publishes its books in a variety of electronic formats. Some content that appears in print may not be available in electronic books.

Set in 9.5/12 pt Palatino by Toppan Best-set Premedia Limited

Disclaimer

Publication of *The ADA Practical Guide to Patients with Medical Conditions* is offered as a resource tool for dentists and physicians, as well as other members of the health care team. It champions consultation with a patient's physician as indicated, in accordance with applicable law. This Practical Guide is not intended nor should be construed to set specific standards of care, or to provide legal or other professional advice, or to restrict a dentist's exercise of professional judgment in any given situation, with any given patient. Dentists should consult with their professional advisors for such advice.

The ADA, publishers, editors, authors and their employees, volunteers and agents disclaim all responsibility with any liability, loss, injury or damage resulting directly or indirectly from the reader's use and application of the information in this Practical Guide and make no representations or warranties with respect to the completeness, accuracy or any other quality of such information, including information or statements about products described herein.

To the extent that the information in this Practical Guide includes links to any web sites, the ADA, publishers, editors, authors, and their employees, volunteers, and agents intend no endorsement of their content and imply no affiliation with the organizations that provide their content. Nor do they make any representations or warranties about the information provided on those sites, which they do not control in any way.

The ADA, editors, and authors have produced this Practical Guide in their individual capacities and not on behalf of or the interest of any pharmaceutical companies or state or federal agencies.

The treatment and pharmacotherapy discussed in this Practical Guide should be undertaken within the bounds of applicable federal and state laws. Many of the proprietary names of the products in this Practical Guide are trademarked and registered in the U.S. Patent Office.

Printed and bound in Singapore by Markono Print Media Pte Ltd

Contents

Contributors — vii

Preface — xi

Acknowledgments — xiii

List of Common Drugs — xv

1. Medical History, Physical Evaluation, and Risk Assessment — 3
2. Cardiovascular Diseases — 25
3. Pulmonary Disease — 43
4. Endocrine and Metabolic Disorders — 69
5. Renal and Urinary Tract Disease — 95
6. Hepatic Disease — 115
7. Gastrointestinal Disease — 127
8. Hematological Disease — 143
9. Bleeding Disorders — 173
10. Autoimmune and Connective Tissue Diseases — 191

11.	HIV/AIDS and Related Conditions	217
12.	Immunological and Mucocutaneous Disease	243
13.	Head and Neck Cancer	257
14.	Neurological Disorders	281
15.	Neurodevelopmental and Psychiatric Disorders	305
16.	Substance Use Disorders	331
17.	Developmental Defects of the Craniofacial Complex and Orthopedic Disorders	357
18.	Geriatric Health and Functional Issues	381
19.	Women's Health	399
20.	Medical Emergencies	425
	Index	437

Companion website

This book is accompanied by a companion website:

www.wiley.com/go/patton

The website includes:
- Webliography
- Powerpoints of all figures and tables from the book for downloading

Contributors

Michael T. Brennan, DDS, MHS
Associate Chairman
Oral Medicine Residency Director
Department of Oral Medicine
Carolinas Medical Center
Charlotte, North Carolina

William M. Carpenter, DDS, MS
Professor and Chair Department of Pathology and Medicine
Pacific Oral & Maxillofacial Pathology
Arthur A. Dugoni School of Dentistry,
University of the Pacific
San Francisco, California

Katharine N. Ciarrocca, DMD, MSEd
Assistant Professor
Department of Oral Rehabilitation
Assistant Professor
Division of Geriatric Dentistry
Department of Oral Health and Diagnostic Sciences
Georgia Health Sciences University
College of Dental Medicine
Augusta, Georgia

Scott S. De Rossi, DMD
Associate Professor of Oral Medicine
Chair Department of Oral Health and Diagnostic Sciences
College of Dental Medicine, Georgia Health Sciences University
Augusta, Georgia

Bhavik Desai, PhD, DMD
Oral Medicine Resident
University of Pennsylvania, School of Dental Medicine
Philadelphia, Pennsylvania

Nancy J. Dougherty, DMD, MPH
Clinical Associate Professor
Director, Postgraduate Program in Pediatric Dentistry
Department of Pediatric Dentistry
New York University College of Dentistry
New York, New York

Joel B. Epstein, DMD, MSD, FRCD(C), FDS RCS (Edin)
Director, Oral Medicine Services, Adjunct Professor
Division of Otolaryngology and Head and Neck Surgery
City of Hope National Medical Center
Duarte, California and
Cedars-Sinai Medical Center
Los Angeles, California

Dena J. Fischer, DDS, MSD, MS
Assistant Professor
Department of Oral Medicine and Diagnostic Sciences
University of Illinois at Chicago
Chicago, Illinois

Robert G. Henry, DMD, MPH
Director of Geriatric Dental Services and Chief of Dentistry
Lexington Department of Veterans Affairs Medical Center and
Clinical Associate Professor
University of Kentucky, College of Dentistry
Lexington, Kentucky

Wendy S. Hupp, DMD
Assistant Professor of Oral Medicine
Department of General Dentistry and Oral Medicine
University of Louisville, School of Dentistry
Louisville, Kentucky

Bassam A. Issa, BDS
Oral Medicine Resident
Department of Oral Medicine
Carolinas Medical Center
Charlotte, North Carolina

Michael Milano, DMD
Clinical Associate Professor
Department of Pediatric Dentistry
School of Dentistry, University of North Carolina
Chapel Hill, North Carolina

Abdel R. Mohammad, DDS, MS, MPH
Professor of Geriatric Dentistry and Oral Medicine
Director of Tobacco Cessation and Geriatric Dentistry Programs
College of Dentistry, The Ohio State University
Columbus, Ohio

Brian C. Muzyka, DMD, MS, MBA
Associate Professor and Director of Hospital Dentistry
East Carolina University School of Dental Medicine
Greenville, North Carolina

Steven R. Nelson, DDS, MS
Private Practice
Oral and Maxillofacial Surgery
Denver, Colorado

Linda C. Niessen, DMD, MPH
Clinical Professor
Department of Restorative Sciences
Texas A&M Health Science Center
Baylor College of Dentistry
Dallas, Texas and
Vice President, Chief Clinical Officer
DENTSPLY International
York, Pennsylvania

Lauren L. Patton, DDS
Professor and Chair, Department of Dental Ecology
School of Dentistry, University of North Carolina
Chapel Hill, North Carolina

Luiz Andre Pimenta, DDS, MS, PhD
Clinical Professor, Department of Dental Ecology
Dental Director, UNC Craniofacial Center
School of Dentistry, University of North Carolina
Chapel Hill, North Carolina

Srinivasa Ramachandra, MD, BDS, FDS RCS (Eng)
Resident, General Surgery
Emory University School of Medicine
Atlanta, Georgia

Terry D. Rees, DDS, MSD
Professor, Department of Periodontics
Director of Stomatology
Baylor College of Dentistry
Texas A and M Health Science Center
Dallas, Texas

Miriam R. Robbins, DDS, MS
Director, Special Needs Clinic
Clinical Associate Professor and Associate Chair
Oral and Maxillofacial Pathology, Radiology and Medicine
New York University, College of Dentistry
New York, New York

Maureen Munnelly Romer, DDS, MPA
Associate Dean, Post-Doctoral Education
Associate Professor & Director, Special Care Dentistry
Arizona School of Dentistry and Oral Health
A.T. Still University
Mesa, Arizona

Steven M. Roser, DMD, MD, FACS
DeLos Hill Professor and Chief, Division of Oral and Maxillofacial Surgery
Emory University, School of Medicine
Atlanta, Georgia

Thomas P. Sollecito, DMD
Professor and Chair of Oral Medicine
University of Pennsylvania, School of Dental Medicine
Philadelphia, Pennsylvania

J. Timothy Wright, DDS, MS
Distinguished Professor and Chair
Department of Pediatric Dentistry
School of Dentistry, University of North Carolina
Chapel Hill, North Carolina

Janet A. Yellowitz, DMD, MPH
Director of Geriatric Dentistry
Associate Professor, Department of Periodontics
School of Dentistry, University of Maryland Baltimore
Baltimore, Maryland

Juan F. Yepes, DDS, MD, MPH, DrPH, MS
Associate Professor, Division of Pediatric Dentistry
Medical Institutional Review Board Vice-Chair
Department of Oral Health Practice
College of Dentistry, Chandler Medical Center
University of Kentucky
Lexington, Kentucky

Preface

In communities around the United States, dental practice is experiencing dramatic change influenced by scientific discoveries, new technologies, evolution of population demographics, changing health behaviors, and differential health-care access. Important trends include the aging and increasing diversity of the U.S. population; continued development of chronic diseases resulting from tobacco use, poor dietary habits, and inactivity; emerging and reemerging infectious diseases influenced by globalization; and growth in pharmaceutical research and drug development. The result is increasing health complexity of patients who seek care to prevent or manage their oral and medical health.

This *Practical Guide* has been developed to assist the health-care team in the safe delivery of coordinated oral health care for patients with medical conditions. Medical conditions included in the *Practical Guide* have been carefully chosen to include both common medical conditions and some less common conditions that present challenges for dental treatment planning. Dental treatment modifications should be considered when medical risk assessment suggests that adverse events may occur during or after dental treatment or for patients with significant health complexity. Many diseases, as well as some medical treatments, have oral manifestations that may reflect the patient's general health status. The dentist is particularly qualified and trained to diagnose and treat these oral conditions.

An advisory consultation between the dentist and physician is often beneficial to share information about the patient's oral and medical status and to coordinate care. Medical information obtained from such a consultation should be considered when developing the patient's treatment options. The chapter authors include contemporary information that can be applied in making evidence-based treatment decisions to assist in managing dental conditions in medically complex patients. It is ultimately the responsibility of the dentist to deliver safe and appropriate patient-focused oral health care.

This *Practical Guide* is an outgrowth of the Oral Health Care Series updated by expert consultants and members of the Oral Health Care Series Workgroup of ADA's Council on Access, Prevention and Interprofessional Relations (CAPIR). The goal of this *Practical Guide* is to provide information on treating patients with medical conditions to advance competent treatment and efficacious oral health outcomes.

There is a commitment to a patient-focused approach in collaboration with the patient's physician and other health-care providers.

In compiling information for this *Practical Guide*, the framework of risks of dental care, use of "Key Questions to Ask the Patient" and "Key Questions to Ask the Physician," and the overall organizational scheme for presentation of information within the chapters was the brainchild of the Oral Health Care Series Workgroup. A major strength of this book is that it is written by both academicians and clinicians who are experts in the content areas.

This *Practical Guide* is organized using a systems approach. With the exception of Chapter 1, "Medical History, Physical Evaluation, and Risk Assessment," Chapter 12, "Immunological and Mucocutaneous Disease," and Chapter 20, "Medical Emergencies," in each chapter, individual disorders are discussed under three major sections: **I. Background** (disease/condition description, pathogenesis/etiology, epidemiology, and coordination of care between dentist and physician), **II. Medical Management** (identification, medical history, physical examination, laboratory testing, and medical treatment), and **III. Dental Management** (evaluation, dental treatment modifications, oral lesion diagnosis and management, risks of dental care, special considerations, and, if applicable, medical emergencies). References and additional recommended readings are included. Key risks or concerns for dental care (*hemostasis, susceptibility to infection, drug actions/interactions*, and the *patient's ability to tolerate the stress of dental care*) are included to prompt the dentist to consider these particular elements of care provision. The *Practical Guide* includes illustrations, boxes, and tables that can be used as quick references.

All medical information gathering begins with a comprehensive medical and dental history. The included "Key Questions to Ask the Patient" and "Key Questions to Ask the Physician" are intended to serve as prompts for discussions held to gather additional disease-specific information. While tables of commonly used medications, drug interactions, and side effects are included in some chapters, the dentist is advised to keep abreast of the constantly changing scope and safety of medications with use of additional drug reference resources such as the *ADA/PDR Guide to Dental Therapeutics* or online resources.

Lauren L. Patton, DDS
University of North Carolina at Chapel Hill

Acknowledgments

I am deeply indebted to the distinguished chapter authors for so graciously sharing their expertise. Their generosity, persistence, and timely contributions have allowed this *Practical Guide* to become a reality under significant time pressure. I am grateful for the many individuals with medical conditions who served as photographic subjects for this *Practical Guide*. Without them, the authors and I would not have developed the clinical expertise that helps to inform our clinical practices. This *Practical Guide* is based on both our clinical experiences and our understanding of the scientific literature.

I wish to acknowledge the background work of the Oral Health Care Series Workgroup members: Steven R. Nelson, DDS, MS; Michael Glick, DMD; William M. Carpenter, DDS, MS; Steven M. Roser, DMD, MD, FACS; and Lauren L. Patton, DDS.

I would also like to acknowledge the ADA CAPIR Director, Lewis N. Lampiris, DDS, MPH, for his vision and advocacy that led to production of this *Practical Guide* and Senior Manager of CAPIR, Sheila A. Strock, DMD, MPH, for her steadfast oversight of the project and review of chapters in concert with the members of the Interprofessional Relations Subcommittee of CAPIR (Greg Baber, DMD; Melanie S. Lang, DDS, MD; David J. Miller, DDS; Todd A. Pankratz, MD, FACOG; Stacey Swilling, DDS; Philip H. Hunke, DDS; and John P. Fisher, DDS) who reviewed each chapter during the editorial process. I wish to thank Ms. Carolyn B. Tatar, Senior Manager of Product Development and Management at the ADA; Ms. Nancy Turner, Development Editor, Wiley-Blackwell, Ames, Iowa; and Ms. Sophia Joyce, Publisher, Health Sciences, Wiley-Blackwell, Oxford, UK, for their guidance, wisdom, and dedication to making this publication a success. The authors and I would also like to thank ADA President William R. Calnon, DDS for his leadership and commitment to the ADA's mission to advance the oral health of the public and focus on raising public awareness of the importance of oral health to overall health.

LLP

List of Common Drugs

Brand Name Drugs

Proprietary Name	Generic Name	Company	Headquarters Location (U.S. Location)	Chapter(s)
Abilify®	Aripiprazole	Bristol-Myers Squibb/ Otsuka America Pharmaceutical, Inc.	Princeton, NJ, USA	15
Aclasta®	Zolendronic acid	Novartis Pharmaceuticals Corp.	East Hanover, NJ, USA	19
Actonel®	Risedronate	Warner Chilcott Laboratories	Rockaway, NJ, USA	19
Adderall	Amphetamine and dextroamphetamine	Shire US, Inc.	Newport, KY, USA	15
Advair Diskus	Fluticasone/salmeterol	GlaxoSmithKline	Research Triangle Park, NC, USA	3
Agenerase	Amprenavir	GlaxoSmithKline	Research Triangle Park, NC, USA	11
Aggrenox	Extended release dipyrimadole and aspirin	Boehringer Ingelheim Pharmaceuticals	Ridgefield, CT, USA	9, 14
Amicar	ε-Aminocaproic acid	Xanodyne Pharmaceuticals	Newport, KY, USA	9

(Continued)

Proprietary Name	Generic Name	Company	Headquarters Location (U.S. Location)	Chapter(s)
Ammonia Inhalant Solution	Strong ammonia solution NF	James Alexander Corp.	Blairstown, NJ, USA	20
Amrix	Cyclobenzaprine	Cephalon, Inc.	West Chester, PA, USA	15
Antabuse	Disulfiram	Duramed Pharmaceuticals, Inc.	Pomona, NY, USA	16
Apidra	Insulin glulisine	Sanofi-Aventis, U.S.	Indianapolis, IN, USA	4
Aptivus	Tipranavir	Boehringer Ingelheim Pharmaceuticals	Ridgefield, CT, USA	11
Aredia	Pamidronate	Novartis Pharmaceuticals Corp.	East Hanover, NJ, USA	8, 19
Aricept	Donepezil	Eisai Co. Ltd and Pfizer	Woodcliff Lake, NJ, USA	18
Arixtra	Fondaparinux	GlaxoSmithKline	Research Triangle Park, NC, USA	9
Artane	Trihexyphenidyl HCL	Pfizer Labs	New York, NY, USA	14
Atelvia	Risedronate	Warner Chilcott Laboratories	Rockaway, NJ, USA	19
Ativan®	lorazepam	Biovail Pharmaceuticals, Inc.	Bridgewater, NJ, USA	3
Atrovent	Ipratropium bromide	Boehringer Ingelheim Pharmaceuticals	Ridgefield, CT, USA	3
Augmentin	Amoxicillin/clavulonate	GlaxoSmithKline	Research Triangle Park, NC, USA	11
Avitene	Microfibrillar collagen hemostat	C.R. Bard Inc./ Davol Inc.	Warick, RI, USA	9, 10
Avonex	Interferon beta-1a	Biogen IDEC, Inc	Cambridge, MA, USA	14
Benadryl	Diphenhydramine	McNeil- PPC, Inc.	Fort Washington, PA, USA	20
Betaseron	Interferon beta-1b	Bayer Healthcare Pharmaceuticals	Montville, NJ, USA	14
Bonefos	Clodronate	Bayer	Canada, EU, Australia	19
Boniva	Ibandonate	Roche Laboratories	Nutley, NJ, USA	19
Botox	Onabotulinumtoxin A	Allergan	Irvine, CA, USA	15
Campral	Acamprosate	Forest Laboratories	St. Louis, MO, USA	16
Carbatrol	Carbamazepine	Shire US, Inc.	Newport, KY, USA	15
Celexa	Citalopram	Forest Laboratories, Inc.	St. Louis, MO, USA	15
Cleocin	Clindamycin	Pfizer Labs	New York, NY, USA	11

Proprietary Name	Generic Name	Company	Headquarters Location (U.S. Location)	Chapter(s)
Clozaril	Clozapine	Novartis Pharmaceuticals Corp.	East Hanover, NJ, USA	15
Cogentin	Benztropine mesylate	Lundbeck Inc.	Deerfield, IL, USA	14
Cognex	Tacrine	Shionogi Inc.	Florham Park, NJ, USA	18
Collaplug	Type 1 bovine collagen hemostat	Zimmer Dental	Carlsbad, CA, USA	10
Combivent	Ipratropium/albuterol	Boehringer Ingelheim Pharmaceuticals	Ridgefield, CT, USA	3
Combivir	Zidovudine and lamivudine	GlaxoSmithKline	Research Triangle Park, NC, USA	11
Complera	Emtricitabine, tilpivirine, and tenofovir	Gilead Sciences, Inc.	Foster City, CA, USA	11
Comtan	Entacapone	Novartis Pharmaceuticals Corp.	East Hanover, NJ, USA	14
Concerta	Methylphenidate	Janssen Pharmaceuticals, Inc.	Titusville, NJ, USA	15
Copaxone	Glatiramir acetate injection	Teva Neuroscience, Inc.	Kansas City, MO, USA	14
Coumadin	Warfarin	Bristol-Myers Squibb	Princeton, NJ, USA	2, 9
Crixivan	Indinavir	Merck & Co., Inc.	Whitehouse Station, NJ, USA	11
Cyklokapron	Tranexamic acid	Pfizer Labs	New York, NY, USA	9
Dantrium	Dantrolene	Proctor & Gamble Pharmaceuticals	Mason, OH, USA	15
Decadron	Dexamethasone	Various		11
Deltasone®	prednisone	Various		11
Depade	Naltrexone	Mallinckrodt Inc. Pharmaceuticals Group	St. Louis, MO, USA	16
Depakene	Valproic acid	Abbott Laboratories	Abbott Park, IL, USA	14
Depakote	Divalproex sodium	Abbott Laboratories	Abbott Park, IL, USA	14
Detrol LA	Tolterodine tartrate	Pfizer Pharmacia & Upjohn	New York, NY, USA	14
Dexedrine	Dextroamphetamine	GlaxoSmithKline	Research Triangle Park, NC, USA	15
Didronel	Etidronate	Warner Chilcott Laboratories	Rockaway, NJ, USA	19

(Continued)

Proprietary Name	Generic Name	Company	Headquarters Location (U.S. Location)	Chapter(s)
Diflucan	Fluconazole	Pfizer Labs	New York, NY, USA	11
Dilantin	Phenytoin	Parke-Davis Division of Pfizer Inc.	New York, NY, USA	14
Ditropan XL	Oxybutynin	Alza Corporation	Palo Alto, CA, USA	14
Edurant	Rilpivirine	Tibotec Pharmaceuticals	Raritan, NJ, USA	11
Effexor	Venlafaxine	Pfizer Labs	New York, NY, USA	15
Effient	Prosugrel	Eli Lilly and Corp.	Indianapolis, IN, USA	9
Elavil	Amitriptyline	AstraZeneca LP	Wilmington, DE, USA	14, 15, 19
Eldepryl	Selegiline	Somerset Pharmaceuticals, Inc.	Tampa, FL, USA	14
Emtriva	Emtricitabine	Gilead Sciences, Inc.	Foster City, CA, USA	11
EpiPen Auto-Injector	Epinephrine	Dey Pharma, L.P.	Napa, CA, USA	20
Epivir	Lamivudine	GlaxoSmithKline	Research Triangle Park, NC, USA	11
Epzicom	Abacavir and lamivudine	GlaxoSmithKline	Research Triangle Park, NC, USA	11
Exelon	Rivastigmine	Novartis Pharmaceuticals Corp.	East Hanover, NJ, USA	18
Famvir	Famciclovir	Novartis Pharmaceuticals Corp.	East Hanover, NJ, USA	11
Fazaclo	Clozapine	Azur Pharma, Inc.	Philadelphia, PA, USA	15
Flagyl	Metronidazole	Pfizer Labs	New York, NY, USA	11
Flexeril	Cyclobenzaprine	McNeil- PPC, Inc.	Fort Washington, PA, USA	15
Fosamax	Alendronate	Merck & Co., Inc.	Whitehouse Station, NJ, USA	19
Fragmin	Dalteprin	Eisai Inc. and Pfizer Inc.	Woodcliff Lake, NJ, USA and New York, NY, USA	9
Fuzeon	Enfuviritide	Hoffman-La Roche Inc./Genentech USA, Inc.	South San Francisco, CA, USA	11
Gablofen	Baclofen	CNS Therapeutics	St. Paul, MN, USA	15
Gelfoam	Absorbable gelatin sponge	Baxter Healthcare Corp. or Pfizer Inc.	Hayward, CA, USA	9, 10, 14
Geodon	Ziparsidone	Pfizer Labs	New York, NY, USA	15

Proprietary Name	Generic Name	Company	Headquarters Location (U.S. Location)	Chapter(s)
Gleevec	Imatinib mesylate	Novartis Pharmaceuticals Corp.	East Hanover, NJ, USA	8
Haldol	Halperidol	Janssen Pharmaceuticals, Inc.	Titusville, NJ, USA	15
Humalog	Insulin lispro	Ely Lilly USA LLC	Indianapolis, IN, USA	4
Instat MHC	Microfibrillar collagen hemostat	Ethicon, Inc., a J & J Company	Somerville, NJ, USA	9
Intelence	Etravirine	Janssen Therapeutics	Titusville, NJ, USA	11
Invirase	Saquinavir	Genentech, Inc.	South San Francisco, CA, USA	11
Isentress	Raltegravir	Merck & Co., Inc.	Whitehouse Station, NJ, USA	11
Kaletra	Lopinavir and ritonavir	Abbott Laboratories	Abbott Park, IL, USA	11
Kaopectate®	bismuth subsalicylate	Chattem, Inc.	Chattanooga, TN, USA	13
Kenalog	Triamcinalone acetonide	Bristol-Myers Squibb	Princeton, NJ, USA	11
Klonopin	Clonazepam	Roche Laboratories	Nutley, NJ, USA	14, 19
Lamictal	Lamotrigine	GlaxoSmithKline	Research Triangle Park, NC, USA	14, 15
Lantus	Insulin glargine	Sanofi-Aventis, U.S.	Bridgewater, NJ, USA	4
Lexapro	Escitalopram	Forest Laboratories, Inc.	St. Louis, MO, USA	15
Lexiva	Fosamprenavir	GlaxoSmithKline	Research Triangle Park, NC, USA	11
Lidex	Fluocinonide	Medicis Pharmceuticals Corp.	Scottsdale, AZ, USA	11
Lioresal	Baclofen	Various		15
Lithobid	Lithium	Noven Therapeutics	Miami, FL, USA	15
Lovenox	Enoxaprin	Sanofi-Aventis, U.S.	Bridgewater, NJ, USA	9
Luvox	Fluvosamine	Jazz Pharmaceuticals	Palo Alto, CA, USA	15
Maalox®	aluminum hydrochloride	Novartis Consumer Health	East Hanover, NJ, USA	13
Mirapex	Pramipexole	Boehringer Ingelheim Pharmaceuticals	Ridgefield, CT, USA	14
Mycelex	Clotrimazole	Janssen Pharmaceuticals, Inc.	Titusville, NJ, USA	11
Mycolog II	Nystatin-triamcinalone acetonide	Various		11

(Continued)

Proprietary Name	Generic Name	Company	Headquarters Location (U.S. Location)	Chapter(s)
Mycostatin suspension	Nystatin	Bristol-Myers Squibb	Princeton, NJ, USA	11
Namenda	Mematine	Forest Laboratories, Inc.	New York, NY, USA	18
Narcan	Naloxone	Endo Pharmaceuticals	Chadds Ford, PA, USA	16
Neurontin	Gabapentin	Pfizer Labs	New York, NY, USA	19
Nicorette	Nicotine polacrilex	GlaxoSmithKline	Research Triangle Park, NC, USA	16
Nizoral	Ketoconazole	Janssen Pharmaceuticals, Inc.	Titusville, NJ, USA	11
Normiflo	Ardeparin	Wyeth-Ayerst Laboratories	Philadelphia, PA, USA	9
Norvir	Ritonavir	Abbott Laboratories	Abbott Park, IL, USA	11
Novantrone	Mitoxantron	EMD Serano, Inc.	Rockland, MA, USA	14
Novolog	Insulin aspart (rDNA) injection	Novo Nordisk	Bagsvaerd, Denmark (Princeton, NJ, USA)	4
Orabase®	preparation for mouth	Colgate-Palmolive Co.	New York, NY, USA	11, 12
Oravig	Miconazole buccal tablet	Strativa Pharmaceuticals	Woodclifff Lake, NJ, USA	11
Parlodel	Bromocriptine	Novartis Pharmaceuticals Corp.	East Hanover, NJ, USA	14
Peridex	0.12% chlorhexidine	Zila, Inc.	Phoenix, AZ, USA	11
Periogard	0.12% chlorhexidine	Colgate-Palmolive	New York, NY, USA	11
Permitil	Fluphenazine	Various		15
Persantine	Dipyridamole	Boehringer Ingelheim Pharmaceuticals	Ridgefield, CT, USA	9
Plavix	Clopidogrel	Sanofi-Aventis, U.S.	Bridgewater, NJ, USA	9, 14
Pradaxa	Dabigatran	Boehringer Ingelheim Pharmaceuticals	Ridgefield, CT, USA	9, 14
Prezista	Darunavir	Janssen Therapeutics	Titusville, NJ, USA	11
Procrit	Epoetin alpha	Amgen Inc.	Thousand Oaks, CA, USA	5
Prolia	Densumab	Amgen Inc.	Thousand Oaks, CA, USA	19
Prolixin	Fluphenazine	Various		15
Proventil	Albuterol FHA inhalation aerosol	Schering-Plough Corp.	Kenilworth, NJ, USA	3, 20
Prozac	Fluoxetine HCL	Lilly USA, LLC	Indianapolis, IN, USA	14, 15
Pulmicort	Budesonide	AstraZeneca LP	Wilmington, DE, USA	3
Qvar	Beclomethasone	Teva Respiratory LLC	Horsham, PA, USA	3

Proprietary Name	Generic Name	Company	Headquarters Location (U.S. Location)	Chapter(s)
Razadyne	Glantamine	Janssen Pharmaceuticals, Inc.	Titusville, NJ, USA	18
Reclast	Zolendronic acid	Novartis Pharmaceuticals Corp.	East Hanover, NJ, USA	19
Rebif	Interferon beta-1a	EMD Serano, Inc.	Rockland, MA, USA	14
Requip	Ropinirole HCl	GlaxoSmithKline	Research Triangle Park, NC, USA	14
Rescriptor	Delaviridine	Pfizer Labs	New York, NY, USA	11
Retrovir	Zidovudine	GlaxoSmithKline	Research Triangle Park, NC, USA	11
ReVia	Naltrexone	Duramed Pharmaceuticals, Inc.	Pomona, NY, USA	16
Reyataz	Atazanavir	Bristol-Myers Squibb	Princeton, NJ, USA	11
Risperdal	Risperdone	Janssen Pharmaceuticals, Inc.	Titusville, NJ, USA	15
Ritalin	Methylphenidate	Novartis Pharmaceuticals Corp.	East Hanover, NJ, USA	15
Sarafem	Fluoxetine HCL	Warner Chilcott Laboratories	Rockaway, NJ, USA	15
Selzentry	Miraviroc	Pfizer Labs	New York, NY, USA	11
Seroquel	Quetiapine	AstraZeneca Pharmceuticals	Wilmington, NC, USA	15
Sinemet CR	Carbidopa/levodopa	Merck & Co., Inc.	Whitehouse Station, NJ, USA	14
Singulair	Montelukast	Merck & Co., Inc.	Whitehouse Station, NJ, USA	3
Skelid	Clodronate	Sanofi Aventis	Bridgewater, NJ, USA	19
Spiriva	Tiotropium	Boehringer Ingelheim Pharmaceuticals	Ridgefield, CT, USA	3
Sporanox	Itraconazole	Janssen Pharmaceuticals, Inc.	Titusville, NJ, USA	11
Stimate	Desmopressin acetate nasal spray	CSL Behring	King of Prussia, PA, USA	9
Strattera	Atomoxetine	Eli Lilly and Corp.	Indianapolis, IN, USA	15
Suboxone	Buprenorphine	Reckitt Benckiser Pharmaceuticals, Inc.	Richmond, VA, USA	16

(Continued)

Proprietary Name	Generic Name	Company	Headquarters Location (U.S. Location)	Chapter(s)
Subutex	Buprenorphine	Reckitt Benckiser Pharmaceuticals, Inc.	Richmond, VA, USA	16
Surgicel	Fibrillar absorbable hemostat	Ethicon, Inc., a J & J Company	Somerville, NJ, USA	9, 10
Sustiva	Efavirenz	Bristol-Myers Squibb	Princeton, NJ, USA	11
Symbicort	Budesonide/formoterol	AstraZeneca LP	Wilmington, DE, USA	3
Symmetrel	Amantadine	Endo Pharmceuticals	Chadds Ford, PA, USA	14
Synthroid	Levothyroxine	Abbott Laboratories	Abbott Park, IL, USA	4
Tapazole	Methimazole	King Pharmaceuticals, Inc.	Bristol, TN, USA	4
Tasmar	Tolcapone	Valeant Pharmceuticals, Inc.	Costa Mesa, CA, USA	14
Tegretol	Carbamazepine	Novartis Pharmaceuticals Corp.	East Hanover, NJ, USA	14, 15
Temovate	Clobetasol proprionate	PharmDerma	Florham Park, NJ, USA	11
Thalomid	Thalidomide	Celgene Corp.	Warren, NJ, USA	11
Thorazine	Chlorpromazine	Various		15
Ticlid	Ticlopidine	Roche Laboratories	Nutley, NJ, USA	9
Tofranil	Imipramine	Mallinckrodt Inc Pharmaceuticals Group	St. Louis, MO, USA	15
Topamax	Topiramate	Janssen Pharmaceuticals, Inc.	Titusville, NJ, USA	14
Trilafon	Perphenazine	Various		15
Trizavir	Zidovudine, abacavir, and lamivudine	GlaxoSmithKline	Research Triangle Park, NC, USA	11
Truvada	Emtricitabine and tenofovir	Gilead Sciences, Inc.	Foster City, CA, USA	11
Valtrex	Valacyclovir	GlaxoSmithKline	Research Triangle Park, NC, USA	11
Ventilin	Albuterol	GlaxoSmithKline	Research Triangle Park, NC, USA	3
Versed	Midazolam	Roche Laboratories	Nutley, NJ, USA	14
Videx	Didanosine	Bristol-Myers Squibb	Princeton, NJ, USA	11
Viracept	Nelfinavir	Agouron Pharmaceuticals	La Jolla, CA, USA	11
Viramune	Nevirapine	Boehringer Ingelheim Pharmaceuticals	Ridgefield, CT, USA	11

Proprietary Name	Generic Name	Company	Headquarters Location (U.S. Location)	Chapter(s)
Viread	Tenofovir	Gilead Sciences, Inc.	Foster City, CA, USA	11
Vivitrol	Naloxone	Alkermes	Cambridge, MA, USA	16
Wellbutrin	Bupropion	GlaxoSmithKline	Research Triangle Park, NC, USA	15
Xarelto	Rivaroxaban	Janssen Pharmaceuticals, Inc.	Titusville, NJ, USA	9
Xgeva	Densumab	Amgen Inc.	Thousand Oaks, CA, USA	19
Zanaflex	Tizanidine	Acorda Therapeutics	Hawthorne, NY, USA	14
Zarontin	Ethosuximide	Pfizer Labs	New York, NY, USA	14
Zelapar	Selegiline	Valeant Pharmceuticals, Inc.	Costa Mesa, CA, USA	14
Zerit	Stavudine	Bristol-Myers Squibb	Princeton, NJ, USA	11
Ziagen	Abacavir	GlaxoSmithKline	Research Triangle Park, NC, USA	11
Zoloft	Sertraline	Pfizer Labs	New York, NY, USA	15
Zometa	Zolendronic acid	Novartis Pharmaceuticals Corp.	East Hanover, NJ, USA	8, 19
Zovirax	Acyclovir	GlaxoSmithKline	Research Triangle Park, NC, USA	11
Zyban	Bupropion	GlaxoSmithKline	Research Triangle Park, NC, USA	15, 16
Zyprexa	Olanzapine	Eli Lilly and Corp.	Indianapolis, IN, USA	15

(Resources: Monthly Prescribing Reference® available at: www.empr.com; company websites)

The ADA Practical Guide to Patients with Medical Conditions

Medical History, Physical Evaluation, and Risk Assessment

Lauren L. Patton DDS

I. Background

The U.S. and global population demographics are constantly changing, chronic diseases are becoming more prevalent, new medications are being developed and brought to the market, and new and reemerging infectious diseases are being identified. These trends result in more patients seeking oral health care who have underlying medical conditions that may alter oral health status, treatment approaches, and outcomes. The challenges of medical history information gathering and risk assessment required for safe dental treatment planning and care delivery will be discussed and presented in a practical manner applicable to day-to-day needs of the general practice dentist. There are four key considerations that serve as a framework for assessing and managing the risks of dental care used in this book, although additional considerations may be relevant for certain medical conditions. The key considerations are hemostasis, susceptibility to infections, drug actions/interactions, and ability to tolerate the stress of dental care. The potential for the dental practice to encounter different types of medical emergencies is related to the patient's medical health, adequacy of management, and stress tolerance.

Four key risks of dental care
- Hemostasis
- Susceptibility to infections
- Drug actions/interactions
- Patient's ability to tolerate dental care

II. Medical History

A medical history can be recorded by the patient in advance of the dental appointment and reviewed by providers seeking clarification of patient responses. In the national shift to electronic health records, medical history, medications, and allergies may be recorded in a number of data collection formats and in a variety of settings, including use of web-based applications. Personal information should be kept private and shared only in compliance with privacy rules.

The ADA Practical Guide to Patients with Medical Conditions, First Edition. Edited by Lauren L. Patton.
© 2012 American Dental Association. Published 2012 by John Wiley & Sons, Inc.

Figure 1.1 ADA Health History Forms. (a) Adult form S500 page 1, copyright 2007; (b) adult form S500 page 2, copyright 2007. Please see companion website (www.wiley.com/go/patton) for full-sized forms.

An example is the American Dental Association (ADA) Health History Form (see Fig. 1.1; available at http://www.ada.org), which is comprised of the following:

- demographic information;
- screening questions for active tuberculosis;
- dental information;
- medical information, including physician contact information;
- hospitalizations, illnesses, and surgeries;
- modified review of systems and diseases survey;
- medications (prescribed, over-the-counter and natural remedies, including oral and intravenous bisphosphonates);
- substance use history, including tobacco, alcohol, and controlled substances;
- allergies;
- a query about prosthetic joint replacements and any prior antibiotic recommendations by a physician or dentist and name and contact phone number of recommending provider;
- a query about the four cardiac disease conditions recommended for antibiotic coverage for prevention of infective endocarditis;
- a query of women about current pregnancy, nursing status, or birth control pills or hormonal therapy.

There is a Child Health/Dental History Form (see Fig. 1.2) also available from the ADA that focuses on inherited, developmental, infectious, and acquired diseases of importance to dental health-care delivery for children.

Family history can facilitate awareness of need to screen for and engage in prevention

Figure 1.2 ADA Child Health/Dental History Form S707, copyright 2006.

efforts for common diseases such as heart disease, cancer, diabetes, and rarer diseases including hemophilia, sickle cell anemia, and cystic fibrosis. The Surgeon General has created a family health history initiative to facilitate family discussion of inherited diseases. This free tool found at https://familyhistory.hhs.gov will allow patients and providers to download the form to gather relevant health information for patients to share with providers. Whether disease etiology derives from genetics, environment, learned behaviors, or a combination of factors, many health conditions, such as propensity to hypertension, may run in families.

III. Physical Evaluation and Medical Risk Assessment

The initial and ongoing assessment of patient medical risk in dental practice has several purposes:

- To minimize risk of adverse events in the dental office resulting from dental treatment.
- To identify patients who need further medical assessment and management.
- To identify patients for whom specific perioperative therapies or treatment modifications will minimize risk, including postponing elective treatment.
- To identify appropriate anesthetic technique, intraprocedure monitoring, and postprocedure management.
- To discuss treatment procedures with patients, outlining risks and benefits, in order to obtain informed consent and determine need for additional anxiolysis.

One of the most common medical risk assessment frameworks is the American Society of Anesthesiologists (ASA) Physical Status Score[1] used to classify patients for anesthesia risk (Table 1.1). A medical risk-related health history is important to detect medical problems in patients. While across all ages most (78%) dental patients are healthy ASA 1 patients, the percentage that is of higher ASA physical status (ASA 2–ASA 6) increases with increasing age.[2] By age 65, only 55% of adults remain healthy ASA 1. Medical conditions such as cardiovascular disease and hypertension account for a high proportion of ASA 3 and ASA 4 patients.

Up to a third of dental patients who answer yes to "Are you in good health?" on verification are found to be medically compromised.[3] In a survey of dental patients completing health history forms based on the ADA Health History Form available at the time, the diseases most inaccurately reported or omitted were blood disorders, cardiovascular disease, and diabetes.[3] The authors concluded that using both a self-administered questionnaire and dialog on the health history might improve communication.

There are several physical signs or clues that indicate a patient who reports having received no medical care might not truly be healthy, but rather simply not accessing medical care:

Table 1.1. American Society of Anesthesiology (ASA) Physical Status Classification, Activity Characteristics/Treatment Risk, and Medical Examples

ASA Physical Status	Activity Characteristics/Treatment Risk	Medical Examples
ASA 1 A normal healthy patient.	• Patient is able to walk up one flight of stairs or two-level city blocks without distress. • Little of no anxiety. • Little or no risk during treatment.	• Healthy 20-year-old.
ASA 2 A patient with mild systemic disease.	• Patient has mild to moderate systemic disease or is a healthy ASA 1 patient who demonstrated a more extreme anxiety and fear toward dentistry. • Patient is able to walk up one flight of stairs or two-level city blocks, but will have to stop after completion of the exercise because of distress. • Minimal risk during treatment.	• ASA 1 with respiratory condition, active allergies, dental phobia, or pregnancy. • Well diet or oral hypoglycemic agent—controlled diabetic. • Well-controlled asthmatic. • Well-controlled epileptic. • Well-controlled hypertensive not on medication.
ASA 3 A patient with severe systemic disease.	• Patient has severe systemic disease that limits activity, but is not incapacitating. • Patient is able to walk up one flight of stairs or two-level city blocks, but will have to stop on the way because of distress. • If dental care is indicated, stress reduction protocol and other treatment modifications are indicated.	• Well-controlled hypertensive on medication. • Well-controlled diabetic on insulin. • Slight chronic obstructive pulmonary disease. • Six or more months ago history of myocardial infarction, cerebrovascular accident, or congestive heart failure.
ASA 4 A patient with severe systemic disease that is a constant threat to life.	• Patient has severe systemic disease that limits activity and is a constant threat to life. • Patient is unable to walk up one flight of stairs or two-level city blocks. Distress is present even at rest. • Patient poses significant risk during treatment. • Elective dental care should be postponed until such time as the patient's medical condition has improved to at least an ASA 3 classification. • Emergent dental care may be best provided in a hospital setting in consultation with the patient's physician team.	• History of unstable angina, myocardial infarction, or cerebrovascular accident in the last 6 months. • Severe congestive heart failure. • Moderate to severe chronic obstructive pulmonary disease. • Uncontrolled hypertension. • Uncontrolled diabetes. • Uncontrolled epilepsy or seizure disorder.
ASA 5 A moribund patient who is not expected to survive without the operation.	• Hospitalized patient in critical condition. • Emergency dental care to eliminate acute oral disease is provided only when deemed a component of lifesaving surgery.	• Terminal illness often of acute onset.
ASA 6 A declared brain-dead patient whose organs are being removed for donor purposes.	• Dental care not warranted.	• Brain-dead.

- age over 40 years,
- obese or cachectic body habitus,
- low energy level,
- abnormal skin coloration,
- poor oral hygiene,
- tobacco smoking.

Often the patient's response to the question "Can you walk up two flights of stairs without stopping to catch your breath?" can indicate general cardiovascular and pulmonary health status.

Vital signs, including blood pressure and heart rate (pulse), should be assessed at each visit. The other vital signs of temperature, respiration rate, and pain score may be useful additional signs of current health. A focused review of systems should allow a cursory review of the patient's recent state of health, focusing on recent changes and tailored to the patient and planned dental procedure(s).

Brief review of systems

- **General:** fever, chills, night sweats, weakness, fatigue
- **Cardiovascular:** reduced exercise tolerance, chest pain, orthopnea, ankle swelling, claudication
- **Pulmonary:** upper respiratory infection symptoms—productive cough, bronchitis, wheezing
- **Hematological:** bruising, epistaxis
- **Neurological:** mental status changes, transient ischemic attacks, numbness, paresis
- **Endocrine:** polydipsia, polyuria, polyphagia, weigh gain/loss

---

Under each medical topic, we present "key questions to ask the patient" to allow improved risk assessment and determination of dental treatment modifications.

Communication with the Patient's Physician

The dentist should consult with the patient's physician to clarify areas of the patient's health that are unclearly communicated by the patient who is a poor historian or where a reported medical condition is monitored and the patient does not have complete information. This includes consultations about current laboratory assessments, prescribed medications and other medical and surgical therapies, and coordination of care. Under each medical topic, we present "key questions to ask the physician" to facilitate improved communication and coordination of care.

Influence of Systemic Disease on Oral Disease and Health

The health history should give the dentist an appreciation of oral conditions that may have a systemic origin and thus require systemic management as an aspect of treatment. Several abnormal signs and symptoms in the facial region, oral structures, and teeth with systemic origin are listed in Table 1.2 and illustrated in Figs. 1.3–1.6.

The astute dental provider also has the opportunity to observe physical and oral conditions that might indicate undiagnosed or poorly managed systemic disease. Examples are oral candidiasis that might indicate a poorly controlled immune suppressing medical condition, significant inflammatory periodontal disease as an indicator of poorly controlled diabetes, gingival enlargements that are leukemic infiltrates, or mucosal pallor indicating an anemia. Tooth erosion in adolescent females might raise suspicion for an eating disorder such as bulimia. Acutely declining oral hygiene and self-care in the elderly might indicate physical disability or

Table 1.2. Facial, Oral, and Dental Signs Possibly Related to Medical Disease or Therapy

	Possible Causative Medical Disease or Therapy
	Facial signs
Cachexia	Wasting from cancer, malnutrition, HIV/AIDS
Cushingoid facies	Cushing syndrome, steroid use
Jaundiced skin/sclera	Liver cirrhosis
Malar rash	Systemic lupus erythematosus
Ptosis	Myasthenia gravis
Taught skin and microstomia	Scleroderma, facial burns
Telangiectasias	Liver cirrhosis
Weak facial musculature	Neurological disorder, facial nerve palsy, tardive dyskinesia, myasthenia gravis
	Oral signs
Bleeding, ecchymosis, petechiae	Thrombocytopenia, thrombocytopathy, hereditary coagulation disorder, liver cirrhosis, aplastic anemia, leukemia, vitamin deficiency, drug induced
Burning mouth/tongue	Anemia, vitamin deficiency, candida infection, salivary hypofunction, primary or secondary neuropathy
Dentoalveolar trauma	Interpersonal violence, accidental trauma, seizure disorder, gait/balance instability, alcoholism
Drooling	Neoplasm, neurologic–amyotrophic lateral sclerosis, Parkinson's disease cerebrovascular accident, cerebral palsy, medications (e.g., tranquilizers, anticonvulsants, anticholinesterases)
Dry mucosa	Drug-induced xerostomia, salivary hypofunction from Sjögren's syndrome, diabetes, or head and neck cancer radiation therapy
Gingival overgrowth	Leukemia, drug induced (phenytoin, cyclosporine, calcium channel blockers)
Hard tissue enlargements	Neoplasm, acromegaly, Paget's disease, hyperparathyroidism
Mucosal discoloration or hyperpigmentation	Addison's disease, lead poisoning, liver disease, melanoma, drug induced (e.g., zidovudine, tetracycline, oral contraceptives, quinolones)
Mucosal erythema and ulceration	Cancer chemotherapy, uremic stomatitis, autoimmune disorders (systemic lupus, Bechet's syndrome), vitamin deficiency, celiac disease, Crohn's disease, drug induced, self-injurious behavior
Mucosal pallor	Anemia, vitamin deficiency

Table 1.2. (*Continued*)

	Possible Causative Medical Disease or Therapy
Nondental source oral/jaw pain	Referred pain (e.g., cardiac, neurological, musculoskeletal) including myofascial and temporomandibular joints, drug induced (e.g., vincristine chemotherapy), primary neoplasms, cancer metastases, sickle cell crisis pain, primary or secondary neuropathies
Opportunistic infections	Immune suppression (from HIV, cancer chemotherapy, hematological malignancy, primary immune deficiency syndromes), poorly controlled diabetes, stress
Oral malodor	Renal failure, respiratory infections, gastrointestinal conditions
Osteonecrosis	Radiation to the jaw, use of bisphosphonates and other bone-modifying agents
Poor wound healing	Immune suppression (from HIV, cancer chemotherapy, primary immune deficiency syndromes), poorly controlled diabetes, malnutrition, vitamin deficiency
Soft tissue swellings	Neoplasms, amyloidosis, hemangioma, lymphangioma, acromegaly, interpersonal violence or accidental trauma
Trismus	Neoplasm, postradiation therapy, arthritis, posttraumatic mandible condyle fracture
Dental signs	
Early loss of teeth	Neoplasms, nutritional deficiency (e.g., hypophosphatemic vitamin-D-resistant rickets, scurvy), hypophosphatasia, histiocytosis X, Hand–Schüller–Christian disease, Papillon–Lefevre syndrome, acrodynia, juvenile-onset diabetes, immune suppression (e.g., cyclic neutropenia, chronic neutropenia), interpersonal violence or other traumatic injury, radiation therapy to the jaw, dentin dysplasia, Trisomy 21-Down syndrome, early-onset periodontitis
Rampant dental caries	Salivary hypofunction from disease (e.g., Sjögren's syndrome), post radiation, or xerogenic medications; illegal drug use (e.g., methamphetamines); inability to cooperate with oral hygiene and diet instructions
Tooth discoloration	Genetic defects in enamel or dentin (e.g., amelogenesis imperfecta, dentinogenesis imperfect), porphyria, hyperbilirubinemia, drug induced (e.g., tetracycline)
Tooth enamel erosion	Gastroesophageal reflux disease, bulimia nervosa

Figure 1.3 Cachexia due to HIV wasting syndrome.

Figure 1.5 Taught facial skin and microstomia due to systemic sclerosis (scleroderma).

Figure 1.4 Cushingoid faces and malar rash due to systemic lupus erythematosus and chronic steroid use.

Figure 1.6 Facial port-wine stain of Sturge–Weber syndrome (encephalotrigeminal angiomatosis).

mental decline with dementia onset. On panoramic radiographs, carotid artery calcifications may be detected that correlate with hypertension, hyperlipidemia, and heart disease, and may warrant patient referral for further medical evaluation.[4] Dental radiographic signs suggestive of systemic disease or therapy are shown in Table 1.3.

Table 1.3. Dental Radiographic Signs Suggestive of Medical Disease or Therapy

Dental Radiographic Signs	Possible Causative Medical Disease or Therapy
Carotid artery calcification	Carotid arteritis, stroke or transient ischemic attack-related disease, hypertension, hyperlipidemia, heart disease
Condyle/temporomandibular joint (TMJ) articular space destruction	Rheumatoid arthritis, osteoarthritis
Marrow hyperplasia, increased spacing of bony trabeculae, generalized radiolucency	Sickle cell anemia, osteopenia, osteoporosis, malnutrition, secondary hyperparathyroidism from renal disease—renal osteodystrophy
Marrow hypoplasia, generalized increased density-radiopacity	Osteopetrosis, Paget's disease, hypoparathyroidism
Reduced cortical bone density	Primary hyperparathyroidism
Resorption of angle of the mandible	Scleroderma
Well-defined radiolucencies not associated with teeth	Neoplasms, multiple myeloma, metastatic cancer

Framework for Key Risks of Dental Care

The scope of dental practice is wide, encompassing aspects of both medicine and surgery. Dental care plans and individual procedures vary in their level of invasiveness and risk to the patient. Systemic health may alter the healing response to surgery, response to and effectiveness of surgical and nonsurgical therapies, and risks of precipitating a medical emergency.

Hemostasis

A bleeding risk assessment must consider both patient-related factors of medical history, medications, review of systems, and physical exam assessment for inherited and acquired defects of hemostasis, as well as procedure-related factors including intensity of the planned surgery. When more than one of the four phases of hemostasis is defective, the clinical bleeding response from surgery is generally more severe than when there is an isolated defect in only one phase of hemostasis.

The four phases of hemostasis
- Vascular
- Platelet
- Coagulation
- Metabolic/fibrinolytic

Oral and physical exam findings indicating increased risk for hemostatic defects include the following:

- skin and mucosal petechiae, ecchymoses, or purpura (see Figs. 1.7–1.9);
- skin and mucosal hematomas (see Fig. 1.10);
- spontaneous gingival hemorrhage (see Fig. 1.11);
- hemosiderin staining of calculus on teeth (see Fig. 1.12);
- jaundice of sclera, mucosa, and skin (see Fig. 1.13);

Figure 1.7 Petechiae and mucosal pallor due to aplastic anemia.

Figure 1.9 Purpura of arm skin due to alcoholic cirrhosis.

Figure 1.8 Petechiae and ecchymoses of tongue and lip due to severe thrombocytopenia.

- spider angioma skin stigmata of severe liver disease (see Fig. 1.14).

Anticoagulant medications (warfarin, low-molecular-weight heparins, dabigatran) and antiplatelet agents (clopidogrel) are commonly prescribed for cardiovascular diseases, and some of the most commonly used over-the-counter analgesic medicines (aspirin, ibuprofen) may alter hemostasis. Dental providers also need to be aware that use of herbal supplements, often not revealed in the health history, can enhance bleeding risk. Four of the top five

Figure 1.10 Hematoma of finger due to severe hemophilia A.

supplements (green tea, garlic, *ginko biloba*, and ginseng) taken by dental patients in a dental-school-based study are reported to enhance bleeding risk.[5]

Weighing against the need to discontinue aspirin therapy for dental extractions, a recent case-control study demonstrated no difference in bleeding outcome from a single tooth extrac-

Figure 1.11 Spontaneous gingival bleeding due to severe thrombocytopenia.

Figure 1.13 Jaundice of sclera of eye due to severe liver cirrhosis.

Figure 1.12 Hemosiderin-stained calculus on teeth from chronic oral bleeding due to severe hemophilia A.

Figure 1.14 Spider angioma of skin due to severe liver disease.

tion for patients on 325 mg daily aspirin compared with those receiving placebo.[6]

Because of the importance of anticoagulation for certain cardiac conditions, the management of dental patients on warfarin has been controversial with a trend toward little or no modification in warfarin use around the time of dental treatment for most procedures except surgical procedures anticipating significant blood loss.[7] In addition, in an attempt to reduce coronary events after coronary artery stent placement, an advisory group involving representatives from dentistry stresses the importance of maintaining 12 months of dual antiplatelet therapy after placement of a drug-eluting stent and educating patients and health-care providers about hazards of premature discontinuation.[8] This advisory statement also recommends postponing elective dental surgery for 1 year, and if surgery cannot be deferred, considering the continuation of aspirin during the perioperative period in high-risk patients with drug-eluting stents.[8]

Local measures to control bleeding such as pressure, local hemostatic materials, epinephrine, electrocautery, surgical stents, and the antifibrinolytic drug (epsilon-aminocaproic acid 25% syrup) may be used to supplement any modification in the dental management plan. Hemorrhage control might be easier to obtain with local measures when a single tooth is extracted compared with a more intense surgery such as removal of all the teeth in an arch.

Susceptibility to Infection

The oral cavity is host to numerous bacteria and fungi raising the concern of local infection and the potential for distant hematogenous spread of oral microorganisms. Expert panel consensus statements or guidelines exist for antibiotic prophylaxis for invasive dental procedures for patients with several medical conditions, including infectious endocarditis,[9] implanted nonvalvular cardiac devices,[10] and other nonvalvular cardiovascular devices.[11] Current controversy exists around the issue of susceptibility to oral site distant infection for patients with total prosthetic joint replacements and the feasibility of prevention by antibiotic coverage for dental appointments.[12] New joint ADA and American Academy of Orthopedic Surgeons (AAOS) guidelines are anticipated in 2012.

A systematic review of patients with eight medical conditions or medical devices who are often given antibiotics prior to invasive dental procedures found little or no evidence to support this practice or to demonstrate that antibiotic coverage prevents distant site infections for any of these eight groups of patients.[13] The conditions and devices reviewed included cardiac-native heart valve disease; prosthetic heart valves and pacemakers; hip, knee, and shoulder prosthetic joints; renal dialysis shunts; cerebrospinal fluid shunts; vascular grafts; immunosuppression secondary to cancer and cancer chemotherapy; systemic lupus erythematosus; and insulin-dependent (type 1) diabetes mellitus.

The general paradigm shift occurring in health-care professional advisory statements and guidelines related to concern about distant site infection resulting from dental treatment is to emphasize the importance of the patient maintaining good oral hygiene and good gingival, periodontal, and dental health as a method of preventing distant site infection rather than using pretreatment antibiotic coverage for many unproven and low-risk conditions or conditions for which treatment of the infection would not be especially morbid.

Drug Actions/Interactions

Patients with complex medical conditions are likely to be on multiple medications for management of their systemic disease. Pharmaceutical agents taken as directed have both therapeutic (desired) effects and adverse (unwanted) effects. Most adverse effects can be anticipated from the known pharmacology of the drug and tend to be tolerable, although unpleasant. Patients should be informed of the most common side effects of medications and given advice at the time of prescription as to how to manage them.

A large U.S. ambulatory adult population-based phone survey in 1998–1999 indicated that most adults (81%) routinely take at least one medication and many take multiple medications with substantial overlap between use of prescription medications, over-the-counter medications, and herbals/supplements, raising concerns about unintended interactions.[14] The top 25 most commonly used prescription and over-the-counter drugs reported in this study are shown in Table 1.4. Vitamins and minerals are taken by 40% and herbals/supplements by 14% of adults. The most commonly used dietary supplements are shown in Table 1.5. Overall, 16% of prescription medication users also used one or more herbals/supplements, with greatest use among middle-aged women.[14]

Table 1.4. Top 25 Most Commonly Used Prescription and Over-the-Counter Drugs, 1-Week Prevalence, by Gender/Age (in Years) (Adapted from Kaufman et al.[14])

Rank	Total Adult, % use	Drug[a]	Men, % Use in Age Group			Women, % Use in Age Group		
			18–44 y	45–64 y	≥65 y	18–44 y	45–64 y	≥65 y
1	23	Acetaminophen	20	16	16	28	25	27
2	17	Ibuprofen	15	13	7	24	22	8
3	17	Aspirin	10	22	39	10	21	23
4	8.1	Pseudoephedrine	8	6	2	12	9	3
5	5.2	**Conjugated estrogens**	0	0	0	1	21	17
6	4.4	Diphenhydramine hydrochloride	4	3	5	5	6	4
7	4.2	**Levothyroxine sodium**	<1	2	4	3	9	13
8	4.2	**Ethinyl estradiol**	0	0	0	14	2	0
9	3.9	Caffeine £	3	2	2	6	5	1
10	3.7	**Hydrochlorothiazide**	1	4	6	1	6	12
11	3.5	Dextromethorphan hydrobromide	4	1	<1	6	3	3
12	3.5	Naproxen	1	3	3	5	4	4
13	2.9	Chlorpheniramine maleate/tannate	2	3	1	4	2	2
14	2.6	**Atorvastatin calcium**	2	7	7	<1	2	3
15	2.6	**Linsinopril**	1	3	7	<1	4	7
16	2.6	**Medroxyprogesterone acetate**	0	0	0	<1	12	4
17	2.5	**Loratadine**	3	2	0	3	4	1
18	2.3	**Furosemide**	<1	2	12	0	2	9
19	2.3	Phenylpropanolamine	2	2	1	3	2	3
20	2.2	Ranitidine hydrochloride	1	5	4	1	2	3
21	2.2	**Atenolol**	<1	2	7	<1	3	8
22	2.1	**Omeprazole**	1	3	5	1	3	3
23	2.1	**Albuterol**	2	1	4	2	3	2
24	1.9	Guanifenesin	2	<1	2	2	2	3
25	1.8	**Hydrocodone**	1	1	<1	3	2	3

[a] Prescription drugs in bold font.
y, years; £, excluding caffeine in food and beverages.

Table 1.5. Top 10 Most Commonly Used Vitamins/Minerals and Herbal/Supplements, 1-Week Prevalence (Adapted from Kaufman et al.[14])

Rank	Total Adult, % use	Dietary Supplements
Vitamin/mineral		
	40	Any use
1	26	Multivitamin
2	10	Vitamin E
3	9.1	Vitamin C
4	8.7	Calcium
5	3.0	Magnesium
6	2.2	Zinc
7	2.2	Folic acid
8	2.1	Vitamin B_{12}
9	1.9	Vitamin D
10	1.8	Vitamin A
Herbal/supplements		
	14	Any use
1	3.3	Ginseng
2	3.2	*Ginko biloba* extract
3	1.9	*Allium sativum* (garlic)
4	1.9	Glucosamine
5	1.3	St. John's wort
6	1.3	*Echinacea augustifolia*
7	1.1	Lecithin
8	1.0	Chondroitin
9	0.9	Creatine
10	0.9	*Serenoa repens* (saw palmetto)

In a subsequent study in 2005–2006 of nationally representative community-swelling older adults (aged 57–85 years) in the United States, 81% used at least one prescription medication, 42% used at least one over-the-counter medication, and 49% used at least one dietary supplement.[15] Twenty-nine percent used at least five prescription medications concurrently. Overall, 4% of these older adults were potentially at risk of having a major drug–drug interaction; half of these involved the use of nonprescription medications. These regimens were most prevalent in older men and nearly half involved concurrent use of anticoagulants.[15]

Drug actions or reactions can be predictable or unpredictable. Common drug interactions in the dental setting can be minor to life threatening. Minor interactions are not absolute contraindications to drug use.

Special precautions are needed when prescribing drugs for patients who are compromised in their ability to metabolize and excrete drugs and drug breakdown products:

- liver disease,
- renal impairment,
- young children,
- the very old.

For such patients, reduced drug dosages, extended intervals between doses, or avoidance of certain drugs may be indicated. Pregnant patients require consideration of teratogenic effects of all drugs, especially during the first trimester during embryogenesis, and some systemic medications can be found in the breast milk of nursing mothers.

Serious adverse effects may result from allergic reactions, overdosage, or drug interactions when certain medications are taken concomitantly. For safe patient management, the dentist must obtain a medication use and allergy history from the patient and have an understanding of the actions and interactions of all medications he or she prescribes. Drug classes used in dentistry and potential interactions with patient medications are shown in Table 1.6.

The dentist must ask about known drug "allergies." If an allergy is reported, the patient should be asked what physical response resulted from taking the medication. True drug allergy is most often an immediate type I immunoglobulin E (IgE)-mediated hypersensitivity involving inflammatory mediators, such as histamine and bradykinin, released from mast cells. This is often not seen at the first exposure to a drug that creates sensitization to the allergen, with the exception of the rare anaphylactoid toxic drug reaction. The inflammatory mediator release in true drug allergy leads to vasodilation, increased capillary permeability, and bronchoconstriction. Symptoms of true allergy include skin rash, pruritus (itching), urticaria (hives), and swelling of the lips, tongue, and throat; angioedema, shortness of breath, and wheezes and stridor; and syncope and cardiovascular collapse in anaphylaxis. True allergy to ester local anesthetics (procaine-novocaine, benzocaine) most often relates to the preservative para-aminobenzoic acid (PABA); however, true allergy to amide local anesthetics (lidocaine, mepivacaine, bupivacaine, prilocaine, articaine) is rare. More common reactions to local anesthetics are vasovagal or to the epinephrine.

Other drug reactions may be known side effects that are predictable negative consequences of a therapeutic dose of the drug, such as nausea and vomiting resulting from narcotics. There are additional known effects from overdosage or sensitivity to drugs, such as apnea and oversedation from benzodiazepines, or delirium from excessive pain medication use or toxicity from use of too much local anesthetic. Drug actions important to dentistry include alteration of hemostasis (anticoagulants and platelet inhibitors), immune suppression (cytotoxic chemotherapy, immunosuppressants, corticosteroids), and ability to withstand treatment (corticosteroids).

Medications taken for systemic disease management may also have oral sequelae, a common one being xerostomia related to salivary hypofunction. Side effects that involve the oral cavity may be first detected by the dentist (e.g., antihypertensive-induced lichenoid drug reaction) or may require management by the dental team (antidepressant/antipsychotic-induced xerostomia, dilantin-induced gingival overgrowth) when alternatives are unavailable. Common or important oral consequences of systemic drugs are shown in Table 1.7.

Ability to Tolerate Dental Care

A patient's ability to withstand dental treatment relates to both physiological and psychological stress that accompanies treatment. One response of the body to stress is release of catecholamines (epinephrine and norepinephrine) from the adrenal medulla into the cardiovascular system that results in an increased workload on the heart.[16] ASA classification[1] can provide a baseline health and stress tolerance status, with ASA 1 patients being the most stress tolerant and ASA 4 patients being the least tolerant, and most likely to need additional stress reduction techniques. Stress reduction should begin before and continue during and after dental treatment.

Physical or physiological stress of dental treatment may relate to the following:

- pain,
- time of day or length of appointment,
- dental chair position,
- use of local anesthetic with or without epinephrine.

Table 1.6. Common Dental Drug Interactions[a]

Patient-Reported Medication	Dentist-Prescribed Drug	Consequence
Antimicrobial drugs		
Alcohol	Metronidazole	Disulfuram-like reaction of nausea, vomiting, headache, flushing
Antacids and iron supplements	Tetracyclines	Loss of antibacterial action of tetracyclines
Atorvastatin, simvastatin, pravastatin	Erythromycin, clarithromycin	Increased statin level precipitating possible muscle weakness and breakdown
Carbamazepine	Erythromycin, clarithromycin, doxycycline, itraconazole, ketoconazole	Increased risk of carbamazepine toxicity
Cyclosporin	Fluconazole, itraconazole, ketoconazole, amphotericin, clarithromycin	Increased risk of nephrotoxicity
Digoxin	Erythromycin, tetracyclines, itraconazole, clarithromycin	Digoxin toxicity
Lithium	Metronidazole, tetracyclines	Increased lithium toxicity
Methotrexate	Penicillins	Methotrexate toxicity
Midazolam and other benzodiazepines	Erythromycin, clarithromycin, ketoconazole, itraconazole	Profound sedation
Oral contraceptives	Amoxicillin, erythromycin, tetracyclines, metronidazole, ampicillin, possibly other antibiotics	Contraceptive failure (low risk) (Patient should discuss with physician additional nonhormonal contraception used during antibiotic use and subsequent week.)
Phenytoin	Fluconazole, ketoconazole, metronidazole	Increased plasma levels of phenytoin
Theophylline	Erythromycin, clarithromycin, ketoconazole, itraconazole	Theophylline toxicity
Warfarin	Erythromycin, metronidazole, tetracyclines, ketaconazole, clarithromycin, cephalosporins	Enhanced anticoagulation effect
Anti-inflammatory drugs		
Alcohol	Aspirin	Increased risk of damage to gastric mucosa
Captopril, other angiotensin-converting enzyme (ACE) inhibitor	Aspirin, ibuprofen	Reduction in antihypertensive effect

Table 1.6. (Continued)

Patient-Reported Medication	Dentist-Prescribed Drug	Consequence
Corticosteroids	Aspirin	Risk of salicylate toxicity on steroid withdrawal, increased risk of damage to gastric mucosa
Cyclosporin	Aspirin, NSAIDs	Increased risk of nephrotoxicity
Digoxin	Aspirin, ibuprofen	Digoxin toxicity
Heparin, warfarin	Aspirin, NSAIDs	Risk of hemorrhage
Insulin, chlorpropamide, other hypoglycemics	Aspirin	Risk of hypoglycemia
Lithium	Ibuprofen, naproxen, celecoxib	Lithium toxicity
Methotrexate	Aspirin, ibuprofen, naproxen	Methotrexate toxicity
Phenytoin	Aspirin, NSAIDs	Increased plasma levels of phenytoin
Valproic acid	Aspirin	Risk of hemorrhage, increased valproate toxicity
Other drugs		
Alcohol, sedative H1 antagonists, neuroleptics, antiepileptics	Diazepam	Excessive sedation, impaired psychomotor skills, possible respiratory depression
Levothyroxine	Epinephrine	Coronary insufficiency in patients with coronary artery disease
Propranolol, other beta-blockers	Epinephrine	Marked hypertension and reflex bradycardia
Tricyclic antidepressants	Epinephrine	Hypertensive reaction and possible cardiac arrhythmias

[a] This list is constantly changing with new medications and new drug interactions and toxicities reported. The dentist should consult with a contemporary electronic drug interaction program, pharmacist, or the treating physician before prescribing drugs. NSAIDs, nonsteroidal anti-inflammatory drugs.

Adequate pain control during the dental procedure is essential for patient comfort and safety. Most medically complex patients will prefer morning appointments when they are more rested and stress tolerant; however, patients with osteoarthritis may prefer short, afternoon appointments. Those with arthritis or skeletal deformities may require frequent positional changes and pillow or other supports. While full supine chair position is comfortable for many patients, those with congestive heart failure will have a limit to how far back they

Table 1.7. Oral Consequences of Systemic Drugs

Oral Manifestation/ Side Effect	Medications with Reported Oral Side Effect
Angioedema	Angiotensin converting enzyme (ACE) inhibitors; H2 blockers
Chemo-osteonecrosis of the jaw	IV bisphosphonates (zolendronic acid, pamidornate, clodronate), oral bisphosphonates (alendronate, ibandronate, risedronate, etidronate, tilurdronate), other bone-modifying agents
Erythema multiforme	Antimalarials, barbiturates, busulfan, carbamazepine, cefaclor, chlorpropamide, clindamycin, codeine, isoniazid, H2 blockers, methyldopa, penicillins, phenylbutazone, phenytoin, rifampin, salicylates, sulfonamides, tetracyclines
Gingival overgrowth	Calcium channel blockers (especially nifedipine and verapamil), cyclosporine, phenytoin
Glossitis/coated tongue	Amoxicillin, nitrofurantoin, tetracyclines, triamterine/hydrochlorothiazide
Lichenoid reactions	ACE inhibitors, allopurinol, chloropropamide, chloroquine, chlorothiazide, dapsone, furosemide, gold salts, methyldopa, NSAIDs, palladium, penicillamine, propranolol, phenothiazines, quinidine, spironolactone, streptomycin, tetracyclines, tolbutamide, triprolidine
Lupus erythematosus-like lesions	Griseofulvin, hydralazine, isoniazid, methyldopa, nitrofurantoin, penicillin phenytoin, primidone, procainamide, rifampin, streptomycin, sulfonamides, tetracyclines, thiouracil, trimethadione
Stomatitis/oral ulceration	Carbamazepine, dideoxycytosine, enalapril, erythromycins, fluoxetine, ketoprofen, ofloxacin, piroxicam, cancer chemotherapeutic agents
Taste alteration	ACE inhibitors, albuterol, benzodiazepines, carbimazole, chlorhexidine, clofibrate, ethionamide, dimethyl sulfoxide, D-penicillamine, gold salts, griseofulvin, guanfacin, levodopa, lincomycin, lithium, methamphetamines, methocarbamol, metronidazole, nicotine, nortriptyline, phenindione, prednisone, sertraline, tranquilizers
Tooth discoloration	Chlorhexidine, nitrofurantoin, tetracyclines
Xerostomia	Anticholinergics, anticonvulsants, antidepressants, antihistamines, antihypertensives, antineoplastics, antiparkinsonians, antipsychotics, antispasmodics, central nervous system (CNS) stimulants, diuretics, gastrointestinals, muscle relaxants, narcotics, HIV protease inhibitors, sympathomimetics, systemic bronchodilators

can be comfortably reclined without having breathing distress, and women in the third trimester of pregnancy may also need the back of the dental chair slightly elevated, with the ability to roll their torso to the left to treat or prevent supine positional hypotension. All patients will have small rises in their systolic and diastolic blood pressure and heart rate when given local anesthetic, with or without epinephrine, for dental treatment, and this effect is more marked in patients with underlying hypertension.[17]

Psychological stress of dental treatment may relate to

- anxiety and
- fear.

Dental anxiety and fear are significant barriers to dental treatment. Stress reduction protocols are procedures and techniques used to minimize the stress during treatment, thus decreasing the risk to the patient.[16] A medical consultation may be needed to help gain information to determine the degree of risk and the modifications that might be helpful. Patient anxiety can be further reduced by the dental provider preoperatively reviewing with the patient the procedure and anticipated postoperative expectations for pain and the intended methods for obtaining adequate postoperative pain control, management of other anticipated consequences of care, and availability of and means of accessing the dentist should unanticipated after-hours questions or concerns arise.

> **Stress reduction considerations**
>
> - **Anxiolytic premedication:** benzodiazepine at bedtime night before appointment and 1 hour prior to appointment
> - **Appointment scheduling:** early in the day
> - **Minimize waiting time:** in waiting room and dental chair
> - **Preoperative and postoperative vital signs:** blood pressure, heart rate and rhythm, respiratory rate, pain score
> - **Sedation during treatment:** iatrosedation (music and video distraction, hypnosis), nitrous oxide/oxygen analgesia or pharmacosedative procedures including oral, inhalational, intramuscular, intranasal or intravenous (minimal or moderate) sedation, or general anesthesia
> - **Treatment duration:** short appointments

IV. Dental Management Modifications

When a medical risk assessment screening is completed, the dental provider develops an awareness of the medical complexity or risk status of the patient and can predict the possible complications related to the planned dental procedures. Complications may vary from minor to major or life threatening. Minor complications can be prevented or managed easily at home or at chair-side, while major complications may require medical management and possible hospitalization. An understanding of the patient's underlying medical condition allows the dental provider to recommend modification before, during, or after the dental procedures in order to safely provide dental care.

Examples of modification *before dental treatment* include the following:

1. antibiotic prophylaxis;
2. scheduling the treatment at a certain time of day or day of the week around medical therapy such as insulin management, chemotherapy, or hemodialysis;
3. altering medication timing or dose, in consultation with the patient's physician;
4. steroid supplementation;
5. preoperative drug use, for example, bronchodilator or hemostasis supportive medications;
6. preoperative blood product administration;
7. verification of last food intake;
8. obtaining day of procedure baseline blood pressure and heart rate;
9. verification of metabolic hemostasis with laboratory tests, such as glycosylated hemoglobin (HbA1C), blood glucose from finger stick, prothrombin time (PT)/international normalized ratio (INR), platelet count, white blood cell count with absolute neutrophil count;
10. obtaining hyperbaric oxygen wound healing enhancement.

Examples of modification *during dental treatment* include the following:

1. stress management with anxiolytic oral agents or nitrous oxide/oxygen,
2. providing physical supports or rest breaks,
3. limiting dosage of local anesthetic,
4. avoiding use of certain medications,
5. maintaining adequacy of pain control,
6. assuring aseptic surgical technique or using preoperative oral antiseptic rinse,
7. application of local hemostatic agents,
8. using supplemental oxygen by nasal cannula.

Examples of modification *after dental treatment* include the following:

1. prescribing therapeutic course of antibiotics,
2. use of postoperative antifibrinolytics,
3. postoperative stress management,
4. maintaining adequacy of pain control,
5. avoiding use of certain medications,
6. assuring appropriate and understood postoperative instructions.

V. Recommended Readings and Cited References

Recommended Readings

Cianco S. The ADA/PDR Guide to Dental Therapeutics, 5th ed. 2009. American Dental Association, Chicago, IL.

Hersh EV. Adverse drug reactions in dental practice: interactions involving antibiotics. J Am Dent Assoc 1999;130(2):236–51.

Hersh EV, Moore PA. Adverse drug interactions in dentistry. Periodontol 2000 2008;46:109–42.

Lockhart PB, Hong CHL, van Diermen DE. The influence of systemic diseases on the diagnosis of oral diseases: a problem-based approach. Dent Clin North Am 2011;55(1):15–28.

Scully C, Bagan JV. Adverse drug reactions in the orofacial region. Crit Rev Oral Biol Med 2004;15(4):221–39.

Cited References

1. American Society of Anesthesiologists. ASA Physical Status Classification System. Available at: http://www.asahq.org/clinical/physicalstatus.htm. Accessed July 4, 2011.
2. Smeets EC, de Jong KJ, Abraham-Inpijn L. Detecting the medically compromised patient in dentistry by means of the medical risk-related history. A survey of 29,424 dental patients in The Netherlands. Prev Med 1998;27(4):530–5.
3. Brady WF, Martinoff JT. Validity of health history data collected from dental patients and patient perception of health status. J Am Dent Assoc 1980;101(4):642–5.
4. Ertas ET, Sisman Y. Detection of incidental carotid artery calcifications during dental examinations: panoramic radiography as an important aid in dentistry. Oral Surg Oral Med Oral Pathol Oral Radiol Endod 2011;112(4):e11–7.
5. Abebe W, Herman W, Konzelman J. Herbal supplement use among adult dental patients in a USA dental school clinic: prevalence, patient demographics, and clinical implications. Oral Surg Oral Med Oral Pathol Oral Radiol Endod 2011;111(3):320–5.
6. Brennan MT, Valerin MA, Noll JL, Napeñas JJ, Kent ML, Fox PC, et al. Aspirin use and postoperative bleeding from dental extractions. J Dent Res 2008;87(8):740–4.
7. Wahl MJ. Myths of dental surgery in patients receiving anticoagulant therapy. J Am Dent Assoc 2000;131(1):77–81.
8. Grines CL, Bonow RO, Casey DE Jr., Grines CL, Bonow RO, Casey DE Jr., et al. Prevention of premature discontinuation of dual antiplatelet therapy in patients with coronary artery stents: a science advisory from the American Heart Association, American College of Cardiology, Society for Cardiovascular Angiography and Interventions, American College of Surgeons, and American Dental Association, with representation from the American College of Physicians. J Am Dent Assoc 2007;138(5):652–5.
9. Wilson W, Taubert KA, Gewitz M, Lockhart PB, Baddour LM, Levison M, et al. Prevention of infective endocarditis: guidelines from the American Heart Association: a guideline from the American Heart Association Rheumatic Fever, Endocarditis and Kawasaki Disease Committee,

Council on Cardiovascular Disease in the Young, and the Council on Clinical Cardiology, Council on Cardiovascular Surgery and Anesthesia, and the Quality of Care and Outcomes Research Interdisciplinary Working Group. J Am Dent Assoc 2008;139(Suppl.):3S–24S. Erratum in: J Am Dent Assoc 2008;139(3):253.
10. Baddour LM, Epstein AE, Erickson CC, Knight BP, Levison ME, Lockhart PB, et al. A summary of the update on cardiovascular implantable electronic device infections and their management: a scientific statement from the American Heart Association. J Am Dent Assoc 2011;142(2):159–65.
11. Baddour LM, Bettmann MA, Bolger AF, Epstein AE, Ferrieri P, Gerber MA, et al. Nonvalvular cardiovascular device-related infections. Circulation 2003;108(16):2015–31.
12. Little JW, Jacobson JJ, Lockhart PB, American Academy of Oral Medicine. The dental treatment of patients with joint replacements: a position paper from the American Academy of Oral Medicine. J Am Dent Assoc 2010;141(6):667–71.
13. Lockhart PB, Loven B, Brennan MT, Fox PC. The evidence base for the efficacy of antibiotic prophylaxis in dental practice. J Am Dent Assoc 2007;138(4):458–74.
14. Kaufman DW, Kelly JP, Rosenberg L, Anderson TE, Mitchell AA. Recent patterns of medication use in the ambulatory adult population of the United States: the Slone survey. JAMA 2002;287(3):337–44.
15. Qato DM, Alexander GC, Conti RM, Johnson M, Schumm P, Lindau ST. Use of prescription and over-the-counter medications and dietary supplements among older adults in the United States. JAMA 2008;300(24):2867–78.
16. Malamed SF. Knowing your patients. J Am Dent Assoc 2010;141(Suppl. 1):3S–7S.
17. Bader JD, Bonito AJ, Shugars DA. A systematic review of cardiovascular effects of epinephrine on hypertensive dental patients. Oral Surg Oral Med Oral Pathol Oral Radiol Endod 2002;93(6):647–53.

Cardiovascular Diseases

Wendy S. Hupp DMD

I. Background

Description of Disease/Condition

Cardiovascular diseases (CVDs) include a wide spectrum of signs and symptoms, and approximately one in three adults in the United States have more than one CVD at a time. In addition, many CVD patients have other systemic diseases that increase the morbidity and mortality of each disease. There are numerous well-known risk factors (see Table 2.1), and evidence is building to connect periodontal disease and chronic inflammation to CVD.[1-3] It is important for patients with CVD to have optimum oral health to reduce the potential for pain that in turn may elevate endogenous epinephrine and add stress to the cardiovascular system. CVD pain may also be confused with pain of dental origin.

Pathogenesis/Etiology

Ischemic heart disease is defined as a lack of oxygen to the heart muscles. It can be caused by coronary artery blockage by atherosclerotic plaque or thrombosis, narrowing because of coronary artery spasm, coronary arteritis, embolism, or shock secondary to hypotension. Other causes of ischemia include tachycardia, hyperthyroidism, catecholamine treatment, cardiac hypertrophy, anemia, advanced lung disease, congenital cyanotic heart disease, and carbon monoxide poisoning.

Coronary artery disease (CAD) specifies inadequate blood supply to the blood vessels in the heart: the left coronary artery (LCA) divides into the left anterior descending (LAD) and left circumflex (LCX) arteries; and the right coronary artery (RCA). See Fig. 2.1. Symptoms may include fatigue, shortness of breath, or none at all.

Angina pectoris (AP) is defined as sudden-onset, substernal, or precordial chest pain due to myocardial ischemia, but without infarction (necrosis). The pain often radiates to the left arm, neck, jaw, or back. Angina is classified as stable, unstable, or Prinzmetal angina:

- *Stable angina* is predictable, induced by exercise or exertion, and lasts for less than 15 minutes.

The ADA Practical Guide to Patients with Medical Conditions, First Edition. Edited by Lauren L. Patton.
© 2012 American Dental Association. Published 2012 by John Wiley & Sons, Inc.

- *Unstable angina* can occur at any time, is more severe, and lasts longer.
- *Prinzmetal angina* occurs at rest, with electrocardiogram (ECG) changes, and is most likely due to spasm of a coronary artery.

Other less common causes of angina include aortic stenosis, arrhythmias, myocarditis, mitral valve prolapse, and hypertrophic cardiomyopathy.

Table 2.1. Risk Factors for Cardiovascular Disease

Modifiable	Nonmodifiable
High blood pressure	Age
Atherosclerosis/dyslipidemia	Sex
Diabetes	Family history
Tobacco smoking	
Obesity/diet	
Inactivity	
Stress	
Alcohol use	

Myocardial infarction (MI), or acute myocardial infarction (AMI), occurs after persistent ischemia leads to irreversible coagulative necrosis of myocardial fibers. The area of infarct loses normal conduction and contraction, and may heal with nonfunctional scar tissue. Most MIs involve the left ventricle, or by extension, to the right ventricle. Symptoms are severe substernal pain that may radiate to the left arm, neck, jaw, or back; shortness of breath; profuse sweating; loss of consciousness; or symptoms may be only very mild discomfort.

MIs are evaluated using two criteria: depth and location. If the infarct involves the full thickness of the ventricular wall, it is termed transmural; a subendocardial infarct is limited to the inner one-third to one-half of the ventricular wall. Location is reported by wall or coronary artery involvement, for example, antero-septal infarct, left ventricular anterior wall infarct, and LAD coronary infarct. Clinical evaluation of patients with MIs by ECG shows two types: those with ST elevation (STEMI) or non-ST elevation (non-STEMI).[4]

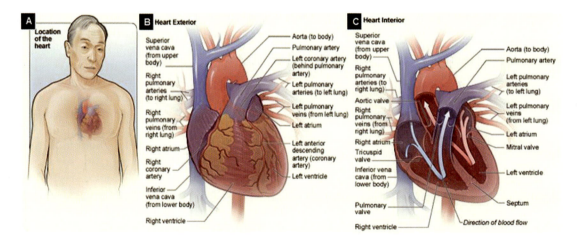

Figure 2.1 The healthy heart. Source: National Heart Lungs and Blood Institute. Available at: http://www.nhlbi.nih.gov/health/health-topics/topics/hhw/anatomy.html. Accessed December 28, 2011. (A) Location of the heart in the body. (B) Front exterior surface of the heart, including the coronary arteries and major blood vessels. (C) Internal cross section of a healthy heart. Blue arrow shows venous blood and red arrow shows arterial blood flow pattern.

Acute coronary syndrome (ACS) is a relatively new term that is gaining favor. It is used to describe patients with unstable angina, STEMI, or non-STEMI. The pain associated with ACS is more severe and prolonged than AP, and signifies a worsening of the CVD.[5]

Hypertension (HTN) is a disease that has been defined as systolic blood pressure (BP) above 140 mmHg and/or diastolic BP above 90 mmHg. HTN is also a risk factor in many diseases, including CVD, stroke, renal failure, and heart failure (HF). The great majority of patients with HTN (90%) have no primary cause, thus the term essential HTN. The remaining 10% have an identified etiology such as pheochromocytoma, aortic regurgitation, renal artery stenosis, and preeclampsia, or are drug-induced by corticosteroids, nonsteroidal anti-inflammatory drugs, or oral contraceptives. Sustained HTN may lead to hypertrophy of the left ventricle to compensate for the elevated pressure. Symptoms may be nonexistent, or cause dizziness or headache, nosebleeds, and fatigue:

- The Seventh Report of the Joint National Committee on Prevention, Detection, Evaluation, and Treatment of High Blood Pressure (JNC 7) published HTN guidelines in 2003.[6] The 8th report is expected to be more evidence based and published in 2012. The term prehypertension was introduced to draw attention to those patients whose BP was at increased risk of developing into HTN. This classification of systolic BP 120–139 mmHg and/or diastolic BP 80–89 mmHg was developed to encourage people to adapt healthy lifestyles. Dentists were specifically included in this report to help with surveillance, as most patients with HTN may have no symptoms. The earlier that patients can be diagnosed and treated, the less the extent of lasting effects[7]:
  - *normal BP for adults* = <120/80 mmHg;
  - *prehypertension* = 120–139/80–89 mmHg;
  - *stage 1 HTN* = 140–159/90–99 mmHg;
  - *stage 2 HTN* = >160/100 mmHg.

Heart failure (HF) occurs when the heart can no longer maintain circulation that is adequate for body tissues to function. Congestive HF describes the clinical signs of pulmonary and/or peripheral edema in addition to the inadequate circulation. Symptoms may include shortness of breath, orthopnea, fatigue, and inability to cope with physical activity.

The pathophysiology has two components:

1. Pump failure (weakness or inefficiency of ventricular contraction)
   - Due to myocardial ischemia or CAD; cardiomyopathy; myocarditis; stiff or rigid ventricles; pericardial effusion or tamponade; or severe rhythm disorders, for example, ventricular tachycardia, atrial fibrillation, or flutter.
2. Increased workload
   - Due to atrial or mitral regurgitation or ventricular septal defect resulting in increased peripheral resistance and increased volume load.
   - Due to anemia, obstructive or restrictive pulmonary disease, or thyrotoxicosis preventing blood from efficiently oxygenating all tissues.

Congenital heart disease or defects are evident from birth. See Fig. 2.2. These are structural problems that range from minor holes between chambers to major malformations that require surgical intervention. Some examples include atrial–septal defects, patent ductus arteriosus, atrioventricular (AV) septal defects, tetralogy of Fallot, transposition of the great arteries, hypoplastic left heart syndrome, and coarctation of the aorta.

Valvular heart disease is characterized as stenosis or insufficiency:

- *Stenosis* means that the opening of the valve is reduced compared with normal. This limits the amount of blood volume that is able to pass through the valve.
  - Some causes are fibrosis of the valve opening secondary to rheumatic heart

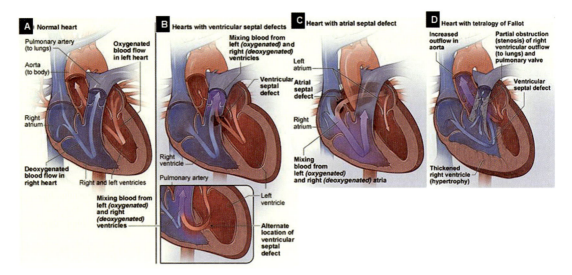

Figure 2.2 Congenital heart defects. (A) Normal heart. (B) Ventricular septal defect. (C) Atrial–septal defect. (D) Tetralogy of Fallot. Source: National Heart Lungs and Blood Institute. Available at: http://www.nhlbi.nih.gov/health/health-topics/topics/chd/types.html. Accessed December 28, 2011.

disease, calcification of the valve leaflets, and congenital malformation of the valve leaflets.
- *Insufficiency* means that the valve fails to close completely. This leads to regurgitation of blood in the reverse direction of normal.
  ○ Some causes are prolapse, ruptured papillary muscles, left ventricular hypertrophy, infective endocarditis (IE), Marfan syndrome, systemic lupus erythematosis, and congenital malformation.

Infective endocarditis (IE) is defined as microbial infection and inflammation of the endocardium including the heart valves. Damage to the valve leaflets may be part of the cause and the result of this condition. Vegetations form on the valves that consist of organisms, usually streptococci or staphylococci, fibrin, and inflammatory cells. Erosions, valve perforations, and abscesses in the myocardium can occur. Symptoms are similar to HF. Most patients recover from the infection, but injury to one or more valves persists. Rarely, other complications result, for example, septic emboli to the brain, spleen, or kidneys. In 2006, approximately 2400 U.S. adults died due to IE.[8]

Dysrhythmia or arrhythmia is a disruption of the electrical impulse generation or conduction in the heart that leads to an abnormal function. The disruption may be due to an area of infarction, ischemia, electrolyte imbalance, or medication. Some examples include atrial fibrillation, tachycardia, paroxysmal supraventricular tachycardia, and ventricular fibrillation. Many patients have no symptoms of arrhythmia; however, some patients have HF secondary to the arrhythmia with symptoms that can be very severe.

Epidemiology

It is estimated that about 86,600,000 U.S. adults (over age 20) have one or more types of CVD. This is approximately one of three adults[8]:

- 40,400,000 are over age 60 years;
- 76,400,000 have high BP;
- 16,300,000 with coronary heart disease;
- 7,900,000 have had an MI;
- 9,000,000 experience AP;
- 5,700,000 have HF;
- 650,000–1,300,000 have congenital cardiovascular defects.[8]

CVD accounts for about 40% of all deaths in the United States, of which 90% result from ischemic heart disease. In 2007, there were 813,800 deaths caused by CVD.[8]

Coordination of Care between Dentist and Physician

Patients with CVD will need elective and urgent dental care. The dentist must be able to ask the right questions of the physician regarding the patient's ability to tolerate the stress of dental treatment, as well as understand the information provided by the physician. Certain medications have oral adverse drug reactions that can be managed by the dentist. Other medications cause increased bleeding. For patients with acute or severe CVD, hospital-based dental care may be necessary.

For some patients, the dentist may observe signs of CVD during a dental appointment. Reviewing the patient's medical history and measuring the BP and assessing the heart rate and rhythm (pulse) may identify contraindications or the need for modifications in the provision of dental care. Moreover, these processes may reveal inadequate control of existing medical conditions or the onset of new problems. The dentist should feel confident in contacting the physician regarding these findings.[9] A patient with poorly controlled CVD, and/or who does not follow his physician's guidance or adhere to prescription medication regimens should not have elective dental care.

II. Medical Management

Identification

People who have CVD may have very distinct signs and symptoms, or conversely may have no awareness of the problem. Many cases of CVD develop very insidiously so that patients are unaware of the severity until a catastrophic event happens. Ideally, everyone would have simple tests related to the cardiovascular system done on a regular basis: BP measurement, ECG, stress test, blood lipids, blood chemistry, and so on. Unfortunately, many U.S. adults have multiple risk factors that increase the incidence and prevalence of CVD including smoking, obesity, poor diet, and physical inactivity.[8]

Medical History

The patient who knows that he or she has CVD should identify his or her specific problems upon review of his or her medical history. Other observations may lead the dentist to understand the severity of the problems, and the degree of control or management of the problem:

- elevated BP,
- irregular or abnormal heart rate,
- abnormal respiratory rate,
- shortness of breath upon exertion,
- patient is uncomfortable in supine position,
- surgical scars,
- prolonged bleeding/easy bruising.

Reviewing the patient's list of medications can lead the discussion to clarify the specifics of the type of CVD. Also, by understanding the pharmacological category of each drug on the patient's list, the dentist can deduce how difficult the CVD is for the physician and patient to manage; that is, a patient who takes four different types of antihypertensive medications has a very difficult time controlling his or her disease.

Figure 2.3 Implantable cardioverter-defibrillator (ICD) and pacemaker. (A) Location and general size of an ICD. (B) Location and general size of a pacemaker. For each device, the wires with electrodes on the ends are inserted into the right atrium and ventricle through the cephalic vein or subclavian vein in the upper chest. Source: National Heart Lungs and Blood Institute. Available at: http://www.nhlbi.nih.gov/health/health-topics/topics/icd/. Accessed December 28, 2011.

Surgical or cardiac procedural history will reveal patients who have received coronary artery angioplasty and stents, coronary artery bypass grafts (CABG), heart valve repair or prosthetic valve replacements, repair of congenital heart defects, removal of excess heart muscle (e.g., ventricular septal myotomy or myectomy), pacemakers or implantable cardioverter-defibrillator (ICD) (as shown in Fig. 2.3), or heart transplantation.

Physical Examination

Many patients with CVD are managed by their primary care physician or by an internist. For more severe cases, a cardiologist and/or cardiothoracic surgeon may be involved. Physical examination by the medical team may include BP, heart rate and rhythm, respiratory rate and volume, chest auscultation, ECG, echocardiography, stress test with or without radioactive agents, radiograph, magnetic resonance imaging, computed tomography (CT), cardiac catheterization, and angiography. Ejection fraction (EF) is a measurement (estimated on echocardiogram or other tests) of the degree of HF. When the left ventricle contracts, there is residual blood remaining in the chamber. Normal EF is 50–70%, and heart transplant may be considered when EF is <25%.

When treating the patient with CVD, the dentist should check the BP and heart rate before any invasive procedures, and before injecting local anesthetic. Comparing these data with baseline values may reveal a disease that is worsening, problems with medication compliance, or development of tolerance to a medication. This information should be shared with the patient, and depending on the severity, a referral to the treating physician or the emergency department is indicated.

Laboratory Testing

Many U.S. adults have less than ideal blood cholesterol and triglycerides that contribute to the formation of atherosclerotic plaques. These patients will have routine blood tests to determine if diet and medication are normalizing these levels. There is little impact on dental care related to blood cholesterol problems.

For a patient who is suspected of having an MI, blood tests are done over several hours to days to measure special markers: cardiac troponin, creatinine kinase, lactate dehydrogenase, and other enzymes.

IE will cause the complete blood count and inflammatory markers (erythrocyte sedimentation rate, homocysteine, etc.) to be abnormal. For many patients, a positive blood culture for bacteria or other infectious agent will also be found.

Patients who are taking warfarin should have monthly blood tests of the prothrombin time (PT)/international normalized ratio (INR). Dentists should be aware of the results of this test within hours to several days before surgical dental procedures. See Chapter 9 for additional discussion of patients receiving anticoagulants.

Medical Treatment

Most patients with CVD take medications by mouth daily. Commonly prescribed medications by pharmacological category are listed in Table 2.2. Other interventions include surgery, for example, CABG, angioplasty, coronary artery stent placement, prosthetic valve replacement, and heart transplantation; and placement of ICDs or pacemakers.

Table 2.2. Common Medications for Cardiovascular Disease and Oral Adverse Drug Reaction/Dental Implication

Cardiovascular Drug Category	Culprit Drug	Oral Adverse Drug Reaction/ Dental Implication and Likelihood of Association
Alpha-adrenergic blockers	Class effect	*Est*: dry mouth
	Methyldopa	*Pos*: lichenoid drug eruption
Beta-adrenergic blockers	Class effect/unspecified	*Est*: dry mouth, angioedema
	Labetolol/unspecified	*Prob*: aphthae/ulcers
	Atenolol, oxprenolol, practolol, propranolol	*Pos*: lichenoid drug eruption
	Propranolol	*Pos*: thrombocytopenia
	Practolol	*Pos*: oculo-mucocutaneous syndrome
	Carvediol	*Pos*: SJS
	Propranolol (sublingual)	*Pos*: mouth paresthesia
Angiotensin-converting enzyme (ACE) inhibitors	Class effect	*Est*: angioedema
	Class effect	*Est*: neutropenia/agranulocytosis
	Captopril, enalapril	*Est*: taste disturbances
	Captopril	*Prob*: aphthae/ulcers; pemphigus
	Captopril, enalapril, lisinopril	*Prob*: scalded mouth syndrome
	Lisinopril	*Prob*: dry mouth
	Captopril	*Pos*: lichenoid drug eruption
Antiotensin II receptor blocker	Losartan	*Prob*: angioedema

(Continued)

Table 2.2. (Continued)

Cardiovascular Drug Category	Culprit Drug	Oral Adverse Drug Reaction/ Dental Implication and Likelihood of Association
Anti-arrhythmics, Class I (sodium channel blockers)	Class effect	*Est*: dry mouth
	Phenytoin	*Est*: gingival overgrowth; hypersensitivity reaction syndrome
	Phenytoin	*Prob*: agranulocytosis; SJS, TEN
	Quinidine	*Prob*: thrombocytopenia
	Quinidine	*Pos*: FDE
Anti-arrhythmics, Class III (potassium channel blockers)	Amiodarone	*Prob*: angioedema
	Amiodarone	*Pos*: taste disturbance
Calcium channel blockers	Class effect	*Est*: gingival overgrowth, dry mouth, taste disturbances
	Diltiazem, verapamil	*Pos*: aphthae/ulcers, EM, SJS, TEN
	Nifedipine, diltiazem	*Pos*: angioedema
	Amlodipine	*Pos*: lichenoid drug eruption
Diuretics	Class effect	*Est*: dry mouth
	Amiloride, furosemide, hydrochlorothiazide	*Prob*: agranulocytosis, thrombocytopenia
	Amiloride, spironolactone	*Prob*: taste disturbance
	Bendrofluazide, furosemide/spironolactone	*Uncertain/Pos*: lichenoid drug eruption
	Hydrochlorothiazide, furosemide	*Pos*: EM, SJS, TEN, drug hypersensitivity reaction
	Unspecified	*Pos*: angioedema
Potassium channel opener	Nicorandil	*Prob*: aphthae/ulcers
Direct-acting peripheral vasodilator	Hydralazine	*Prob*: lupus erythematosus
Lipid regulators (statins)	Simvastatin	*Pos*: cheilitis, lichenoid drug eruption
Platelet inhibitors	Aspirin	*Prob*: FDE
	Aspirin	*Pos*: angioedema
Anticoagulants	Warfarin, dabigatran, rivaroxaban	*Est*: impaired hemostasis

Est, established drug reaction; *Prob*, probable drug reaction; *Pos*, possible drug reaction; SJS, Stevens–Johnson syndrome; TEN, toxic epidermal necrolysis; FDE, fixed drug reaction; EM, erythema multiforme.
Modified from Torpet et al.[10]

III. Dental Management

Evaluation

Identifying the underlying cardiac condition and related symptoms, medical management approaches taken by the patient and physician, and level of control is an important first step in dental treatment planning.

Dental Treatment Modifications

Several classification systems are used by physicians when evaluating patients with CVD. Understanding these classifications will help

> **? Key questions to ask the patient**
>
> - For all patients with CVD:
>   - Do you ever have prolonged bleeding or easy bruising?
>   - Have you ever had open-heart surgery? When and what kind?
>   - Have you ever had infective or bacterial endocarditis?
> - For the patient with coronary artery disease (angina pectoris, post MI, stent, CABG):
>   - Do you ever have chest pain? Does it occur spontaneously or at night? When did it last occur? How often does it occur? Has there been a change in the frequency of your chest pain? What brings it on? Makes it stop?
>   - Do you have difficulty walking a city block without stopping?
>   - How long ago was your MI, CABG, last cardiac catheterization/stenting?
>   - When was your last cardiac evaluation and what is your present status?
>   - Are you taking a blood thinner?
> - For the patient with congestive heart failure:
>   - Do you need to sleep with pillows or have your head elevated?
>   - Do your ankles ever get swollen?
>   - Are you taking a water pill?
>   - Do you get light-headed or dizzy?
> - For the patient with hypertension:
>   - How long have you had high blood pressure? Is your high blood pressure controlled or uncontrolled? What does your blood pressure normally run?
>   - What blood pressure medications do you routinely take? Did you take your blood pressure pills this morning?
> - For the patient with an arrhythmia:
>   - What type of arrhythmia do you have?
>   - What signs and symptoms do you have and does stress make it worse?
>   - Do you have a pacemaker or implanted cardioverter-defibrillator?
>   - Are you on a blood thinner?
> - For the patient with valvular heart disease:
>   - What type of surgery did you have?
>   - Do you have a prosthetic heart valve? If so is this mechanical requiring Coumadin® or other anticoagulant or bioprosthetic (bovine, porcine)?
> - For the patient with a heart transplant:
>   - When was your transplant?
>   - Are you taking antirejection immune suppressant drugs?
>   - Is the heart healthy?

Key questions to ask the physician

Generally address the specific kind of anesthesia planned (e.g., general vs. local—2% lidocaine with 1:100,000 epinephrine) as well as any surgery that may be performed so that hemostasis can be addressed.

- For all patients with CVD:
  - What is the specific diagnosis?
  - Is the patient able to tolerate the stress of the proposed dental treatment?
  - What medications have been prescribed?
  - What are the pertinent lab test results (EF, INR)?
- For the patient with angina pectoris:
  - Is the angina well controlled or worsening despite medication?
- For the patient with history of MI:
  - When was the MI?
  - Was any surgery performed?
- For the patient with CABG or stents:
  - When was the surgery?
- For the patient with hypertension:
  - What is the blood pressure goal?
    (If uncontrolled, report the findings and determine if the patient should be sent to the emergency room or the physician's office.)
- For the patient with valvular heart disease:
  - Has there been a prosthetic valve placed? If so, is this mechanical or bioprosthetic? Is the patient on Coumadin®? What is the last INR? If surgery is planned, when is the next scheduled INR?
- For the patient with a heart transplant:
  - Does the patient need antibiotic premedication?
  - Does the patient need steroid supplementation due to antirejection medication?

---

the dentist determine the patient's ability to tolerate the stress of dental treatment.

- *All Patients*:
  - The American Society of Anesthesiologists (ASA) developed a physical status classification system to predict the risk of general anesthesia. This scale has been applied to the provision of dental care[11] (see Table 1.1).
- *HTN*:
  - Stage of HTN and BP measurements at the time of treatment in the dental office affect recommendations for deferring or continuing elective and emergency dental care. See Table 2.3.
- *AP*:
  - The Canadian Cardiovascular Society (CCS) published guidelines to classify the severity of AP.[12] This is a functional classification, relying on the patient's ability to perform certain activities. The recommendations for provision of dental care are given below:
    - Class 1: Ordinary physical activity does not cause angina; no special precautions for dental care.

Table 2.3. Outpatient Dental Care Guidelines for the Adolescent or Adult Patient with Hypertension[a]

Patient Age (Years)	BP Level (mmHg)	Elective Dental Care	Emergency Dental Care
Adult (>18)	<160/100	No modification	No modification
Adult (>18)	>160/100[b]	Repeat measurement 1. If lowered or within written guidelines from physician ⇨ proceed. 2. If confirmed ⇨ no elective dental treatment and patient seeks consultation with physician.	Repeat measurement 1. If lowered or within written guidelines from physician ⇨ proceed. 2. If confirmed SBP 160–180 and/or DBP 100–109 where dental symptoms and pain contribute to HTN ⇨ initiate emergency care with BP monitoring every 10–15 minutes during procedure; consider anxiety reduction techniques. 3. If confirmed SBP >180 and/or DBP >109 ⇨ dentist seeks consultation with physician before proceeding.
Adolescent (10–17)	<140/90	No modification	No modification
Adolescent (10–17)	140–160/90–100	Repeat measurement 1. If lowered or within written guidelines from physician ⇨ proceed. 2. If confirmed ⇨ no elective dental treatment and patient seeks consultation with physician.	Repeat measurement 1. If lowered or within written guidelines from physician ⇨ proceed. 2. If confirmed SBP 140–160 and/or DBP 90–100 where dental symptoms and pain contribute to HTN ⇨ initiate emergency care with BP monitoring every 10–15 minutes during procedure; consider anxiety reduction techniques.
Adolescent (10–17)	>160/100[b]	Same as above for adolescent with BP 140–160/90–100.	Repeat measurement 1. If lowered or within written guidelines from physician ⇨ proceed. 2. If confirmed SBP >160 and/or DBP >100 ⇨ dentist seeks consultation with physician before proceeding.

[a] BP measurement should begin after the patient has been at rest a minimum of 5 minutes, with proper BP cuff size for patient (too small a cuff falsely elevates BP), with the patient in a sitting or supine position, and the patient's bare arm extended at heart level.
[b] Patients with SBP >180 and/or DBP >110 should be referred to their physician as soon as possible or sent for urgent medical evaluation if symptomatic.
HTN, hypertension; BP, blood pressure; mmHg, millimeters of mercury; SBP, systolic BP; DBP, diastolic BP.

- Class 2: Angina with vigorous activity; elective dental care okay, consider treatment modification.
- Class 3: Angina with mild exertion (angina occurs when walking one- to two-level blocks at normal pace or climbing a flight of stairs at normal pace); elective dental care with treatment modification—limit anesthetic with epinephrine.
- Class 4: Angina occurs at any level of physical exertion; urgent dental care only—hospital-based dental care indicated, where vital sign monitoring can be provided.
- *HF*: The American College of Cardiology/American Heart Association (AHA) published guidelines for diagnosis and management of HF in 2009.[13] Stage A and B patients are at risk of experiencing HF, and Stage C and D patients are defined as already having HF. Routine dental care can usually be provided for most Stage A and Stage B patients, and for many in Stage C. For more advanced stages of HF, dental care should be provided in hospital-based dental clinic.[14]
  - Stage A = high risk of HF, no structural heart damage or symptoms of HF.
  - Stage B = structural heart disease, no signs or symptoms of HF.
  - Stage C = structural heart disease, prior or current symptoms of HF.
  - Stage D = refractory HF requiring specialized interventions.
- *Cardiac Dysrhythmias/Arrhythmias*: Arrhythmias can be divided into three risk levels (major, intermediate, and minor) by the risk that the patient may have MI, HF, or death.[15] The physician should be consulted regarding the specific diagnosis of the arrhythmia, and if the condition is adequately controlled.
  - *Major risk*: third-degree AV block, symptomatic ventricular arrhythmias, supraventricular arrhythmias with uncontrolled ventricular rate.
  - *Intermediate risk*: first- or second-degree AV block.
  - *Minor risk*: atrial fibrillation, premature atrial beats, sinus bradycardia in a young individual, asymptomatic ectopic beats.

  Arrhythmias are treated with medications such as beta-blockers, calcium channel blockers, and cardiac glycosides. If necessary, a surgically implanted pacemaker and/or ICD may help manage the condition. These electronic devices have been used for many years, and the newer units have been made to tolerate exposure to other instruments, such as electronic apex locators and pulp testers.[16] However, electrosurgery units, ultrasonic cleaners, and scaling devices still pose a risk for many of these patients.[15]
- *MI*: Patients who have recently had an MI, with or without surgical intervention, should not receive elective dental care within the first 30 days. If urgent care is needed, the cardiologist should be consulted, and the care should be provided in a hospital-based clinic where vital sign monitoring can be provided. After 30 days, if the patient has no symptoms, elective care can be provided with caution. It is recommended that anesthetic with epinephrine be limited to two carpules.[3,17,18] Patients diagnosed with ACS or who have persistent symptoms after 30 days post MI should be treated the same as AP patients.[19]
- *Valvular Cardiomyopathy or End-Stage HF*: Patients with very severe CVD may need to have a prosthetic valve replacement or heart transplant. The dentist should be consulted before these surgeries, if possible, to eliminate any potential sources of infection. Excellent oral hygiene should be stressed, and potential oral problems with medications should be discussed. For example, anticoagulation with warfarin will increase postsurgical bleeding risk and gingival overgrowth is a potential side effect of the antirejection medication cyclosporine.

Risks of Dental Care

Hemostasis

Antiplatelet medications (aspirin, clopidogrel, prasugrel, ticlopidine, aspirin/dipyridamole sustained release) and anticoagulants (warfarin, heparin, dabigatran, rivaroxaban) may be prescribed for patients with CVD. These patients may have prolonged bleeding after surgical procedures, but many studies have demonstrated that use of local hemostatic agents are preferable to discontinuing the medications.[20-24] For patients who have had coronary artery stents placed, discontinuation of antiplatelet agents greatly increases the risk of stent thrombosis, MI, or death during the first 12 months after placement.[25] Any suggested modification of anticoagulant regimen in the CVD patient for dental surgery should be done in consultation and on advice of the patient's physician.

Susceptibility to Infection/Antibiotic Prophylaxis

Antibiotic premedication is indicated for patients with high risk of developing IE. The AHA and the American Dental Association have worked together to review the evidence of these risks, and the most recent guidelines were published in 2007 (see Table 2.4).[26] It should be specifically noted that patients with implanted electronic devices such as pacemakers, cardioverters, and defibrillators, do not need to have antibiotic premedication prior to invasive dental care.[27] Similarly, patients who have had coronary artery stents or CABG surgery do not need antibiotic premedication prior to dental procedures.[28]

A patient who has had a heart transplant may be taking antirejection drugs, for example, tacrolimus, cyclosporine, azathioprine, and prednisone. The cardiologist should be consulted regarding potential need for supplemental

Table 2.4. Summary of AHA Infective Endocarditis Antibiotic Premedication Guidelines

Cardiac conditions associated with the highest risk of adverse outcome from endocarditis for which prophylaxis with dental procedures is recommended

- Prosthetic cardiac valve
- Previous infective endocarditis
- Congenital heart disease
  - Unrepaired cyanotic conditions
  - Completely repaired with prosthetic material within the first 6 months after the repair
  - Incompletely repaired with prosthetic material
- Cardiac transplantation patients who develop valvulopathy

Dental procedures for which antibiotic prophylaxis is recommended

- All dental procedures that involve the manipulation of gingival tissue or the periapical region of teeth or perforation of the oral mucosa
- This does *not* include
  - routine anesthetic injections through noninfected tissue,
  - dental radiographs,
  - placement or removal of prosthodontic or orthodontic appliances,
  - adjustment of appliances,
  - shedding of deciduous teeth,
  - bleeding from trauma to the lips or oral mucosa.

Table 2.5. Antibiotic Prescriptions (Single Dose 30–60 Minutes before Dental Procedure)

Route of Administration	Antibiotic	Adult Dosage	Child Dosage
Oral	Amoxicillin	2 g	50 mg/kg
Penicillin allergic	Clindamycin	600 mg	20 mg/kg
	Cephalexin	2 g	50 mg/kg
	Azithromycin	500 mg	15 mg/kg
Unable to take oral meds	Ampicillin or cefazolin	2 g IM or IV	50 mg/kg IM or IV
	Ceftriaxone	1 g IM or IV	50 mg/kg IM or IV
Penicillin allergic	Cefazolin or ceftriazone	1 g IM or IV	50 mg/kg IM or IV
	Clindamycin	600 mg IM or IV	20 mg/kg IM or IV

Adapted from Wilson et al.[26]

corticosteroids for stressful dental procedures, as well as the potential for antibiotic premedication if the "new" heart is developing any valvulopathy[26] (Table 2.5).

Drug Actions/Interactions

Beta-blockers are prescribed for many patients with CVD. For patients who are taking a nonselective beta-blocker, for example, propranolol, it is recommended that the amount of epinephrine-containing local anesthesia be limited to two to three carpules per appointment to avoid a rapid elevation in BP.[11,29] In a systematic review, the use of epinephrine-containing local anesthetic in uncontrolled hypertensive patients, on average, slightly elevated systolic BP 15.3 mm, diastolic BP 2.3 mm, and heart rate 9.3 beats per minute compared with 11.7, 3.3, and 4.7, respectively for anesthesia without epinephrine.[30] A limit of two to three carpules of anesthetic with lidocaine per appointment for patients with CVD is supported by JNC 7 and others.[7,29] Retraction cord containing epinephrine is not recommended for any patient with CVD, although no evidence is available to support this recommendation.[30]

Many other medications for CVD can cause oral adverse effects (see Table 2.2). For some patients, the dentist can consult with the physician to see if another medication is appropriate so that the deleterious side effects can be avoided. The dentist should never advise the patient to discontinue a medication without consulting the prescribing physician.

Patient's Ability to Tolerate Dental Care

For patients with CVD, it is important to reduce anxiety and pain related to a dental procedure as the stress could provoke a release of endogenous epinephrine and norepinephrine. A patient with stable angina may report an episode of chest pain, and cardiac dysrhythmias may develop as a patient's heart rate increases.[11] In patients who are recovering from a recent MI, CABG, valve replacement, or other cardiac surgery, the heart may be even more sensitive to these catecholamines. However, the epinephrine used in local anesthetic appears to be tolerated in most patients with CVD, with many studies that show the benefit of extending the duration of anesthesia is greater than the potential risk.[29,30]

Anxiolytic drugs, nitrous oxide/oxygen analgesia, or sedation protocols might be of benefit to the anxious patient with CVD;

however, in the CHF patient receiving conscious sedation with intravenous agents, fluid overload must be avoided. Scheduling appointments in the afternoon may increase tolerance to dental treatment. Patients with CHF may also feel as though they struggle for breath when fully reclined in the dental chair, making a semisupine chair position preferable. For patients with severe CHF, supplemental oxygen should be available.

Medical Emergencies

Recognition

Dental patients with CVD are at higher risk of MI, especially if pain and anxiety are present. Knowing the patient's medical history is the first step in preventing medical emergencies. The dentist should assure that the patient is taking his medications as prescribed, and vital signs should be measured before any treatment begins. If there are questions about the medical history, a consultation with the physician is indicated.

If a dental patient starts to experience difficulty breathing, irregular heartbeat, or chest pain, it must be considered that the CVD has become acute, and there could be a life-threatening situation. For many of these patients, the acute situation is MI that must be managed quickly before heart muscle is permanently damaged.

Management Protocol

Many states are requiring that dental offices be equipped with automated external defibrillators. In a medical emergency, the dental team must assess the patient's signs and symptoms, perform basic life support measures (cardiopulmonary resuscitation or CPR), and pursue emergency medical service (EMS), call 9-1-1, as fast as possible. For a patient who has been prescribed nitroglycerine for AP, it is suitable to have the patient try at least one dose while sitting in the dental chair before EMS is called. If the pain does not resolve, the patient is likely to be having an MI, and must be transported to the hospital. EMS personnel will benefit from good record-keeping during the first stages of the emergency, that is, document vital signs, the time that the patient takes the nitroglycerine, and other observations of the patient's status.

It is strongly recommended that dental offices have a plan for dealing with patients who have medical emergencies, and that the personnel involved practice this plan periodically. Any emergency medications, including oxygen should be checked periodically for readiness. Refer to Chapter 20.

IV. Recommended Readings and Cited References

Recommended Readings

Haas SF. Preparing dental office staff members of emergencies: developing a basic action plan. J Am Dent Assoc 2010;141(Suppl. 1):8S–13S.

Little JW, Falace DA, Miller CS, Rhodus NL. Dental Management of the Medically Compromised Patient, 7th ed. Chapters 2–6. 2008. Mosby Elsevier, St. Louis, MO.

Reed KL. Basic management of medical emergencies: recognizing a patient's distress. J Am Dent Assoc 2010;141(Suppl. 1):20S–4S.

Cited References

1. Friedewald VE, Kornman KS, Beck JD, Genco R, Goldfine A, Libby P, et al. The American Journal of Cardiology and Journal of Periodontology Editors' consensus: periodontitis and atherosclerotic cardiovascular disease. Am J Cardiol 2009; 104(1):59–68.
2. Demmer RT, Desvarieux M. Periodontal infections and cardiovascular disease: the heart of the matter. J Am Dent Assoc 2006;137(Suppl. 1): 14S–20S.
3. Minassian C, D'Aiuto F, Hingorani AD, Smeeth L. Invasive dental treatment and risk for vascular

events: a self-controlled case series. Ann Intern Med 2010;153(8):499–506.
4. Moe KT, Wong P. Current trends in diagnostic biomarkers of acute coronary syndrome. Ann Acad Med Singapore 2010;39(3):210–5.
5. Grech ED, Ramsdale DR. Acute coronary syndrome: unstable angina and non-ST segment elevation myocardial infarction. BMJ 2003;326(7401):1259–61.
6. Chobanian AV, Bakris GL, Black HR, Cushman WC, Green LA, Izzo JL Jr., et al. Seventh report of the Joint National Committee on Prevention, Detection, Evaluation, and Treatment of High Blood Pressure. Hypertension 2003;42(6):1206–52.
7. Herman WW, Konzelman JL, Prisant LM; Joint National Committee on Prevention, Detection, Evaluation, and Treatment of High Blood Pressure. New national guidelines on hypertension: a summary for dentistry. J Am Dent Assoc 2004;135(5):576–84.
8. Roger VL, Go A, Lloyd-Jones DM, Adams RJ, Berry JD, Brown TM, et al. Heart disease and stroke statistics—2011 update: a report from the American Heart Association. Circulation 2011;123(4):e18–209.
9. Glick M, Greenberg BL. The potential role of dentist in identifying patients' risk of experiencing coronary heart disease events. J Am Dent Assoc 2005;136(11):1541–6.
10. Torpet LA, Kragelund C, Reibel J, Nauntofte B. Oral adverse drug reactions to cardiovascular drugs. Crit Rev Oral Biol Med 2004;15(1):28–46.
11. Malamed SF. Knowing your patients. J Am Dent Assoc 2010;141(Suppl. 1):3S–7S.
12. Campeau L. Grading of angina pectoris. Circulation 1976;54(3):522–3.
13. Jessup M, Abraham WT, Casey DE, Feldman AM, Francis GS, Ganiats TG, et al. 2009 Focused update: ACCF/AHA guidelines for the diagnosis and management of heart failure in adults—a report of the American College of Cardiology Foundation/American Heart Association Task Force on practical guidelines, developed in collaboration with the International Society for Heart and Lung Transplantation. Circulation 2009;119(14):1977–2016.
14. Herman WW, Ferguson HW. Dental care for patients with heart failure: an update. J Am Dent Assoc 2010;141(7):845–53.
15. Rhodus NL, Little JW. Dental management of the patient with cardiac arrhythmias: an update. Oral Surg Oral Med Oral Pathol Oral Radiol Endod 2003;96(6):659–68.
16. Wilson BL, Broberg C, Barmgartner JC, Harris C, Kron J. Safety of electronic apex locators and pulp testers in patients with implanted cardiac pacemakers or cardioverter/defibrillators. J Endod 2006;32(9):847–52.
17. Niwa H, Sato Y, Matsuura H. Safety of dental treatment in patients with previously diagnosed acute myocardial infarction or unstable angina pectoris. Oral Surg Oral Med Oral Pathol Oral Radiol Endod 2000;89(1):35–41.
18. Silvestre FJ, Miralles L, Tamarit C, Gascon R. Dental management of the patient with ischemic heart disease: an update. Med Oral 2002;7(3):222–30.
19. Little JW, Falace DA, Miller CS, Rhodus N. Dental Management of the Medically Compromised Patient, 7th ed. 2008. Mosby Elsevier, St. Louis, MO.
20. Blinder D, Manor Y, Martinowitz U, Taicher S, Hashomer T. Dental extractions in patients maintained on continued oral anticoagulant: comparison of local hemostatic modalities. Oral Surg Oral Med Oral Pathol Oral Radiol Endod 1998;88(2):137–40.
21. Blinder D, Manor Y, Martinowitz U, Taicher S. Dental extractions in patients maintained on oral anticoagulant therapy: comparison of INR value with occurrence of postoperative bleeding. Int J Oral Maxillofac Surg 2001;30(6):518–21.
22. Napeñas JJ, Hong CH, Brennan MT, Furney SL, Fox PC, Lockhart PB. The frequency of bleeding complications after invasive dental treatment in patients receiving single and dual antiplatelet therapy. J Am Dent Assoc 2009;140(6):690–5.
23. Van Dierman DE, Aartman IHA, Baart JA, Hoogstraten J, van der Waal I. Dental management of patients using antithrombotic drugs: critical appraisal of existing guidelines. Oral Surg Oral Med Oral Pathol Oral Radiol Endod 2009;107(5):616–24.
24. Wahl MJ. Myths of dental surgery in patients receiving anticoagulant therapy. J Am Dent Assoc 2000;131(1):77–81.
25. Grines CL, Bonow RO, Casey DE Jr., Gardner TJ, Lockhart PB, Moliterno DJ, et al. Prevention of premature discontinuation of dual antiplatelet

therapy in patients with coronary artery stents: a science advisory from the American Heart Association, American College of Cardiology, Society for Cardiovascular Angiography and Interventions, American College of Surgeons, and American Dental Association, with representation from the American College of Physicians. J Am Coll Cardiol 2007;49(6):734–39.
26. Wilson W, Taubert KA, Gewitz M, Lockhart PB, Baddour LM, Levison M, et al. Prevention of infective endocarditis. Guidelines from the American Heart Association. A guideline from the American Heart Association Rheumatic Fever, Endocarditis, and Kawasaki Disease Committee, Council on Cardiovascular Disease in the Young, and the Council on Clinical Cardiology, Council on Cardiovascular Surgery and Anesthesia, and the Quality of Care and Outcomes Research Interdisciplinary Working Group. Circulation 2007;116(15):1736–54.
27. Baddour LM, Epstein AE, Erickson CC, Knight BP, Levison ME, Lockhart PB, et al. A summary of the update on cardiovascular implantable electronic device infections and their management: a scientific statement from the American Heart Association. J Am Dent Assoc 2011;142(2):159–65.
28. Baddour LM, Bettmann MA, Bolger AF, Epstein AE, Ferrieri P, Gerber MA. Nonvalvular cardiovascular device-related infections. Circulation 2003;108(16):2015–31.
29. Brown RS, Rhodus NL. Epinephrine and local anesthesia revisited. Oral Surg Oral Med Oral Pathol Oral Radiol Endod 2005;100(4):401–48.
30. Bader JD, Bonito AJ, Shugars DA. A systematic review of cardiovascular effects of epinephrine on hypertensive patients. Oral Surg Oral Med Oral Pathol Oral Radiol Endod 2002;93(6):647–53.

Pulmonary Disease

Miriam R. Robbins DDS, MS

I. Background

Description of Disease/Condition

The prime function of the lungs is respiration to oxygenate tissues and remove carbon dioxide. Obstructive lung diseases are characterized by decreased expiratory flow rates and include asthma, chronic obstructive pulmonary disease (COPD), and cystic fibrosis (CF). Restrictive lung diseases are characterized by a decrease in the compliance of the lungs, the chest wall, or both, and are often due to pulmonary fibrosis or neuromuscular diseases affecting the respiratory muscles.

Asthma

Asthma is a chronic, potentially life-threatening, inflammatory disorder of the airways associated with airway hyperresponsiveness to stimuli resulting in bronchial edema and narrowing of bronchial airways. It is marked by episodic exacerbations that lead to recurrent episodes of wheezing, breathlessness, chest tightness, and coughing that result in variable and often reversible airflow limitation.

COPD

COPD is a term used to describe preventable respiratory disorders that involve airway obstruction that is not fully reversible. Examples of COPD are chronic bronchitis, peripheral airway disease (bronchiolitis), and emphysema. These often present with overlapping symptoms, the most characteristic being cough and sputum production that may precede the development of chronic and progressive dyspnea.

CF

CF is an autosomal recessive disorder. Most carriers are asymptomatic. CF is a disease of exocrine gland function that primarily involves the upper and lower airways, pancreas, and gastrointestinal and reproductive systems. CF is diagnosed by measuring electrolyte levels in sweat, particularly chloride. Production of

The ADA Practical Guide to Patients with Medical Conditions, First Edition. Edited by Lauren L. Patton.
© 2012 American Dental Association. Published 2012 by John Wiley & Sons, Inc.

abnormally thick mucus in the lungs leading to chronic respiratory infections and pancreatic enzyme insufficiency leading to malnutrition are common occurrences.

Restrictive Lung Diseases

Restrictive lung diseases are characterized by a decrease in the total volume of air that the lungs are able to hold. It can be caused by a decrease in the elasticity of the lungs themselves, weakness of the chest wall muscles during inhalation, or conditions that increase the size of the abdomen and limit movement of the diaphragm.

Tuberculosis (TB)

TB is an infectious and communicable disease caused by *Mycobacterium tuberculosis*. Its transmission is person to person through the inhalation of infectious respiratory droplets that become airborne when a person with active TB disease of the lungs speaks, coughs, sneezes, or sings.

Obstructive Sleep Apnea[1] (OSA)

Obstructive sleep apnea syndrome (OSAS) is characterized by partial or complete upper airway obstruction during sleep, causing apnea and hypopnea, coupled with daytime symptoms, most often excessive sleepiness.

- *Apnea* is the cessation of airflow at the nose or the mouth for at least 10 seconds.
- *Hypopnea* is a 30–50% reduction in airflow for at least 10 seconds and oxygen desaturation of at least 2–4%.
- The *apnea-hypopnea index (AHI)* is the number of apneas and hypopneas per hour of sleep.
- OSAHS is obstructive sleep apnea/hypopnea syndrome.
    - Mild cases have an AHI of 5–14.
    - Moderate cases have an AHI of 15–30.
    - Severe cases have an AHI >30.

Patients with moderate to severe OSA have significantly increased mortality. Even mild-to-moderate OSA (AHI 5–15/hour) increases the risk for hypertension, stroke, myocardial infarction and injury due to motor vehicle accidents.

Lung Cancer

Lung cancer forms in tissues of the lungs, usually in the cells lining air passages. The two main types are small cell lung cancer and non-small-cell lung cancer.

Lung Transplantation

Lung transplantation can prolong and improve the quality of life for patients with severe end-stage pulmonary disease. The majority of lung transplants are performed for patients with severe COPD/emphysema, idiopathic pulmonary fibrosis, CF, and pulmonary arterial hypertension.

Pathogenesis/Etiology

Asthma

Exposure to a trigger produces release of histamine and cytokines that result in bronchospasm, hypersecretion of mucus, and diminished ciliary motion.

There are two main types of asthma, categorized by the trigger stimulus:

- Extrinsic (or allergic) asthma
    - Accounts for over 50% of asthma (>90% in children)
    - Triggered by activation of mast cells and histamine degranulation following exposure to allergens such as dust, pet dander, mold, and pollen
- Intrinsic (or nonallergic/idiopathic) asthma
    - Tends to occur after the age of 30
    - Triggered by respiratory irritants (e.g., tobacco smoke and air pollution), respira-

Table 3.1. Classification of COPD Severity

Stage	Pulmonary Function Test Findings	Symptoms
I: Mild	Mild airflow limitations FEV_1/FVC <70% FEV_1 ≥80% predicted	+/− Chronic cough and sputum production; patient unaware of abnormal lung function
II: Moderate	Worsening airflow limitations FEV_1/FVC <70% FEV_1 between 50% and 80% predicted	Dyspnea on exertion, cough, and sputum production; patient usually seeks medical care because of symptoms
III: Severe	Further worsening of airflow limitations FEV_1/FVC <70% FEV_1 between 30% and 50% predicted	Increased SOB, reduced exercise capacity, fatigue, repeated exacerbations impact quality of life
IV: Very severe	Severe airflow limitations FEV_1/FVC <70% FEV_1 <30% predicted or FEV_1 <50% predicted plus chronic respiratory failure	Cor pulmonale (right heart failure), quality of life impaired, life-threatening exacerbations

FEV_1, forced expiratory volume in 1 second; FVC, forced vital capacity; FEV, forced expiratory volume; SOB, shortness of breath. Adapted from Global Strategy for the Diagnosis, Management and Prevention of COPD, Global Initiative for Chronic Obstructive Lung Disease (GOLD).[8]

tory infections, exercise, cold air, anxiety and stress, and gastroesophageal reflux disease (GERD)[2]

A subtype of intrinsic asthma is induced by aspirin and other nonsteroidal anti-inflammatory (NSAID) medications. This is not an allergic reaction but appears to be the result of these medications' effect on cyclooxygenase.[3]

About 10% of asthma sufferers will have both extrinsic and intrinsic triggers. Symptoms are frequently worse at night or in the early morning. Pulmonary function testing generally shows airflow limitations that reverse with bronchodilator therapy.

COPD

COPD is a progressive disease associated with an abnormal inflammatory response to noxious agents, such as tobacco smoke or occupational/environmental pollution. Chronic inflammation causes narrowing of the small airways that decreases airway flow and destroys lung parenchyma and alveolar walls. This leads to decreased elastic recoil, diminishing the ability of the airways to remain open during expiration. Airflow limitation and lung function are best measured by spirometry, which measures the amount (volume) and/or speed (flow) of air that can be inhaled and exhaled. Classification of the severity of impairment is listed in Table 3.1.

Worldwide, the most significant cause of COPD is cigarette smoking:

- Approximately 20% of current smokers and 14% of former smokers have some degree of clinically significant COPD.[4]
- The degree of severity of COPD increases as the number of cigarettes smoked per day and the duration of smoking increases.
- Smoking cessation, even when significant airflow limitation is present, can lead to improvement in lung function and can slow or halt disease progression.

There are genetic factors that modify risk:

- A hereditary deficiency of alpha-1 antitrypsin, commonly seen in people of northern European descent, leads to accelerated development of emphysema and decrease in lung function in both smokers and nonsmokers, although smoking increases the risk significantly.[5]

Bacterial colonization may play a significant role in airway inflammation and the pathogenesis and progression of COPD. Respiratory tract infections have been associated with acute exacerbations of this condition.

COPD is characterized by a specific pattern of inflammation involving neutrophils, macrophages, and lymphocytes.

Bronchitis
- Airflow obstruction is the result of chronic inflammation of the bronchioles resulting in
    - hyperplasia of the mucous-producing glands,
    - edema of the mucosa,
    - secretions resulting in narrowing of the airways.
- The lungs become poorly ventilated leading to hypoxemia, cyanosis, CO_2 retention, and polycythemia.

Emphysema
- Airflow obstruction that hinders expiration develops when there is an irreversible enlargement of the bronchioles and alveoli.
- Inflammatory mediators attract activated neutrophils that release proteases that break down connective tissue components and lead to destruction of alveolar walls resulting in enlarged air spaces and loss of elastic recoil of the lungs.

COPD results in progressive dyspnea and hypercapnia with increasing exacerbations and debilitation. COPD and its comorbidities must be treated continuously to control symptoms, improve quality of life, reduce exacerbations, and possibly reduce mortality. Death results mainly from cardiovascular diseases and respiratory failure in advanced COPD.

Restrictive Lung Diseases

Common causes include idiopathic pulmonary fibrosis, radiation fibrosis, scleroderma, sarcoidosis, eosinophilic pneumonia, scoliosis, myasthenia gravis, muscular dystrophy, and obesity. These underlying diseases are often progressive.

TB

The lungs are the most common site of TB infection. Once an airborne droplet containing TB bacillus is inhaled, it travels through the lungs to the terminal bronchi and alveoli. In hosts with healthy immune systems, the majority of the bacilli are destroyed. The ones not immediately destroyed can enter the bloodstream and spread throughout the body infecting other sites, or remain in the alveolus. Within 2–6 weeks, the bacilli are engulfed by macrophages that form a barrier shell, called a granuloma that keeps the bacilli contained and prevents systemic dissemination, resulting in latent TB infection (LTBI).

Asymptomatic LTBI occurs in 90% of those infected with the bacilli, with only a 10% lifetime chance of progressing to TB disease. Patients with LTBI are not infectious and cannot spread organisms to others. Progression from LTBI to TB disease occurs when the immune system cannot prevent the TB bacilli from multiplying. Coinfection with HIV is the strongest risk factor for progressing to active TB disease, and TB is one of the leading causes of death among people infected with HIV worldwide. Other risk factors for developing active TB disease include diabetes, chronic and end-stage renal failure, hematological malignancies, and malnutrition.[6]

OSA

OSA is caused by a narrowed upper airway and increased collapse of the muscles and soft tissues. As the muscles and tongue relax during sleep, they can partially occlude the opening to the airway and cause increased resistance to airflow. Risk factors include obesity, smoking and alcohol use, having hypertension, or any anatomical deviation that narrows the dimensions of the upper airway including deviated nasal septum and enlarged turbinates, elongated soft palate and uvula, retrognathic mandible, enlarged tongue, and redundant parapharyngeal folds. Sleep apnea can affect multiple family members, suggesting a possible genetic basis.

Lung Cancer

Most lung cancers fall into three pathological types: squamous cell carcinoma, adenocarcinoma, and small-cell (oat-cell) carcinoma. Thoracic symptoms can include cough, hemoptysis, wheezing, and pleural pain. Extrathoracic signs and symptoms are due to metastasis, which is common to the liver, adrenal glands, brain, and bone. Nonspecific signs include anorexia, weight loss, weakness, and fatigue.

Epidemiology
Asthma

Prevalence, hospitalizations, and fatal asthma exacerbations have all increased in the United States over the past 20 years. Centers for Disease Control and Prevention (CDC) statistics show 34 million or 1 in 9 Americans have been diagnosed with asthma during their lifetimes, with 12.3 million having experienced an asthma attack in the previous year. In 2008, asthma was responsible for 1.6 million emergency department visits and almost half a million hospitalizations.[7]

COPD

It is the fourth leading cause of chronic morbidity and mortality in the United States, and is projected to rank fifth in 2020 in burden of disease worldwide.[8]

CF

CF is the most common lethal inherited disease among Caucasians (occurring in the United States in 1:3200–3500 newborns)[9] and the most common cause of obstructive airway disease in patients under 30 years. End-stage lung disease is the principal cause of death 90% of the time[9] with the average life expectancy around 37 years.

TB

The CDC recently estimated that one-third of the world's population is infected with TB, with 9 million developing active TB disease each year, and nearly 2 million TB-related deaths annually. Most of these cases are in Southeast Asia and Sub-Saharan Africa. In the United States, TB has shown a steady decline, with the number of reported TB cases in 2010 (11,182) the lowest recorded since 1953.[10]

OSA

An estimated 18 million Americans have sleep apnea. It affects all ages, although the incidence is highest in middle-aged persons. It is more common among men. The incidence and prevalence depend on the criteria used to define the syndrome. As many as 40–60% of all adults age 60 or older have some form of sleep-related breathing disorder, most commonly snoring, which is a significant risk factor for OSA. In a random sample of employed Americans aged 30–60 years, 9% of women and 24% of men had AHI scores of 5 or higher accompanied with complaints of daytime sleepiness.[11] The incidence of OSAS in children is 1–3%.

Lung Cancer

Lung cancer is the leading cause of cancer deaths in the United States, with over 160,000 deaths annually, and the second leading site of new cancers for both genders after prostate cancer for men and breast cancer for women.[12] Smokers are 10–20 times more likely to get lung cancer. Smoking is the principal cause of about 90% of lung cancer in men and almost 80% in women, followed by asbestos and silica exposures. Most patients are clinically asymptomatic until late in the disease course, resulting in a mean survival time of 9 months after diagnosis.

Lung Transplantation

A total of 30,673 lung transplants were done worldwide between 1995 and 2010.[13] Lung transplant patients have the highest mortality rate of organ recipients. Survival rates for all types of lung transplants are 79% at 1 year, 64% at 3 years, 53% at 5 years, and 30% at 10 years.[13]

Coordination of Care between Dentist and Physician

Many dental patients with these pulmonary diseases can receive the full range of dental treatments with minor adjustment, but in those patients with more severe disease, the consequences of airway obstruction and the subsequent hypoxic state may require modification for safe delivery of dental care. Important aspects of care coordination include the dentist gaining an understanding of the pulmonary disease severity, importance of controlling oral bacteria that can be aspirated, awareness of triggers and medications to avoid, and the potential spread of infectious pulmonary conditions. Dentists also play a role in the management of OSA by fabrication of oral appliances.

II. Medical Management

Identification

Obstructive and restrictive lung diseases have different etiologies, but often have overlapping symptoms. A thorough medical history coupled with a comprehensive physical exam, review of systems and review of current and past use of tobacco products are the key to accurate diagnosis of pulmonary diseases. A nonspecific sign of significant cardiopulmonary disease is clubbing of the fingers and bluish fingernails as shown in Fig. 3.1.

Medical History/Physical Examination

Asthma

Asthma has a wide spectrum of clinical severity. The intensity of airflow obstruction determines the severity of an acute event and the frequency and severity of airflow obstruction between episodes determines the severity of the disease. Symptoms used to assess level of asthmatic control are shown in Table 3.2.

Most patients have mild to moderate asthma and function normally with minimal to no symptoms between attacks, although individ-

Figure 3.1 Clubbing of the fingers in a 22-year-old with advanced cystic fibrosis.

Table 3.2. Assessment of Asthma Control

Symptom	Controlled (All of Below)	Partially Controlled (Any Present in Any Week)	Uncontrolled
Daytime symptoms	Twice or less per week	More than twice a week	Three or more features of partially controlled asthma present in any week
Limitations of actions	None	Any	
Nocturnal symptoms	None	Any	
Need for rescue medications	Twice or less per week	More than twice a week	
Lung function (PEF or FEV_1)	Normal	<80% predicted	

PEF, peak expiratory flow.

ual attacks can still produce moderate to severe symptoms. See Table 3.3 for the classification of asthma severity. Attacks occur in paroxysms with rapid onset of chest tightness and airflow obstruction, dyspnea with decrease in forced expiratory volume in 1 second (FEV_1), coughing, wheezing, tachypnea, and tachycardia. Status asthmaticus is a prolonged, severe asthma attack that does not respond to bronchodilator therapy leading to fatigue, cyanosis, tachycardia, and pulsus paradoxus (decrease in systolic blood pressure >15 mmHg with inspiration), and ultimately resulting in respiratory failure and death if not reversed.

Features that are associated with increased risk of adverse events include poor clinical control and/or frequent exacerbations despite high-dose medications, presence of nocturnal symptoms, need for emergency room visits, low FEV_1, and cigarette smoking.

COPD

COPD has an insidious onset. Clinical features include chronic cough that eventually progresses to dyspnea on exertion. For the diagnosis and assessment of COPD, spirometry is the gold standard. The presence of FEV_1/forced vital capacity (FVC) <70% confirms the presence of airflow limitation that is not fully reversible, with FEV_1 serving to quantify the degree of airflow impairment. Both chronic bronchitis and emphysema show marked decrease in the FEV_1/FVC ratio.[14]

Arterial blood gas analysis looking at levels of hypoxia and hypercapnia can be used to individualize the diagnosis, prognosis, and treatment regimen. In chronic bronchitis, chest radiographs may show prominent vascular markings and bronchial thickening, while in emphysema, there are marked signs of hyperinflation (flattened diaphragm on the lateral chest film and an increase in the volume of the retrosternal air space) and a relatively small heart.

Two clinically distinct types of COPD patients exist, although many patients with COPD have elements of both diseases:

Emphysema (pink puffers) usually presents in later years (>60 years of age) with progressive dyspnea and weight loss, but little cough or sputum production. Patients often have a "barrel chest" due to chest wall enlargement and hyperinflation of the lungs. There is no difficulty with inspiration, but expiration may be assisted with pursed lips and use of accessory respiratory muscles. The chest may be hyper-resonant, heart sounds are muffled, and expiratory wheezing may be heard.

Table 3.3. Classification of Asthma

	Symptoms	Nocturnal Symptoms	Pulmonary Function	Treatment Acute	Treatment Chronic
Mild intermittent	Brief exacerbations ≤2 days/week, good exercise tolerance	≤2 nights/month	Normal between exacerbations FEV_1 ≥80% predicted	Short-acting β_2 agonist as needed (needed <2 days/week)	None
Mild persistent	>2 times/week but <1 time/day, episodes may affect activity level	3–4 nights/month	FEV_1 ≥80% predicted	Short-acting β_2 agonist (needed >2 days/week, but not daily)	Daily inhaled anti-inflammatory like low-dose inhaled steroid or cromolyn, nedocromil, or theophylline
Moderate persistent	>Once/day, episodes affect activity	>1 night/week, but not every night	FEV_1 60–80% predicted	Short-acting β_2 agonist (needed daily)	Medium-dose inhaled steroid OR low-dose inhaled steroid AND long-acting β_2 agonist OR leukotriene inhibitor
Severe persistent	Continual symptoms, limited activity	Frequent/nightly	FEV_1 ≤60% predicted	Short-acting β_2 agonist (needed multiple times daily)	Medium- or high-dose steroids AND long-acting β_2 agonist AND/OR systemic steroids, theophylline, or leukotriene inhibitor

Adapted from the National Asthma Education and Prevention Program.[2]

Chronic bronchitis (blue bloaters)	Emphysema (pink puffers)
Overweight	Thin with barrel chest
Productive cough/mucopurulent sputum	Dry cough/little sputum
Inspiratory/expiratory wheeze	Expiratory wheeze
Mild dyspnea	Severe dyspnea
Frequent infections	Infrequent infections
Enlarged heart	Enlarged chest and small heart
Severe hypoxia/hypercapnia	Mild hypoxia/hypocapnia
Polycythemia	Normal hematocrit
Cor pulmonale common	Cor pulmonale rare
Respond to bronchodilators	Poor response to bronchodilators

Chronic bronchitis (blue bloaters) presents at younger age (around 50 years of age). Symptoms include a chronic cough with sputum production and expectoration, weight gain, and episodic dyspnea. Chronic hypoxia leads to cor pulmonale (right-sided heart failure), which can lead to edema and cyanosis. Patients have difficulty with inspiration and expiration and chronic rhonchi and wheezing may be present.

Restrictive Lung Diseases

Symptoms include cough, dyspnea on exertion, wheezing, and chest pain. Pulmonary function tests show a decreased FVC and normal FEV. Patients with early interstitial restrictive lung disease may have normal arterial blood gas values, and cyanosis does not occur until the process is advanced. On physical exam, there is decreased chest wall movement, increased use of accessory muscles, and rapid, shallow breathing.

TB

Symptoms:

- LTBI: asymptomatic
- Active TB disease: general malaise, weakness, weight loss, fever, night sweats, and lymphadenopathy
- Pulmonary TB disease: chronic cough (present for more than 3 weeks), chest pain, and hemoptysis
- TB infections of other organs: symptoms specific to the organ affected

Diagnosis relies on a tuberculin skin test (TST) or TB blood test, chest X-rays, and microscopic

Comparison of latent and active tuberculosis (TB)

Latent TB infection (LTBI)	TB disease
M. tuberculosis in the body Tuberculin skin test (Mantoux or purified protein derivative [PPD]) usually +	
Chest X-ray normal	Chest X-ray abnormal
Sputum/smear/culture negative	Sputum/smear/culture may be positive
No symptoms	Symptoms
Not infectious; has inactive TB bacteria	Infectious; has active TB bacteria
Needs preventive treatment in order to prevent active TB disease	Needs treatment to treat active TB disease

Figure 3.2 Mantoux tuberculin skin test and positive result. Source: http://www.cdc.gov/tb.

examination and culture of bodily fluids. A positive TST or interferon-gamma release assay (IGRA) blood test can only tell that the patient has been infected with TB bacilli. It cannot tell if the person has LTBI or active TB disease. Microscopic identification of acid-fast bacilli (AFB) in sputum samples and chest X-rays are used to determine if a patient is infectious. Definitive diagnosis is based on culture or direct molecular tests that positively identify M. tuberculosis in bodily fluids; however, cultures can take several weeks to grow:

- Mantoux TST: the most useful and reliable method of determining infection.
  - Intradermal injection of 0.1 mL of tuberculin purified protein derivative (PPD) usually on the inside of the forearm.
  - Skin reaction is measured in millimeters (mm) of induration (not erythema) 48–72 hours after administration.
    - A positive test depends on this measurement and the person's risk factors for TB. For a person with no known risk factors, the induration must measure ≥15 mm, while HIV-positive patients or those in recent contact with a person with TB disease only need a 5-mm reaction.[10] See Fig. 3.2.
- IGRAs: whole blood tests that measure a person's immune reactivity to M. tuberculosis. (e.g., QuantiIFERONE® Gold In-Tube test [QFT-GIT], Cellestis Inc., Valencia, CA).
  - Not widely used because of their expense.
  - Useful to screen patients with a history of receiving the bacilli Calmette-Guerin (BCG) vaccine.
- BCG: a vaccine for TB that is used in countries with a high TB prevalence primarily to prevent TB meningitis in children.
  - It is not currently used in the United States because of the variable effectiveness of the vaccine against pulmonary TB and the low risk of infection.
  - Previous vaccination with the BCG vaccine can cause false-positive TST but does not affect the results of the QFT-GIT.

Positive tests require a radiographic examination and sputum culture to rule out active

Table 3.4. Pulmonary Function Changes in Obstructive and Restrictive Disease

Measure	Obstructive Disorders	Restrictive Disorders
FEV_1/FVC	<Predicted	≥Predicted
FEV_1	Always reduced	May be normal or reduced
FVC	Usually reduced	Reduced
TLC	Normal or increased	Always reduced
RV	Normal or increased	Reduced

FEV_1, 1-second forced expiratory volume; FVC, forced vital capacity; RV, residual volume; TLC, total lung capacity. Adapted from http://www.merckmanuals.com/.

disease.[15] A chest X-ray is used to detect pulmonary lesions including infiltrates, cavitations, and hilar adenopathy. These lesions may suggest TB but cannot be used to definitively diagnose TB. A negative chest X-ray can rule out TB disease in an asymptomatic patient with a positive TST. Likewise, the presence of AFB in a sputum smear often indicates TB disease but does not confirm a diagnosis until the culture is positively identified. However, a positive culture is not necessary to begin treatment if other tests are suggestive of disease.

OSA

The most common symptoms of OSAS are snoring, excessive daytime sleepiness, nocturnal snorting and gasping, and witnessed apneic episodes. Nonrestorative sleep that leaves patients feeling mentally dull, groggy, and confused upon waking is a common finding. Other nocturnal symptoms include restlessness, diaphoresis, awakenings with a sensation of choking or dyspnea, esophageal reflux with subsequent heartburn and laryngospasm, frequent nocturia, dry mouth, drooling, and, rarely, enuresis.

The overnight polysomnogram (or sleep study) is the standard diagnostic test for OSA. It is a comprehensive recording of the physiological changes that occur during sleep including brain activity (EEG), eye movements (EOM), muscle activity (EMG), heart rhythm (ECG), respiratory airflow, and effort and changes in blood oxygen levels.

Laboratory Testing

Pulmonary diseases are characterized by airflow limitations that are best evaluated using spirometry. See Table 3.4. Spirometry is the most reproducible, standardized, and objective way of measuring airflow limitation. It is the recording of a forced, rapid, and complete exhalation from a point of maximum inhalation. The exhaled volume is recorded as the FVC and the volume of FVC exhaled in the first second is the FEV_1. Normally, the ratio of FEV_1 to the FVC should exceed 70% in older adults and 85% in young adults. The degree of airflow obstruction generally correlates with the severity of the symptoms and associated physical findings, and is used to classify the severity of the patient's disease.

Chest radiographs, including posteroanterior (PA) and lateral views, are useful to differentiate different types of pulmonary diseases. Helpful laboratory studies include complete blood count, arteriole blood gases (ABG) looking at levels of pCO_2 and pO_2 to assess the degree of hypoxia present, and sputum examination to look for contributing organisms.

Medical Treatment

Asthma

Patients are instructed to avoid triggering agents. Pharmacological management is divided into maintenance drugs (taken chronically to control and prevent asthma symptoms) and rescue drugs (which relieve acute symptoms). Common medications to treat asthma and COPD are shown in Table 3.5:

- *Rescue medications* are most effectively delivered through a metered-dose inhaler (MDI). These first-line drugs are rapidly acting, short-acting (duration) β_2 agonists (sometimes given in combination with an anticholinergic agent) that are given at the onset of symptoms or before exposure to aggravating stimuli. They effectively relax bronchial smooth muscle causing immediate bronchodilatation.
- *Maintenance medications* include such second-line drugs as anti-inflammatory (steroid and nonsteroid) medications that relieve the inflammation that provokes bronchospasm and causes increased mucus, and long-acting bronchodilators designed to keep the airways open for prolonged periods. Nonsteroid drugs include mast cell stabilizers (cromolyn sodium and nedocromil) and leukotriene inhibitors. Steroids included inhaled and systemic forms. Oral xanthines such as theophylline cause smooth muscle relaxation and suppression of the inflammatory response of the airways to stimuli, and are considered third-line drugs added for patients with hard to control symptoms.

COPD

COPD is incurable. Key aspects of management are prevention (smoking cessation and elimination of environmental pollutants) and early intervention. Pharmacological therapy is used to prevent and control symptoms, reduce the frequency and severity of exacerbations, and improve health status and exercise tolerance. Medications alone do not modify the long-term decline in lung function.[8]

Medications used in the management of COPD are generally introduced in a stepwise fashion and added as the severity of the symptoms progresses:

- First-line drugs for symptom relief: anticholinergics that block bronchoconstriction and β_2 agonist bronchodilators that alter smooth muscle tone; usually delivered via inhaler on

Table 3.5. Common Medications to Treat Asthma/COPD

Short-acting β_2 agonists	Albuterol (Proventil®, Ventilin®), levalbuterol, metaproterenol, pirbuterol
Long-acting β_2 agonists	Arformoterol, formoterol, salmeterol
Anti-cholinergics	Ipratropium bromide (Atrovent®), tiotropium (Spiriva®)
Methylxanthines	Theophylline
Mast cell stabilizers	Cromolyn, nedocromil
Corticosteroids (inhaled)	Beclomethasone (Qvar®), budesonide (Pulmicort®), fluticasone, mometasone
Corticosteroids (systemic)	Dexamethasone, fludrocortisone, methylprednisolone, prednisone
Leukotriene receptor antagonists	Montelukast (Singulair®), zafirlukast, zileuton
Combination inhalers	Fluticasone/salmeterol (Advair Diskus®), ipratropium/albuterol (Combivent®), budesonide/formoterol (Symbicort®)

an as-needed basis in short-acting form or on a regular basis to help prevent or reduce symptoms in long-acting form.
- Second-line drugs: inhaled corticosteroids usually combined with a long-acting β_2 agonist in a single inhaler.
- Theophylline: a methylxanthine medication added to inhaled therapies for patients with more severe disease.
- Antibiotic therapy: used when clinical signs of airway infection such as mucopurulent sputum occurs.

Other ancillary measures include the following:

- annual influenza vaccine and pneumococcal vaccine every 5 years for patients over 65 or with FEV_1 <40%;
- use of long-term, low-flow oxygen therapy, with severe COPD;
- lung volume reduction surgery for emphysema to reduce hyperinflation and improve the mechanical efficiency of the lungs;
- lung transplantation in very advanced COPD may improve functional capacity and quality of life but is often prohibitively expensive.[8]

CF

Treatment includes:

- chronic antibiotics to prevent and treat lung and sinus infections;
- inhaled medications including β_2 agonists;
- steroids to help open the airways and decrease inflammation;
- DNAse enzyme therapy to thin mucus and make it easier to cough up;
- oxygen therapy, as needed;
- manual chest percussions (chest physical therapy or PT) and postural drainage several times daily to loosen mucus and make it easier to expectorate;
- diet high in protein and calories taken with pancreatic enzymes and fat-soluble vitamins to help absorb fats and protein to maintain weight and prevent malnutrition;
- lung transplantation.

Restrictive Lung Diseases

Treatment depends on the severity of the disease and the underlying cause:

- oxygen therapy and continuous positive airway pressure (CPAP) for patients with hypoxemia;
- inhaled and systemic corticosteroids and immunosuppressive agents for inflammatory etiologies;
- lung transplantation if there is substantial damage to lung parenchyma;
- correction of spinal deformities or bariatric surgery if related to scoliosis or obesity.

TB

Preventive Treatment for LTBI

Treatment for those with LTBI greatly reduces the risk of progression to TB disease and should be initiated once active TB disease has been ruled out. Treatment usually consists of a 9-month regimen of daily isoniazid (INH) for a minimum of 270 doses for most patients or rifampin daily for 4 months for a minimum of 120 doses.[6]

Treatment for Active TB Disease

Patients with TB disease usually receive multidrug regimens for 6–12 months, consisting of an initial phase of 2 months treatment with four drugs, usually isoniazid, rifampin, ethambutol, and pyrazinamide. This is followed by a continuation phase of 4–7 months of treatment with isoniazid and rifampin. Patients with good clinical response to the medications generally become noninfectious after 3 weeks of treatment. Case management, including directly observed therapy, is often mandatory for patients undergoing treatment for active disease. In order for a patient to be considered cured or noninfectious, there must be three consecutive AFB-negative sputum smears.

OSA

Management of OSA includes diet modification and weight loss, positional sleep therapy, CPAP, nocturnal oral sleep apnea devices, and a variety of surgical procedures aimed at enlarging the posterior airway space and stabilizing the airway against collapse. No medications are presently available for primary treatment.

CPAP (where positive airflow delivered via a nasal or oral mask maintains upper airway patency) is considered the first-line treatment for most patients with OSA, and routine use increases as the severity of the OSA increases. Pressure sores from the nasal mask, claustrophobia, nasal congestion, and dry mouth and eyes are side effects that may lead to poor compliance.[16]

Lung Cancer

Treatment can include surgical resection (for small tumors), radiotherapy for more advanced or not surgically resectable tumors, and multiple agent chemotherapy for small-cell tumors and combined with radiotherapy for the most advanced tumors. Non-small-cell lung cancer tumors are not very sensitive to most chemotherapy regimens, and therefore, chemotherapy alone is used only as palliation. Overall 5-year survival rate for all forms of lung cancer is 14%.[12]

Lung Transplantation

Patients undergoing lung transplants will be on lifelong immunosuppressant medications to prevent organ rejection, putting them at higher risk of infections. Other side effects of antirejection medications can include hypertension, diabetes, osteoporosis, adrenal suppression, poor wound healing, and malignancies. Patients may suffer bouts of acute or chronic rejection. Acute rejection often responds to therapy with increased doses of immunosuppressant medications. Chronic rejection, which results in scarring of the lungs' airways following inflammation, is irreversible and occurs in approximately 50% of all lung transplant patients.

III. Dental Management

Evaluation

Patients presenting with cough, shortness of breath, and wheezing, and using supplemental oxygen by nasal cannula with a mobile oxygen tank should raise suspicion of pulmonary disease.

For the patient carrying a diagnosis of a specific pulmonary condition, the following questions will assist the dentist in medical assessment and risk management related to dental care.

Key questions to ask the patient with asthma

- What type of asthma do you have (e.g., allergic, infectious, stress induced, drug induced, exercise induced)?
- If drug induced, which drugs have been triggers for you (e.g., aspirin, NSAIDs, food preservatives)?
- How severe is your asthma? How often do you have asthma attacks? What do you do to resolve the attacks?
- What treatment are you receiving? Do you use a systemic or inhaled steroid?
- Do you have your bronchodilator with you? You should bring it to each appointment.
- Has this ever been insufficient to stop an attack so that you needed epinephrine injection?

Key questions to ask the asthmatic patient's physician

- Are there medications that should be avoided for this patient because they trigger asthma attacks?
- What is the severity level of the patient's asthma?
- Has the patient's asthma been so bad the patient has needed epinephrine or an emergency department visit?
- Is the patient on corticosteroids? If so, is the patient likely to be adrenally suppressed?

Key questions to ask the patient with COPD

- Do you have emphysema or bronchitis?

Exposure to risk factors:
- Do you smoke?
- If yes, how many cigarettes/how much tobacco per day?
- Would you like to quit smoking?

Disease progression and complications:
- How much can you do before you get short of breath?
- Have you had to reduce your activities because of your breathing or any other symptom?
- Has your breathlessness or any of your symptoms worsened, improved, or stayed the same since your last medical visit?
- Have you experienced any new symptoms since your last medical visit?
- Has your sleep been disrupted by breathlessness or other chest symptoms?
- Are there any other medical problems for which you are currently receiving treatment?

Monitor pharmacotherapy and other medical treatment:
- What are the names, doses, and schedule of medicines that you take?
- Has your treatment been effective in controlling your symptoms?
- Has your treatment caused you any problems?
- Do you require supplemental oxygen?

Monitor exacerbation history:
- What causes your symptoms to get worse?
- What did you do to control the symptoms?
- Have you ever experienced difficulty breathing during dental treatment?

Key questions to ask the patient with COPD's physician

- Is the patient on home oxygen therapy?
- Is the patient's COPD stable?
- What is the patient's baseline oxygen saturation level (on pulse oximeter) on room air or on supplemental oxygen?
- Does the patient have frequent bacterial infections?
- Does the patient have hypertension or heart failure?
- Has the patient been on corticosteroids and is the patient adrenally suppressed?
- Is nitrous oxide/oxygen inhalation analgesia safe for this patient?

Key questions to ask the patient with CF

- What medications are you taking for your CF?
- How often do you have CF exacerbations?

Key questions to ask the CF patient's physician

- What is the severity of the patient's CF?
- Is the patient going to receive a lung transplant?

Key questions to ask the patient with TB

- Is it pulmonary TB or does it involve other areas of your body?
- Is your TB active? Have you had recent night sweats, frequent cough, fever, fatigue, weight loss, chest pain, or cough that produces blood in the sputum or mucopurulent sputum?
- When was your TB diagnosed? When did you start TB treatment?
- What types of anti-TB medications are you taking?

> **Key questions to ask the TB patient's physician**
>
> - Does the patient have active TB?
> - Has the patient been anergy tested?
> - How long has the patient been on anti-TB medications? Is it a multidrug-resistant strain of TB?
> - Is the patient now considered noninfectious based on three consecutive negative AFB sputum samples? If not, how much longer do you anticipate before the patient is noninfectious?

> **Key questions to ask the patient with OSA**
>
> - How is your OSA managed?
> - Are you on a CPAP?

> **Key questions to ask the OSA patient's physician**
>
> - Is there a role for a nighttime oral positioning device for this patient?
> - Is office-based moderate conscious sedation contraindicated in this patient?

Dental Treatment Modifications

Asthma

Elective care should only be performed on asymptomatic or well-controlled patients. The presence of asthmatic symptoms, such as wheezing or coughing, warrants reappointment. Symptomatic patients presenting for emergency care should be given the minimal care needed to address the urgent condition with follow-up treatment once symptoms have resolved.

It is important to educate asthmatic patients about dental disease and increased caries risk, and to adopt caries-preventive measures including use of daily fluoride supplements, chewing xylitol gum, and regular dental maintenance visits. Controversy exists over the relationship between asthma and increased caries risk, but no strong evidence suggests a causal link.[17,18]

> **Dental management of asthma patient**
> - Only treat when patient is asymptomatic
> - Determine triggers and/or precipitating events
> - Assess level of control, frequency of attacks, medications used
> - Have patient take all medications as scheduled before appointment
> - Have patient bring rescue bronchodilator (e.g., albuterol) metered-dose inhaler to each appointment
> - Give prophylactic puff or H_1 histamine blocker prior to appointment as needed
> - Use a stress reduction protocol
> - Consider use of nitrous or short-acting benzodiazepine
> - Use rubber dam to decrease exposure to aerosols if tolerated
> - Recognize signs of acute attack and be prepared to treat
> - Educate patients about oral side effects of medications
> - Have patients rinse mouth out after using steroid inhalers
> - Implement a caries prevention program, including regular recalls and use of topical fluoride supplements and xylitol gum

COPD

- In patients with adequate respiratory capacity and limited cardiovascular comorbidities, most dental treatments can be safely delivered with little to no modifications.
- Patients presenting with dyspnea at rest, cyanotic changes, or the presence of an acute respiratory infection are not good candidates for elective dental care and should be rescheduled.
- Patients who are stable and have adequate breathing can be treated with care taken not to further compromise the airway.

CF

No specific treatment modifications are needed. Regular dental maintenance appointments should be scheduled and the oral cavity monitored for signs of candida if the patient is on inhaled steroids.

Restrictive Lung Diseases

Prior to dental treatment, consideration must be given to the degree of respiratory compromise and to the underlying cause.

TB

The CDC places most dental offices in the minimal risk category for potential occupational exposure to TB. However, all offices should have a written protocol for identifying, managing, and referring patients with active disease. All oral health-care providers should be periodically screened using TST. Dental management of the TB patient is based on the potential infectivity of the patient.

Lung Cancer

Prechemotherapy:

1. Dental evaluation:
   a. Hard and soft tissue exam to determine potential sources of infection that might delay treatment or cause posttreatment complications.
   b. Teeth with acute abscesses, symptomatic periapical pathology and severe periodontal involvement should be carefully evaluated for immediate treatment or extraction, depending on the time before the initiation of the chemotherapy.
   c. Sources of soft tissue irritation, such as fractured teeth, defective restorations, or ill-fitting prostheses should be removed.

Pulmonary Disease

> **Dental management of patients with history of tuberculosis (TB)**
>
> Patients with active TB disease
> - Palliative care with medications if hospital setting is not available.
> - Any urgent care involving aerosols must be done in an isolation setting with negative pressure ventilation and appropriate personal respiratory protection, often in a hospital setting
>
> Patients with symptoms suggestive of TB disease
> - Refer immediately to physician for evaluation
> - If coughing, give patient a surgical mask and place in an isolated area until transportation can be arranged
>
> Patient with past history of TB disease
> - Careful medical history and review of systems (ROS)
> - Establish that patient has been adequately treated and has had negative sputum cultures and chest X-ray demonstrating patient is noninfectious
> - Consult with physician if follow-up evaluation is questionable or symptoms of active disease present
> - Provide routine dental care if there has been appropriate medical follow-up and no signs of clinically active disease
>
> Patient with history of LTBI
> - Medical history and ROS
> - Verify medical evaluation to rule out active disease
> - Determine that patient received prophylactic therapy with isoniazid for at least 6 months
> - Treat as routine patient

2. Preventive care:
   a. Topical fluorides for patients with heavily restored dentition or gingival recession and root exposure since xerostomia can be a transient side effect of chemotherapy.
3. Intense oral hygiene instruction, including
   a. education about the importance of maintaining excellent oral hygiene and the benefits of controlling plaque;
   b. instruction to brush after every meal with a soft bristle toothbrush and mild toothpaste;
   c. use of nonalcoholic mouth rinses;
   d. encouragement to floss daily unless the platelets drop to <30,000.

During chemotherapy:
a. Dental treatment should only be done after consultation with the patient's oncologist to coordinate treatments with the patient's optimal hematological status.
b. Frequent recalls to help maintain a clean oral cavity and reinforce patient education can be useful in preventing or minimizing oral complications.

Lung Transplantation

Pretransplant:

- Comprehensive dental exam.
  a. Eradicate active oral disease and eliminate any potential source of infection.
  b. Patients should be informed of the potential risks of systemic infection from the oral cavity.
  c. Individual assessment as to the extent and severity of dental disease present, the cost of maintaining the dentition, the patients' motivation to keep their teeth, and the physical ability to maintain good oral hygiene should be performed.

i. Poorly motivated patients with extensive dental disease might benefit from extraction of extensively decayed or severely periodontally involved teeth, even if it means full mouth extractions.
ii. Patients with good oral health should be instructed in the need for a more aggressive preventive regimen including more frequent recare visits.
- Treatment: all active dental disease should be addressed.
   a. Teeth with active caries should be restored or extracted and all periapical pathology treated.
   b. Preventive oral hygiene including daily toothbrushing and flossing should be reinforced.

First 3–6 months posttransplant or until the transplanted organ is stable and functional and the proper level of immunosuppression has been achieved:

- No elective dental treatment should be performed.
- The need for antibiotic prophylaxis prior to dental treatment should be made on an individual basis after consultation with the transplant surgeon.

Stable, posttransplant:

- Routine dental procedures can be performed with an emphasis on prevention and preventing infection.
- The oral cavity should be monitored for signs of opportunistic infections.
- Patients with significant signs and symptoms of rejection should only have urgent dental care provided.

Oral Lesion Diagnosis and Management

Asthma

Oropharyngeal candidiasis: a side effect of use of nebulized corticosteroids, due to topical effects on the oral mucosa. See Fig. 3.3. Only 10–20% of the dose from an inhaler actually reaches the lungs, while the rest remains in the oropharynx.[19] Use of a spacer device attached to the inhaler can decrease the local effect of steroids in causing oral candidiasis by maximizing the lung deposition. Patients should be advised to rinse their mouth out immediately after use. Periodic monitoring for candidiasis is indicated and treatment with topical antifungals as needed.

Figure 3.3 Oral candida infections from a steroid inhaler.

CF

Patients' diet necessary to maintain adequate caloric intake often involves eating foods high in carbohydrates and sucrose. However, pancreatic enzymes and vitamins might actually strengthen the enamel and make the teeth more caries resistant.[20] Additionally, the use of long-term antibiotics and salivary buffering capabilities of the pancreatic enzymes may confer some protection against the development and progression of dental caries. Altered amounts of calcium and phosphate in the saliva can lead to higher calculus formation and a higher incidence of enamel defects.[21]

 ## Risks of Dental Care

Hemostasis

There are no significant concerns regarding hemostasis related to pulmonary disease unless the patient is receiving myelosuppressive chemotherapy for lung cancer.

Susceptibility to Infection

COPD

While no study has established that periodontal disease influences the occurrence of COPD, several studies have demonstrated a statistical association between the two conditions,[22] and aspiration of oral bacteria may exacerbate COPD or contribute to recurrent respiratory tract infections.[23]

Asthma, Restrictive Lung Disease, COPD, Lung Transplant

Postoperative antibiotics following surgical procedures might be necessary in patients on systemic steroids due to increased risk of postoperative infection.

Drug Actions/Interactions

Asthma

- Theophylline users: macrolide antibiotics (erythromycin and clarithromycin) and azole antifungals should be avoided in patients taking theophylline because of an increased risk of theophylline toxicity. Aspirin and other NSAIDs should be avoided in susceptible patients.

COPD

- Avoid respiratory depressing drugs such as barbiturates and narcotics.
- Avoid antibiotics including erythromycin, clarithromycin, and ciprofloxacin and the azole antifungals in patients taking theophylline, since they can elevate the concentration of theophylline to a toxic level.

TB

Avoid acetaminophen in patients currently taking isoniazid as drug-induced hepatotoxicity may be an issue.

Patient's Ability to Tolerate Dental Care

Asthma

The chief concern during delivery of dental care is prevention of an acute attack. Patient risk status should be carefully evaluated based on frequency and precipitating factors for attacks, types of pharmacotherapy, degree of control elicited by careful review of systems and presence of current symptoms, functional limitations, presence of nocturnal symptoms, and length of time since an emergency room visit.

- Patients with severe asthma and low oxygen saturation (<90% by pulse oximeter) or those with sudden onset of unprovoked attacks might need to receive dental care in a hospital setting.

- For patients with nocturnal asthma symptoms or patients who used morning nebulizers, late morning/early afternoon appointments are preferable.

It should be confirmed that the patient has taken his or her most recent scheduled dose of medication, and the patient's own short-acting β_2 agonist MDI should readily be available in the operatory (check to make sure it is not expired).[24] If the patient does not use a rescue inhaler, one should be taken from the emergency kit.

Adjunctive anxiolytic therapy including nitrous oxide or short-acting benzodiazepines can be useful in reducing stress in anxious patients, particularly during potentially stimulating events such as anesthesia administration or tooth extraction.

Prophylactic use of the rescue inhaler prior to initiation of treatment may be useful in preventing an attack. H_1-blocking antihistamine blockers (such as diphenhydramine) can also be used prophylactically in patients with extrinsic asthma.[24]

Reduction or elimination of agents known to be triggers for the patient should be attempted:

- Avoid materials with irritating odors (disinfectants, methylacrylate).
- Use a dental dam to reduce exposure to particulate matter like tooth enamel dust and prophy paste.
- Carefully position cotton rolls and suction tips.
- For latex-sensitive patients, nonlatex gloves and dental dams should be used.
- Cold operatory temperatures should also be avoided.
- Patients who experience respiratory discomfort when fully reclined should be treated in a semisupine position.

COPD

- Patients should be treated in a semisupine or upright position to prevent orthopnea.

- Rubber dams, while useful in preventing aspiration of aerosols and tooth/material particles, may be contraindicated in patients with more severe disease or those patients who mouth-breathe.
- There is no contraindication to local anesthetics, but limit epinephrine if significant cardiovascular disease is present.
- Stress reduction including use of low-dose oral lorazepam (Ativan®) or nitrous oxide delivered at an overall rate of 3 L/min can be used with caution in anxious patients.
- Nitrous oxide should be avoided in patients with severe COPD or emphysema because of increased chance of diffusion hypoxia.
- If supplemental oxygen is needed, low flow rates of 2–3 L/min should be used. Patients with long-standing or severe COPD are stimulated to breathe not by hypercarbia but hypoxia, and high flow oxygen (>5 L/min) may suppress the patient's drive to inhale.

Asthma, Restrictive Lung Disease, COPD

The possibility of adrenal suppression in patients receiving oral corticosteroid therapy is extremely low. For most routine dental and simple surgical procedures, increasing the dose of steroids is not needed.

Restrictive Lung Diseases

Patients should be treated in a semisupine position to prevent orthopnea.

Medical Emergencies

Asthma

To manage an asthma attack in the office:

- Stop dental treatment; remove the dental dam and any cotton rolls and saliva evacuators.
- Note the time that the attack began.
- Raise the back of the dental chair and allow the patient to assume the position where the patient feels the most comfortable.

- Administer the short-acting β_2 agonist (repeat as needed) and administer low-flow oxygen (3–4 L/min) by nasal cannula or face mask.
- If the patient does not respond to this treatment or the condition deteriorates, activate the emergency response system and administer 0.3–0.5 mL (0.01 mL/kg of body weight in children) of epinephrine 1:1000 subcutaneously.[25] Arrange for transport to an emergency medical facility.

Special Considerations

OSA

Oral Appliances

OSA device therapy may be an option for patients that cannot tolerate CPAP and has been shown to decrease AHI in most cases, although not as effectively as CPAP. Oral sleep appliances have a higher rate of acceptance and compliance than CPAP and have a lower rate of morbidity than surgery. The American Academy of Sleep Medicine (AASM) currently recommends dental devices only for patients with mild-to-moderate OSA who are not appropriate candidates for CPAP or who have not been helped by it.[26] Currently, there are over 30 U.S. Food and Drug Administration (FDA)-approved OSA devices and another 20 that are approved only for snoring.[27]

There are two basic types of oral appliances:

Tongue-retaining devices directly engage the tongue and pull it forward usually utilizing some type of suction device.[27] These devices are not currently approved by the FDA for treatment of OSA (see Fig. 3.4).

Mandibular advancement devices are acrylic appliances that are fitted to the maxillary and mandibular dentition and reposition the mandible forward. They may be constructed as a single, nonadjustable device or as two separate pieces that are connected to allow adjustable vertical opening and anterior repositioning as necessary to effectively dilate the airway (see Fig. 3.5).

Figure 3.4 Tongue-retaining device. (courtesy of Dr. Kenneth Fleisher)

Figure 3.5 Herbst appliance.

Oral appliances are generally well tolerated, but they are not without adverse effects. Many of these are short term and easily corrected. They include nighttime muscle and tooth pain, temporomandibular joint pain, dry lips, excessive salivation, gingival irritation, and minor changes in occlusion in the morning upon immediate removal. More serious and permanent changes include loosening of teeth, further damage to periodontally involved teeth, and permanent occlusal changes including labioversion of the maxillary teeth and repositioning of the man-

Figure 3.6 Malocclusion from oral appliance (courtesy of Dr. Kenneth Fleisher).

dible in a downward, forward position resulting in an open posterior bite[28] (see Fig. 3.6).

Patients should be closely monitored every 6 months following fabrication of an oral sleep appliance to monitor fit, patient comfort, and compliance, and to check for unanticipated tooth movement and undergo a polysomnogram with the oral appliance in place to evaluate its effectiveness.[26]

IV. Recommended Readings and Cited References

Recommended Readings

Kacmarek R, Dimas S The Essentials of Respiratory Care, 4th ed. 2005. Elsevier Mosby, St. Louis, MO.

Rhodus NL, Miller CS, eds. Clinician's Guide Treatment of Medically Complex Dental Patients, 4th ed. 2009. The American Academy of Oral Medicine, Edmonds, WA.

Robbins MR. Oral care of the patient receiving chemotherapy. In: Oral Cancer: The Dentist's Role in Diagnosis, Management, Rehabilitation and Prevention. Ord RA, Blanchart RH, eds. 2000. Quintessence Publishing, Carol Stream, IL.

Cited References

1. AASM. Sleep-related breathing disorders in adults: recommendations for syndrome definition and measurement techniques in clinical research: the report of an American Academy of Sleep Medicine Task Force. Sleep 1999;22(5): 667–89.
2. National Asthma Education and Prevention Program. Expert Panel Report 3: guidelines for the diagnosis and management of asthma. NIH Pub. No. 07–4051. Bethesda, MD: National Heart, Lung, and Blood Institute, National Institutes of Health. 2007. Available at: http://www.nhlbi.nih.gov/guidelines/asthma/. Accessed November 20, 2011.
3. Szczeklik A, Stevenson DD. Aspirin-induced asthma: advances in pathogenesis, diagnosis,

and management. J Allergy Clin Immunol 2003; 111(5):913–21.
4. Stavem K, Aaser E, Sandvik L, Bjornholt JV, Erikssen G, Thaulow E, et al. Lung function, smoking and mortality in a 26 year followup of healthy middle aged males. Eur Respir J 2005; 25(4):618–25.
5. Stoller JK, Aboussouan LS. Alpha1antitrypsin deficiency. Lancet 2005;365(9478):2225–36.
6. CDC. Core curriculum on tuberculosis: what the clinician should know. Centers for Disease Control and Prevention (CDC), Division of Tuberculosis Elimination, 5th ed. 2011. Available at: http://www.cdc.gov/tb/education/corecurr/. Accessed November 20, 2011.
7. Akinbami LJ, Moorman JE, Liu X. Asthma prevalence, health care use, and mortality: United States, 2005–2009. National health statistics reports; no. 32. 2011. Hyattsville, MD: National Center for Health Statistics. Available at: http://www.cdc.gov/nchs/data/nhsr/nhsr032.pdf
8. Global Strategy for the Diagnosis, Management and Prevention of COPD, Global Initiative for Chronic Obstructive Lung Disease Revised 2011. 2011. Available at: http://www.goldcopd.org/. Accessed March 14, 2012.
9. Davies JC, Alton EW, Bush A. Cystic fibrosis. BMJ 2007;335(7632):1255–9.
10. CDC. Reported Tuberculosis in the United States, 2010. Atlanta, GA: U.S. Department of Health and Human Services, CDC, October 2010. Available at: http://www.cdc.gov/TB/statistics/reports/2010/default.htm. Accessed November 20, 2011.
11. Young T, Palta M, Dempsey J, Skatrud J, Weber S, Badr S. The occurrence of sleep-disordered breathing among middle-aged adults. N Engl J Med 2003;328(17):1230–5.
12. U.S. Cancer Statistics Working Group. United States Cancer Statistics: 1999–2006 Incidence and Mortality Web-Based Report. Atlanta (GA): Department of Health and Human Services, Centers for Disease Control and Prevention, and National Cancer Institute. 2010. Available at: http://www.cdc.gov/uscs. Accessed November 20, 2011.
13. Christie JD, Edwards LB, Kucheryavaya AY, Benden C, Dobbels F, Kirk R, et al. The Registry of the International Society for Heart and Lung Transplantation: Twenty-Eighth Official Adult Lung and Heart-Lung Transplant Report. J Heart Lung Transplant 2011;30(10):1071–32.
14. National Institute for Clinical Excellence (NICE). Chronic obstructive pulmonary disease: national clinical guideline for management of chronic obstructive pulmonary disease in adults in primary and secondary care. Thorax 2004; 59(Suppl. I):1–232.
15. American Thoracic Society (ATS) and CDC. Diagnostic standards and classification of tuberculosis in adults and children. Am J Respir Crit Care Med 2000;161(4 Pt 1):1376–95.
16. Giles TL, Lasserson TJ, Smith B, White J, Wright JJ, Cates CJ. Continuous positive airways pressure for obstructive sleep apnea in adults. Cochrane Database Syst Rev 2006;(3):CD001106:1–80.
17. Maupomé G, Shulman JD, Medina-Solis CE, Ladeinde O. Is there a relationship between asthma and dental caries? A critical review of the literature. J Am Dent Assoc 2010;141(9):1061–74.
18. Alavaikko S, Jaakkola MS, Jaakkola JJK. Asthma and caries: a systematic review and meta-analysis. Am J Epidemiol 2011;174(6):631–41.
19. Han ER, Choi IS, Kim HK, Kang YW, Park JG, Lim JR, et al. Inhaled corticosteroid-related oral problems in asthmatics. J Asthma 2009;46(2): 160–4.
20. Kinirons MJ. Increased salivary buffering in association with a low caries experience in children suffering from cystic fibrosis. J Dent Res 1983; 62(7):815–7.
21. Narang A, Maguire A, Nunn JH, Bush A. Oral health and related factors in cystic fibrosis and other chronic respiratory disorders. Arch Dis Child 2003;88(8):702–7.
22. Scannapieco FA, Bush RB, Paju S. Associations between periodontal disease and risk for nosocomial bacterial pneumonia and chronic obstructive pulmonary disease. A systematic review. Ann Periodontol 2003;8(1):54–69.
23. Zhou X, Wang Z, Song Y, Zhang J, Wang C. Periodontal health and quality of life in patients with chronic obstructive pulmonary disease. Respir Med 2011;105(1):67–73.
24. Steinbacher DM, Glick M. The dental patient with asthma. An update and oral health considerations. J Am Dent Assoc 2001;132(9):1229–39.
25. Malamed SF. Medical Emergencies in the Dental Office, 5th ed. 2000. Mosby, St. Louis, MO, pp. 168–99, 209–23.

26. Kushida CA, Morganthaler T, Littner M, Alessi CA, Bailey D, Coleman J Jr., et al. Practice parameters for the treatment of snoring and obstructive sleep apnea with oral appliances: an update for 2005. Sleep 2006;29(2):240–3.
27. Ferguson KA, Cartwright R, Rogers R, Schmidt-Nowara W. Oral appliances for snoring and obstructive sleep apnea: a review. Sleep 2006;29(2):244–62.
28. Martínez-Gomis J, Willaert E, Nogues L, Pascual M, Somoza M, Monasterio C. Five years of sleep apnea treatment with a mandibular advancement device. Side effects and technical complications. Angle Orthod 2010;80(1):30–6.

Endocrine and Metabolic Disorders

Terry D. Rees DDS, MSD

Endocrine and metabolic disorders of particular importance to dentistry include disorders of the pancreas, adrenal glands, and thyroid gland, and as such, this chapter is divided into three sections.

Section 1. Pancreatic Diseases

I. Background

Description of Disease

Diabetes Mellitus (DM)

DM is a hormonal metabolic disorder of multiple etiologies characterized by chronic hyperglycemia resulting from deficiencies in insulin secretion or function or both.

Pancreatic Cancer

The pancreas is a major endocrine and digestive organ that produces hormones, including insulin, glucagon, and somatostatin, and secretes pancreatic juice containing digestive enzymes that assist the absorption of nutrients and digestion in the small intestine. Cancer of the pancreas has a median survival of 6–12 months. This grim outcome largely relates to the aggressiveness of the malignancy, difficulty in establishing early diagnosis, low rate of resection, and lack of an effective chemotherapy agent to treat the tumor.

Pathogenesis/Etiology

DM

Sustained hyperglycemia adversely affects all body tissues. Classic complications of DM include retinopathy, nephropathy, neuropathy, macrovascular disease (cardiovascular, cerebrovascular, peripheral vascular), altered wound healing, and possibly increased incidence and severity of periodontal diseases. These effects may become more profound in diabetics who smoke or have other major medical conditions.

The ADA Practical Guide to Patients with Medical Conditions, First Edition. Edited by Lauren L. Patton.
© 2012 American Dental Association. Published 2012 by John Wiley & Sons, Inc.

Classification:

- *Type 1 DM* is immune mediated. The autoimmune response usually occurs in children and young adults accounting for 5–10% of all diabetics. Individuals with type 1 DM require insulin supplementation for life. Undiagnosed type 1 DM is associated with the classic symptoms of polydipsia (excessive thirst), polyurea (frequent urination), and polyphagia (excessive hunger), and if untreated, it can lead to ketoacidosis, coma, or death.
- *Type 2 DM* is characterized by impaired insulin resistance, and it may be associated with low, normal, or increased insulin production. It occurs most commonly in adults and is associated with obesity or the metabolic syndrome. Increasing obesity and reduced physical activity among children have resulted in a markedly increased incidence of type 2 DM in younger individuals.
- *Gestational DM* may affect 7% of pregnant females in the United States resulting in more than 200,000 new cases annually.[1] It is defined as increased insulin resistance that develops during pregnancy. Gestational DM is more common in women who are obese and who are at increased risk for other adverse pregnancy outcomes. It may lead to significant perinatal morbidity and mortality, as well as obesity and diabetes in the offspring. After delivery, most women return to a normoglycemic state but 30–50% will subsequently develop type 2 DM within 10 years.
- *Prediabetes (increased risk for DM):* Glucose levels are higher than normal but not high enough for a diagnosis of DM.
- *Metabolic syndrome:* The presence of certain risk factors increases the likelihood of developing type 2 DM. These include a positive family history, obesity, and a cluster of factors sometimes referred to as the metabolic syndrome (dyslipidemia, hypertension, visceral obesity; abnormal coagulation factors; and endothelial dysfunction). These factors collectively increase insulin resistance, induce hyperinsulinemia, and impair glucose tolerance.
- *Impaired glucose tolerance (IGT):* Affected individuals are usually normogylcemic but may develop hyperglycemia after large glucose intake.
- *Impaired fasting glucose (IFG):* Glucose levels respond normally after food consumption but fasting glucose levels remain somewhat elevated.
  - Both IGT and IFG are associated with increased insulin resistance. Type 2 DM may develop in 40–50% of affected individuals within 10 years of onset. Type 2 DM may sometimes be prevented if treatment is initiated in individuals who have IGT or IFG.[2]

Pancreatic Cancer

Ductal adenocarcinoma accounts for >80%. Most arise in the pancreatic head and act in a highly aggressive manner with frequent invasion of the vascular, lymphatic, and perineural tissue. In most instances, it affects the exocrine (digestive enzyme producing) portion of the pancreas, but the endocrine (insulin producing) portion may be affected as well. Causes remain unknown, with smoking, DM, and genetics being likely risks.[3]

Epidemiology

DM

DM has reached epidemic proportions in the United States and around the world, and its impact is worsened by the fact that many diabetics are unaware that they have the disease. U.S. statistics are reported annually by the Centers for Disease Control and Prevention (CDC):

- *Incidence*: In 2010, 1.9 million Americans >20 years of age were newly diagnosed with DM.
- *Prevalence*: In the United States, 25.8 million children and adults (8.3% of the U.S. population) had DM of which 7.0 million were undiagnosed. Prediabetics (persons at risk) were estimated at 79 million people.
- *Race/Ethnicity*: Minority populations are at higher risk. DM occurs in 7.1% of non-Hispanic whites, 8.4% of Asian-Americans, 11.8% Hispanics, and 12.6% non-Hispanic blacks.
- *Mortality*: DM is the seventh leading cause of death in the United States.

Pancreatic Cancer

It is the fourth leading cause of mortality from cancer, primarily because <20% of patients present with localized potentially curable tumors.[3] Individuals of both sexes and all races may be affected. For 2011, there are estimated to be 44,030 new cases and 37,660 deaths from pancreatic cancer.

Coordination of Care between Dentist and Physician

DM

The dentist should review the patient's medical history, take vital signs, and evaluate for oral signs and symptoms of undiagnosed or inadequately controlled DM. If the patient has severe periodontal disease, the physician should be reminded that periodontal therapy *may* improve metabolic control and allow adjustments in drug dosages. Medical consultation may be necessary to determine health status and if planned dental treatment can be safely and effectively accomplished. The physician should provide laboratory test results to the dentist on request and make the dentist aware of any diabetic complications that may be present. On occasion, the physician may need to adjust the patient's DM medications to insure sustained metabolic control before, during, and after surgical procedures.[4]

Pancreatic Cancer

Because of the aggressive nature and current unavailability of effective screening tools, the dentist is unlikely to be asked to provide definitive elective treatment for the patient with active pancreatic cancer. However, emergency dental care may be needed. If so, the physician should be queried about planned medical treatment and when it is to be accomplished. Optional dental treatment should be coordinated so as not to interfere with planned surgery, radiation therapy, or chemotherapy.

II. Medical Management

Identification/Medical History/ Physical and Laboratory Examination

DM

The American Diabetes Association and World Health Organization recognize four suitable tests to diagnose DM. Plasma glucose can be measured in a fasting state, randomly (nonfasting), or 2 hours after consumption of a measured quantity of glucose. Abnormal findings must be present on two separate occasions to establish the diagnosis. See Table 4.1.

Determination of glycated hemoglobin (HbA1c) percentage has recently been added as a diagnostic tool for DM with an HbA1c ≥6.5% indicating DM. HbA1c is also used to monitor long-term metabolic control because it evaluates blood glucose levels over a period of 30–90 days.[5,6]

Table 4.1. American Diabetes Association Diagnostic Criteria for Diabetes Mellitus

Diagnostic Test	Test Result Diagnostic Criteria
Fasting plasma glucose	≥126 mg/dL (7.0 mmol/L)
Random plasma glucose	≥200 mg/dL (11.1 mmol/L)
2-hour plasma glucose (after 75 oral glucose load)	≥200 mg/dL (11.1 mmol/L)
HbA1c (glycated hemoglobin)	≥6.5%

Glycated hemoglobin (HbA1c) test of diabetes mellitus metabolic status	
Normal range	<6%
Good control	<7%
Moderate control	7–8%
Poor control	>8%

Pancreatic Cancer

- *Screening*: Currently, it is neither advisable nor cost-effective to screen the general population for pancreatic cancer, but it is customary to screen individuals who are at high risk. A mechanism for early diagnosis is badly needed and the use of salivary biomarkers offers great promise as one such mechanism.[7]
- *Diagnosis*: Diagnosis is usually based on physical examination and evaluation of signs and symptoms (weight loss, jaundice, abdominal bloating and pain, malaise, diarrhea, nausea, elevated blood sugar). Specific tests include computed tomography (CT), ultrasound, endoscopy and possibly needle biopsy.

Medical Treatment

DM

A primary goal of diabetes care management is to maintain an HbA1c ≤7% so as to reduce microvascular and neuropathic complications.[8]

Type 1 DM requires insulin supplementation. Insulins are classified as rapid, short, intermediate, or long acting. Each class induces variable onset of peak activity and duration. See Table 4.2. Patients frequently use a combination of the various types in order to maintain a normal or near-normal level of plasma glucose.

Type 2 DM may be treated with weight loss, exercise, and oral antidiabetic medications that improve carbohydrate metabolism, decrease insulin resistance, or increase insulin production. See Table 4.3. Over time, individuals with type 2 DM may experience a reduction in insulin production and consequently require insulin supplementation.

- *Prognosis*: Prognosis is good for diabetics who respond adequately to insulin, oral antidiabetic medications, weight loss, and exercise. However, diabetes affects multiple organs, and even with treatment, diabetics are at increased risk for blindness, kidney failure, heart disease, stroke, limb amputation, and peripheral neuropathy. Diabetics who maintain rigid control of their blood glucose at normal or near-normal levels are much less likely to experience these complications.[5]

Pancreatic Cancer

It can be cured if diagnosed early and surgical removal is complete. Chemotherapy, radiation therapy, and targeted therapy may enhance and prolong life.

Table 4.2. Standard Insulins and Insulin Analogs

Insulin	Onset	Peak	Duration
Standard			
Regular	30–60 minutes	2–3 hours	8–10 hours
NPH	2–4 hours	4–10 hours	12–18 hours
Lente (zinc insulin)	2–4 hours	4–12 hours	12–20 hours
Ultra Lente (extended)	6–10 hours	10–16 hours	18–24 hours
Analogs			
Lispro (Humalog®)	5–15 minutes	30–90 minutes	4–6 hours
Aspart (NovoLog®)	5–15 minutes	30–90 minutes	4–6 hours
Glargine (Lantus®)	2–4 hours	None	20–24 hours
Glulisine (Apidra®)	20–30 minutes	30–90 minutes	1–2.5 hours

Table 4.3. Oral Antidiabetic Medications

Medication Class/Drugs	Action

Sulfonylureas
  Glyburide
  Glipzide
  Glimepiride
	Stimulate insulin secretion

Meglitides
  Repaglinide
  Nategline
	Stimulate rapid insulin secretion

Biguanides Metformin	Block liver production of glucose

Thiazolidinediones
  Rosiglitazone
  Proglitazone
	Improve insulin sensitivity

Alpha-glucosides
  Acarbose
  Meglitol
	Slow carbohydrate absorption

Combination agents	Multipurpose

III. Dental Management

Evaluation

DM

Diabetics require a complete medical history supplemented by careful questioning regarding their status.

It is often prudent to discuss the patient's medical status with the physician and obtain medical input before performing invasive dental therapy, particularly in the poorly controlled diabetic.

Pancreatic Cancer

Patients and their physicians should be queried regarding the course of treatment and the patient's overall health status.

Dental Treatment Modifications

DM

The well-controlled diabetic can usually be managed conventionally to include most surgical procedures.

- Maintenance of a normal postsurgical diet is important. If this is not possible, dietary supplements should be recommended.
- Occasionally, it may be necessary for the patient's physician to modify insulin protocols to insure a stable postoperative outcome. Patients may require reduction of insulin dose immediately prior to oral surgical procedures that will result in reduced calorie oral intake so as to prevent unintended hypoglycemia.

Key questions to ask the diabetic patient

- What type of diabetes do you have?
- How old were you when diabetes was diagnosed? How long has it been since the diagnosis?
- What medications do you take?
- How do you monitor your blood sugar levels?
- How often do you see your doctor about your diabetes? When was the last visit to your doctor?
- How does your doctor monitor your blood sugar levels?
- What was the most recent HbA1c (A1C) result?
- Do you ever have episodes of very low or very high blood sugar?
- Do you ever find yourself disoriented, agitated, and anxious for no apparent reason?
- Do you have any mouth sores or discomfort?
- Does your mouth feel dry?
- Do you have any other medical conditions related to your diabetes, such as heart disease, high blood pressure, history of stroke, eye problems, numbness of limbs, kidney problems, delays in wound healing, history of severe gum disease? If so, what?

Key questions to ask the diabetic patient's physician

- What medications does the patient take? Is the patient compliant with the prescribed drug regimen?
- Does the patient have a history of diabetic hyperglycemic or hypoglycemic crisis?
- What are the most recent laboratory findings for the patient, in particular the HbA1c?
- Does the patient have other medical problems that might affect dental care?
- Do you feel prophylactic antibiotics are indicated prior to dental procedures?

Key questions to ask the pancreatic cancer patient

- When was your cancer diagnosed?
- What treatments have you had or are proposed?
- Do you have other medical conditions related to your cancer such as DM, thyroiditis, Addison's disease, or Cushing's disease?
- During your cancer therapy have you developed any problems with excessive or prolonged bleeding?

> **? Key questions to ask the pancreatic cancer patient's physician**
>
> - What is the course of treatment for this patient? What are the adverse effects of the treatment?
> - Does the patient have other medical problems that might affect dental treatment?
> - Do you feel the patient will be able to tolerate the dental treatment without difficulty?
> - Are any special precautions indicated during dental treatment?
> - Are there contraindications to use of local anesthetics, parenteral conscious sedation, oral sedation, or antibiotics?
> - Is the patient likely to have excessive or prolonged bleeding following an invasive dental procedure?
> - Do you feel prophylactic antibiotics are indicated prior to dental treatment?

Marginally or poorly controlled diabetics should be treated with caution. Elective dental treatment should be avoided until the patient is stabilized. If the patient has associated medical complications, apply appropriate steps necessary in management. Patients should be encouraged to maintain excellent oral hygiene and comply with recall appointments. If dental caries is a potential problem, fluoride-containing, caries-preventive agents are appropriate. Xerostomia should be managed on a case-by-case basis.

It is well known that in patients with poor glycemic control, surgical stress promotes hyperglycemia through the release of various hormones and inflammatory cytokines, possibly predisposing them to poor wound healing, surgical site infections, and even diabetic ketoacidosis. However, glycemic control has not been shown to influence the rate of postextraction epithelialization and thus healing in diabetic patients.[9] Dental implants can usually be successfully placed in well-controlled diabetics and possibly in moderately controlled individuals. However, implant placement in poorly controlled diabetics has an unpredictable prognosis and, if possible, should be avoided.[10]

Pancreatic Cancer

- Elective dental treatment is not indicated during cancer treatment.

Oral Lesion Diagnosis and Management

DM

Oral manifestations of undetected or poorly controlled DM are common. See Fig. 4.1. They may include xerostomia, burning mouth (possibly due to neuropathy), delayed wound healing, increased incidence and severity of infections, enlargement of parotid salivary glands, gingivitis, and periodontitis.[11] Conversely improved periodontal health may facilitate metabolic control.[12] The effect of DM on caries risk is unclear. Candidiasis is a frequent secondary infection in the presence of xerostomia and among denture wearers.[13]

Pancreatic Cancer

Some evidence suggests that poor oral health may slightly, but significantly, increase risk for pancreatic and other cancers. However, a cause–effect relationship has not been established, and individuals with oral infection share some risk factors (smoking and possibly genetic similarities) with those with pancreatic cancer. At any rate, cohorts of individuals with pancreatic cancer can be expected to have more tooth loss and periodontal disease than the general population.[14,15]

Risks of Dental Care

Hemostasis

DM: No major concern.
Pancreatic Cancer: If extractions or other oral surgical procedures are necessary, the patient may be at risk of excessive bleeding if actively undergoing myelosuppressive chemotherapy.

Susceptibility to Infection

DM: Antibiotic coverage should be considered for emergency surgical procedures required to treat acute oral infection. For surgical therapy, ask the patients to bring their glucometer to the appointment if they have one and have them take and record their preoperative plasma glucose level prior to the procedure.
Pancreatic Cancer: Emergency treatment should be the minimum required to eliminate the oral problem. For this reason, antibiotic

Figure 4.1 Oral signs of undiagnosed/uncontrolled diabetes mellitus. (a) Xerostomia; (b) chronic candidiasis; (c) multiple periodontal abscesses; (d) severe periodontal disease; (e) rapidly progressive alveolar bone loss over a 2-year period of time.

Figure 4.1 (Continued)

therapy may be the treatment of choice for immediate management of most oral infections. If on cytotoxic chemotherapy, consider potential immune suppression.

Drug Actions/Interactions

DM: Prescribing systemic corticosteroids may decrease the effectiveness of oral hypoglycemic agents and may enhance blood glucose levels; topical steroids with low systemic absorption should not be of concern. Large doses of nonsteroidal anti-inflammatory drugs (NSAIDs) or aspirin may increase the hypoglycemic effect of insulin or oral hypoglycemic drugs.

Pancreatic Cancer: If on cytotoxic chemotherapy, consider potential myelosuppression.

Patient's Ability to Tolerate Dental Care

DM: Surgical patients are best scheduled in the morning after a normal meal and after using normal insulin or oral antidiabetic medications. Insulin-using patients should be queried about last food intake to assure blood sugar levels will be adequately maintained until next meal time. Adhere to office stress reduction protocols, obtain profound local anesthesia, and provide analgesics as necessary for postoperative discomfort.

Pancreatic Cancer: A stress reduction protocol should be followed. Procedures should be short and the area(s) of treatment small. Obtain profound anesthesia if necessary using local anesthetics with vasoconstrictors after medical clearance.

Medical Emergencies

Be prepared to manage diabetic emergencies. Although rare, *hyperglycemia* can be life threatening and is seen far less frequently in type 2 diabetics. Both type 1 and type 2 diabetics are much more likely to experience *hypoglycemia* during dental treatment in this era of "tight" glycemic control.[16]

Recognition and management of diabetic emergencies

Hyperglycemia

- Onset is usually slow, and consequently, ketoacidosis and hyperglycemic crisis are rare in the dental office.
- Signs include mental disorientation, sweating, coma, and even death.
- Patients with ketoacidosis require medical treatment, so activate the emergency medical system, administer oxygen, monitor vital signs, and perform cardiopulmonary resuscitation if needed.

Hypoglycemia

- DM patients are far more likely to experience a hypoglycemic emergency in the dental office.
- Signs include disorientation, agitation, anxiety, sweating, seizures, loss of consciousness, and death.
- If the patient can take food by mouth, give approximately 15 g of carbohydrate (4–6 oz of fruit juice, 3–4 tsp sugar, glucose tablet).
- If the patient is unable to take food by mouth and no IV access is present, give 1 mg glucagon intramuscularly or subcutaneously.
- The patient should respond fully within 15 minutes but should be monitored for at least 1 hour.
- Be prepared to activate the emergency medical system if necessary.
- If the patient recovers uneventfully from a hypoglycemic crisis, it is advisable to notify the patient's physician of the event.

Section 2. Adrenal Diseases

I. Background

Description of Condition

The adrenal cortex produces more than 50 steroids, but the principal products are:

- glucocortisol (cortisol)—maintains homeostasis by regulating many essential functions such as digestion and metabolism, the immune system, blood glucose levels, and the reactions of the body to stress;
- mineralocorticoid (aldosterone)—regulates kidney function and helps control blood pressure and appropriate levels of blood minerals.

The adrenal cortex is regulated by pituitary adrenocorticotrophic hormone (ACTH), which, in turn, is regulated by the release of corticotropic releasing hormone (CRH) from the hypothalamus. The hypothalamus–pituitary–adrenal (HPA) function is sustained by a biofeedback mechanism that is controlled by blood levels of cortisol.

Several diseases or disorders may interfere with normal adrenal function resulting in hormone insufficiency or excessive cortisol production.

Pathogenesis/Etiology

Adrenal Insufficiency (AI)

- *Primary AI (Addison's disease)* occurs when the adrenal glands are destroyed by granulomatous diseases, hemorrhage, idiopathic atrophy, or most often, due to development of autoimmune adrenocortical antibodies.
- *Secondary AI* results when the hypothalamic–pituitary axis fails to produce sufficient quantities of ACTH. The most frequent etiological factor is iatrogenic administration of glucocorticoids in treatment of various systemic disorders, leading to adrenal atrophy.
- *Acute AI (adrenal crisis)* may manifest as progressive adrenal failure usually occurring in association with a physically or emotionally stressful event.
- *Chronic AI* may develop progressively over several years leading to a characteristic yellow-brown (bronzing) cutaneous hyperpigmentation caused by the increased production of ACTH.

Cushing's Syndrome (CS)

CS represents an excess of circulating corticosteroids. This may be induced by tumors of the adrenal or pituitary gland but most often results from administration of glucocorticoids in treatment of a variety of medical conditions. Glucocorticoid replacement therapy is typically given in doses to match normal daily secretory rate of cortisol, which is about 20 mg/day. This can be accomplished by using either short-acting (cortisone, hydrocortisone) or long-acting (prednisone, dexamethasone) agents. See Table 4.4. Over time, adrenal atrophy occurs and the individual may become unable to adequately manage emotional or physical stress, potentially leading to an adrenal crisis.[17]

Epidemiology

Incidence of primary AI is approximately 50:1,000,000 persons. However, secondary AI incidence is 150–180:1,000,000 most often due to long-term medical use of corticosteroids. Six million Americans may have undiagnosed AI related to steroid withdrawal, which may only become clinically significant during times of physiological or emotional stress.

Coordination of Care between Dentist and Physician

As a rule, dental treatment should not be performed on individuals with known or suspected AI without prior medical consultation. The physician should be informed of the nature

Table 4.4. Characteristics and Relative Potencies of Glucocorticoids

Glucocorticoid	Approximate Equivalent Dose/ Anti-Inflammatory Effectiveness (mg)	Daily Dose above which HPA Axis Suppression Is Possible[a] (mg)		Half-Life (Biologic) Hours
		Male	Female	
Short acting				
Cortisone	25	25–35	20–30	8–12
Hydrocortisone (cortisol)	20	20–30	15–20	8–12
Intermediate acting				
Methylprednisolone	4	7.5–10	7.5	18–36
Prednisolone	5	7.5–10	7.5	18–36
Prednisone	5	7.5–10	7.5	18–36
Triamcinolone	4	7.5–10	7.5	18–36
Long acting				
Betamethasone	0.6	1–1.5	2.5–5	36–54
Dexamethasone	0.8	1–1.5	1–1.5	36–54

[a] Intended as a guide only. The dose in an individual depends on total body surface area.
HPA, hypothalamic–pituitary–adrenal.
Adapted from Dubois.[18]

of the planned dental therapy and queried regarding the current health status of the patient, the degree of control achieved by current medical treatment, and any precautions or requirement for supplemental corticosteroids during dental treatment. The physician in turn should inform the referring dentist regarding the results of laboratory tests, any medications that have been prescribed for the patient, and the presence of other collateral diseases or disorders.

II. Medical Management

Identification/Medical History/ Physical and Laboratory Examination

A screening test for random plasma cortisol levels may identify individuals who require further adrenal function evaluation. Plasma ACTH levels and ACTH-stimulating tests are diagnostically useful but time-consuming and, therefore, only appropriate for individuals with mild symptoms for whom medical treatment decisions can be delayed. Testing for anti-adrenal antibodies is important since approximately 80% of primary AI is caused by an autoimmune stimulus. CT abdominal scan and other special tests are useful in investigating for possible tumors.

Common signs of chronic AI include bronze-colored hyperpigmentation of the skin, most noticeable on sun-exposed body surfaces. Other common complaints include weakness, fatigue, and hypotension, especially orthostatic hypotension. Insufficiency of aldosterone may result in loss of extracellular fluid volume leading to compensatory loss of plasma from blood vessels (hypovolemia), an increase in total body potassium (hyperkalemia) and acidosis.[17]

Common signs of CS may include upper body weight gain, and unusual fat deposition in the back of the neck (buffalo hump) and face (moon face), but other features are usually present including facial hirsutism, easy bruising, weakness and fatigue, hypertension, elevated blood glucose, decreased sex drive, and secondary osteoporosis.

Medical Treatment

AI

AI is usually treated by administration of systemic corticosteroids. If possible, the dosage should be carefully balanced depending on endogenous cortisol production since an excess of exogenous steroids may lead to adrenal atrophy.

Prognosis:

- Acute AI—dismal prognosis if undetected and/or untreated.
- Chronic AI—may lead normal lives if lifelong adequate corticosteroid replacement therapy is provided. On rare occasions, borderline or subclinical autoimmune Addison's disease may spontaneously remiss, although a reduced life expectancy and increased risk for oral cancer has been reported in autoimmune AI.[19]

Cushing's Disease

Cushing's disease is CS caused by pituitary corticotroph tumors producing excessive secretion of corticotropin. Adrenal adenomas and carcinomas can also produce CS. Treatment involves surgical removal of the tumor.[20]

III. Dental Management

Evaluation

AI patients and their physicians should be queried regarding the course of medical treatment and the patient's overall health status.

Dental Treatment Modifications

- Be alert for signs and symptoms of AI.
- Do not treat individuals with known or suspected AI without medical consultation.

Oral Lesion Diagnosis and Management

- *Oral Mucosal Hyperpigmentation*: The oral cavity in patients with chronic AI may

---

Key questions to ask the adrenal insufficiency patient

- How long has it been since your diagnosis? How often do you see your doctor about your condition?
- What signs and symptoms caused your physician to test you? Do you have any of those signs and symptoms now?
- Do you have any disorders related to your adrenal dysfunction such as DM, hypertension, osteoporosis, gastrointestinal ulcers, and slow healing?
- What medications do you take? What dosage? Has the dosage changed recently?

Key Questions

Key questions to ask the adrenal insufficiency patient's physician

- What medications does the patient take? What dosage? How long?
- Is the patient compliant with the prescribed drug regimen?
- Has the patient ever presented with an adrenal crisis?
- Do you feel the patient needs corticosteroid supplementation for dental treatment?
- Do you feel the patient needs prophylactic antibiotic coverage for dental procedures?

present with bluish-black mottling of oral mucosa, palate, and lips (Fig. 4.2).[21,22]

- *Osteoporosis-Related Periodontal Disease*: There is no increased risk for caries, and susceptibility to periodontal diseases does not appear to be markedly increased despite long-term corticosteroid therapy. However, osteoporosis often associated with long-term steroid supplementation may accelerate bone loss if periodontal disease is present.

Risks of Dental Care

Hemostasis

- Not a major concern.

Susceptibility to Infection

- There is no clear evidence concerning the need of antibiotic prophylaxis prior to dental treatment for patients on chronic corticoste-

Figure 4.2 Composite view of AI-associated oral hyperpigmentation.

roid therapy. Patients being treated with systemic corticosteroids may be susceptible to systemic toxemias in the presence of localized oral infections so prophylactic antibiotics may be indicated in these cases. No antibiotic prophylaxis is warranted if the daily steroid dose is <10 mg prednisone.[23]

Drug Actions/Interactions

- Chronic glucocorticoid therapy may predispose to oral candidiasis or oral herpes recurrence.

Patient's Ability to Tolerate Dental Care

- Use a stress reduction protocol for dental treatment, long-acting local anesthetics, and good postoperative pain control.
- Patients on long-term steroid therapy, with theoretical adrenal suppression, do not require supplementary "steroid cover" for routine dentistry under local anesthesia, including minor surgical procedures. In addition, patients on long-term daily corticosteroid therapy, the equivalent of 10 mg of prednisone or more, usually have an adequate level of corticosteroid reserve. If a patient with HPA suppression has recently tapered off the exogenous steroid, a preprocedure steroid dose for a stressful dental procedure might be warranted. Corticosteroid supplementation may be beneficial during the operative and postoperative period for dentistry performed under general anesthesia.[24,25]

Medical Emergencies
Adrenal Crisis

Dental treatment or oral infections have been anecdotally reported to precipitate adrenal crisis on very rare occasions.[26,27]

- Be prepared to manage medical emergencies. In acute adrenal crisis, administer 100 mg of hydrocortisone intravenously or

---

Steroid supplementation guidelines for dental patients with adrenal insufficiency*

- **Negligible risk**
  - Using topical or inhaled steroids or previous history of regular steroid use.
    - No supplementation required for routine dental procedures.
  - Taking daily systemic steroids at dose below level for HPA axis suppression or alternate day therapy.
    - No supplementation required for routine dental procedures.
  - Taking daily systemic steroids at dose above level for HPA axis suppression.
    - No supplementation required for routine dental procedures.
- **Mild risk**
  - Taking daily systemic steroids and minor oral surgery (e.g., a few simple extractions, biopsy, minor periodontal surgery) lasting <1 hour is planned.
    - Ensure that the patient takes 25 mg of hydrocortisone equivalent prior to procedure.
- **Moderate-major risk**
  - Taking daily systemic steroids (or has low adrenal reserve) and major oral surgery (e.g., multiple extractions, quadrant periodontal surgery, osseous or bony impaction extractions), procedures >1 hour in duration, use of general anesthesia, anticipated significant blood loss.
    - The glucocorticoid target is 50–100 mg/day of hydrocortisone equivalent the day of surgery and the first postoperative day.

* Infection, stress, and pain increase the risk of adrenal crisis in susceptible patients.
Key: HPA, hypothalamic–pituitary–adrenal.
Adapted from Miller et al.[25]

Signs and symptoms of adrenal failure	
Hypotension	Headache
Lethargy	Confusion
Nausea and vomiting	Syncope
Abdominal pain	Fever
Hypoglycemia	Seizures
Hypovolemic shock	Cardiovascular collapse
Coma and death	

intramuscularly. Be prepared to perform basic life support and activate the emergency medical system.

Section 3. Thyroid Diseases

I. Background

Description of Diseases

Thyroid hormones play a major role in growth and development in infancy and childhood, and on cellular turnover and energy metabolism in adults. See Table 4.5. Gland function is controlled by the HPA feedback mechanism. Circulating thyroid hormone levels regulate hypothalamus release of thyrotropin-releasing hormone (TRH). TRH acts on the anterior pituitary gland to produce thyroid-stimulating hormone (TSH) causing the thyroid to release hormones as needed. When this feedback mechanism malfunctions, it may result in either deficiency or excess of thyroxine (T4) that may seriously affect body functions.

Although thyroid malfunction can occur in infants resulting in developmental abnormalities, the dentist is most likely to encounter individuals who develop thyroid malfunction later in life.

The most common cause of thyroid disease worldwide is iodine deficiency leading to formation of goiters and to hypothyroidism. In developed nations, however, most thyroid diseases are of autoimmune etiology. Most Americans afflicted with thyroid diseases are unaware of their condition. See Table 4.6:

A. *Hyperthyroidism: Diseases Associated with Excess Circulating Thyroid Hormones*
   - *Thyrotoxicosis* is an inclusive term that identifies excess thyroid hormone levels regardless of cause and with or without frank hyperthyroidism.
   - *Graves' disease (diffuse toxic goiter)* is an autoimmune disorder, more common in women, in which immunoglobulins are directed against TSH receptors, allowing for retention of excessive quantities of TSH. It is the most common cause of hyperthyroidism. The elevated TSH level induces overproduction of T4, resulting in formation of diffuse toxic goiters. Signs and symptoms can be quite varied,

Table 4.5. Hormones Secreted by the Thyroid and Their Normal Ranges

Hormone/Test	Normal Range	Function
Thyroxine (T4)	4.5–11.2 mcg/dL	This iodine-rich hormone is primarily protein bound in blood, and it acts as a prohormone for T3.
Triiodothyronine (T3)	100–200 ng/dL	T3 is largely free in blood and four times more active in life functions than T4.
Calcitonin	<10 pg/mL	Calcitonin interacts with parathyroid hormone to regulate serum calcium and phosphorus levels.

Table 4.6. Characteristics of Thyroid Diseases

Category	Hypothyroidism	Hyperthyroidism
General	Weakness, lethargy, hoarse voice, weight gain	Fatigue and weakness
Metabolic	Cold intolerance, decreased basal metabolic rate, weight gain	Heat intolerance, increased appetite, weight loss
Central nervous system	Slurring of words, sleep apnea, decreased concentration, mental slowness	Tremor, emotional lability, nervousness, sleep disturbances
Skin	Decreased sweating, coarse hair, nonpitting edema (myxedema)	Excessive perspiration, warm moist skin, fine hair or alopecia
Cardiac/pulmonary	Dyspnea, bradycardia, diastolic hypertension	Dyspnea, palpitations and tachycardia (associated with widened pulse pressure)
Other	Macroglossia, salivary gland enlargement, chronic constipation, muscle cramps and pain, cretinism (children)	Menstrual dysfunction, enlargement of thyroid gland, proptosis or exophthalmos

ranging from rosy skin to significant eye involvement. If untreated, exophthalmos may occur and may progress to vision loss. Graves' disease can be successfully treated, but once ophthalmopathic changes have occurred, they tend to remain.

B. *Hypothyroidism: Disorders Associated with Reduced Circulating Thyroid Hormones*
- *Iodine insufficiency* is the most common cause of hypothyroidism worldwide, especially in undeveloped countries. Iodine is stored in the thyroid and is required to manufacture thyroid hormones. Abnormal enlargement of the thyroid or goiters tend to develop in an effort to compensate for the deficiency. Goiters may remain permanent if the deficiency exceeds 5 years' duration.
- *Hashimoto's thyroiditis*, an autoimmune inflammatory thyroid condition, with possible genetic propensity, is the most common cause of hypothyroidism in developed countries. It may initially increase T4 output, but ultimately leads to hypothyroidism.
- *Congenital hypothyroidism (cretinism)* can cause severe developmental deformities and mental deficiencies in children, but these can be prevented if the abnormality is detected early in infancy. In medical practice, it has become standard practice to perform thyroid function tests neonatally in order to detect and correct the deficiency. Early treatment may result in normal growth and development and mental acuity.
- *Myxedema* results from prolonged untreated hypothyroidism. Facial changes of myxedema are characterized by a dull expression, puffy eyelids, coarse skin, dry hair, dysgeusia, and an enlarged tongue. Mental and physical activities are slowed, and lethargy is a dominant feature.

C. *Thyroid Cancer*
- There are four histological types of thyroid cancer: papillary, follicular, medullary, and anaplastic. The papillary and

follicular forms are well differentiated, and they progress slowly. They are very responsive to treatment and have a very high survival rate.

Pathogenesis/Etiology

Hyperthyroidism occurs when the gland produces an excessive quantity of circulating biologically active T4. Untreated hyperthyroidism can lead to severe complications, including acute life-threatening thyroid crisis or "storm," resulting in coma and death. Fortunately, thyroid storm rarely occurs and is most likely in patients who have a long history of hyperthyroidism or in those with one or more goiters.

Hypothyroidism results from a deficiency of thyroid hormone production, or resistance to thyroid hormone action. In addition to Hashimoto's thyroiditis, other precipitating factors may include iron-deficiency anemia, or acquired conditions such as thyroidectomy, previous treatment with radioactive iodine, excessive ingestion of antithyroid drugs, or use of lithium or other drugs. There are several metabolic manifestations of hypothyroidism, and secondary cardiovascular effects may be severe. The heart may become dilated and enlarged and cardiac output is diminished, but there appears to be no increased risk for morbidity. However, on rare occasions, in elderly individuals with severe dysfunction, hypothyroidism may induce coma, which has a high mortality rate.

> **Signs of thyroid crisis or storm**
> Restlessness
> Nausea and vomiting
> Abdominal pain
> Fever
> Profuse sweating
> Tachycardia and arrhythmias
> Pulmonary edema
> Congestive heart failure
> Coma with severe hypotension
> Death

Thyroid Cancer

There are four histological types:

- *Papillary*—80%; this tends to develop between the ages 30 and 50 years.
- *Follicular*—15%; this usually occurs in individuals >40 years.
- *Medullary*—3%; this progresses slowly but is more likely to metastasize.
- *Anaplastic*—2%; this is very aggressive and often invades esophageal tissue resulting in a very low survival rate.

Risk factors include women >40 years, previous radiation exposure especially in childhood, and a family history of thyroid cancer or goiters.

Epidemiology

Hyperthyroidism

Hyperthyroidism occurs in 80/100,000/year in females and 8/100,000/year in males.[28] It can occur in people of all ages but generally peaks in the third decade.

Hypothyroidism

Hypothyroidism incidence is estimated to be 350/100,000/year in females and 80/100,000/year in males.[28] The prevalence of spontaneous hypothyroidism is between 1% and 2% of adults, more common in older women and 10 times more common in women than in men. It is estimated that 8% of women (10% of women >55 years old) and 3% of men have asymptomatic subclinical hypothyroidism, most with Hashimoto's thyroiditis, a chronic autoimmune thyroiditis.[29]

Thyroid Cancer

Thyroid cancer represents 1% of all malignancies, making it the most common malignant endocrine tumor. It occurs in all races and occurs more often in females (3:1) than males.[30] The incidence has more than doubled since the early 1970s. The National Cancer Institute projects 48,020 new cases in 2011 with 1740 deaths for an overall incidence of 0.5–10/100,000/year.

Coordination of Care between Dentist and Physician

Hyperthyroidism and Hypothyroidism

The dentist should remain alert for signs and symptoms of undiagnosed or inadequately controlled thyroid diseases. The dentist should refer the patient for medical consultation if signs or symptoms of thyroid hypofunction are evident or if the patient develops new unexplained oral conditions such as macroglossia or dysgeusia. If these are present, elective dental treatment should be delayed until medical consultation is obtained. The physician in turn should provide information regarding the current degree of control for the patient, laboratory test results, medications, and other collateral disorders.

Thyroid Cancer

Dentists can play a major role in early detection of thyroid cancer by performing neck palpation during the dental examination. Any palpable thyroid nodule should be referred for medical evaluation. Once the diagnosis has been established, the physician should be queried about planned treatment and when it is to be accomplished. Any necessary dental treatment should be coordinated with the physician and, when possible, should be accomplished before cancer therapy begins, especially if the patient will receive external radiation and/or chemotherapy.

II. Medical Management

Identification/Medical History/Physical and Laboratory Examination

Hyperthyroidism

A screening test for TSH and/or thyroxine (T4) may be the first indication that an abnormality is present; triiodothyronine (T3) is also often elevated. More sophisticated tests may follow. A low TSH level and a high free T4 concentration may signify hyperthyroidism.

Hypothyroidism

Laboratory evaluation will reveal elevated serum levels of TSH and reduced levels of T4. In subclinical myxedema, TSH levels may remain within normal limits. A large majority of individuals with overt hypothyroidism will be affected by Hashimoto's autoimmune disease and circulating thyroid autoantibodies will be present.

Thyroid Cancer

Diagnosis begins with careful physical examination to detect thyroid nodules. It may be followed by measurement of TSH in blood, by ultrasound examination, and by local or full-body thyroid scan using radioactive iodine. The definitive diagnosis, however, is achieved by fine-needle biopsy or surgical biopsy.

Medical Treatment

Hyperthyroidism: Surgical thyroidectomy is often the treatment of choice although the patient will require lifelong thyroid hormone supplementation. Antithyroid drugs can be used to block hormone synthesis, and Graves' disease is usually treated with radioactive iodine or thyroidectomy. Prognosis is good

> **Drugs used to treat hyperthyroidism**
>
> Propylthiouracil (PTU) (risk of serious hepatic injury)
> Carbimazole (a prodrug that converts internally into methimazole)
> Methimazole (Tapazole®)
> Radioactive iodine 131 (for killing of thyroid gland tissues)

when appropriately diagnosed and treated. In the elderly, signs and symptoms of hyperthyroidism may mimic symptoms of aging and go undiagnosed and untreated.[31]

- *Thyrotoxic crisis (thyroid storm)* represents the major complication of the disease, and this may result in significant morbidity and mortality if untreated.

Hypothyroidism: Drugs containing sodium levothyroxin simulate thyroxine and represent the most common therapy for hypothyroidism. Initial levothyroxine (Synthroid®) doses are 50–100 µg and titrated to individual need, with dosages monitored and changed according to variations in weight and age of the patient. Prognosis is good if treated early. Treatment must be sustained, with interruptions resulting in recurrence of symptoms. Untreated individuals are at risk of myxedema coma with its high mortality rate.

Thyroid Cancer

Treatment will often include partial or complete thyroidectomy, TSH suppression, and/or ablative radioactive iodine therapy (I^{131}). In more advanced cases, external radiation therapy or chemotherapy may be necessary with multikinase inhibitors.[32]

 ## III. Dental Management

Evaluation

Hyperthyroidism

Medical risks should be carefully assessed and patients and their physicians queried regarding the course of medical treatment and the patient's overall health status.

Hypothyroidism

Patients with a history of hypothyroidism should be questioned about the status of their disease and unresolved concerns about medical risk should be discussed with the patient's physician. Vital signs should be taken, and most recent laboratory tests for thyroid function should be acquired if extensive stressful dental therapy is anticipated.

> **Key questions to ask the hyperthyroid patient**
>
> - How long has it been since your diagnosis? How often do you see your doctor about your condition?
> - What signs and symptoms caused your physician to test you? Do you have any of those signs and symptoms now?
> - Do you have any disorders related to your thyroid dysfunction such as heart disease, respiratory disease, diabetes, anemia, osteoporosis, high or low blood pressure?
> - What medications do you take? What dosage? Has the dosage changed recently?

Endocrine and Metabolic Disorders 89

Key questions to ask the hyperthyroid patient's physician

- Does the patient have any remaining thyroid hyperfunction?
- How has the patient been treated? Antithyroid medications? Surgical ablation? Radioactive iodine therapy? External radiation? Chemotherapy?
- Does the patient have acquired *hypo*thyroidism?
- Does the patient have any associated systemic disorders?
- What medications does the patient take?
- Do you feel antibiotics are needed for dental treatment?

Key questions to ask the hypothyroid patient

- When were you first diagnosed?
- What signs or symptoms did you have that caused your physician to test you?
- How often do you see your physician?
- Have you fainted or passed out at any time since you last saw your physician?
- What medications do you take? Has your physician increased or decreased your medication dosage recently? If so, why?
- Do you currently have other medical problems such as anemia or heart disease?
- Do you find yourself weaker and more lethargic than you were a few months ago?
- What type of problems are you having in your mouth? Enlarged tongue, dry mouth, swollen salivary glands?

Key questions to ask the hypothyroid patient's physician

- What medications does the patient take? What dosage? How long? To your knowledge, is the patient compliant with the prescribed drug regimen?
- Is the patient's thyroid status stable?
- Has the patient ever presented with a hypothyroid crisis?
- Does the patient have any other medical problems that might affect dental care?
- Do you feel the patient needs prophylactic antibiotic coverage for dental procedures?

Thyroid Cancer

Neck palpitation is an important component of the routine dental examination. The detection of a localized nodule on the gland requires medical referral. Cancer patients and their physicians should be queried regarding their course of treatment and overall health status.

Dental Treatment Modifications

Hyperthyroidism

- Neck palpation to check for nodules or goiter should be a routine component of an initial dental examination.
- If untreated or poorly controlled hyperthyroidism is present or suspected, the patient should not receive elective treatment until the condition is successfully medically managed.
- If there is a question of a patient being under adequate control, it is best to consult with the managing physician who may want to check the appropriate thyroid hormone levels.
- Be aware that patients currently or previously treated for *hyperthyroidism* are at risk for *hypothyroidism*, which may go unrecognized.

Hypothyroidism

- Patients with well-controlled hypothyroidism require no special precautions for routine or emergent dental treatments in the absence of other medical problems.
- Be alert for signs and symptoms of undetected or inadequately controlled hypothyroidism.
- Elective dental treatment should be deferred pending medical consultation if the patient is not adequately controlled.

Thyroid Cancer

- When possible, good oral health should be established prior to cancer therapy and maintained postoperatively with frequent recall appointments.
- After thyroid ablation, dental management protocols for hypothyroidism should be considered because patients will have iatrogenic thyroid hypofunction until therapeutic drug levels are achieved.
- Use a xerostomia management protocol if needed—salivary stimulants, salivary substitutes, topical fluoride, bland dentifrice, dietary modifications.

Oral Lesion Diagnosis and Management

Hyperthyroidism

- An occasional ectopic lingual thyroid nodule or tumor may occur in the posterior dorsum of the tongue.
- Chronic thyrotoxicosis may be associated with an increased risk of osteoporosis, which may have an effect on the incidence and severity of periodontal disease.
- Dental caries has been reported to occur more frequently.
- Development of the teeth and jaws may be accelerated and premature loss of deciduous dentition may occur.

Hypothyroidism

- Untreated neonatal hypothyroidism may result in altered development of the jaws, delayed tooth eruption, malocclusion, thick lips, and a protruding tongue.
- In older children and adults, uncontrolled hypothyroidism may be associated with macroglossia, glossitis, salivary gland enlargement, and increased risk for dental caries and periodontal diseases.
- Treatment of hypothyroidism has been of occasional benefit in managing burning mouth syndrome.[33]
- An association between oral lichen planus and hypothyroidism has been reported.[34]

Thyroid Cancer

- On rare occasions, primary thyroid cancer has been reported in lingual thyroid nodules.
- Radioactive iodine therapy can induce transient salivary gland sialadenitis, xerostomia, nausea and vomiting, altered taste sensation, and pain.[35,36]
- External radiation is usually not directed at the jaws, but some radiation effect and the effects of chemotherapy may add to the severity of oral complications.

 Risks of Dental Care

Hemostasis

- Hyperthyroidism and hypothyroidism pose no greater risk for altered hemostasis. Treatment of thyroid cancer rarely involves myelosuppressive chemotherapy drugs.

Susceptibility to Infection

Hyperthyroidism

- Acute infections should be treated with appropriate antibiotics, but antibiotic prophylaxis is usually not required for dental procedures including surgeries.

Hypothyroidism

- Untreated or inadequately controlled hypothyroidism patients may be more susceptible to infections and may require appropriate antibiotic therapy.

Thyroid Cancer

- Patients with current or history of thyroid cancer have no greater risk of infection.

Drug Actions/Interactions

Hyperthyroidism

- Antithyroid agents, methimazole and propylthiouracil, have the potential to cause bone marrow suppression and can cause mouth sores, sialadenopathy, taste loss, delayed wound healing, and gingival bleeding.

Hypothyroidism

- Individuals taking levothyroxine-type medication may experience an exaggerated response to drugs that affect central nervous system (CNS) function (narcotics, tranquilizers, and barbiturates). When possible, their use should be avoided and effects should be carefully monitored if they are required.

Patient's Ability to Tolerate Dental Care

Hyperthyroidism

- Use vasoconstrictors with caution in patients with nonmedically uncontrolled hyperthyroidism as it can exacerbate symptoms of tachycardia, dyspnea, and fatigue. For patients under control, there are no special precautions.
- Monitor vital signs and use a stress reduction protocol as patients with poorly controlled hyperthyroidism are at risk of thyroid storm. Conscious sedation may be indicted to control anxiety, but some oral sedatives may potentiate antithyroid drugs.

Hypothyroidism

- Dentists should have heightened awareness of possible lethargy, although well-medicated patients should have no problem withstanding dental treatment.

Medical Emergencies

- *Hypothyroidism*: Be prepared to manage an office emergency. In theory, acute oral infections, trauma, stress, or surgery may precipitate coma in uncontrolled hypothyroidism but that is not likely. The emergency medical

> **Management of hyperthyroid crisis**
>
> 1. Activate the emergency medical system
> 2. Prevent hyperthermia. One method is to keep the patient cool with cold towels.
> 3. Administer IV or injectable hydrocortisone (100–300 mg) and IV hypertonic glucose if equipment is available.
> 4. Monitor vital signs and be prepared to administer cardiopulmonary resuscitation if necessary.

system should be activated if the patient becomes progressively less responsive and cardiopulmonary support should be provided as necessary.

- *Hyperthroidism*: Be alert in detecting suspected clinical manifestations of thyroid crisis. Be prepared to take emergency measures and seek medical support.

IV. Recommended Readings and Cited References

Section 1. Pancreatic Diseases

Recommended Reading

Mealey BL, Ocampo GL. Diabetes mellitus and periodontal disease. Periodontol 2000 2007;44: 127–53.

Cited References

1. Gestational Diabetes. A Guide for Pregnant Women. Eisenberg Center at Oregon Health & Science University. Comparative Effectiveness Review Summary Guides for Consumers. Rockville, MD: Agency for Healthcare Research and Quality (US); 2005. AHRQ Comparative Effectiveness Reviews. 2009 Aug 5.
2. DeFronzo RA, Abdul-Ghani M. Type 2 diabetes can be prevented with early pharmacological interventional. Diabetes Care 2011;34(Suppl. 2): S202–9.
3. Hidalgo M. Pancreatic cancer. N Engl J Med 2010;362(17):1605–17.
4. Mealey BL. The interactions between physicians and dentists in managing the care of patients with diabetes mellitus. J Am Dent Assoc 2008; 10(Suppl.):4s–7s.
5. American Diabetes Association. Standard medical care in diabetes. Diabetes Care 2010; 33(Suppl. 1):s11–s61.
6. World Health Organization. Use of Glycated Haemoglobin (HbA1c) in the Diagnosis of Diabetes Mellitus. 2011. World Health Organization, Geneva Switzerland.
7. Zhang L, Farrell JJ, Zhou H, Elashoff D, Akin D, Park N-H, et al. Salivary transcriptomic biomarkers for detection of resectable pancreatic cancer. Gastroenterology 2010;138(3):949–57.
8. American Diabetes Association. Executive summary: standards of medical care in diabetes. Diabetes Care 2010;33(Suppl. 1):s4–10.
9. Aronovich S, Skope LW, Kelly JP, Kyriakides TC. The relationship of glycemic control to the outcomes of dental extractions. J Oral Maxillofac Surg 2010;68(12):2955–61.
10. Javed F, Romanos GE. Impact of diabetes mellitus and glycemic control on the osseointegration of dental implants: a systematic literature review. J Periodontol 2009;80(11):1719–30.
11. Lamster IB, Lalla E, Borgnakke WS, Taylor GW. The relationship between oral health and diabetes mellitus. J Am Dent Assoc 2008;139(10 Suppl.): 19s–24s.
12. Taylor GW, Borgnakke WS. Periodontal disease: associations with diabetes glycemic control and complications. Oral Dis 2008;14(3):191–203.
13. Dorocka-Bobkowska B, Zozulinska-Ziolkiewicz D, Wierusz-Wysocka B, Hedzelek W, Szumala-Kakol A, Budtz-Jörgensen E. Candida-associated denture stomatitis in type 2 diabetes mellitus. Diabetes Res Clin Pract 2010;90(1):81–6.
14. Michaud DS, Joshipura K, Giovannucci E, Fuchs CS. A prospective study of periodontal disease and pancreatic cancer in US male health professionals. J Natl Cancer Inst 2007;99(2):171–5.
15. Meyer MS, Joshipura K, Giovannucci E, Michaud DS. A review of the relationship between tooth loss, periodontal disease and cancer. Cancer Causes Control 2009;19(9):895–907.
16. Mealey BL, Rees TD, Rose LF, Grossi S. Systemic factors impacting the periodontium. Chapter 31.

In: Periodontics Medicine, Surgery and Implants. Rose LF, Mealey BL, Genco RJ, Cohen DW, eds. 2004. Elsevier Mosby, St. Louis, MO.

Section 2. Adrenal Diseases

Recommended Readings

Arlt W, Allolio B. Adrenal insufficiency. Lancet 2003;361(9372):1881–93.

Oelkers W. Adrenal insufficiency. N Engl J Med 1996;335(16):1206–12.

Cited References

17. Reddy P. Clinical approach to adrenal insufficiency in hospitalized patients. Int J Clin Pract 2011;65(10):1089–66.
18. Dubois EFL. Clinical potencies of glucocorticoids: what do we really measure? Curr Resp Med Rev 2005;1(1):103–8.
19. Bensing S, Brandt L, Tabaroj F, Sjoberg O, Milsson B, Ekbom A, et al. Increased death risk and altered cancer incidence pattern in patients with isolated or combined autoimmune primary adrenocortical insufficiency. Clin Endocrinol (Oxf) 2008;69(5):697–704.
20. Orth DN. Cushing's syndrome. N Engl J Med 1995;332(12):791–803.
21. Erickson QL, Faleski EJ, Koops MK, Elston DM. Addison's disease: the potentially life-threatening tan. Cutis 2000;66(1):72–4.
22. Nieman LK, Chanco Turner ML. Addison's disease. Clin Dermatol 2006;24(4):276–80.
23. Radfar L, Somerman M. Glucocorticoids. In: ADA/PDR Guide to Dental Therapeutics, 5th ed. Cianco SG, ed. 2009, pp. 155–91. ADA, Chicago, IL.
24. Gibson N, Ferguson JW. Steroid cover for dental patients on long-term steroid medication: proposed clinical guidelines based upon a critical review of the literature. Br Dent J 2004;197(11):681–5.
25. Miller CS, Little JW, Falace DA. Supplemental corticosteroids for dental patients with adrenal insufficiency. Reconsideration of the problem. J Am Dent Assoc 2001;132(11):1570–9.
26. Scheitler L, Tucker WM, Christian D. Adrenal insufficiency; report of a case. Spec Care Dentist 1984;4(1):22–4.
27. Milenkovic A, Markovic D, Zdravkovic D, Peric T, Milenkovic T, Vukovic R. Adrenal crisis provoked by dental infection: case report and review of the literature. Oral Surg Oral Med Oral Pathol Oral Radiol Endod 2010;110(3):325–9.

Section 3. Thyroid Diseases

Recommended Readings

Brent GA. Clinical practice. Graves' disease. N Engl J Med 2008;358(24):2594–605.

Little JW. Thyroid disorders. Part 1: hyperthyroidism. Oral Surg Oral Med Oral Pathol Oral Radiol Endod 2006;101(3):276–84.

Little JW. Thyroid disorders. Part II: hypothyroidism and thyroiditis. Oral Surg Oral Med Oral Pathol Oral Radiol Endod 2006;102(2):148–53.

Little JW. Thyroid disorders. Part III: neoplastic thyroid disease. Oral Surg Oral Med Oral Pathol Oral Radiol Endod 2006;102(3):275–80.

Pinto A, Glick M. Management of patients with thyroid disease. J Am Dent Assoc 2002;133(7):849–58.

Vanderpump MP. The epidemiology of thyroid disease. Brit Med Bull 2011;99:39–51.

Cited References

28. McGrogan A, Seaman HE, Wright JW, de Vries CS. The incidence of autoimmune thyroid disease: a systematic review of the literature. Clin Endocrinol 2008;69(5):687–96.
29. Vanderpump MP, Tunbridge WM. Epidemiology and prevention of clinical and subclinical hypothyroidism. Thyroid 2002;12(10):839–47.
30. Schlumberger MJ. Papillary and follicular thyroid carcinoma. N Engl J Med 1998;338(5):297–306.
31. Mitrou P, Raptis SA, Dimitriadis G. Thyroid disease in older people. Maturitas 2011;70(1):5–9.
32. Carter WB, Tourtelot JB, Savell JG, Lilienfeld H. New treatments and shifting paradigms in differentiated thyroid cancer management. Cancer Control 2011;18(2):96–103.
33. Femiano F, Lanza A, Buonaiuto C, Gombos F, Nunziata M, Cuccurullo L, et al. Burning mouth syndrome and burning mouth in hypothyroidism:

proposal for a diagnostic and therapeutic protocol. Oral Surg Oral Med Oral Pathol Oral Radiol Endod 2008;105(1):e22–7.
34. Siponen M, Huuskonen L, Laara E, Salo T. Association of oral lichen planus with thyroid disease in a Finnish population: a retrospective case-control study. Oral Surg Oral Med Oral Pathol Oral Radiol Endod 2010;110(3):319–24.
35. Mandel L, Liu F. Salivary gland injury resulting from exposure to radioactive iodine. Case reports. J Am Dent Assoc 2007;138(12):1582–87.
36. Grewal RK, Larson SM, Pentlow CE, Pentlow KS, Gonen M, Qualey R, et al. Salivary gland side effects commonly develop several weeks after initial radioactive iodine ablation. J Nucl Med 2009;50(10):1605–10.

Renal and Urinary Tract Disease

William M. Carpenter DDS, MS

I. Background

Renal and urinary tract diseases encompass a number of different entities, but the major individual disease process affecting the oral cavity and dental treatment is renal or kidney disease. Kidney disease is a major public health problem throughout the world, and as it progresses, results in a concomitant decrease in kidney function and is associated with complications in nearly all organ systems. It is linked to poor health outcomes and increasing medical expenditures.

Description of Disease/Condition

Kidney disease and kidney failure can be classified broadly as acute or chronic renal failure (CRF). CRF leads to the deterioration of nephrons and the functional unit of the kidney, and includes a broad spectrum of disease processes. CRF is defined as a progressive loss of kidney function and the development of systemic complications, namely cardiovascular disease.

Acute renal failure (ARF) is characterized by a sudden loss of kidney function, as evidenced by oliguria or anuria and an increase in blood urea nitrogen (BUN) or serum creatinine.

There are numerous causes of ARF, which can be classified as

- diminished kidney perfusion (prerenal);
- glomerular, vascular, or tubulointerstitial/ acute tubular necrosis (renal);
- obstruction of the urinary tract (postrenal).

Pathogenesis/Etiology

The most common causes of CRF are diabetes mellitus (34%), hypertension (25%), and chronic glomerulonephritis (16%). Other common causes include systemic lupus erythematosus, neoplasms, polycystic kidney disease, and acquired immune deficiency syndrome (AIDS) nephropathy. A variety of hereditary and environmental factors may contribute to the disease process as well.

The progression to end-stage renal disease (ESRD) begins with an initially asymptomatic

The ADA Practical Guide to Patients with Medical Conditions, First Edition. Edited by Lauren L. Patton.
© 2012 American Dental Association. Published 2012 by John Wiley & Sons, Inc.

stage known as "diminished kidney reserve." This stage is characterized by a 10–20% decline in glomerular filtration rate (GFR) and a mildly elevated creatinine level. Diminished kidney reserve progresses to "renal insufficiency" where nitrogenous products begin to accumulate in the blood and the GFR continues to decline (20–50% of normal). "Renal failure" is the final stage of the disease process in which the kidney can no longer maintain its excretory, metabolic, and endocrine functions beyond the normal compensatory mechanisms. This stage involves multisystem organ involvement including endocrine, neuromuscular, cardiovascular, gastrointestinal, hematological, and dermatological manifestations.

Patients with kidney disease have a variety of metabolic abnormalities such as impaired excretory capacity, fluid and electrolyte imbalance, moderate-to-severe hypertension, anemia, bleeding problems, skeletal abnormalities, and altered drug metabolism. Medical management of kidney disease has improved considerably during the past decade. Presently, preventive health care is improving and conservative care is initiated as early in the progression of the disease as possible, with the goals to retard disease progression and preserve the patient's quality of life. When kidney disease can no longer be treated by conservative medical management, dialysis is initiated, and if necessary, kidney transplantation is performed.[1]

Epidemiology

In the United States, more than 20 million people (10% of adults) have some form of CRF.[2] The largest growth in the CRF population has occurred among Medicare patients.

The overall incident rate of ESRD has increased dramatically since 1992. Approximately 548,000 patients in the United States have irreversible ESRD, and the point prevalence rate is 1752 per 1 million U.S. residents.[2] ESRD occurs more commonly in African-, Native-, and Asian-Americans, and patients from ages 45–64 years. Specifically, African-Americans have the highest incident rates, at 982 per million population in 2002. Additionally, the rate of new ESRD cases remains higher for males than females. Treatment of ESRD patients in the United States in 2008 involved dialysis (382,343) or transplant (17,413), and numbers are predicted to increase in the future. Nearly 60,000 Americans die annually as a result of ESRD, most with cardiovascular complications.[2]

Coordination of Care between Dentist and Physician

Patients with kidney disease may have significant oral and dental complications, either directly related to kidney failure, from systemic complications arising from their kidney disease, or as untoward sequelae from various treatment modalities, including pharmacotherapy, dialysis, and/or transplant. Adequate pretreatment dental evaluation and dental treatment with proper consideration for the patient's kidney status and related problems can prevent significant complications. Coordination of care between the dentist and physician cannot be overemphasized to ensure proper medical and dental care and overall health optimization, tailored to each individual patient.

II. Medical Management

Most dentists will encounter CRF with more frequency in their patient population, but a general understanding of ARF is necessary for dentists who may be consulted to examine or treat a hospitalized patient undergoing treatment for ARF.

Identification

The National Kidney Foundation (NKF) defines CRF as either kidney damage for ≥3 months or

> **NKF definition of chronic kidney disease**
>
> Kidney damage for ≥3 months, as defined by structural or functional abnormalities of the kidney, with or without decreased GFR, manifested by either
>
> - pathological abnormalities or
> - markers of kidney damage, including abnormalities in the composition of the blood or urine or abnormalities in imaging tests
>
> or
> GFR <60 mL/min/1.73 m² for ≥3 months, with or without kidney damage.
>
> Key: NKF, National Kidney Foundation; GFR, glomerular filtration rate.
> *Source*: National Kidney Foundation. Am J Kidney Dis 2002;39(Suppl. 1):S1–S266.

a GFR of <60 mL/min/1.73 m² for ≥3 months. CRF follows a predictable course and is categorized based on clinical and laboratory findings.[3]

Medical History

In 2002, the Kidney Disease Outcome Quality Initiative (K/DOQI) of the NKF published clinical guidelines and a classification system for chronic kidney disease (CKD).[3-5] Staging of the disease is based on the level of kidney function, regardless of the underlying etiology or disease process, and allows dentists and physicians to discuss kidney disease with more clarity than ever before. This also allows patients the opportunity to take greater control of their disease and understand their own progression when the classification is based on their GFR.[3] See Table 5.1.

Patients with CKD require a complete medical evaluation to determine the specific type of kidney disease (diagnosis), comorbid conditions, severity of the disease (based on level of kidney function), risk for further loss of kidney function, and development of complications, either directly related to the loss of kidney function or from systemic organ involvement. K/DOQI also published guidelines for risk factors for CKD, treatment guidelines, and disease outcomes.[2,6-8] Many of the susceptibility, initiation, progression, and end-stage factors can be determined through a thorough medical history and physical exam. Certain clinical and sociodemographic factors that have been implicated in the development and progression of CKD can be elicited during routine health-care visits. If these factors are present, further medical testing for the presence of albuminuria or diminished GFR should be performed.[1]

Physical Examination

Clinical manifestations of kidney disease and of uremia (excessive urea and other nitrogen compounds in the blood due to loss of kidney function) include nocturia, fatigue, altered mental status, peripheral neuropathy, nausea, vomiting, anorexia, and pruritus. Other common findings are hypertension, fluid and electrolyte abnormalities, anemia, and osteodystrophy. It is important to note that uremia is a serious medical syndrome, due in part to the various systemic complications that can develop. For example, uremic patients can have qualitative platelet abnormalities, may develop pericarditis, become encephalopathic with mental status changes, have immune suppression, and can develop a dermatological condition known as "uremic frost."[9,10] Many dentists may never encounter a patient with uremic syndrome since most patients with kidney failure undergo dialysis, prior to such manifestations.

Laboratory Testing

Some general guidelines for medical assessment of the patient with kidney disease are listed below[11,12]:

- The degree of kidney function should be estimated by assessment of serum creatinine (the breakdown product of creatine phosphate in muscle that ends up in blood), creatinine

Table 5.1. NKF Classification of Chronic Kidney Disease and Clinical Features

Stage	Description[a]	GFR (mL/min/1.73 m^2)	U.S. Prevalence,[b] # Affected (%)	Clinical Features	Action Plan[c]
—	At increased risk for CKD	>60 (with risk factors for CKD)	[d]	DM, autoimmune diseases, systemic infections, drug exposure, neoplasia, family history, HTN	Screening, reduction of risk factors for CKD
1	Kidney damage with normal or elevated GFR	≥90	5.9 million (3.3)	Micro-albuminuria (DM 5–10 years, retinopathy, rising blood pressure), albuminuria (DM 10–15 years, retinopathy, HTN), cysts, proteinuria, + RBCs, ± WBCs, ± hydronephrosis	Diagnosis and treatment, treatment of comorbid conditions, interventions to slow disease progression, reduction of risk factors for CVD
2	Kidney damage with mildly decreased GFR	60–89	5.3 million (3.0)		Estimation of disease progression
3	Moderately decreased GFR	30–59	7.6 million (4.3)	DM, HTN, CVD, DM complications (retinopathy), HTN complications	Evaluation and treatment of disease complications
4	Severely decreased GFR	15–29	400,000 (0.2)		Preparation for kidney replacement therapy (dialysis, transplantation)
5	Kidney failure	<15 (or dialysis)	300,000 (0.1)	DM, DM complications (retinopathy), CVD, uremia	Kidney replacement therapy if uremia is present

[a] For stages 1 and 2, kidney damage was estimated by a ratio of greater than 17 mg of albumin to 1 g of creatinine in men or greater than 25 mg of albumin to 1 g of creatinine in women on two untimed (spot) urine tests.
[b] Prevalence age ≥20 for stages 1 through 4 are based on data obtained from the Third National Health and Nutrition Examination Survey (1988–1994) (Sources: Jones CA et al. Am J Kidney Dis 1988;32(6):992–9; for stage 5, from the U.S. Renal Data Survey, NIDDK, 1998).
[c] Includes actions from preceding stages.
[d] Prevalence of persons at increased risk for CKD has not been estimated accurately.
NKF, National Kidney Foundation; GFR, glomerular filtration rate; CVD, cardiovascular disease; HTN, hypertension; DM, diabetes mellitus; RBCs, red blood cells; WBCs, white blood cells. CKD, chronic kidney disease; defined as either kidney damage or a GFR <60 mL per minute per 1.73 m^2 for ≥3 months. Kidney damage is defined as pathological abnormalities or markers of damage, including abnormalities in blood or urine tests or imaging studies.
Adapted from the National Kidney Foundation. Am J Kidney Dis 2002;39(Suppl. 1):S1–S266.

clearance, BUN (BUN is the waste product of protein metabolism), and other factors. Progressive reduction in creatinine clearance is a direct reflection of diminishing renal capacity. The BUN level is also a reflection of renal function and increases during progressive renal failure. See Table 5.2.
- Patients with CKD usually have chronic anemia due to the inability of the kidney to produce sufficient erythropoietin (EPO) to stimulate bone marrow production of red blood cells. Patients may be taking iron, vitamin B_{12}, and folic acid supplements, and EPO (Procrit®) injections thrice weekly to achieve a target hemoglobin of 10–12 g/dL. Hematocrit or hemoglobin should be measured before administering general anesthesia or intravenous sedation, before beginning dental procedures that might cause significant blood loss, or before prescribing narcotics.
- Patients with CKD usually have qualitative and quantitative platelet deficiencies. The platelet count, prothrombin time/international normalized ratio, and partial thromboplastin time should be measured before surgery.
- Hypertension is often associated with CKD. Blood pressure determination, before and during dental treatment, may be indicated and, when significantly elevated, appropriate medical referral should be considered.
- Abnormalities such as metabolic acidosis, fluid overload, and hyperkalemia can exist. Measurement of serum electrolytes and an electrocardiogram may be indicated prior to dental treatment. Elective dental treatment should be deferred when these abnormalities are present.

Medical Treatment

Medical treatment for CKD begins with therapy for the specific underlying etiology; recognition and treatment of comorbid conditions; intervention to slow the loss of kidney function; measurements to prevent and treat cardiovascular disease and other systemic complications; and preparation for kidney failure and replacement of kidney function, by dialysis or transplantation if necessary.

First-line medical treatment may include angiotensin-converting enzyme (ACE) inhibitors to decrease the progression to kidney failure, in both diabetic and nondiabetic patients. Protein restriction has also been advocated as a preventive measure to slow the progression, once diagnosed with renal insufficiency. Other pharmacological agents employed in kidney disease include diuretics, potassium-binding resins to treat hyperkalemia, phosphate binders to prevent the development of renal osteodystrophy (elevated parathyroid hormone and subsequent calcium mobilization), sodium bicarbonate for acidosis, EPO for anemia, and fresh frozen plasma (FFP) or cryoprecipitate for bleeding diathesis.

CKD may progress to CRF, and thus, dialysis must be initiated to artificially filter the blood. This decision is usually made when the serum creatinine is chronically above 20 mg/dL, the creatinine clearance is below 20 mL/min, serum BUN is greater than 100 mg/dL, volume overload, refractory acidosis, and refractory hyperkalemia are present. The NKF guideline[7] recommends discussion of options for treatment, including kidney transplantation, peritoneal dialysis (PD), hemodialysis (HD) in the home or in-center, and conservative treatment, when patients reach CKD stage 4 (estimated GFR <30 mL/min/1.73 m^2) and initiation at least by stage 5 (estimated GFR <15 mL/min/1.73 m^2). Over 382,000 patients receive dialysis in the United States at a cost of more than $39 billion dollars a year.[2] Dialysis can be performed by either PD, HD, or, in the acute setting, continuous renal replacement therapy (CRRT):

HD: Removal of toxins and excess fluids is accomplished via extracorporeal circulation of blood through a dialyzer (artificial kidney). Treatment is usually performed three times per week for 3–4 hours. See Figs. 5.1 and 5.2. A vascular access is established via an arteriovenous (AV) fistula, vascular graft, or indwelling vascular catheter. Typically, an

Table 5.2. Serum Chemistry Laboratory Changes in Chronic Kidney Disease (CKD)

Laboratory Test	Normal Range	Normal Values in CKD	Signs/Symptoms of Abnormality
Serum creatinine	0.7–1.4 mg/dL	Increased generally 12–20 mg/dL (*depends on muscle mass*)	Fatigue, dehydration, mental confusion, shortness of breath
Blood urea nitrogen (BUN)	7–21 mg/dL	Increased but <100 mg/dL (*depends on protein intake*)	Fatigue, insomnia, nausea, dry or itching skin, urine-like body odor and breath
Creatinine clearance	85–150 mL/min	<10 mL/min	
Serum calcium (Ca^{++})	8.5–10.5 mg/dL	Same but goal is <10	Low: cataracts, depression, hair loss, muscle twitching/cramping, seizures High: fatigue, muscle weakness, mental changes, thirst
Serum phosphorus (PO_4)	2.5–4.5 mg/dL	Increased but goal 3.5–5.5 mg/dL	High: causes elevated PTH by lowering Ca^{++}, bone fractures
Serum sodium (Na^+)	135–145 mmol/L	Same—decreased	Thirst resulting in drinking more with fluid gain, elevated blood pressure, shortness of breath
Serum potassium (K^+)	3.6–5.0 mEq/L	Same—increased but <6.0 mEq/L	Few until >7 mEq/L, then weakness preceding cardiac arrest
Serum chloride (Cl^-)	95–108 mEq/L	Same	Low: hyperexcitable nervous system, low blood pressure, shallow breathing, tetany High: deep breathing, fatigue, muscle weakness
Serum albumin	3.5–5.0 g/dL	Goal >4.0 g/dL	Weight loss, poor appetite, medication side effects
Parathyroid hormone level (PTH)	10–65 pg/mL	Stage 3; 35–70 pg/mL Stage 4; 70–110 pg/mL Stage 5; 150–300 pg/mL	Early: asymptomatic Late: itching, bony changes on X-ray, fractures

Modified from Dialysis Lab Tests at a Glance. Available at: http://www.esrdnetworks.org.

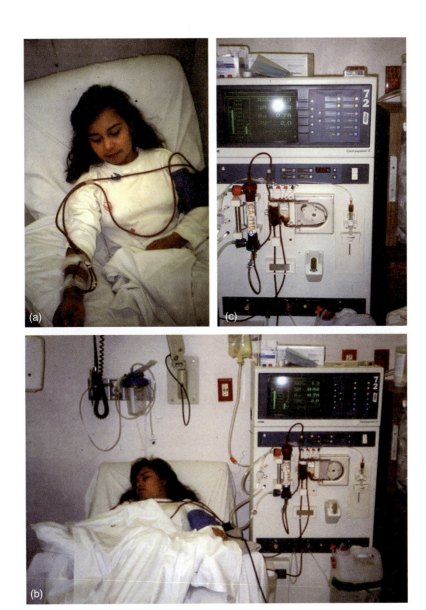

Figure 5.1 Hemodialysis. (a) Hemodialysis taking place through the shunt in the right arm. (b) Patient undergoing hemodialysis at an outpatient dialysis center. Typically, heparin is used as an anticoagulant during dialysis. (c) Hemodialysis machine. Exchange occurs across a semipermeable membrane into a dialysate with electrolyte composition mimicking extracellular fluid that allows fluid volume and waste products (uremic toxins) from the patient's plasma to diffuse out of the blood while retaining other cellular elements of the blood.

indwelling catheter is used for short-term dialysis in the patient with ARF, and AV fistulas or grafts are reserved for patients with long-term or indefinite dialysis needs. See Fig. 5.3.

PD: Placement of a catheter into the abdominal cavity, which facilitates filtration through the drainage of toxins:
- Intermittent PD needs frequent exchanges of dialysate, usually three times per week for 10–12 hours.
- Continuous ambulatory peritoneal dialysis (CAPD) requires four changes of 2–3 L of dialysate per day. This is usually performed by the patient at home.
- Continuous cycling peritoneal dialysis (CCPD) utilizes a programmed machine that performs the dialysate exchanges during the night. CCPD accounts for approximately 10% of all PD, while CAPD accounts for almost all the remaining 90%.

CRRT: Access is obtained either by AV or venovenous route, and the body's blood is pumped through a filter and cleansed with a dialysate and excess fluid is removed from the body. CRRT is used temporarily in the intensive care unit (ICU) for a hospitalized patient with CKD requiring temporary dialysis until their kidneys have recovered from injury, trauma, or other cause of acute failure. Dentists are unlikely to treat these patients, as this form of dialysis is in the acute setting and typically in the hospitalized patient.

The 1- and 5-year survival rates of patients on dialysis are 79.6% and 34.5%, respectively.[2] The annual, per-person costs for PD patients were almost $20,000 lower than for HD patients in 2007, yet in 2008 only 7% of U.S. dialysis patients were using PD, based on largely nonmedical factors.[13] Mortality rates for patients on PD in the United States have been driven down to rates comparable with patients on HD, improving the prospect of future growth in use of this modality.

Figure 5.2 Hemodialysis machine with a computer hookup.

(a)

(b)

(c)

Figure 5.3 Hemodialysis access shunts. Blood pressure measurement should not be taken in the arm with the shunt. (a) Vascular access site. (b) Arteriovenous (AV) fistula for hemodialysis access. (c) Enlargement of the arm veins secondary to a surgically created AV fistula for hemodialysis.

Table 5.3. Transplantation Immunosuppressant Medications

Medication	Action	Oral Side Effects/Dentally Relevant Toxicities
Glucocorticoids	Glucocorticoid receptor agonists, receptor-independent effects	Angioedema, moon face, oral candidiasis and oral herpes simplex virus, anemia, neutropenia, possible adrenal suppression
Cyclosporine	Calcineurin inhibitor	Gingival overgrowth
Tacrolimus	Calcineurin inhibitor	Gingival overgrowth (lower incidence than cyclosporine)
Sirolimus, everolimus	Target of rapamycin inhibitors	Mouth ulcers, delayed wound healing, thrombocytopenia
Mycophenolate mofetil	Purine synthesis inhibitor	Neutropenia, mild anemia
Azathioprine	Antimetabolite	Leukopenia, bone marrow depression
Daclizumab, basiliximab	Anti-CD25 antibody	Rare mouth ulcers, oral candidiasis, gingival overgrowth, thrombocytopenia
Horse or rabbit antithymocyte globulin	Polyclonal antithymocyte globulin	Thrombocytopenia, leukopenia

Adapted from Hallorhan PF. N Engl J Med 2004;351(26): 2715–29.

However, diabetic patients treated with PD have a significantly higher risk for mortality compared with those on HD.[13]

Almost half of all hemodialyzed patients with ESRD die from cardiovascular causes, such as cardiac arrest, acute myocardial infarction, other cardiovascular causes, and cerebrovascular disease. Other causes with relatively high mortality rates include septicemia and malignancies.

Kidney Transplantation: Another option, with other advantages and problems is kidney transplantation. Although kidneys are the most commonly transplanted organ, this option is hampered by a lack of available donor organs. Two types of donors are living and cadaveric donors. Approximately 17,000 renal transplants are performed each year in the United States, with over 87,000 patients on the wait list.[2] The recipient mounts an immune response against the antigens expressed by the donor-grafted organ, leading to the need for lifelong immune suppressive medications to prevent graft rejection. Human leukocyte antigen (HLA) typing facilitates the matching process between donor and recipient, because the closer the genetic identity, the less likely rejection is to occur. Immunosuppressive drugs are used for induction (intense immunosuppression in the first days posttransplant), maintenance, and reversal of established rejection, and are the key to successful allograft function.[14] See Table 5.3.

III. Dental Management

Evaluation

Numerous factors to be considered before dental treatment include:[15,16]

- minimizing patient morbidity and increasing quality of life by eliminating sources of oral infection;
- decreasing patient discomfort and morbidity by preventing or minimizing the complications resulting from oral mucosal disease occurring in ESRD patients;
- preventing the AV HD shunt from becoming infected;
- minimizing the risk of endocarditis.

Coordination of care between dentists and physicians should begin with a consultation with the primary care physician regarding:

- underlying cause of ESRD (diabetes, hypertension, etc.);
- recent coagulation values (heparin is commonly used during hemodialysis);
- consideration of antibiotic prophylaxis for HD patients prior to dental treatment (to protect patient from potential endocarditis and endarteritis);
- timing of dental visit (preferably on a non-HD day).

Dental Treatment Modifications

CKD Patients

The specific management of patients with CKD prior to dental treatment includes the following:

Key questions to ask the patient

- What type of kidney disease do you have?
- How is your kidney disease treated?
- What are the signs and symptoms of your kidney disease?
- What are the laboratory values associated with your medical conditions?
- Are you on an anticoagulant, or do you have any increased bleeding tendencies?
- What types of medications are you not able to take?
- Are you on dialysis? If so, is this hemodialysis or peritoneal dialysis?
- If hemodialysis, what is your dialysis schedule? And, where is your shunt?
- Have you ever had a transplant, or are you on a transplant list?
- Have you ever had infective endocarditis?

Key questions to ask the physician

- What is the severity of the patient's kidney disease?
- What medications are being prescribed for the patient's kidney disease?
- What are the patient's most recent laboratory values?
- Is the patient on hemodialysis? If so, what is his/her schedule?
- Is the patient on the transplant list?
- If the patient has cyclosporine-induced gingival overgrowth, is there a substitute medication that can be tried?
- Has the patient had infective endocarditis/endarteritis or is the patient at risk?

Dental Evaluation

Since CRF patients have an increased susceptibility to infection as the result of decreased leukocyte function and leukopenia, an examination to eliminate oral and dental sources of infections is recommended. Oral changes seen in these patients include uremic stomatitis, oral malodor, metallic taste, reduced salivary function, pallor of oral mucosa due to anemia, white patches called "uremic frost," and tooth mobility.

Treatment Considerations

- Patients with CRF have impaired metabolism of drugs normally excreted by the kidney. Adjustments of the dosages and intervals of these drugs must be considered.[17,18] See Table 5.4. Additionally, drugs that are nephrotoxic or that significantly affect acid–base or electrolyte balance should be used with caution.
- Patients with a uremic bleeding diathesis should have local hemostatic measures taken to prevent bleeding after surgical procedures (microfibrillar collagen application, absorbable gelatin sponge, topical thrombin and sutures). Effective dialysis can often correct uremic bleeding. Patients with serious bleeding problems or those who require major surgery may be treated with preoperative intranasal desmopressin acetate (DDAVP). Platelet transfusions should be used with extreme caution as they are highly immunogenic, causing sensitization against potential transplants and future platelet transfusions. Use of cryoprecipitate may be considered in refractory cases, in consultation with a hematologist. See Chapter 9.
- When there is significant suppression of leukocyte function, broad-spectrum antibiotic prophylaxis is recommended before dental procedures that may present a risk of infection.
- If residual renal function is diminishing rapidly, elective dental treatment should be delayed until dialysis is instituted and the patient is medically stable.

HD Patients

Medical Evaluation

In addition to the foregoing precautions described under CKD, HD patients have these additional considerations:
- The AV shunt should not be used for venipunctures or for administration of medication.
- The arm must not be used for measuring blood pressure.

Dental Evaluation

Dental evaluation is similar to that described under CKD. In addition, dialysis patients may develop renal osteodystrophy due to secondary hyperparathyroidism and vitamin D deficiency. This condition includes the following oral signs and symptoms: tooth mobility, radiographic changes, loss of lamina dura, bone demineralization, decreased trabeculation, "ground glass" appearance, radiolucent giant cell lesions (brown tumors), soft tissue calcifications, and spontaneous bone fractures. See Figs. 5.4 and 5.5.

Treatment Considerations

Patients are generally dialyzed according to a regular schedule, usually on alternate days, for example, Monday, Wednesday, and Friday; or Tuesday, Thursday, and Saturday. During dialysis, patients are heparinized to prevent blood clotting during the procedure. Dental treatment can be performed without increased risk of bleeding from heparin on nondialysis days because of the short half-life of heparin. In patients who have had regional heparinization for dialysis, dental treatment can be performed later on the day of dialysis, if required. However, the dentist may still have to be concerned about bleeding since some centers keep dialysis patients continuously anticoagulated with warfarin,

Table 5.4. Dentally Prescribed Medication Adjustment for Patients with Kidney Disease

Adjustment of Maintenance Dose Intervals (in Hours), Total Dose, or Timing with Dialysis for Adult Patients in Renal Failure

Drug	Usual Dosage Normal Renal Function	Mild Renal Failure (GRF > 50)	Moderate Renal Failure (GRF 10–50)	Severe Renal Failure (GRF < 10)	Hemodialysis (HD)	Peritoneal Dialysis
Antibiotics						
Amoxicillin	250–500 mg q8	8	8–12	24	Dose after HD	250 mg q12
Ampicillin	250 mg–2 g q6	6	6–12	12–24	Dose after HD	250 mg q12
Cephalexin	250–500 mg q6	6–8	8–12	12–24	Dose after HD	12–24
Clindamycin	150–450 mg q6	a	a	a	a	a
Doxycycline	100 mg q12	a	a	a	a	a
Erythromycin	250–500 mg q6	a	a	a	a	a
Metronidazole	250–500 mg q8-12	a	a	a	Dose after HD	a
Penicillin VK	500 mg q6	a	a	a	a	a
Tetracycline	250–500 mg q6-12	8–12	12–24	24		
Vancomycin	500 mg–1.25 g q12	1 g q12-24	1 g q24-96	1 g q4-7 days	1 g q4-7 days	1 g q4-7 days
Analgesics						
Acetaminophen	650 mg q4	4	6	8		
Aspirin	650 mg q4	4	4–6	Avoid use	Dose after HD	a
Ibuprofen	400–800 mg q8	a	a	a	a	a
Ketorolac	30–60 mg load; 15–30 mg q6	100%	50%	25–50%	a	a
Local anesthetics	Individualized	a	a	a	a	a

Narcotics

Codeine	30–60 mg q4-6	a	75%	No data
Meperidine	50–100 mg q3-4	a	75%	Avoid
Morphine	20–25 mg q4	a	75%	No data
Propoxyphene	65 mg q6-8	a	Avoid	Avoid

Barbiturates

Pentobarbital	30 mg q6-8	a	a	a
Secobarbital	30–50 mg q6-8	a	a	a

Benzodiazepines

Midazolam	Individualized	a	50%	a
Diazepam[a]	2–10 mg q6-24	a	a	a
Lorazepam	1–2 mg q8-12	a	a	a
Triazolam	0.25–0.50 mg qhs	a	a	a

Others

Dexamethasone	0.75–9.0 mg q24	a	a	a
Diphenhydramine	25 mg q6-8	a	a	a
Prednisone	5–60 mg q24	a	a	a
Fluconazole	100–400 q24	a	50%	Dose after HD	50%
Acyclovir	5–10 mg/kg q8	q12-24	50% q24	Dose after HD	50% q24

[a] No adjustment needed. Adapted from Aronoff GR et al. Drugs Prescribing in Renal Failure: Dosing Guidelines for Adults, 4th ed. 1999. American College of Physicians. Philadelphia, PA.

Figure 5.4 Panoramic radiograph showing "ground glass" appearance of renal osteodystrophy in a 44-year-old woman with a 10-year history of CKD due to focal segmental glomerulosclerosis on hemodialysis.

Figure 5.5 Periapical radiographs showing loss of lamina dura and "ground glass" appearance of renal osteodystrophy in a 36-year-old male with type 1 diabetes and ESRD on hemodialysis awaiting a kidney/pancreas transplant.

or because the uremic bleeding may not be fully corrected by dialysis[19]:
- Patients with AV fistulas appear to present a low risk of infection from transient bacteremias during dental procedures. An analysis of the evidence base for the practice of antibiotic premedication of patients with HD shunts to protect the patient from distant site infection of the shunt is lacking evidence to support this practice.[20] In studies of patients with infective endocarditis, HD dependence and related increased *Staphylococcus aureus* infection has raised concern.[21] While there is no clear consensus on this topic, some dentists and physicians may choose to use prophylactic antibiotics based on individual patient concerns and profes-

sional judgment. The American Heart Association standard regimen[22] is considered adequate, but alternate regimens may be chosen. Use of intravenous vancomycin during dialysis is preferred by some clinicians because it provides prophylaxis for up to 7 days. Since some antibiotics are dialyzed, reduced dosages may not always be necessary. The specific antibiotics and dosages should be selected in consultation with the patient's nephrologist.

PD Patients

- In patients receiving long-term PD, a permanent transcutaneous catheter is placed into the peritoneal cavity. There is no evidence that dental procedures need to be modified or antibiotic prophylaxis is necessary prior to dental treatment to prevent infection of this catheter.

Transplant Patients

Medical Evaluation

The recent history should be evaluated for evidence of increased susceptibility to infection:
- Results of a recent complete blood cell count should be obtained to detect the effect of immunosuppressive drugs.
- Adrenal suppression, secondary to long-term corticosteroid therapy, must be considered.

Dental Evaluation

- Before renal transplantation, all dental, periodontal and pericoronal sources of bacteremia should be identified and treated. Currently, the risk of retaining moderately periodontally involved teeth in renal transplant patients is unknown.
- Posttransplantation patients should have dental evaluations and dental prophylaxis

Figure 5.6 Recurrent herpetic lesion of the left nostril following immunosuppression in a kidney transplant patient.

every 3–6 months, depending on their dental and periodontal status.
- Oral mucosal lesions suggestive of herpes simplex, candidiasis or other infections should be evaluated and diagnosed as indicated. These infections may lead to severe or disseminated disease in these immunosuppressed patients and must be detected early in order that antiviral, antibacterial, or antifungal therapy can be instituted. See Fig. 5.6.
- Immunosuppressed transplant patients have an increased risk of cancer. Therefore, patients should be observed for enlarged cervical lymph nodes and suspicious oral mucosal lesions.

Treatment Considerations

- Immunosuppressive drugs used may mask early signs or symptoms of oral infections.
- For patients receiving adrenal suppressive doses of corticosteroids, supplementation may be necessary for stressful dental procedures.
- Prophylactic antibiotics may be recommended for indicated dental procedures. Preoperative topical antiseptic application of chlorhexidine to the surgical site may also reduce the likelihood of infection.
- For herpes simplex mucosal lesions, systemic acyclovir is indicated.

Figure 5.7 Gingival enlargement in the maxillary anterior area secondary to cyclosporine for immunosuppression in a kidney transplant patient.

- Candidiasis may be treated with nystatin or clotrimazole. More resistant fungal infections may require fluconazole, ketoconazole, itraconazole, or amphotericin B. Some of these drugs are potentially nephrotoxic, and they should be used with caution and in consultation with the nephrologist.
- Gingival overgrowth may develop in patients taking cyclosporine. See Fig. 5.7. Meticulous oral hygiene may minimize this complication with gingivectomy being occasionally of benefit.
- If gingival overgrowth is present, the dentist should communicate this to the physician who might alter the immunosuppressant maintenance regimen to tacrolimus or mycophenolate mofetil.
- No elective dental treatment should be performed in the immediate posttransplant period.

Special Considerations

Hospitalized immunosuppressed patients are susceptible to infections, particularly with methicillin-resistant *Staphylococcus aureus* (MRSA) and gram-negative bacilli such as *Klebsiella* and *Pseudomonas*. Therefore, culture of infections is necessary to identify the specific organisms involved in these life-threatening infections, in order to administer the appropriate antibiotics.

Follow-Up and Long-Term Care

Because these patients as a group are more susceptible to the consequences of oral/dental disease, they are best followed in a manner that permits the prevention of oral disease and/or allows its early diagnosis and treatment.

Regular contact with the patient's physician is necessary because the treating dentist must have current knowledge of the patient's overall condition.

Renal, Bladder, and Prostate Cancer

There are several malignant neoplasms of the kidney. The most prevalent is renal cell carcinoma, which originates from the tubular or ductal epithelial cells and makes up 80–90% of the cases, accounting for 30,000 cases per year in the United States. The second most common type is transitional cell carcinoma (5–10%), which originates in the pelvis or calyces. This type is associated with bladder cancer in half of the cases. The third type of malignancy of the kidney is Wilms' tumor (nephroblastoma), which makes up 85% of pediatric renal malignancies, 98% occurring before the age of 10 years. The prevalence is 1 in 10,000, making it the most common abdominal solid tumor of children.

Cancers of the urinary tract are most common in the bladder. These cancers occur in older patients and are rare under age 50. These neoplasms of the transitional epithelium were formerly called transitional cell carcinoma but are now termed urothelial cancers.

Prostate cancer is now the most frequent type of cancer in the U.S. male with 220,000 new cases and 30,000 deaths annually. Three-fourths of the cases occur in 60- to 80-year-olds.

As with all of these cancers, treatment is dependent on the stage and often involves combination treatment. In advanced cases, metastasis may occur and the jaws or oral mucosa may be affected. The dentist must be aware of this and also be familiar with dental management of the cancer patient undergoing antineoplastic chemotherapy. See Chapter 13.

 ## Risks of Dental Care

Hemostasis

Patients with ESRD are at risk for bleeding as a result of the platelet abnormalities, defects in the platelet–vessel wall interaction, uremic toxins in the blood, abnormal production of nitric oxide, anemia, and possible drug treatments.[23] Uremic bleeding is most likely to occur if they are inadequately dialyzed. This is at greatest risk at day 2 from HD or if on ineffective PD or no dialysis. Acute postsurgical bleeding episodes resulting from uremic bleeding can be managed by assuring adequacy of dialysis and using desmopressin nasal spray at a dose of 3 µg/kg, generally one spray per nostril. Alternatively, desmopressin can be given subcutaneously or intravenously.

Patients on HD are likely to have heparin used during the dialysis session that will create a coagulopathy for the subsequent 6–8 hours or, less commonly, may be chronically anticoagulated with warfarin. Treating the patient on an "off" day removes the concern about heparin in the dialysate causing bleeding. Patients on warfarin should be managed as described in Chapter 9.

Susceptibility to Infection

Post kidney transplant patients on immune suppressants may have increased susceptibility to infections and should be closely monitored.

Drug Actions/Interactions

Drug choice and dose should be carefully considered. Doses of many drugs excreted by the kidney require dose and/or schedule adjustment for patients in renal failure to prevent drug accumulation and drug toxicity. The goal is to maintain a serum level associated with the intended therapeutic response observed in patients with normal renal function. Table 5.4 lists maintenance dose intervals for patients in moderate and severe renal failure as compared with normal renal function. Oral side effects and toxicities of transplant immunosuppressive medications, such as cyclosporine, which may cause gingival overgrowth, are shown in Table 5.3.

Patient's Ability to Tolerate Dental Care

Few limitations exist in stress tolerance.

Special Considerations for the Renal Transplant Recipient

There is some evidence that untreated dental inflammation and infections may be a possible risk factor for infection and rejection in patients undergoing a kidney transplant, although there is not much published literature on this topic.[24] The dentist should inform patients and their families about the necessity of dental treatment, with particular emphasis on its relationship to their disease. It is critical that patients be advised of the circumstances under which they should contact the dentist between regularly scheduled appointments. Patient information handouts are helpful complements to verbal instruction; a sample of a patient instruction sheet follows.

> **Patient instruction sheet**
>
> - You have been referred to the dentist for dental services by your physician because you are either awaiting a kidney transplant or have recently received one.
> - Because transplant patients are more likely to get infections in the mouth or jaws, we need to examine you and treat you for all potential areas of infection. You should be seen by your dentist on a routine basis.
> - If you should develop pain or a sore area in your mouth, please call your dentist or physician as soon as possible.

IV. Recommended Readings and Cited References

Recommended Readings

De Rossi SS, Cohen DL Chapter 15. Renal disease. In: Burket's Oral Medicine, 11th ed. Brightman VJ, Greenberg MS, Glick M, Ship JA, eds. 2008. J.B. Lippincott Co., Philadelphia, PA, pp. 363–83.

Proctor R, Kumar N, Stein A, Moles D, Porter S Oral and dental aspects of chronic renal failure. J Dent Res 2005;84(3):199–208.

Suthanthiran M, Strom TB Renal transplantation. N Engl J Med 1994;331(6):365–76.

Cited References

1. Levey AS, Coresh J, Balk E, Kausz AT, Levin A, Steffes MW, et al. National Kidney Foundation practice guidelines for chronic kidney disease: evaluation, classification, and stratification. Ann Intern Med 2003;139(2):137–47.
2. National Institute of Diabetes and Digestive and Kidney Diseases, National Institutes of Health. Kidney and Urologic Disease Statistics for the United States. NIH Publication No. 11-3895. August 2011. Available at: http://kidney.niddk.nih.gov/KUDiseases/pubs/kustats/index.aspx. Accessed December 23, 2011.
3. National Kidney Foundation. K/DOQI clinical practice guidelines for chronic kidney disease: evaluation, classification and stratification. Am J Kidney Dis 2002;39(Suppl. 1):S1–S266.
4. Jones CA, McQuillan GM, Kusek JW, Eberhardt MS, Herman WH, Coresh J, et al. Serum creatinine levels in the US population: Third National Health and Nutrition Examination Survey. Am J Kidney Dis 1998;32(6):992–9.
5. U.S. Renal Data System. USRDS 1998 Annual Data Report, National Institutes of Health, National Institute of Diabetes and Digestive and Kidney Diseases. Bethesda, MD. 1998.
6. National Kidney Foundation. KDOQI™ clinical practice guidelines and clinical practice recommendations for diabetes and chronic kidney disease. Am J Kidney Dis 2007;49(Suppl. 2): S1–S180.
7. National Kidney Foundation. KDOQI clinical practice guidelines and clinical practice recommendations for 2006 updates: hemodialysis adequacy, peritoneal dialysis adequacy and vascular access. Am J Kidney Dis 2006;48(Suppl. 1): S1–S322.
8. U.S. Renal Data System. USRDS 2004 Annual Data Report: Atlas of End-Stage Renal Disease in the United States, National Institutes of Health, National Institute of Diabetes and Digestive and Kidney Diseases, Bethesda, MD. 2004.
9. Johnson CA, Levey AS, Coresh J, Levin A, Lau J, Eknoyan G Clinical practice guidelines for chronic kidney disease in adults: part I. Definition, disease stages, evaluation, treatment, and risk factors. Am Fam Physician 2004;70(5):869–76.
10. Weigert AL, Schafer AI Uremic bleeding: pathogenesis and therapy. Am J Med Sci 1998; 316(2):94–104.
11. Johnson CA, Levey AS, Coresh J, Levin A, Lau J, Eknoyan G Clinical practice guidelines for chronic kidney disease in adults: part II. Glomerular filtration rate, proteinuria, and other markers. Am Fam Physician 2004;706(6): 1091–7.
12. Dialysis Lab Tests at a Glance. Available at: http://www.esrdnetworks.org/resources-conditions-for-coverage/esrd-update-transitioning-to-new-esrd-conditions/DialysisLabTestsAt-a-Glance-FINAL-PinkSZEdit.pdf/view. Accessed December 23, 2011.
13. Mehrotra R, Chiu YW, Kalantar-Zadeh K, Bargman J, Vonesh E Similar outcomes with hemodialysis and peritoneal dialysis in patients with end-stage renal disease. Arch Intern Med 2011;171(2):110–8.

14. Halloran PF Immunosuppressive drugs for kidney transplantation. N Engl J Med 2004; 351(26):2715–29.
15. Little JW, Falace DA, Miller CS, Rhodus NL Dental Management of the Medically Compromised Patient, 7th ed. 2008. Mosby, St. Louis, MO.
16. Rhodus NL, Miller CS Clinician's Guide to Treatment of Medically Complex Dental Patients, 4th ed. 2009. American Academy of Oral Medicine, Edmonds, WA.
17. Munar MY, Singh H Drug dosing adjustments in patients with chronic kidney disease. Am Fam Physician 2007;75(10):1487–96.
18. Aronoff GR, Berns JS, Brier ME, Golper TA, Morrison G, Singer I, et al. Drugs Prescribing in Renal Failure: Dosing Guidelines for Adults, 4th ed. 1999. American College of Physicians, Philadelphia, PA. Available at: http://www.kdp-baptist.louisville.edu/renalbook/. Accessed December 23, 2011.
19. De Rossi SS, Glick M Dental considerations for the patient with renal disease receiving hemodialysis. J Am Dent Assoc 1996;127(2):211–9.
20. Lockhart PB, Loven B, Brennan MT, Fox PC The evidence base for the efficacy of antibiotic prophylaxis in dental practice. J Am Dent Assoc 2007;138(4):458–74.
21. Cabell CH, Jollis JG, Peterson GE, Corey GR, Anderson DJ, Sexton DJ Changing patient characteristics and the effect on mortality in endocarditis. Arch Intern Med 2002;162(1):90–4.
22. Wilson W, Taubert KA, Gewitz M, Lockhart PB, Baddour LM, Levison M, et al. Prevention of infective endocarditis: guidelines from the American Heart Association: a guideline from the American Heart Association Rheumatic Fever, Endocarditis, and Kawasaki Disease Committee, Council on Cardiovascular Disease in the Young, and the Council on Clinical Cardiology, Council on Cardiovascular Surgery and Anesthesia, and the Quality of Care and Outcomes Research Interdisciplinary Working Group. Circulation 2007;116(15):1736–54.
23. Galbusera M, Remuzzi G, Boccardo P Treatment of bleeding in dialysis patients. Semin Dial 2009;22(3):279–86.
24. Segelnick SL, Weinberg MA The periodontist's role in obtaining clearance prior to patients undergoing a kidney transplant. J Periodontol 2009; 80(6):874–7.

Hepatic Disease

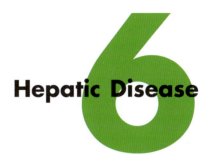

Juan F. Yepes DDS, MD, MPH, DrPH, MS

I. Background

Description of Disease/Condition

Viral Hepatitis

Virally induced hepatitis can be caused by hepatitis A, B, C, D, or E strains and results in inflammation and destruction of the liver. It can present as acute or chronic persistent disease.

Alcoholic Liver Disease (ALD)

Alcoholic cirrhosis is the terminal stage of ALD, where fibrosis and scarring has resulted in severe liver dysfunction. It is one of the main causes of death among alcohol abusers. Excessive alcohol intake can lead to fatty liver, hepatitis, and cirrhosis. Alcoholic hepatitis has a sudden onset typically following decades of heavy alcohol use (mean intake of 100 g per day) and is characterized by acute or chronic inflammation and parenchymal necrosis of the liver.[1]

Hepatocellular Carcinoma

Malignant neoplasms of the liver that arise from parenchymal cells are called hepatocellular carcinomas. Hepatocellular carcinomas are associated with cirrhosis in 80% of cases.

Pathogenesis/Etiology

Viral Hepatitis

The five currently classified hepatitis viruses vary in transmission mode from primarily percutaneous (hepatitis B virus [HBV], hepatitis C virus [HCV], hepatitis D virus [HDV]) to primarily fecal–oral (hepatitis A virus [HAV], hepatitis E virus [HEV]). Characteristics are shown in Table 6.1.

HAV and HEV generally have clinical and morphological features of acute icteric hepatitis. Onset is usually insidious, with an initial prodromal phase lasting a few days and a variable combination of flu-like symptoms: fever, mild chills, abdominal pain, anorexia, nausea,

The ADA Practical Guide to Patients with Medical Conditions, First Edition. Edited by Lauren L. Patton.
© 2012 American Dental Association. Published 2012 by John Wiley & Sons, Inc.

Table 6.1. Characteristics of Hepatitis Viruses: Pathogenesis/Etiology/Disease Course

	HAV	HBV	HCV	HDV	HEV
Classification	Picornavirus	Hepadnavirus	Flaviviridae family	Small defective RNA virus, infects with HBV	Calicivirus or alpha-virus family
Mode of transmission	Fecal–oral, *rarely*: percutaneous	Percutaneous, sexual, perinatal	Percutaneous, *rarely*: sexual, perinatal	Percutaneous, sexual, perinatal	Fecal–oral
Prophylaxis	Ig, vaccine	HBIg, vaccine	None	None (HBV vaccine for susceptible)	None
Incubation days	15–50	30–180	15–160	21–140	14–63
Clinical features					
Chronic infection	No	1–10%, up to 90% in neonates	80–90%	Common	No
Carrier state	No	Yes	Yes	Yes	No
Severity of symptoms	Usually mild, age dependent	Moderate	Asymptomatic to mild	May be severe	Usually mild
Fulminant hepatitis	<0.1%	1%	Rare	Up to 20% in superinfection	10–20% in pregnant women
Hepatocellular carcinoma	No	Yes	Yes	?	No

Adapted from *Harrison's Manual of Medicine*; Fauci AS, Braunwald E, Kasper DL, et al. eds. 2009; New York, NY: The McGraw Hill Companies; 1264 pgs. Table 161-1.
HAV, hepatitis A virus; HBV, hepatitis B virus; HCV, hepatitis C virus; HDV, hepatitis D virus; HEV, hepatitis E virus; Ig, immune globulin.

vomiting, and diarrhea. HAV viral particles are replicated only in hepatocytes and gastrointestinal epithelial cells and are released into the blood and bile. The damage of the liver cells results from a cell-mediated immune response.[2] Peak infectivity correlates with the greatest viral excretion in the stool during the 2 weeks before the onset of jaundice or elevation of the liver enzymes.[3]

HBV and HCV infections are usually diagnosed several years and decades after acquisition on routine blood testing or after blood donation. Approximately 25% of patients with HCV infection will have hepatic fibrosis that can end in cirrhosis,[4] on average 20 years after infection,[5] while the other 75% have different degrees of hepatic inflammation. Factors that contribute to the development of cirrhosis are unclear; it may be genetic factors or the consumption of alcohol. If cirrhosis develops, the annual incidence of hepatocellular carcinoma is 1–4%.[6]

Clinical expression of HDV, that can infect only individuals who have HBV, is wide, and although it sometimes follows a benign course, the disease is clinically important. Studies have shown that most patients with HBV coinfected with HDV or HCV have more severe liver disease and more rapid progression to cirrhosis.[7]

ALD

Rather than being caused singularly by ethanol toxicity in hepatocytes, ALD is currently considered to be a multifactorial disease, where gender, genetic, and nutritional factors influence the disease progression to cirrhosis. The key process in the pathophysiology is the oxidative stress, inflammation, alterations in cytokine secretion, and fibrosis.[8] Secondary abnormalities include malnutrition and impaired hepatic regeneration.

Epidemiology

Viral Hepatitis

HAV, HBV, and HCV are the most common types, with the Centers for Disease Control and Prevention (CDC) estimating that there are 80,000 new infections each year and an estimated 4.4 million Americans are living with chronic hepatitis, many being unaware of their infection.[9] See Table 6.2 for characteristics of acute hepatitis infections.

Risk factors for HAV include close personal contact with an infected person, men who have sex with men, travel outside the United States, illicit drug use, known food-borne outbreaks (fresh produce or food handlers), and contact with a child or employee in a child care center.[9] Studies performed in the United States have not shown an occupational risk for health-care workers.[3]

The prevalence of HBV infection in the United States is 0.4%, with an estimated 0.8–1.4 million persons chronically infected. With the implementation of vaccination programs in 1991, the incidence of new infections in the United States has declined by approximately 82% to 1.5 per 100,000 in 2009.[9]

HCV is a common problem in the United States with an estimated prevalence of 1.8% (of which approximately 75% are chronic infections), involving approximately 2.7 million people, excluding high-risk groups, such as inmates, institutionalized, and homeless persons.[10]

In the United States, the prevalence of HDV and HEV are low and HDV is confined to high-risk groups, such as intravenous drug users, while outbreaks of HEV infection have rarely been observed. Vaccination programs for HBV, increased awareness of HDV and its mode of transmission, and better preventive measures (e.g., use of disposable needles) have probably contributed substantially to the decline in HDV in different regions of the world.

Table 6.2. Acute Hepatitis Virus Infection Epidemiology (2009) in the United States

	HAV	HBV	HCV
Acute cases	1987	3371	781
Incidence rate per 100,000	0.6	1.1	0.3
New infections	21,000	38,000	16,000
% with jaundice	68.8	79.9	74.7
% hospitalized	39.3	46.7	56.2
% died	0.9	1.3	0.4

Source: Centers for Disease Control and Prevention. Available at: http://www.cdc.gov/hepatitis/Statistics/2009Surveillance/Commentary.htm#bkgrndl.

ALD

Cirrhosis mortality rates are higher in men than women and higher in Hispanics than Caucasians or African-Americans.[11] Cirrhosis mortality is also associated with poverty, and factors such as less nutritional diets, exposure to environmental toxins, and greater stress may aggravate alcohol effects in the liver of disadvantaged populations. Finally, genetic factors influence both patterns of heavy drinking and physiological vulnerability to alcohol effects.[8] True prevalence of ALD is difficult to estimate as many adults consume some level of alcohol; however, in the United States in 2009, 30,444 deaths were estimated to have resulted from chronic liver disease and cirrhosis, making this the 12th leading cause of death.[12]

Hepatocellular Carcinoma

Incidence and mortality rates for hepatocellular carcinoma are rising rapidly in the United States because of the increased prevalence of cirrhosis associated with HCV infection in younger patients resulting in up to 4% of patients with cirrhosis developing cancer each year.[13] In developed countries, risk factors for hepatocellular carcinoma in patients known to have cirrhosis are male gender, age over 55 years, non-Caucasian ethnicity, anti-HCV positivity, and platelet count <75,000.

Coordination of Care between Dentist and Physician

In general, diseases of the liver have several implications for a patient receiving dental care, including potential increased bleeding risk and altered metabolism of medications, requiring dose adjustment or avoidance. The medical history is essential for a correct assessment of the potential risk. The medical history must include questions regarding jaundice, cancer, autoimmune disorders, surgeries, history of alcohol intake, recreational drug use, sexual history, and bleeding tendencies.[14] It is important to discuss details of the liver disease with the physician in order to have a better understanding of the patient's medical status and degree of control. Dentists can encourage chronic alcohol users with ALD to seek counseling and support services, such as Alcoholics Anonymous (see Chapter 16).

II. Medical Management

Identification

Patients with chronic liver disease may be able to self-identify on the health history. Liver dysfunction in viral hepatitis and ALD can progress over time requiring identification of current functional status, which is critically important to help gauge coagulation status and ability of the liver to metabolize medications. Patients with acute hepatitis from viral, bacterial, or parasitic infection; autoimmune disorders; and reactions to alcohol, medications, and toxins, require prompt identification of the causative agent to facilitate patient treatment.

Medical History/Physical Examination

Viral Hepatitis

- *HAV*: The presence and severity of symptoms with HAV infection is related with the patient's age, including nonspecific and flu-like symptoms, persistent fever, severe pruritus, jaundice, diarrhea, and weight loss. Chronic infection does not occur with HAV.
- *HBV*: The symptoms of acute HBV infection are nonspecific and include fatigue, poor appetite, nausea, vomiting, abdominal pain, low-grade fever, jaundice, and dark urine.[15] Clinical signs include liver tenderness, hepatomegaly, and splenomegaly. Acute

HBV infection typically lasts for 2–4 months. Approximately 30–50% of children 5 years and older and adults are symptomatic; infants, children younger than 5 years, and immunosuppressed adults are more likely to be asymptomatic.[16] In adults with healthy immune systems, approximately 95% of acute infections are self-limited, with patients recovering and developing immunity.[17] Fewer than 5% of adults acutely infected with HBV progress to chronic infection, defined as disease lasting longer than 6 months. A small number (1%) develop acute hepatic failure and may die or require immediate liver transplantation.[18]

- *HCV*: The majority of acute and chronic HCV cases are asymptomatic, and patients rarely know when they acquired the infection.[10] Nonspecific symptoms such as fatigue, vague right upper quadrant discomfort, and pruritus may be noted. HCV infection may progress to cirrhosis with the consequent development of complications such as bleeding, hepatocellular carcinoma, and liver failure. Extrahepatic manifestations of HCV are uncommon and include renal disease, lichen planus, seronegative arthritis, and some neurological conditions.[19]

ALD

The clinical presentation of ALD can vary from an asymptomatic patient who may have an enlarged liver to a critically ill individual who dies quickly or a patient with end-stage cirrhosis. A recent period of heavy drinking, complaints of anorexia and nausea, and the demonstration of hepatomegaly and jaundice strongly suggest the diagnosis. See Fig. 6.1. Abdominal pain and tenderness, splenomegaly, ascites, fever, and encephalopathy may be present.

Hepatocellular Carcinoma

The presence of hepatocellular carcinoma may be unsuspected until there is deterioration in

Figure 6.1 Jaundiced skin and sclera in a 39-year-old with end-stage alcoholic cirrhosis.

the condition of a cirrhotic patient who was stable. Weakness and weight loss are associated symptoms. The sudden appearance of ascites, which may be bloody, suggests portal or hepatic vein thrombosis by a tumor or bleeding from a necrotic tumor. Physical examination may show tender enlargement of the liver with occasionally a palpable mass.

Laboratory Testing

Viral Hepatitis

HAV

- HAV immunoglobulin M (IgM) test (preferred confirmatory test for acute HAV infection)[20]
  - Serum antibodies IgM usually can be detected 5–10 days before symptom onset, and the level remains elevated for 4–6 months.[3]
- Elevated liver enzymes
- Elevated bilirubin levels

HBV

- Hepatitis B surface antigen (HBsAg)
  - Indicates currently infectious, with acute or chronic infection

- Hepatitis B surface antibody (HBsAb)
  - Indicates recovery or successful immunization
- Hepatitis B core antibody (HBcAb)
  - Indicates previous or ongoing infection
- IgM antibody to HBc antigen (IgM anti-HBc)
  - Indicates acute infection, acquired in the last 6 months

HCV

- Enzyme immunoassay to detect antibodies to multiple HCV antigens
- Hepatitis C RNA virus by polymerase chain reaction (PCR) detects quantity of the virus itself in the blood (quantification of the virus).

HDV

- Anti-HDV immunoglobulin G (IgG) antibodies (only if HBsAg positive)
  - Persists after HDV infection has cleared
- Serum HDV RNA with sensitive real-time PCR assay
  - Confirms active infection
- HDV genotyping
  - Patients with HDV genotype 1 are at a high risk for developing end-stage disease.[21]

HEV

- Serological essays for identification of anti-HEV antibody of IgM or IgG class
- PCR for detection of the virus in stool or serum

Liver Enzymes

- Aspartate aminotranferase (AST) or serum glutamic-oxaloacetic transaminase (SGOT); normal range: 5–40 units/L serum
- Alanine aminotransferase (ALT) or serum glutamic-pyruvic transaminase (SGPT); normal range: 7–56 units/L serum

Medical Treatment

Viral Hepatitis

HAV

Treatment is supportive and includes appropriate rest when necessary.[2] Balanced nutrition and avoidance of hepatoxins such as alcohol and acetaminophen are recommended. No specific antiviral therapy is currently available.[3] About 30% of symptoms require hospitalization for dehydration, severe prostration, coagulopathy, encephalopathy, or other evidence of hepatic acute failure.[3] Caregivers should observe strict contact precautions during the infection period. Healthy adults are noninfectious by 2 weeks after the onset of the disease, but children and immune-compromised persons may remain infectious for up to 6 months.

Immunoglobulin administered intramuscularly provides short-term protection (3–5 months) through passive transfer of HAV antibody. Immunoglobulin administered as prophylaxis within 2 weeks after exposure to HAV is 69–89% effective in preventing symptomatic infection.[22] Two types of inactivated whole virus vaccines for HAV are available in the United States.[3] The first dose provides immunity in 37% of persons within 2 weeks, in 90% of persons within 4 weeks, and in 100% of persons at 26 weeks.[23] The second dose provides persistent immunity projected to last at least 20 years.

HBV

The objectives for treatment of chronic HBV infection are to reduce the inflammation of the liver; prevent liver failure and cirrhosis; and reduce the risk of hepatocellular carcinoma by reducing or suppressing HBV replication.[15] It is important to differentiate patients who are hepatitis B e antigen (HBeAg) positive and those who are HBeAg negative because of viral mutation. Seroconversion (from HBeAg positive to HBeAg negative) predicts long-term reduction in viral replication, and it is used to monitor the response to the treatment. Chronic infection of HBV can go through four different phases that directly affect the therapeutic decisions. Patients in the first phase (active), with elevated hepatic enzymes, are candidates for treatment with the best anticipated response.

HCV

Recent advances in medical treatment now permit clearance of HCV in the majority of the patients.[24] A decision about whether to treat must be made on an individual basis, taking in consideration patient motivation, severity of the disease, potential for response to the treatment, and anticipated adverse events. The current standard of care for treatment involves use of interferon alpha 2a or 2b in combination with ribavirin.[19] Interferon alpha is administered subcutaneous once weekly. Ribavirin is administered orally in divided doses. Response rates of 54–56% are to be expected. Common adverse effects associated with interferon therapy are fatigue, headaches, myalgias, fever and chills, insomnia, nausea, anorexia, weight loss, alopecia, irritability, depression, neutropenia, and thrombocytopenia. Absolute contraindications to treatment are decompensated liver disease, pregnancy, active autoimmune disease, severe depression, poorly controlled diabetes mellitus, seizures, coronary artery disease, and heart failure.[25]

HDV

The accepted practice for treatment of chronic HDV is subcutaneous injections of interferon every week for at least 48 weeks. This treatment is considered in patients with active replication of HDV RNA and histological evidence of disease activity, with no contraindications to interferon therapy.

HEV

Current recommendations for the treatment of HEV infection are similar to the recommendations for HAV infection.

ALD

The most important treatment of ALD is the abstinence of alcohol. The use of corticosteroids for the treatment of ALD should be offered consistent with the U.S. guidelines for the treatment of ALD.[26] Nutritional supplementation is important because protein-calorie malnutrition is almost always present. The severity of the malnutrition correlates with the survival of the patient. It is important to attempt an intake of about 2000 calories per day to correct these deficiencies and promote the hepatic repair process in individuals with severe ALD.

Hepatocellular Carcinoma

Surgical resection of solitary hepatocellular carcinomas may result in cure if liver function is preserved. Treatment of underlying chronic viral hepatitis may lower postsurgical recurrence rates.

Liver Transplantation

Liver transplantation is used for patients with decompensated HCV infection with reinfection of the graft, but comparable survival rates with other patients receiving liver transplants. It may also be appropriate for small unresectable tumors in a patient with advanced cirrhosis, with reported 5-year survival rates of up to 75%.[27] Liver transplantation may also be required for autoimmune chronic hepatitis that is refractory to anti-inflammatory and immunosuppressive therapy.[28]

The Model for End-Stage Liver Disease (MELD) score, introduced in 2002 as a replacement of the Child–Tucotte–Pugh classification, is the basis for organ allocation among candidates for liver transplantation in the United States and serves as an objective scale of disease severity for chronic liver disease.[29] It is derived from measurements of serum bilirubin, the international normalized ratio (INR) of prothrombin time (PT), and serum creatinine to evaluate pretransplantation renal function.

III. Dental Management

Evaluation

It is difficult to identify potential or actual carriers of HBV, HCV, and HDV. Therefore, all patients with a history of viral hepatitis must be treated as though they are potentially infectious. Recommendations for infection control practices in dentistry published by the CDC and the American Dental Association (ADA) have become the standard of care for preventing cross infection in dental practice. This document published in 2003 recommends that all dental care workers who provide patient care should receive vaccination against HBV and should implement standard precautions during the care of all dental patients.[30] Additionally, these guidelines discuss the management of occupational exposures to blood-borne pathogens, including postexposure prophylaxis (PEP) for work exposures to HBV, HCV, and human immunodeficiency virus (HIV).[30] (See Chapter 11, Table 11.4.)

Most patients who are infected by HBV, HCV, and HDV are unaware that they have hepatitis. The majority of these cases are symptomatic and difficult to identify by the symptoms because they are similar with upper respiratory infections. In case that the patient reports a history of hepatitis or other liver disease, detailed information from the patient may be useful for the dentist to determine the type of disease and severity.

Key questions to ask the patient

- What type of liver disorder do you have?
- What is the underlying cause of your liver disease?
- What type of treatment are you receiving for your liver disease?
- What types of medications are you taking?
- What types of medications have you been told you cannot take?
- What are the signs and symptoms of your liver disorder?
- What are the laboratory values associated with your medical conditions?
- Do you have any increased bleeding tendencies?
- Do you drink any alcoholic beverages?

Key questions to ask the physician

- What is the severity of the patient's liver disorder?
- What medications are being prescribed for the patient's liver disease?
- Is the patient being treated for other medical conditions?
- What are the patient's most recent laboratory values (complete blood count [CBC], PT/INR, PTT, liver enzymes)?

Dental Treatment Modifications

For chronic and advanced liver disease, emergency dental care and elective dental treatment can be provided depending on the medical status and type/extent of dental care needed. For the rare patient with acute hepatitis, only emergency dental care should be provided. For the more prevalent HBV/HCV carrier with laboratory tests indicating infection without evidence of significant liver dysfunction, no modifications in the treatment plan may be necessary.

Oral Lesion Diagnosis and Management

Oral lesions in patients with significant liver disease may relate to the bleeding diatheses and include hematomas, ecchymoses, petechiae, and spontaneous bleeding of the gingiva and mucosal tissues. See Fig. 6.2. Jaundice can affect the oral mucosa. Immune-suppressed post-liver transplant patients can develop oral candidiasis and other opportunistic infections. See Fig. 6.3.

Risks of Dental Care

Hemostasis

Abnormal bleeding is associated with hepatitis and cirrhosis/end-stage liver disease. Vitamin-K-dependent clotting Factors II, VII, IX, and X are synthesized in the liver, and the production is affected in patients with severe liver disease. Factors I and V are also affected. Additionally, thrombocytopenia could be present in patients with splenomegaly associated with chronic liver disease. Before surgical procedures, patients with liver disease must have a careful evaluation of their capacity for hemostasis, and testing should include at minimum a platelet count, PT/INR, and partial thromboplastin time (PTT) tests. Platelet count should be above 50,000 and INR below 2.0–3.5 for surgical procedures depending on the extent of surgery; nonsurgical dental procedures may be safely performed in the higher INR ranges (below 4.0) and lower platelet counts. If laboratory values are critically altered, consultation with the physician will help the dentist interpret the results and delineate the treatment plan to minimize the potential for bleeding complications. This may include either or both, platelet transfusions to correct the thrombocytopenia and fresh frozen plasma (FFP) to correct the factor-related coagulopathy. Vitamin K injections the week prior to dental surgery may be helpful. Intraoperative hemostatic agents, such as microfibrillar collagen hemostat or absorbable gelatin sponge, should be used in extraction sites when hemostasis is impaired. Recently, the use of intranasal desmopressin

Figure 6.2 Severe intraoral spontaneous bleeding in a patient with end-stage cirrhosis.

Figure 6.3 Candida infection secondary to the use of steroids in a patient recipient of a liver transplant.

(DDAVP) has been suggested to be effective at restoring hemostatic capacity in patients undergoing dental extractions as a cost-effective alternative to FFP transfusion.[31]

Susceptibility to Infection

The patient with viral hepatitis being actively treated with interferon may have neutropenia and warrant antibiotic prophylaxis. Patients who have received a liver transplant and are on immunosuppressive medications may be at increased risk of infection and warrant more aggressive management of dental infections and consideration for antibiotic prophylaxis depending on the stage of transplant engraftment, although routine prophylaxis prior to dental treatment for posttransplant patients is not recommended.

Drug Actions/Interactions

Generally, for short periods of time, normal therapeutic doses of drugs can be used except when liver function is severely compromised. If necessary, alternative drugs not metabolized in the liver can be selected or doses and intervals adjusted. Extreme caution should be used in prescribing medications that are metabolized in the liver for patients with severe liver disease.

- *Analgesics/Pain Control*
  - Aspirin, ibuprofen, and other nonsteroidal anti-inflammatory drugs (NSAIDs) should be avoided as they are extensively metabolized by the liver and result in increased bleeding risk due to antiplatelet effects and ulcerogenicity.
  - Acetaminophen is relatively safe if limited to <4 g/day for acute pain management.
  - Codeine, hydroxycodone, and oxycodone are conjugated in the liver and should be used at increased dose intervals and for short-term use only.
  - Morphine is safe, while meperidine should have increased dosing intervals.
  - Local anesthetics, while metabolized in the liver, are safe if they are used within the suggested doses. Doses should be kept below 7 mg/kg when combined with epinephrine (13 cartridges of 1.8 mL 2% lidocaine 1:100,000 epinephrine).
- *Sedative/Anxiolytics*
  - Benzodiazepines require reduced dosages and increased intervals.
  - Barbiturates and propofol should be slowly titrated to desired effect, with prolonged recovery anticipated.
- *Antibiotics*
  - Beta-lactam antibiotics (penicillin, amoxicillin, ampicillin, cephalexin, cefazolin, ceftriaxone) are predominantly handled by renal excretion; thus, these can be used safely in patients with liver failure.
  - Metronidazole must be avoided in patients who actively ingest alcohol as this interaction will create a disulfiram-like reaction of flushing, headache, tachycardia, shortness of breath, severe nausea and vomiting, mental confusion, and possible circulatory collapse. It is liver metabolized and should be used with caution and with increased dose intervals with severe disease (acute hepatitis or cirrhosis).
  - Clindamycin, aminoglycosides (streptomycin, gentamycin), vancomycin, and macrolides (erythromycin, azithromycin, clarithromycin) should be avoided in severe liver disease.
  - Tetracycline, minocycline, and doxycycline undergo hepatic metabolism and recycling, so these should be used with caution, at reduced dosage, and increased dose intervals.

Patient's Ability to Tolerate Dental Care

While local anesthetics are considered safe in normal doses and maintain the same duration of action locally as in patients without liver disease, total dose is a concern for some patients. With significant liver disease, it may be prudent to treat one quadrant at a time to minimize total dose.[32] Avoid mouthwashes with high alcohol content in the patient with ALD.

Special Considerations

HBV infection is a well-recognized risk for health-care personnel making vaccination essential for dental providers. Health-care personnel's occupational risk of acquiring HBV is related to the extent of percutaneous injury and HBeAg status of the source person. Risk of clinical hepatitis from a needlestick injury with HBsAg-positive, HBeAg-negative blood is 1–6%, with serological evidence of HBV infection at 23–37%, compared with an injury with HBsAg-positive and HBeAg-positive blood resulting in clinical hepatitis for 22–31%, with serological evidence of HBV infection in 37–62% cases.[33]

Fortunately, HCV is rarely transmitted occupationally and in these cases most often from hollow-bore needles. HCV seroconversion after percutaneous exposure to HCV-positive source patient blood is estimated at 1.8%.[33] The OraQuick® HCV Antibody Test (OraSure technologies, Inc., Bethlehem, PA) was recently approved as the first rapid point of care test for HCV antibodies allowing increased opportunities to detect HCV outside of traditional settings.[33]

IV. Recommended Readings and Cited References

Recommended Readings

Douglas LR, Douglass JB, Sieck JO, Smith PJ. Oral management of the patient with end-stage liver disease and the liver transplant patient. Oral Surg Oral Med Oral Pathol Oral Radiol Endod 1998;86(1):55–64.

Lauer GM, Walker BD. Hepatitis C virus infection. N Engl J Med 2001;345(1):41–52.

Lee SR, Kardos KW, Schiff E, et al. Evaluation of a new, rapid test for detecting HCV infection, suitable for use with blood or oral fluid. J Virol Methods 2011;172(1–2):27–31.

Little JW, Rhodus NL. Dental treatment of the liver transplant patient. Oral Surg Oral Med Oral Pathol 1992;73(4):419–26.

Cited References

1. Lucey MR, Mathurin P, Morgan TR. Alcoholic hepatitis. N Engl J Med 2009;360(26):2758–69.
2. Cuthbert JA. Hepatitis A: old and new. Clin Microbiol Rev 2001;14(1):38–58.
3. Centers for Disease Control and Prevention. Chapter 8. Hepatitis A; Chapter 9. Hepatitis B. In: Epidemiology and Prevention of Vaccine-Preventable Diseases, 12th ed. Atkinson W, Wolfe S, Hamborsky J, eds. 2011, pp. 101–38. Public Health Foundation, Washington DC. Available at: http://www.cdc.gov/vaccines/pubs/pinkbook/default.htm
4. Freeman AJ, Dore GJ, Law MG, et al. Estimating progression to cirrhosis in chronic hepatitis C virus infection. Hepatology 2001;34(4 Pt 1):809–16.
5. Tong MJ, El-Farra NS, Reikes AR, Co RL. Clinical outcomes after transfusion-associated hepatitis C. N Engl J Med 1995;332(22):1463–6.
6. Bruno S, Silini E, Crosignani A, et al. Hepatitis C virus genotypes and risk of hepatocellular carcinoma in cirrhosis: a prospective study. Hepatology 1997;25(3):754–8.
7. Peters MG. Special populations with hepatitis B virus infection. Hepatology 2009;49(5 Suppl.):S146–55.
8. Addolorato G, Russell M, Albano E, Haber PS, Wands JR, Leggio L. Understanding and treating patients with alcoholic cirrhosis: an update. Alcohol Clin Exp Res 2009;33(7):1136–44.
9. Centers for Disease Control and Prevention. *Viral hepatitis*. Available at: http://www.cdc.gov/hepatitis/HBV/HBVfaq.htm. Accessed March 13, 2012.
10. Alter HJ, Seeff LB. Recovery, persistence, and sequelae in hepatitis C virus infection: a perspective on long-term outcome. Semin Liver Dis 2000;20(1):17–35.
11. Chen CM, Yoon YH, Yi HY, Lucas DL. Alcohol and hepatitis C mortality among males and

females in the United States: a life table analysis. Alcohol Clin Exp Res 2007;31(2):285–92.
12. Kochanek KD, Xu JQ, Murphy SL, et al. Deaths: Preliminary Data for 2009. National Vital Statistics Reports, Vol. 59, No. 4. 2011. National Center for Health Statistics, Hyattsville, MD.
13. Rustgi VK. The epidemiology of hepatitis C infection in the United States. J Gastroenterol 2007;42(7):513–21.
14. Golla K, Epstein JB, Cabay RJ. Liver disease: current perspectives on medical and dental management. Oral Surg Oral Med Oral Pathol Oral Radiol Endod 2004;98(5):516–21.
15. Wilkins T, Zimmerman D, Schade RR. Hepatitis B: diagnosis and treatment. Am Fam Physician 2010;81(8):965–72.
16. Mast EE, Weinbaum CM, Fiore AE, et al. A comprehensive immunization strategy to eliminate transmission of hepatitis B virus infection in the United States: recommendations of the Advisory Committee on Immunization Practices (ACIP) Part II: immunization of adults. MMWR Recomm Rep 2006;55(RR-16):1–33.
17. Lok AS, McMahon BJ. Chronic hepatitis B. Hepatology 2007;45(2):507–39.
18. Petrosillo N, Ippolito G, Solforosi L, Varaldo PE, Clementi M, Manzin A. Molecular epidemiology of an outbreak of fulminant hepatitis B. J Clin Microbiol 2000;38(8):2975–81.
19. Hoofnagle JH. Course and outcome of hepatitis C. Hepatology 2002;36(5 Suppl. 1):S21–9.
20. Center of Disease Control and Prevention. Positive test results for acute hepatitis A virus infection among persons with no recent history of acute hepatitis: United States, 2002–2004. MMWR Morb Mortal Wkly Rep 2005;54:453–6.
21. Marsh JW, Finkelstein SD, Demetris AJ, et al. Genotyping of hepatocellular carcinoma in liver transplant recipients adds predictive power for determining recurrence-free survival. Liver Transpl 2003;9(7):664–71.
22. Bianco E, De Masi S, Mele A, Jefferson T. Effectiveness of immune globulins in preventing infectious hepatitis and hepatitis A: a systematic review. Dig Liver Dis 2004;36(12):834–42.
23. Sonder GJ, van Steenbergen JE, Bovee LP, Peerbooms PG, Coutinho RA, van den Hoek A. Hepatitis A virus immunity and seroconversion among contacts of acute hepatitis A patients in Amsterdam, 1996–2000: an evaluation of current prevention policy. Am J Public Health 2004; 94(9):1620–6.
24. Fried MW, Shiffman ML, Reddy KR, et al. Peginterferon alfa-2a plus ribavirin for chronic hepatitis C virus infection. N Engl J Med 2002; 347(13):975–82.
25. Flamm SL. Chronic hepatitis C virus infection. JAMA 2003;289(18):2413–7.
26. McCullough AJ, O'Connor JF. Alcoholic liver disease: proposed recommendations for the American College of Gastroenterology. Am J Gastroenterol 1998;93(11):2022–36.
27. Seeff LB. Introduction: the burden of hepatocellular carcinoma. Gastroenterology 2004;127(5 Suppl. 1):S1–4.
28. Krawitt EL. Autoimmune hepatitis. N Engl J Med 2006;354(1):54–66.
29. Brown RS Jr., Kumar KS, Russo MW, et al. Model for end-stage liver disease and Child-Turcotte-Pugh score as predictors of pretransplantation disease severity, posttransplantation outcome, and resource utilization in United Network for Organ Sharing status 2A patients. Liver Transpl 2002;8(3):278–84.
30. Kohn WG, Collins AS, Cleveland JL, Harte JA, Eklund KJ, Malvitz DM. Guidelines for infection control in dental health-care settings—2003. MMWR Recomm Rep 2003;52(RR-17):1–61.
31. Stanca CM, Montazem AH, Lawal A, Zhang JX, Schiano TD. Intranasal desmopressin versus blood transfusion in cirrhotic patients with coagulopathy undergoing dental extraction: a randomized controlled trial. J Oral Maxillofac Surg 2010;68(1):138–43.
32. Haas DA. An update on local anesthetics in dentistry. J Can Dent Assoc 2002;68(9):546–51.
33. Centers for Disease Control and Prevention. Recommendations for prevention and control of hepatitis C virus (HCV) infection and HCV-related chronic disease. MMWR 1998;47(RR-19): 1–39.

Gastrointestinal Disease

Brian C. Muzyka DMD, MS, MBA

I. Background

The general impact of gastrointestinal (GI) disorders is often underestimated. Diseases of the GI tract are frequently misdiagnosed, untreated, or undertreated. Approximately 70 million Americans are diagnosed with GI disorders accounting for more than 105 million physician visits per year. GI diseases are associated with significant morbidity, mortality, and decreased quality of life. This chapter will review the more common GI disorders.

Description of Disease/Condition

Dyspepsia

Dyspepsia is classically described as an episodic or recurrent pain or discomfort arising from the proximal GI tract. Dyspepsia is a group of symptoms associated with heartburn, weight loss, regurgitation, indigestion, bloating, early satiety, and gastroesophageal reflux. Therefore, prevalence of dyspepsia cannot be accurately estimated due to lack of a standardized definition. In an effort to further refine the term dyspepsia, an international panel of clinical investigators published a consensus opinion and the term functional dyspepsia is now preferred:

- Functional dyspepsia is the presence of gastroduodenal symptoms without any causative organic, systemic, or metabolic disease.
- Functional dyspepsia has been separated into two distinct subgroups:
    - postprandial distress syndrome (postprandial fullness and early satiety);
    - epigastric pain syndrome (constant non-meal-related pain).

Gastroesophageal Reflux Disease

Gastroesophageal reflux disease (GERD) is an excessive retrograde movement (reflux) of acid-containing gastric secretions or bile and acid-containing secretions from the duodenum and stomach into the esophagus, causing troublesome symptoms and/or complications. The condition of gastroesophageal reflux is experienced occasionally by most people, especially after meals. Typical symptoms of GERD include heartburn, regurgitation, and dysphagia. Atypical symptoms include noncardiac chest

The ADA Practical Guide to Patients with Medical Conditions, First Edition. Edited by Lauren L. Patton.
© 2012 American Dental Association. Published 2012 by John Wiley & Sons, Inc.

pain, aspiration, asthma, hoarseness, and pneumonia. Complications include Barrett's esophagus, which is the premalignant lesion that links GERD and the most rapidly increasing cancer of the GI tract, esophageal adenocarcinoma. Erosion of the teeth may also occur.

Peptic Ulcer Disease

Peptic ulcer disease (PUD) is ulceration of the stomach or duodenum, the first section of the small intestine. Ulcerations are caused by decreased protective mucosal factors or by various mucosal damaging mechanisms.

Inflammatory Bowel Disease

Inflammatory bowel disease (IBD) is a chronic condition that includes ulcerative colitis (UC) and Crohn's disease (CD) and is characterized by acute flare-ups separated by periods of quiescence. Remission can occur without therapy. More recently, the less common microscopic colitis has been categorized as a type of IBD[1]:

- *UC* is an inflammatory disorder resulting in ulcerations of the lining of the colon and rectum. UC patients typically present with mild-to-moderate diarrhea without constitutional symptoms. The number of bowel movements increases with severity of UC and constitutional symptoms such as dehydration, fatigue, fever, and weight loss are more likely to occur. With rectal involvement, there are frequent small, more urgent, bloody stools.
- *CD* is an inflammatory disease of the bowel more commonly affecting the terminal ileum, the most distant part of the small intestine. CD symptoms also include diarrhea, fatigue, weight loss, and abdominal pain. With mild CD, abdominal pain can be vague, diarrhea intermittent, and no weight loss noted.

Irritable Bowel Syndrome

Irritable bowel syndrome (IBS) is an inclusive term for multiple potential physiological issues including disturbed central nervous system (CNS) pain processing, mucosal inflammation, abnormal colon motility, and anxiety disorders. Discussion of IBS is beyond the scope of this chapter. But it is important to note that IBS is much more prevalent than IBD, and IBD patients are frequently mislabeled with a diagnosis of IBS.

Pseudomembranous Colitis

Pseudomembranous colitis (PC) is an inflammation of the colon associated with antibiotic use. It is generally caused by *Clostridium difficile*, a gram-positive, anaerobic, spore-forming bacteria. *C. difficile* releases an enterotoxin (toxin A) and a cytotoxin (toxin B) that cause mucosal inflammation and lead to apoptosis.[2]

Celiac Disease

Celiac disease (gluten-sensitive enteropathy) is a chronic digestive disease characterized by small intestine malabsorption. Individuals with celiac disease have an abnormal immune reaction to gliadin, the alcohol-soluble fraction of gluten. Gluten is found in wheat and related species including rye and barley. Gluten is a source of protein in many parts of the world and is also used as an additive to foods low in protein or as a meat substitute.[3]

An immunologically mediated inflammatory response occurs when gliadin is ingested. As a result, the villi, the tiny, fingerlike protrusions lining the small intestine, are damaged or destroyed. Malabsorption results from the immunomodulated process and diarrhea may occur. Some individuals may have subtle symptoms or are asymptomatic.

Gastric Cancer

Gastric cancer is an adenocarcinoma of the stomach. Approximately 15% of gastric cancers occur in the upper part of the stomach while 40% of cancers develop in the middle part and 40% develop in the lower part of the stomach. Anatomically, the location of gastric cancer is related to differing vascular supply sources.

Colorectal Cancer

Colorectal cancer is a complex disease where genetic changes are often associated with progression from a premalignant lesion (adenoma) to invasive adenocarcinoma in the lower GI tract. Approximately 10% of adenomas will progress to adenocarcinomas, and this process may take up to 10 years. Adenocarcinomas make up the majority of colon and rectal cancers. Other rarer rectal cancers include lymphoma, sarcoma, and carcinoid adenocarcinoma.

Pathogenesis/Etiology

Functional Dyspepsia

Dysmotility has been the prime focus of research in functional dyspepsia. Visceral hypersensitivity also plays a role in 30–40% of patients with functional dyspepsia. The role of aberrant cerebral processing of visceral stimuli and visceral events is also being explored in functional dyspepsia. The evidence to date does not suggest a significant genetic contribution to functional dyspepsia.

GERD

The pathophysiology of GERD is multifactorial. The normal highly efficient barrier between stomach and esophagus becomes weakened in GERD. Patients with GERD have defective esophageal peristalsis; more frequent and prolonged transient lower esophageal sphincter relaxation; abnormal gastric emptying resulting in increased gastric pressure; and esophagitis and mucosal damage from gastric hydrochloric acid, bile salts, and pancreatic enzyme refluxate, with resultant dysmotility. Some will have hiatal hernias, *Helicobacter pylori* infection, and Barrett's esophagus.[4]

PUD

The damaging mechanisms associated with *PUD* include the following:

- Infection by *H. pylori* bacteria:
  - Fecal–oral infection with *H. pylori* is higher in populations who have a lower standard of living than routinely seen in industrialized countries. In the United States, approximately 40% of duodenal ulcer patients are infected with *H. pylori*. Successful eradication of *H. pylori* is associated with elimination of ulcer recurrence. This is the strongest evidence to support the role of *H. pylori* as an etiology of PUD.
- Increasing and widespread use of both non-steroidal anti-inflammatory drugs (NSAIDs) and aspirin:
  - In *H. pylori*-negative patients, the use and overuse of NSAIDs and aspirin is the most common cause of PUD.
- Idiopathic causes and hypersecretory causes are less common.

IBDs (CD and UC)

A key feature in the pathogenesis of IBD is a failure to downregulate the immune system and control local GI inflammation. The exact etiology of UC is unknown and the disease appears to be multifactorial. Environmental factors, immune dysfunction, smoking, NSAID use, low levels of antioxidants, psychological stress, consumption of milk products, and a genetic predisposition have all been proposed as causes of UC. First-degree relatives of IBD patients have a 10% lifetime risk of developing UC. The genetic component in the pathogenesis of CD has been identified as the gene NOD2 located on chromosome 16q12 and is related to the immune response to bacteria activating inflammatory cell signals.

A variety of immunological changes occur in IBD. T-lymphocyte cell subsets accumulate in the lamina propria of the affected area of the colon and are cytotoxic to colon epithelium. An increase in number of B lymphocytes and plasma cells, and an increase in the production of immunoglobulin G (IgG) and immunoglobulin E (IgE) follow. A small proportion of patients with UC develop smooth muscle and anticytoskeletal antibodies.

Microscopically, there is an inflammatory infiltrate of the lamina propria, crypt branching, and erosion of the tiny villi in the intestines that absorb nutrients. The ulcerated areas are eventually covered by granulation tissue. This leads to the formation of inflammatory polyps also known as pseudopolyps.[1]

PC

PC is associated with increased GI colonization with *C. difficile*. *C. difficile* can be found in 2–3% of healthy adults and up to 70% of healthy infants. *C. difficile* forms heat-resistant spores that persist in the environment for months to years. In hospital and other health-care facilities, outbreaks may occur as a result of contamination with these spores. Colonization occurs by the fecal–oral route, and as many as 30% of hospitalized adults are colonized with *C. difficile*. Normal gut flora resists colonization and overgrowth with *C. difficile*. In PC, the antibiotic disruption of the normal colon flora allows *C. difficile* overgrowth.

Many antibiotics may be responsible for *C. difficile* overgrowth, but third-generation cephalosporins are implicated most frequently. Third-generation cephalosporins have an intramuscular or intravenous route of administration with the exception of cefixime, which has an oral route of administration. Cefixime is used to treat community-acquired pneumonia, sinusitis, pharyngitis, and urinary tract infections. Third-generation cephalosporins including cefixime are not typically used to treat odontogenic infections. Immunosuppression is also a predisposing factor for *C. difficile* colitis.

Celiac Disease

Celiac disease is a multifactorial, multisystem disorder with a genetic predisposition. The majority of persons with celiac disease have the human leukocyte antigen (HLA) DQ2 haplotype found on chromosome 6. Interestingly, approximately 40% of general populations also have this haplotype but do not express the disease. Presence of this halpotype is required for the expression of celiac disease but not all who have this haplotype express disease. Relatives of individuals with celiac disease have a higher incidence of the disease than the general population. First-degree relatives have a prevalence rate of 10%. Environmental factors associated with celiac disease are ingestion of the gliadin found in gluten chiefly from wheat, rye, and barley. Some individuals also show sensitivity to oats. Grains not associated with celiac disease activity include rice, corn, sorghum, buckwheat, amaranth, quinoa, and millet.[3]

In susceptible individuals, exposure of small intestine mucosa to gluten triggers an inflammatory reaction causing villi destruction. Additionally, an immunological response occurs resulting in large numbers of CD8+ T lymphocytes, B lymphocytes, and other lymphocytes. As a result, various immunoglobulins, cytokines, interferons, tumor necrosis factor, and other inflammatory mediators are secreted with an end result of villous atrophy. The Marsh criteria are used to characterize abnormalities noted in the small bowel biopsy specimens. Marsh 0 represents a pre-infiltrative or normal stage, while Marsh 4 represents hypoplastic lesions as seen in T-cell lymphoma.[5,6]

Gastric Cancer

Gastric cancer can be subdivided using the Lauren classification for adenocarcinomas into two different histology subtypes. These subtypes have different genetic and biological patterns and treatment options:

- The intestinal type (IT) of gastric cancer is structurally similar to colon cancer with formation of gland-like tubular structures. This type of cancer is usually preceded by chronic gastritis and intestinal metaplasia. IT gastric cancer is more closely linked to environmental and dietary risk factors. This was the most common form of cancer in areas with a high incidence of gastric cancer and is now declining worldwide.

- The diffuse type (DT) of gastric cancer lacks glandular structure and instead consists of poorly differentiated, discohesive cells that infiltrate the wall of the stomach and secrete mucus. DT gastric cancer is associated with a worse prognosis and occurs at a younger age than the intestinal form. This subtype can result in a rigid thickened stomach.
- Approximately 5% of gastric cancers are lymphomas.

A multiple step model (the Correa pathway) has been proposed in the development of IT gastric cancer. In this model, preneoplastic changes eventually lead to the development of gastric cancer. Specifically, alterations in the DNA are caused by chronic inflammation, which in tandem with imbalanced epithelial cell proliferation and apoptosis in a local environment of atrophy and achlorhydria, colonization of intestinal bacteria that have nitrate reductase activity leads to the formation of carcinogenic nitrosamines. The development of gastric cancer has been attributed to loss of specialized glandular cell types such as parietal and chief cells (corpus-predominant atrophy), and this appears to be the critical initiating step in cancer progression.[7]

Other risk factors include use of alcohol and tobacco, ingestion of food additives (nitrosamines), smoked foods, and occupational exposure to heavy metals, rubber, and asbestos.

Colorectal Cancer

Three mechanisms in the development of colon and rectal carcinoma have been described:

1. adenomatous polyposis coli (*APC*) gene adenoma–carcinoma mechanism;
2. UC dysplasia;
3. hereditary nonpolyposis colorectal cancer (HNPCC) mechanism.

The majority of colorectal cancers (75%) develop in people with no known risk factors. The remaining 25% occur in people with risk factors such as familial history of colorectal polyps or cancer. Relative risk for the development of colorectal cancer is 2.42 when a first-degree relative has the diagnosis and 4.25 when more than one first-degree relative is affected. Other significant risk factors include genetic conditions such as HNPCC, IBD, and familial adenomatous polyposis. The incidence of colorectal cancer in patients with CD is up to 20 times greater than that of the general population.

A high-fat, low-fiber diet has been associated with the development of colorectal cancer while a high-fiber diet may have a protective role. Smoking and alcohol intake increase the risk for the development of colon cancer. Colon cancer can be detected; therefore, routine screening is indicated especially in individuals with high risk for disease development.

Epidemiology
Functional Dyspepsia

Functional dyspepsia is not life-threatening, and it has not been shown to be associated with any increase in mortality. Prevalence rates of 23–25.8% are reported in the United States. The impact of dyspepsia on patients and healthcare services has been shown to be significant. In European and North American populations sampled, 20% of people with dyspeptic symptoms had sought medical care, more than 50% were using medication most of the time, and approximately 30% reported their symptoms resulted in missed school or work.

GERD

GERD is common, with prevalence in Western populations estimated at 10–15% of adults, and is increasing among children. Obesity, prior use of NSAIDs, increasing age, smoking, and other GI and cardiac conditions are risk factors. Higher rates are seen among Hispanic-Americans than Caucasian-Americans and lowest rates are among Asian-Americans.[8]

PUD

Approximately 4.5 million Americans annually are affected by PUD, and 10% of the U.S. population at some point in time has evidence of a duodenal ulcer. *H. pylori*-positive patients have a 20% lifetime prevalence. The proportion of people with *H. pylori* infection increases steadily with age. The hospitalization rate for PUD is approximately 30 patients per 100,000 cases. The prevalence of PUD shows similar occurrences in males and females.

IBD

It is estimated that as many as 1.4 million persons in the United States are affected by IBD, divided approximately equally between UC and CD. It is diagnosed more often in Caucasians, and there is no specific gender predilection. IBD has a bimodal presentation. Most IBD patients are diagnosed around ages 15 and 25; there is a second peak around age 55 and 65 years. The incidence of UC and CD is 1.5–8 new cases per 100,000 in the United States yearly.[9]

PC

PC caused by *C. difficile* infection primarily occurs in hospitalized patients. Up to 20% of hospitalized patients are affected, causing as many as 3 million cases of diarrhea and colitis per year. The incidence of *C. difficile* in hospitalized patients was reported to be 84/100,000 in 2005. Less than 20,000 cases per year are diagnosed in nonhospitalized patients.

Celiac Disease

It is most prevalent in western Europe and the United States and approximately 1% of the U.S. population is affected. There is no age predilection, but women have a slightly higher incidence. Because of the difficulty in diagnosis, celiac disease is underdiagnosed in most affected people.

Gastric Cancer

It is the fourth most common cause of cancer-related death in the world. In the United States, incidence of gastric cancer is lower than it is worldwide. Unfortunately, most patients present with advanced disease, which contributes to the relatively high mortality rate of the disease.

Using data from the American Cancer Society Cancer Facts & Figures, 2011, it is estimated that 21,520 men and women (13,120 men and 8,400 women) will be diagnosed with and 10,340 men and women will die of gastric cancer in 2011 in the United States. Asian and Pacific Islander males and females have the highest incidence of gastric cancer, followed by black, Hispanic, white, American Indian, and Inuit populations. The overall 5-year relative survival rate is 26.3%.[10]

Colorectal Cancer

It is the third leading cause of cancer deaths in both males and females in the United States but was relatively rare before we became an industrial society. Diet may have an etiological role, especially diet with high fat content. Both colon and rectal cancer incidences and mortality rates have been decreasing from the 1980s. Decreased incidence and mortality rates are primarily the result of increased screening and detection and removal of colorectal polyps. The most recent data by the American Cancer Society estimates 101,340 new cases of colon cancer and 39,870 new cases of rectal cancer in 2011. Of the total colorectal cancers, 50.9% (71,850) are expected in men and 49.1% (69,360) are expected in women. Approximately 49,380 deaths from colorectal cancer are expected to occur in 2011.[10] The majority of colorectal cancers still occur in industrialized countries. Most colon cancers occur after the age of 50.

Coordination of Care between Dentist and Physician

Collaboration between dentists and physicians is strongly advocated to prevent or ameliorate possible adverse oral effects from both endogenous and exogenous acids, and to promote adequate saliva production in patients with GERD. Medical management for UC may effect provision of dental care. Dentists detecting signs and symptoms of PC may require physician management if discontinuation of the presumptive offending antibiotic does not resolve symptoms.

II. Medical Management

Identification/Medical History/Physical Exam/Laboratory Testing

GI disorders may present with symptoms of abdominal or back pain, nausea and vomiting, heartburn, burping, belching, appetite loss, diarrhea, bloody or tarry stools, or with no symptoms at all. They are typically diagnosed based on clinical manifestations, radiographic findings, endoscopic exam with pathological findings or other imaging techniques and occasional supportive laboratory tests. Patients should be able to report the existence of GI disorders and treatment received on the health history.

It is estimated that up to 60% of unexplained cases of PUD are associated with unrecognized NSAID use. Alcohol may increase the risk of ulcer complications in these NSAID users. Smoking may also increase the risk of PUD and ulcer complications through impairment of gastric mucosal healing.

Many rectal cancers produce no symptoms and are discovered as a result of routine screening. The most common symptom of rectal cancer is bleeding. Diarrhea and abdominal pain can also occur. Visibly undetectable loss of blood occurs in approximately 25% of colorectal cancer and is found through the fecal occult blood test. Back pain or urinary symptoms are usually signs of tumor invasion or compression of a nerve trunk. A digital rectal exam is performed to determine if a tumor can be palpated. Rigid proctoscopy is also performed to identify the exact location of the tumor.

Medical Treatment

Medical therapies for GI disorders range from diet modification, medications to relieve symptoms or treat underlying etiology, or surgery and/or radiation. Currently, there is no clinical consensus for the pharmacological management of dysgeusia.

Dyspepsia

Diagnosis

- Symptoms present for the last 3 months with onset at least 6 months before diagnosis.
- Nonendoscopic laboratory testing for *H. pylori* with the stool antigen test; a radiolabeled urea breath test or a quantitative assay for antibodies to serum immunoglobulin G (IgG).

Treatment

- Determine if cardiac, hepatobiliary, or medications are the cause.
- If no apparent cause, assess for alarm features (vomiting, bleeding or anemia, unexplained weight loss, abdominal mass, dysphagia).
- If alarm features are present in those age <50 years old, upper endoscopy is indicated.
- If age >50 years old without alarm features, evaluate for NSAID or aspirin use and discontinue.
- If aspirin or NSAIDs are not used and major symptom is heartburn or regurgitation, treat as if GERD.

Modified from Schwartz.[11]

GERD

Diagnosis

- Upper GI endoscopy with biopsies
- Esophagram
- Esophageal acid (pH) testing
- Esophageal motility testing
- Gastric emptying studies

Treatment

- Lifestyle change with weight loss, diet modification (avoid chocolate, peppermint, alcohol, caffeine, fatty foods, citric or spicy foods), smoking, lying flat after eating
- Antacids
- Medications: histamine antagonists (cimetidine, ranitidine, nizatidine, famotidine); proton pump inhibitors (omeprazole, esomeprazole, lansoprazole, pantoprazole, rabeprazole); pro-motility drugs (metoclopramide)
- Surgery: laparoscopic Nissen fundoplication
- For Barrett's esophagus: radiofrequency ablation and endoscopic mucosal resection

Modified from Schwartz.[11]

Peptic ulcer disease (PUD)

Diagnosis

- Exam may be normal.
- Epigastric tenderness, blood loss symptoms including tachycardia, pallor, hypotension, hematemesis, melena, or anemia may occur.
- Endoscopy with histological exam for *H. pylori* (preferred), upper GI barium studies, stool antigen test, urea breath test.

Treatment

- Avoid alcohol, NSAIDs, aspirin, and tobacco
- If *H. pylori* negative:
  - H_2-receptor antagonists (ranitidine or famotidine)
  - Proton pump inhibitors (PPI) (esomeprazole, lansoprazole, omeprazole, pantoprazole)
- If *H. pylori* positive:
  - A 10-day sequential therapy for eradication of *H. pylori* has been suggested. It consists of 5 days of treatment with a PPI and one antibiotic (usually amoxicillin) followed by a 5-day treatment with a PPI and two other antibiotics.
  - A 5-day course of PPI and one antibiotic (usually amoxicillin) followed by
  - 5-day course of PPI and clarithromycin and amoxicillin or
  - PPI and amoxicillin and metronidazole or
  - PPI and clarithromycin and metronidazole.

Modified from Schwartz.[11]

Inflammatory bowel disease (IBD) (UC and CD)

Diagnosis

- History of abdominal tenderness and enlargement (distension)
- Bloody diarrhea, fever, dehydration, weight loss, night sweats
- Extraintestinal manifestations include hepatic disease, iritis, uveitis, arthritis, erythema nodosum, atrophic glossitis, and aphthous stomatitis (vitamin B_{12} and folate malabsorption/deficiency)
- Anemia decreased hemoglobin/hematocrit from blood loss
- Imaging is generally not used. A double-contrast barium enema may reveal small pseudopolyps and superficial ulceration.
- Proctosigmoidoscopy or colonoscopy will reveal characteristic mucosal changes.

Treatment

- Medications to control inflammation and pain. Depending on severity from mild to severe:
    - aminosalicylates (5-aminosalicylic acid [5-ASA] including mesalamine, sulfasalazine, balsalaside);
    - corticosteroids;
    - immunomodulators (azathioprine, methotrexate, 6-mercaptopurine, cyclosporine);
    - biologics/antitumor necrosis factor (TNF) agents (infliximab, adalimumab, certolizumab pegol)
- Medications include antibiotics and antidiarrheal agents
- Nutrition supplements
- Surgery (a portion of the intestine or the entire colon may need to be removed)

Pseudomembranous colitis/*C. difficile*

Diagnosis

- Suspect in any patient with diarrhea:
    - who has received antibiotics within the previous 60 days
    - when diarrhea occurs 72 hours or more after hospitalization
- Enzyme-linked immunosorbent assay (ELISA) testing is used to identify *C. difficile* toxins A and B.
- A sudden increase in white blood cells >30,000 mm^3 may indicate fulminant colitis.
- Radiographic films of the abdomen are not sensitive enough for diagnosis.
- Because of potential risk for perforation, contrast enemas should be avoided.
- Computed tomography (CT) findings are not specific but will show suggested features and are often used.

Treatment

- The severity of the *C. difficile* infection will impact treatment decisions.
- Asymptomatic carriers: no treatment necessary.
- Mild diarrhea without fever or abdominal pain: discontinuance of the causative antibiotic.
- Moderate diarrhea for 10 days: oral metronidazole or vancomycin.
- Severe diarrhea is treated with intravenous vancomycin.
- Relapse, occurring 3 days to 3 weeks after treatment occurs in up to 25% of cases.

Celiac disease

Diagnosis

- Clinical signs and symptoms may include
    - children: weight loss, dyspepsia, failure to thrive, dental enamel defects;
    - adults: weight loss, fatigue, diarrhea, iron-deficiency anemia, and less commonly infertility, neurological issues, osteoporosis.
- Biopsy of the small bowel is the gold standard for the diagnosis of celiac disease.
- Iron, folic acid, and vitamin B_{12} deficiency may occur.
- Immunoglobulin A (IgA) antibodies to smooth muscle endomysium and tissue transglutaminase (IgA tissue transglutaminase TTG) antibodies using enzyme-linked immunosorbent assay (ELISA) are used for serological diagnosis.
- Anti-gliadin antibodies (gluten-free diet monitoring not for screening).

Treatment

- Maintain a gluten-free diet.
- Avoid lactose-containing products that can worsen GI symptoms.

Gastric cancer

Diagnosis

- Clinical signs and symptoms may include weight loss, dysphagia, dyspepsia not relieved with antacids, nausea, postprandial fullness
- Abdominal mass, epigastric pain
- Blood in stools, anemia
- Upper endoscopy with biopsy will confirm diagnosis. Endoscopic ultrasonography in combination with CT scanning and operative lymph node dissection can be used in staging of the tumor.
- Abdominal CT scan to evaluate for metastasis

Treatment

- Preoperative treatment with epirubicin, cisplatin, and fluorouracil (decrease tumor size and improve overall survival significantly)
- Gastrectomy and regional lymph node dissection
- Postoperative adjuvant chemotherapy using 5-fluorouracil and leucovorin

For inoperable gastric cancer

- Palliative resection
- Palliative chemotherapy (5-fluorouracil, adriamycin, and mitomycin C)

> **Colorectal cancer**
>
> **Diagnosis**
>
> - Clinical signs and symptoms may include fatigue and weight loss.
> - Iron-deficiency anemia, diarrhea, rectal bleeding, change in bowel habits, abdominal pain
> - Colonoscopy, sigmoidoscopy, and biopsy of suspicious lesions
> - Positron emission tomography (PET) scans are being used more frequently for staging and assessment of colorectal cancers.
>
> **Treatment**
>
> - Surgery (colectomy or colostomy)
> - Chemotherapy
> - Radiation therapy
> - Targeted therapy in which specific molecules involved in tumor growth and progression are disrupted.

Because of the possibility of developing PC from antibiotics prescribed by the dentist, the dentist should be able to recognize the possibility of *C. difficile* infection in at-risk populations and refer these patients for further workup and treatment if PC is suspected. *C. difficile*-related PC symptoms may include fever, dehydration and electrolyte imbalance, and abdominal tenderness. Important risk factors are hospitalization, age 60 and older, and use or recent use of antibiotics.

III. Dental Management

Evaluation

The patient with GI disease should have routine dental care with consideration given to the patient's underlying disease and impact on oral mucosa, dentition, and tolerance of dental care.

? Key questions to ask the patient

- What type of disorder do you have?
- Do you have any signs or symptoms associated with your disease?
- What type of medications do you take?
- Have you experienced any oral side effects with your disease?
- Are you uncomfortable in a reclining position?

? Key questions to ask the physician

- What medications is the patient taking?
- Should aspirin and NSAIDs be avoided?
- Are there any other medical concerns about the patient that you would like to share?

Dental Treatment Modifications

PUD

Patients undergoing antibiotic therapy for *H. pylori* PUD should have routine dental prophylaxis, because dental plaque and oral secretions may serve as a reservoir for *H. pylori* reinfection and ulcer relapse after antibiotic therapy.

Symptomatic IBD

Patients may avoid dental care because of frequent abdominal symptoms including diarrhea. IBD patients have been noted to experience more dental health problems especially dental caries. Remineralization and prevention protocols should be considered in caries-susceptible individuals.[12]

Oral Lesion Diagnosis and Management

PUD

- Oral dryness and oral complications associated with reduced salivary flow may occur.
- Palatal enamel erosion from persistent regurgitation of gastric acid may be found.
- Atrophic glossitis and angular cheilitis from gastric ulcer bleeding-induced iron-deficiency anemia can occur. These changes may occur early even without overt iron-deficiency anemia. Several investigators have noticed an association between oral candida and iron deficiency. Deficiency of iron, folic acid, or vitamin B_{12} alone does not promote oral mucous membrane growth of *Candida albicans*. In some susceptible individuals, iron or folic acid deficiency may facilitate *C. albicans* hyphal epithelial invasion.[13]

Celiac Disease

Celiac disease can progress to nutritional deficiencies when left untreated. Patients with celiac disease should be evaluated by a medical nutritionist.[14]

Dental enamel defects in the permanent dentition of children may be due to celiac disease. Defects such as discoloration, hypoplasia, and hypomineralization can occur and tend to appear symmetrically and be chronologically distributed. These defects may look similar to dental fluorosis. Dental enamel defects are more commonly noted when celiac disease occurs before 7 years of age. These defects are not noted in celiac patients who have developed the disease as adults. It is thought that immune-mediated damage is responsible for the enamel defects.

Recurrent aphthous ulcers, atrophic glossitis, and dry mouth may also be symptoms of celiac disease. The exact cause of aphthous ulcers in celiac disease is unknown; however, it may be related to hematinic deficiency, with low serum iron, folic acid, and vitamin B_{12} due to malabsorption in patients with untreated celiac disease.

GERD

- Dental erosion with possible thermal sensitivity occurs in some individuals. There is a strong association between GERD and dental erosion (see Fig. 7.1). In adults, the severity of the dental erosion is correlated with GERD symptoms. In patients with GERD, use of remineralization protocols such as fluoride varnish or gels and casein phosphopeptide-amorphous calcium phosphate (CPP-ACP) alone or in combination should be used.[15]
- Patients may complain of dysgeusia (bad taste).
- Mucosal erythema and atrophy may be noted during the intraoral exam.[16]

IBD (UC and CD)

- Major and minor aphthous stomatitis has been reported in patients with active UC, but their appearance may be coincidental (see

Figure 7.1 Dental erosion from gastroesophageal reflux disease in a 59-year-old white male. (a) Collapsed arch with loss of vertical dimension of occlusion. (b) Mandibular arch with occlusal surface erosion. (c) Maxillary arch with severe erosion of maxillary anterior teeth.

Figure 7.2 Aphthous ulcerations on the buccal and labial mucosa of a patient being treated for inflammatory bowel disease.

Figure 7.3 Pyostomatitis vegetans in a patient with inflammatory bowel disease. Note the multiple white and yellow pustules and surrounding erythema on the attached gingiva (courtesy of R. Epifanio, DDS).

Fig. 7.2). However, aphthous ulcers may result from iron, folic acid, and vitamin B_{12} deficiencies known to exist with UC.
- Other nonspecific forms of cutaneous ulcerations have been reported. Pyoderma gangrenosum (an uncommon cutaneous ulcerative condition of uncertain etiology) may occur.
- Pyostomatitis vegetans, characterized by erythematous, thickened oral mucosa with multiple pustules and superficial erosions may also occur (see Fig. 7.3). These ulcerations chiefly affect the labial gingival and the buccal and labial mucosa. These lesions appear similar to aphthous ulcers and may be mistaken for them. Pyostomatitis vegetans is a specific marker of UC. It has been suggested that the cross-reacting antigens in the bowel and skin are responsible for this manifestation. The oral lesions can be managed with local therapies utilizing chlorhexidine gluconate or other antiseptic mouthwashes and topical corticosteroids.[17]
- Cobblestone appearance of buccal mucosa may occur with CD (see Fig. 7.4).

Figure 7.4 Cobblestone appearance of buccal mucosa in a patient with Crohn's disease (courtesy of R. Epifanio, DDS).

Figure 7.5 Oral candida on the buccal mucosa of a patient on corticosteroids.

 Risks of Dental Care

Hemostasis

Gastric and Colorectal Cancer: Patients actively undergoing chemotherapy are at risk for thrombocytopenia related to cytotoxic chemotherapy-related myelosuppression.[18]

Susceptibility to Infection

IBD (UC or CD): Corticosteroids are also used to control inflammation. Corticosteroids can cause side effects such as weight gain, diabetes, hypertension, decrease in bone mass, and an increased risk of infection including oral candidiasis (see Fig. 7.5). They are not recommended for long-term use but are effective short term. Immune system suppressors such as azathioprine and infliximab are also used. Consulting with the patient's gastroenterologist is warranted prior to extensive dental surgical procedures.

Gastric and Colorectal Cancer: Patients actively undergoing chemotherapy are at risk for immune suppression related to cytotoxic chemotherapy-related myelosuppression.[18]

Drug Actions/Interactions

PUD: Avoid recommending over-the-counter drugs or prescribing medications containing NSAIDs or aspirin. Be aware of the reduction in the efficacy of antibiotics, such as erythromycin, tetracycline, and doxycycline, if given within 1 hour of antacids containing calcium, magnesium, or aluminum salts.

Use of antacids containing bismuth subsalicylate may lead to development of black hairy tongue (lingua villosa nigra), a painless brownish-black coating of the dorsal surface of the tongue (see Fig. 7.6). Black hairy tongue is a benign disorder caused by defective desquamation and reactive hypertrophy of the filiform papillae. Treatment for black hairy tongue includes brushing the dorsal

Figure 7.6 Black hairy tongue (lingua villosa nigra); a painless brownish-black coating of the dorsal surface of the tongue may result from use of bismuth-containing compounds used in the treatment of peptic ulcer disease.

Figure 7.7 Lichenoid drug reaction on the labial mucosa of a patient being treated with sulfasalazine for ulcerative colitis.

surface with a soft toothbrush. Topical retinoids have been used for treatment of more resistant forms.

IBD (UC or CD): Avoid recommending over-the-counter or prescribing medications containing NSAIDs or aspirin. Instead, acetaminophen-containing products should be recommended and prescribed as indicated.

Most people with UC are first treated with the anti-inflammatory mesalamine or similar drugs that may cause aphthous ulcers (see Fig. 7.2). Other IBD drug-related oral lesions include oral lichenoid drug reaction from NSAIDs or sulfasalazine (see Fig. 7.7); candidiasis from corticosteroids or bacteriostatic effect of sulfasalazine; hairy leukoplakia from corticosteroids or other immunosuppressants; gingival overgrowth from cyclosporine; and macrocytic anemia from sulfasalazine.

Patient's Ability to Tolerate Dental Care

IBD (UC or CD): Elective dental care should be scheduled during periods of remission with emergency care only during exacerbations of GI disease.

GERD: Patients may request dental chair positioning at a 45 degree angle to minimize gastric retrograde flow when undergoing dental treatment.

PUD: Minimize stress that can exacerbate symptoms. Address potential anemia if there is a recent history of ulcer perforation. Anemia (decreased hemoglobin levels) leads to hypoxia and can cause nonspecific symptoms such as weakness, fatigue, and shortness of breath on exertion. To compensate, cardiac output may be increased leading to symptoms of palpitations or angina. Blood pressure and pulse should be recorded when treating a patient suspected of having an underlying anemia and nonemergent treatment deferred for patient with tachycardia. Narcotics depress the respiratory center in the brain and should be used with caution in patients with anemia.

Medical Emergencies

Risk of medical emergencies is low for patients with GI disease.

IV. Recommended Readings and Cited References

Recommended Readings

Boivirant M, Cossu A. Inflammatory bowel disease. Oral Dis 2012;18(1):1–15.

Kornbluth A, Sachar DB. Practice Parameters Committee of the American College of Gastroenterology. Ulcerative colitis practice guidelines in adults: American College of Gastroenterology, Practice Parameters Committee. Am J Gastroenterol 2010;105(3):501–23.

Rashid M, Zarkadas M, Anca A, Limeback H. Oral manifestations of celiac disease: a clinical guide for dentists. J Can Dent Assoc 2011;77:b39.

Siegel MA, Jacobson JJ. Inflammatory bowel diseases and the oral cavity. Oral Surg Oral Med Oral Pathol Oral Radiol Endod 1999;87(1):12–4.

Cited References

1. Krasteva A, Panov V, Krasteva A, Kisselova A. Oral cavity and systemic disease-inflammatory bowel disease. Biotechnol Biotechnol Equip 2011;25(2):2305–9.
2. Kuehne SA, Cartman ST, Heap JT, Kelly ML, Cockayne A, Minton NP. The role of toxin A and toxin B in Clostridium difficile infection. Nature 2010;467(7316):711–3.
3. Green PH, Cellier C. Celiac disease. N Engl J Med 2007;357(17):1731–43.
4. Herbella FA, Patti MG. Gastroesophageal reflux disease: from pathophysiology to treatment. World J Gastroenterol 2010;16(30):3745–9.
5. Marsh M. Gluten, major histocompatibility complex, and the small intestine. A molecular and immunobiologic approach to the spectrum of gluten sensitivity ("celiac sprue"). Gastroenterology 1992;102(1):330–54.
6. Oberhuber G, Granditsch G, Vogelsang H. The histopathology of coeliac disease: time for a standardized report scheme for pathologists. Eur J Gastroenterol Hepatol 1999;11(10):1185–94.
7. Fox JG, Wang TC. Inflammation, atrophy, and gastric cancer. J Clin Invest 2007;117(1):60–9.
8. Vakil N. Disease definition, clinical manifestations, epidemiology and natural history of GERD. Best Pract Res Clin Gastroenterol 2010;24(6):759–64.
9. Fatahzadeh M. Inflammatory bowel disease. Oral Surg Oral Med Oral Pathol Oral Radiol Endod 2009;108:e1–e10.
10. American Cancer Society. Cancer Facts & Figures. 2011. American Cancer Society. Available at: http://www.cancer.org/acs/groups/content/@epidemiologysurveilance/documents/document/acspc-029771.pdf. Accessed October 8, 2011.
11. Schwartz MD. Dyspepsia, peptic ulcer disease, and esophageal reflux disease. West J Med 2002;176(2):98–103.
12. Singhal S, Dian D, Keshavarzian A, Fogg L, Fields JZ, Farhadi A. The role of oral hygiene in inflammatory bowel disease. Dig Dis Sci 2011;56(1):170–5.
13. Rennie JS, MacDonald DG, Dagg JH. Iron and the oral epithelium: a review. J R Soc Med 1984;77(7):602–07.
14. Murray JA. The widening spectrum of celiac disease. Am J Clin Nutr 1999;69(3):354–65.
15. Ranjitkar S, Smales RJ, Kaidonis JA. Oral manifestations of gastroesophageal reflux disease. J Gastroenterol Hepatol 2012;27(1):21–7.
16. Lazarchik DA, Filler SJ. Effects of gastroesophageal reflux on the oral cavity. Am J Med 1997;103(5A):107S–13S.
17. Femiano F, Lanza A, Buonaiuto C, Perillo L, Dell'Ermo A, Cirillo N. Pyostomatitis vegetans: a review of the literature. Med Oral Patol Oral Cir Bucal 2009;14(3):E114–7.
18. Macdonald JS, Smalley SR, Benedetti J, Hundahl SA, Estes NC, Stemmermann GN, et al. Chemoradiotherapy after surgery compared with surgery alone for adenocarcinoma of the stomach or gastroesophageal junction. N Engl J Med 2001;345(10):725–30.

Hematological Disease

Bhavik Desai PHD, DMD
Thomas P. Sollecito DMD

I. Background

This chapter addresses diseases of the white blood cells (leukemias, lymphomas, multiple myeloma [MM]), red blood cells (RBCs) (anemias), and patients requiring hematopoietic stem cell (bone marrow) transplants (HSCTs).

Description of Disease/Condition

Leukemia

Leukemia refers to a group of hematological malignancies characterized by the abnormal proliferation or increased life span of immature white blood cells in the bone marrow and peripheral blood.

Leukemia can be divided into two main types: lymphocytic leukemia and myeloid leukemia. Lymphoid precursor cells developing in lymphatic tissue give rise to T lymphocytes and B lymphocytes. Myeloid cells are derived from the bone marrow and differentiate into erythrocytes, polymorphonuclear leukocytes, monocytes, eosinophils, basophils, and platelets.[1] Of these main types, there are various subtypes of leukemia based on the predominant malignant cell/precursor cell type seen. Leukemia is also classified depending on duration and onset of diseases as acute or chronic.[2]

Acute Lymphocytic Leukemia (ALL)

- It is often an early childhood disease with the mean age of occurrence being 2–4 years.
- It is the most common leukemia in children, but can be seen at any age.
- Most cases involve B-cell malignant proliferation, followed by T-cell lymphocytic leukemia.
- Proliferating immature lymphoblasts may accumulate in the lymph nodes, liver, and spleen, in addition to peripheral blood and bone marrow.[3]

Chronic Lymphocytic Leukemia (CLL)

- It is characterized by the abnormal proliferation of certain types of lymphocytes, mostly CD5+ B lymphocytes.[2] CD refers to a specific

The ADA Practical Guide to Patients with Medical Conditions, First Edition. Edited by Lauren L. Patton.
© 2012 American Dental Association. Published 2012 by John Wiley & Sons, Inc.

marker known as *cluster of differentiation*. CD 5 is found on cell surfaces of T and B lymphocytes.
- It can manifest with little or no signs or symptoms other than mild lymphadenopathy.
- It may often be an incidental finding during a routine complete blood count (CBC).

Acute Myeloid Leukemia (AML)

- It involves uncontrolled proliferation of clonal myelocytic leukocytes in the bone marrow and peripheral circulation.
- An accepted guideline for reaching a diagnosis of AML is the presence of at least 30% blast cells in peripheral blood.[2]

Chronic Myeloid Leukemia (CML)

- It is the neoplasm of mature myeloid leukocytes.
- Genetic basis is the reciprocal translocation (referred to as the *Philadelphia chromosome*) of the cellular gene ABL from chromosome 9 to the BCR gene on chromosome 22.[2]

Anemia

Anemia is defined as the decrease in the oxygen-carrying capacity of blood. Anemia can be caused by either a decreased production of RBCs, increased destruction of RBCs, increased demand for iron, or formation of abnormal erythrocytes in place of physiological cells. Normal hemoglobin consists of two pairs of globin chains (α and β, δ or γ).

Based on the underlying etiopathogenesis, anemias are classified as:

- blood loss anemia;
- iron-deficiency anemia;
- anemia of chronic disease[4];
- hemolytic anemias: glucose-6 phosphate dehydrogenase deficiency (G6PD)-induced nonimmune or autoimmune anemias;
- hemoglobinopathies such as sickle cell anemia (SCA) or thalassemia[5];
- hypoproliferative anemias: folate- or B_{12}-deficiency anemia, pernicious anemia, aplastic anemia (AA).

Anemias can also be classified based on size of RBCs as:

- *microcytic* (mean corpuscular volume <80 micron): iron deficiency, thalassemia;
- *normocytic* (mean corpuscular volume 80–100 micron): SCA, G6PD deficiency, AA, blood loss anemia;
- *macrocytic* (mean corpuscular volume >100 micron): pernicious anemia, folate deficiency, B_{12} deficiency.

Iron-Deficiency Anemia

- This is the most common type of anemia.
- It is classified as a microcytic anemia.
- It is caused by low iron ingestion, excessive blood loss, or increased demand for iron.

G6PD Anemia

- It is associated with an inherited deficit of the enzyme G6PD that is needed for the biochemical hexose monophosphate (HMP) shunt pathway. On erythrocytes, it facilitates the conversion of carbohydrates into energy.
- It is classified as a normocytic hemolytic-type anemia associated with the increased rate of destruction of RBCs in response to oxidative stress.

SCA

- It is classified as an inherited hemoglobinopathy resulting from structurally deficient hemoglobin protein, which impedes its oxygenation capacity and ability to circulate throughout capillary beds. Typical hemoglobin levels are 6–9 g/dL in SCA.[5]

Thalassemia

- It is classified as a hemoglobinopathy sometimes manifesting as a microcytic hemolytic anemia.
- Thalassemias are a group of hereditary disorders resulting from decreased produc-

tion of globin chains of the hemoglobin molecule.

Vitamin B$_{12}$- and Folate-Deficiency Anemia

- It is classified as hypoproliferative macrocytic anemia.
- Together they constitute megaloblastic anemia.
- Megaloblastic anemia refers to the anemic state wherein RBCs are macrocytic, or larger than normal.

AA

- This is a rare condition resulting in complete suppression of bone marrow and the consequent depletion of all hematopoetic cell lines.[6]

Lymphoma

Lymphoma refers to a group of heterogeneous malignancies of lymphoid tissue or precursors of lymphoid tissue in the body. Lymphomas occur across the spectrum of lymphoid cell types—B cell, T cell, mucosa-associated lymphoid tissues (MALTs) and natural killer (NK) cells. The most common classifications of lymphomas are Hodgkin's lymphoma and non-Hodgkin's lymphoma (NHL).

Hodgkin's Lymphoma

- This is a lymph node neoplasm involving overproliferation of B lymphocytes.
- The defining histological feature is the presence of a distinct cell type called Reed–Sternberg giant cell.[2]

NHL

- Most cases of NHL involve B cells, followed by T-cell neoplasms and NK cell neoplasms.
- While NHL is a widespread disease and can involve multiple organ systems, initial stages of the malignancy have a favorable prognosis.[2]

Multiple Myeloma (MM)

- This is a malignancy involving the overproliferation of abnormal immunoglobulin-secreting plasma cells.
- The consequent abnormal immunoglobulin fragments accumulate in the bone marrow.
- Sequelae of MM can be osteolysis, bone marrow suppression, bleeding disorders, and renal dysfunction.[7]

Pathogenesis/Etiology

Leukemia

- *ALL*: Pathogenesis involves excessive proliferation and circulation of immature lymphoblasts as opposed to the normal ratio of blood elements. Causes remain speculative. Environmental, genetic, viral and infectious etiologies have been entertained as possible causes. ALL is more frequent in patients with Down syndrome, and increased detection of the Philadelphia chromosome has been linked with ALL.[8]
- *CLL*: As in ALL, there is an overproliferation of immature lymphocytes, but at a slower rate. Although unknown, inheritance and exposure to environmental carcinogens have been postulated as potential causes of CLL.[9]
- *AML*: AML exhibits a rapid onset of increased numbers of immature myeloid blast leukocytes in circulation. Underlying genetic or environmental mechanisms leading to an uncontrolled proliferation of myeloid cells remain unclear, but AML occurrence in younger people is often spontaneous. In the elderly, it may arise as a sequel to a myelodysplastic state of the bone marrow.[2,3]
- *CML*: Blast phase comprises over 20–30% leukemic cells in the bone marrow. The exact mechanism triggering the genetic translocation that leads to CML is unknown but some association has been claimed to radiation exposure and chemicals.

Anemia

- *Iron-Deficiency Anemia*: Decreased availability of iron impedes normal erythrocytosis, and resultant systemic effects of the disease are a consequence of tissue hypoxia:
  - *Low iron consumption* is associated with poor socioeconomic strata and poor dietary habits.
  - *Excessive blood loss* due to
    - heavy menses in women;
    - slow blood loss as seen in malignant gastrointestinal ulcers.
  - *Increased iron demand* due to
    - parturition or pregnancy in women;
    - sequel of chronic diseases:
      - autoimmune diseases (systemic lupus erythematosus [SLE], Crohn's disease, rheumatoid arthritis, or ulcerative colitis);
      - chronic liver disease (hepatitis or cirrhosis);
      - hematological malignancies (leukemias and lymphomas).[10]
- *G6PD Anemia*: Affected individuals have a faulty HMP shunt during the glycolytic pathway of glucose metabolism in RBCs thereby impeding RBCs' ability to manage an oxidative state.[10] The obstructed HMP shunt pathway leads to the accumulation of toxic oxidants inside RBCs that result in methemoglobinemia and aggregate to form Heinz bodies. Heinz bodies circulate through the spleen and liver with difficulty and are removed through hemolysis. Hemolytic episodes in affected individuals can be triggered by the exposure of the bloodstream to oxidative substances such as drugs (sulfonamides, antimalarials, aspirin, dapsone, phenacetin, and vitamin K), fava beans, and during infectious states of the body.
- *SCA*: At decreased pH or lowered oxygen tension, RBCs with this defective structure become sickle shaped. Sickle-shaped RBCs are rigid, eventually leading to stasis of blood flow. See Fig. 8.1. Sluggishly flowing blood accumulates in the spleen and erythrocytes are destroyed by hemolysis. This slow-circulating blood further depletes oxygen tension, leading to further sickling of RBCs—this vicious cycle can cause sickle-cell crisis in patients. Sickle cell crisis can be the consequence of oxygen-lowering states of the body such as dehydration, hypoxia, acidosis, or hypotension. SCA is an autosomal recessive disorder that needs the presence of both copies of the recessive gene (homozygous state) to manifest itself. Sickle-cell trait on the other hand does not result in the disease and is a heterozygous state involving one defective gene and a functional gene together in a pair. See Fig. 8.2. The structural deficiency of SCA stems from the substitution of a valine group with glutamic acid on position 6 of the beta chain of hemoglobin.[10]
- *Thalassemia*: In thalassemia major, at the cellular level, RBCs become more permeable secondary to aggregation of excessive number of defective globin chains. These RBCs are removed from circulation by phagocytosis or hemolysis. Compensatory production of RBCs occurs by expansion of bone marrow compartments and extramedullary erythropoiesis, but is usually insufficient. In alpha-thalassemia there is a depleted production of alpha chains. Beta-thalassemia is characterized by either a decreased production of beta-globin chains or a complete absence of these chains based on the gene mutations involved. Beta-thalassemia minor patients are heterozygous individuals who carry the trait while homozygous individuals have beta-thalassemia major or Cooley's anemia, a fulminant type of congenital hemolytic anemia. Across the spectrum from thalassemia minor to major symptoms may vary from presence of mild or no symptoms in thalassemia minor to profound hemolytic anemia and its accompanying manifestations.[10]

Figure 8.1 (A) The figure shows normal red blood cells flowing freely in a blood vessel. The inset image shows a cross section of a normal red blood cell with normal hemoglobin. (B) This shows abnormal, sickled red blood cells blocking blood flow in a blood vessel. The inset image shows a cross section of a sickle cell with abnormal (sickle) hemoglobin forming abnormal strands. *Source*: National Heart, Lung, and Blood Institute; National Institutes of Health; U.S. Department of Health and Human Services. Available at: http://www.nhlbi.nih.gov/health/health-topics/topics/sca/.

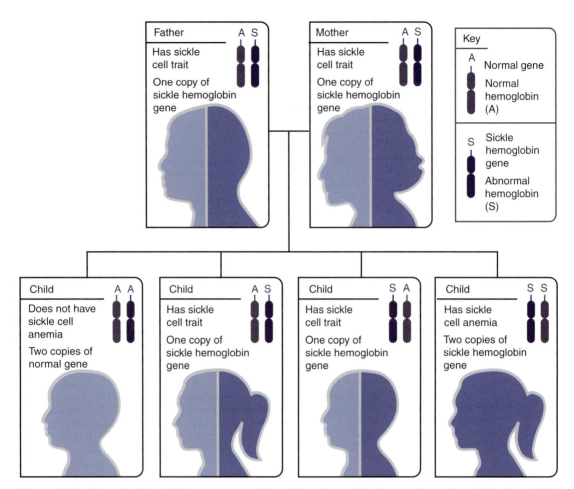

Figure 8.2 Example of an inheritance pattern for sickle cell trait. The image shows how sickle hemoglobin genes are inherited. A person inherits two hemoglobin genes—one from each parent. A normal gene will make normal hemoglobin (A). A sickle hemoglobin gene will make abnormal hemoglobin (S). When both parents have a normal gene and an abnormal gene, each child has a 25% chance of inheriting two normal genes; a 50% chance of inheriting one normal gene and one abnormal gene; and a 25% chance of inheriting two abnormal genes. *Source:* National Heart, Lung, and Blood Institute; National Institutes of Health; U.S. Department of Health and Human Services. Available at: http://www.nhlbi.nih.gov/health/health-topics/topics/sca/causes.html.

- *Vitamin B_{12}- and Folate-Deficiency Anemia*: Vitamin B_{12} and folic acid are both vital ingredients for erythrocytosis within the bone marrow. A deficiency in either of these components results in decreased production of erythrocytes, resulting in anemia. Strict B_{12} deficiency is rare and occurs in those observing an exclusive vegetable-based diet. B_{12} deficiency occurs most commonly secondary to deficiency of intrinsic factor in the gastrointestinal tract, and is referred to as *pernicious anemia*. Intrinsic factor in the gastric mucosa binds to vitamin B_{12}, protecting the latter from proteolysis and facilitating its migration across the ileal mucosa for absorption. Vitamin B_{12} deficiency may also occur as a side effect of certain medications, celiac disease, sprue, or Crohn's disease. Folic acid deficiency is observed in individuals whose diets are poor in leafy vegetables and fruits or with faulty absorption of folic acid, such as in chronic alcoholics and substance abusers. Rarely, genetic defects in folate metabolism may cause folate-deficiency anemia. Absorption of folate is also impaired as a result of cancer chemotherapy drugs.[10]

- *AA*: Bone marrow suppression as seen in AA causes significant leukopenia and anemia and their sequelae.[6] This severe pancytopenia observed in otherwise healthy adults has a rapid onset and progression. AA is an idiopathic condition. Chemicals, radiation, chemotherapy, and autoimmune diseases have been implicated in some cases as etiological agents of AA. While true AA is a disease of young adulthood and old age, a rare autosomal recessive disease called Fanconi's anemia has an earlier age of onset affecting infants and young children.[11]

Lymphoma

- *Hodgkin's Lymphoma*: Overproduction and aggregation of B lymphocytes usually occurs in mediastinal, cervical, and inguinal lymph nodes, although other nodes may be affected. While the exact cause of Hodgkin's disease is unknown, a strong association with the Epstein–Barr virus (EBV) has been reported. Other risk factors include occurrence of the disease among family members and individuals with acquired immune deficiency syndrome (AIDS).
- *NHL*: At the genetic level, malignant proliferation of B and T lymphocytes has been attributed to chromosomal translocations within immunoglobulin and T-cell receptor loci within these cells, respectively. The exact etiology of NHL remains unknown; however, genetic factors and environmental exposure to radiation, chemicals, herbicides, and chemotherapy have been implicated as potential causes. *Helicobacter pylori*, EBV, Kaposi's sarcoma herpesvirus, and retroviruses are several infectious agents reported with increased incidence of lymphoma. Patients with autoimmune disease, posttransplant status, and human immunodeficiency virus (HIV) are also at an increased risk of developing NHLs.[12]

MM

- While the exact etiology of MM remains speculative, radiation and chemical exposure, and pesticides have been hypothesized as potential causes of proliferation of plasma cells and the accumulation of abnormal immunoglobulin proteins in the bone marrow.

Epidemiology

Leukemia

The epidemiology of leukemias is shown in Table 8.1. Most cases of leukemia occur in older adults with the predominant types being CML and AML. The 5-year survival rate of leukemia has increased to 55% over the time frame of 1999–2006. More males than females are diagnosed with leukemia. Leukemia causes one-third of all cancer deaths in children under age 15 years.

Anemia

- *Iron-Deficiency Anemia*: Annual incidence in the United States is 5–11% in women and 2–5% in men.[11] Higher incidence abounds in developing countries. Men usually do not tend to lose iron in physiological states; hence, even mild anemia in men warrants prompt evaluation.
- *G6PD Anemia*: The X-linked G6PD deficiency is the world's most common enzyme disorder afflicting about 400 million people

Table 8.1. Epidemiology of Leukemia in the United States (2010)

Type of Leukemia	Annual Incidence (Number of New Cases)	Percentage of All Leukemias (%)	Annual Deaths	Mean Age
Acute lymphocytic leukemia	5,330	12	1,420	2–5 years
Chronic lymphocytic leukemia	14,990	35	4,390	>60 years
Acute myeloid leukemia	12,330	29	8,950	63 years; most after age 40
Chronic myeloid leukemia	4,870	11	440	60 years[a]
Other leukemia	5,530	13	6,640	
Total	43,050	100	21,840	

[a] Prognosis is less favorable when it occurs at younger ages.
Adapted from The Leukemia and Lymphoma Society Facts 2010–2011.

globally, especially those of Mediterranean, Middle Eastern, and Asian descent.[11] This deficiency is thought to impart some degree of resistance to malaria.

- *SCA*: Eight to ten percent of African-Americans carry the sickle cell trait and up to 0.15% have SCA.[11] Sickle cell trait imparts some degree of resistance to malaria and is endemic in several parts of Africa.
- *Thalassemia*: Thalassemia is more prevalent among population groups of the Middle East, Mediterranean and South Asia. The high prevalence of thalassemia among these groups has been postulated to be related to some degree of protection against malaria similar to the sickle cell trait.
- *Vitamin B_{12}- and Folate-Deficiency Anemia*: The incidence of folate- and B_{12}-deficiency-related anemias is not as high in developed countries as in other parts of the world. Folate- and B_{12}-deficiency anemias are common in older individuals with about 2% of the population over age 60 exhibiting some form of undiagnosed megaloblastic anemia.
- *AA*: AA is rare and has been reported to occur with an incidence rate of about 2 per million population in the United States and the Western world.

Lymphoma

- *Hodgkin's Lymphoma*: It is seen in a younger patient population with peak incidence in early adulthood, age 25–35 years. Men are affected more than women in a 3:2 ratio. An estimated 9000 Americans per year are diagnosed with Hodgkin's lymphoma.[9]
- *NHL*: It comprises over 85% of lymphomas. Around 66,000 new cases of NHL are diagnosed in the United States each year and almost 20,000 deaths are attributed to it. It is a disease of adults over 65 years old.[9]

MM

- About 15,000 new cases of MM are diagnosed each year in the United States with a median age of 65 years and a slightly higher ratio of incidence in males.[9]

Coordination of Care between Dentist and Physician

When a dental professional suspects that a patient has a hematological disease based on history, examination, or laboratory findings, prompt referral to the primary physician is warranted for diagnosis and management of the underlying disease.

In all hematological malignancies, a dentist may be called upon by the primary team to eliminate sources of odontogenic infection prior to chemotherapy or radiotherapy and to manage oral complications associated with the disease and treatment. Dental clearance prior to HSCT is essential because infection can be life threatening in patients with severe neutropenia. Additional coordination between the dentist and oncologist is required to ensure patients in remission are medically stable to receive routine dental care with respect to their hematological status.

Oral manifestations of MM in the maxilla, mandible, and oral soft tissues are managed by the oncologist with chemotherapy and localized radiation if indicated.

II. Medical Management

Identification/Medical History/ Physical Examination

Leukemia

Medical considerations for patients with leukemias are shown in Table 8.2.

Anemia

Medical considerations for patients with anemias are shown in Table 8.3.

Lymphoma

Medical considerations for patients with lymphomas are shown in Table 8.4. Malignant enlargement in NHL may be initially limited to only few a components of the lymphatic system, including intraoral tumors particularly in the tonsil region of Waldeyer's ring (for 5–10% of all NHLs, representing one-third of all extra-nodal sites),[14] but may have spread to multiple lymph nodes, liver, and spleen at the time of diagnosis.

MM

- Presenting signs of patients with MM include fatigue, weight loss, recurring infections and fever, bony pain, peripheral neuropathy, and increased incidence of bone fractures. Physical examination may reveal pallor, fever, and decreased neurological responses upon nerve examination. Neurological symptoms in MM are a result of infiltration of nerves by malignant cells.
- Accumulation of abnormal immunoglobulin proteins in the bone marrow results in bone marrow suppression, extensive bone destruction, predisposition to infections, and pathological bone fractures. Renal failure may occur secondarily to hypercalcemia and deposition of monoclonal light chains in renal tubules. Easy and prolonged bleeding is often a sequela of the disease due to the interference of the immunoglobulins with the normal clotting mechanisms.[7]

Laboratory Testing

The CBC and differential of the white blood cells is often the first blood test to screen for a hematological abnormality and to help guide a differential diagnosis. See Table 8.5.

Leukemia/Anemia/Lymphoma

Laboratory testing ranges from blood tests, such as CBC with differential blood smears, bone marrow biopsy and immunotyping, cytogenetic studies, lymph node biopsies, chest radiographs, and additional scans. See Tables 8.2–8.4.

Table 8.2. Medical Considerations for Patients with Leukemia

	Medical History	Physical Examination	Laboratory Testing	Medical Treatment
Acute lymphocytic leukemia	*Sudden onset* Chills of unknown origin, easy bleeding, fatigue, recurring infections, anemia	Fever, pallor, lymphadenopathy, hepatomegaly, splenomegaly	CBC: ≥20% lymphoblasts in peripheral blood smear, thrombocytopenia Immunotyping[a]: Detection of nuclear enzyme Tdt, CD10, CD19, CD22	Chemotherapy agents include alkylating agents, antimetabolites, enzymes, mitosis inhibitors, and supportive medication including antibiotics and steroids HSCT
Chronic lymphocytic leukemia	*Slow onset* Fatigue, anorexia, unexplained weight loss, night sweats, recurring infections, delayed healing, bleeding tendency	Fever, lymphadenopathy	CBC: Presence of >5000 mature lymphocytes/mL in peripheral blood Immunotyping may detect CD3, CD5, CD19, CD20, or CD 23 marker positive B lymphocytes	Cyclophosphamide, vincristine, doxorubicin, and prednisone Specific monoclonal antibodies such as rituximab, alemtuzumab, and ofatumumab
Acute myeloid leukemia	*Sudden onset* Rigors, easy bleeding, fatigue, anorexia and weight loss, recurring infections, sternal pain	Fever, pallor, hepatomegaly, splenomegaly, lymphadenopathy	CBC: At least 20% immature myeloblasts Immunotyping: Myeloblasts positive for CD13, CD33, CD34, CD65, and CD117 markers Bone marrow biopsy: presence of myeloblasts	Alkylating agents such as busulfan, cisplatin, carboplatin, daunorubicin, cyclophosphamide, and chlorambucil HSCT
Chronic myeloid leukemia	*Slow onset until disease progresses to blast stage* Fatigue, weakness, weight loss, infections, spontaneous bleeding	Fever, hepatomegaly, splenomegaly, lymphadenopathy	CBC: Total leukocytes >50,000/mL Cytogenetics[b]: Presence of Philadelphia chromosome in 90% patients Bone marrow biopsy—presence of immature blasts	Imatinib mesylate (Gleevec®) is effective against CML with the BCR-ABL gene mutation HSCT

[a] Immunotyping refers to the laboratory technique involved in the detection of cell surface proteins with specific immunological characteristics.
[b] Cytogenetics refers to a very specific branch of molecular genetics involved in the study of structure and function of chromosomes.
CBC, complete blood count; HSCT, hematopoietic stem cell transplant.

Table 8.3. Medical Considerations for Patients with Anemias

	Medical History	**Physical Examination**	**Laboratory Testing**	**Medical Treatment**
Iron deficiency anemia	Fatigue, dyspnea, stomatodynia	Pallor on skin and oral mucosa Depapillated atrophic tongue Koilonychia (spoon-shaped nails) Blue sclera Failure to thrive in children	CBC: Lowered hemoglobin count Blood smear: Microcytic hypochromic red blood cells	Address underlying cause if applicable; oral ferrous sulfate 200 mg TID Parenteral iron therapy Vitamin C supplements may aid iron absorption
G6PD-deficiency anemia	Oxidative crisis: Dyspnea, fatigue	Jaundiced skin Yellow sclera Pallor/icterus on oral mucosa Splenomegaly	G6PD screening Indirect bilirubin levels elevated	Prescreening and avoidance of oxidative medication and other triggers
Sickle cell anemia	Sickle cell crisis: Chest, abdominal and bone pain, nausea, vomiting, infections	Pallor/jaundice Frequent skin ulcers Infants: Swelling associated with small joints of hands and feet Dental hypoplasia/delayed eruption Step-ladder appearance of alveolar bone on dental X-rays	Sickledex test, in high-risk populations Hemoglobin electrophoresis Indirect bilirubin levels for hemolysis evaluation	Treatment is palliative (intravenous fluid, oxygen therapy, narcotic pain control, antibiotics as needed) Hydroxyurea increases hemoglobin F^a and reduces crisis rate and hospitalizations Blood transfusions in case of sickle cell crisis Allogeneic HSCT is an option in severe recalcitrant cases

(Continued)

Table 8.3. (Continued)

	Medical History	Physical Examination	Laboratory Testing	Medical Treatment
Thalassemia (major and minor)	Minor: May be asymptomatic Major: Symptoms from mild to severe	Major: Diagnosed within a year by severe jaundice, pallor, growth retardation, splenomegaly Minor: "Chipmunk facies" Bimaxillary protrusion with spacing of teeth Cranial nerve palsies Thin cortical plates and spongy marrow	Peripheral smear shows hypochromic, microcytic red blood cells Hemoglobin electrophoresis shows elevated levels of hemoglobin F[a] DNA analysis of prenatal fluid shows presence of disease	Major: Transfusions to maintain Hgb levels at least 10 mg/dL are crucial for survival Minor: No intervention necessary; genetic counseling advised
Vitamin B_{12}-and folate-deficiency anemia	Weakness, irritability, fatigue, sensory deficit: Ataxia and tingling/numbness in extremities, oral burning	Failure to thrive in children Pernicious anemia: Premature graying hair, vitiligo and blue eyes, atrophic glossitis, glossodynia, angular cheilitis	CBC, vitamin B_{12} levels, folate levels Schilling's test[b]	Vitamin B_{12} supplements are effective in B_{12}-deficient anemia and pernicious anemia Folate-deficient anemia is treated with replacement therapy
Aplastic anemia	History of recurring severe infections, fatigue, weakness	Severe jaundice or pallor Developmental retardation in Fanconi's anemia; gingival hyperplasia and spontaneous oral bleeding Oral mucosal pallor and petechiae	Bone marrow biopsy Erythropoietin levels	Immunosuppressive therapy Epoetin alfa[c] HSCT Management of infections and other symptoms

[a] Fetal hemoglobin whose production is otherwise normally curbed at birth.
[b] Schilling's test: A specific test for pernicious anemia that involves ingestion of radiolabeled vitamin B_{12} by the subject and detection of excreted levels of vitamin B_{12} in urine.
[c] Epoetin alfa is recombinant human erythropoietin and can induce erythrocyte production in the bone marrow.
References: (1) Little et al.[11]; (2) Mawardi et al.[12]; (3) Lanzkron et al.[13]
CBC, complete blood count; HSCT, hematopoietic stem cell transplant; TID, three times a day.

Table 8.4. Medical Considerations for Patients with Lymphomas

	History	Clinical Examination	Diagnosis	Medical Management
Hodgkin's lymphoma	Fever, night sweats, weight loss, fatigue Respiratory distress, dysphagia, and pain are possible	Enlarged lymph nodes: Mediastinal, cervical, axillary, or inguinal Pruritis	Lymph node biopsy or bone marrow aspirate: Presence of distinct Reed–Sternberg giant cells	Combination of chemotherapy and radiation to affected nodes Untreated disease results in death from bone marrow failure or infection Less aggressive early-stage disease may be treated with radiation alone
Non-Hodgkin's lymphoma	Fever, weight loss, fatigue, chest discomfort, night sweats, malaise, visceral pain, persistent cough, spontaneous bleeding, recurrent infections	Mediastinal lymphadenopathy, pleural effusion, hepatomegaly, splenomegaly	CBC: Anemia, thrombocytopenia, leukopenia Lymph node biopsy or aspirate for histopathology Chest X-rays CT scan if suspected bony involvement	Diffuse large B-cell lymphoma is treated with combination chemotherapy Radiotherapy may be an adjunct Specific monoclonal antibodies targeting antigens found on malignant lymphocytes HSCT

References: (1) Little et al.[2]; (2) Mawardi et al.[11]
CBC, complete blood count; HSCT, hematopoietic stem cell transplant.

Table 8.5. Normal Complete Blood Cell (CBC) Count and Differential White Blood Cell (WBC) Count[a] and Disease-Related Changes

Blood Cell Type	Normal Reference Range	May be Increased in:	May be Decreased in:
Red blood cells[b] (RBCs)	M: 4.3–5.7 million cells/μL F: 3.8–5.1 million cells/μL	Polycythemia, congenital heart disease, pulmonary disease, smoking, dehydration, renal disease with high erythropoietin production	Anemias, hemorrhage, bone marrow failure, erythropoietin deficiency due to renal disease, hemolysis, acute leukemia, malnutrition, multiple myeloma
Hemoglobin[b] (HgB)	M: 13.5–17.5 g/dL F: 12.0–16.0 g/dL	See RBC	See RBC
Hematocrit[b] (HCT)	M: 39–49% F: 35–45%	See RBC	See RBC
Platelets	150,000–400,000/mm^3	Polycythemia, leukemia, severe hemorrhage	Thrombocytopenia purpura, aplastic anemia, acute leukemia, acute disseminated intravascular coagulation
White blood cells (WBCs)[c]	4,500–11,000 cells/μL	Leukemia, infections, inflammation, severe burns, severe emotional or physical stress (see below differential)	Autoimmune/collagen vascular disease, 25% with acute leukemia, bone marrow failure, disease of liver or spleen (see below differential)

Differential WBC

Neutrophils segmented (PMNs)	54–62%	3,000–5,800/mm^3	Acute bacterial infection, inflammatory disease, CML, bone marrow disorders, hemorrhage, diabetic acidosis, glucocorticoid use	Chemotherapy, aplastic anemia, leukemias, radiation therapy, widespread bacterial or viral infection
Neutrophils bands	3–5%	150–400/mm^3	Acute bacterial infection, acute leukemia, myeloproliferative diseases	CLL
Lymphocytes	23–33%	1,200–3,000/mm^3	CLL, viral infections, radiation therapy, multiple myeloma	HIV infection, lupus, acute leukemia, CML, sepsis, radiation exposure
Monocytes	3–7%	285–500/mm^3	Viral or parasitic infection, inflammatory disorders, tuberculosis, monocytic leukemia, Hodgkin's disease, lipid storage disease	Leukemia, bone marrow failure
Eosinophils	1–3%	50–250/mm^3	Allergic disorders, CML, parasitic disease, inflammatory disorders, infections, bone marrow disorders, pernicious anemia, collagen vascular disease	
Basophils	0–0.75%	15–50/mm^3	CML, chronic inflammation, hypersensitivity reaction to foods, radiation therapy	Acute allergic reaction

[a] Normal ranges vary with each laboratory.
[b] Varies with altitude.
[c] WBC normal range for infants (8,000–15,000/mm^3) and children age 4–7 years (6,000–15,000/mm^3).
F, female; M, male; absolute neutrophil count (ANC) = WBC × (%PMNs + % Bands).
References: (1) American Academy of Pediatric Dentistry[15]; (2) Elin[16].
PMN, polymorphonuclear leukocytes.

MM

Laboratory investigation to diagnose MM includes serum and urine protein electrophoresis, which reveal the presence of abnormal immunoglobulin bands. Bone marrow biopsy samples when studied under immunohistochemistry may reveal presence of abnormal light immunoglobulin chains. A fraction of MM patients excrete light chain immunoglobulin proteins in urine, known as Bence-Jones proteins. Radiographic and computed tomography (CT) scan examination of bones reveals presence of osteolysis.[7]

Medical Treatments

Leukemia

Diagnosis and treatment of leukemia has significantly advanced over the last decade. Today, persistent remissions and even complete cure for leukemia is now increasing in frequency. See Table 8.2.

Anemia

Medical considerations: See Table 8.3.

Lymphoma

Medical considerations: See Table 8.4.

MM

Chemotherapy for MM often involves a standard regimen of melphalan and prednisone or dexamethasone alone, although other cytotoxic agents such as bortezomib, thalidomide, and lenalidomide are also used in management of MM. Osteolysis associated with MM is controlled with bisphosphonate therapy, such as intravenous injection of Aredia® (pamidronate) or Zometa® (zolendronic acid or zolendronate), which is essential in preventing skeletal morbidity.[17] Solitary lesions in the bone or soft tissue are also managed by external beam radiation.[7]

HSCT

- HSCT is used to achieve long-term remission in patients with hematological malignancies, such as leukemia or lymphoma and other diseases.
- It involves transplantation of marrow or blood-derived hematopoietic stem cells.[18] Cell source can be bone marrow, peripheral blood, or placental or umbilical cord blood.
- Transplant type can be:
  - *Allogeneic* (stem cells come from a relative [genetically similar but not identical donor, typically a sibling] or unrelated matched donor). Matching is performed using three or more loci of the major histocompatibility complex genes that encode for HLA polypeptides. A sibling has a 25% chance of being an HLA identical match, if the same HLA paternal and maternal gene were inherited. Even when there is an identical major HLA match, mismatched minor histocompatibility antigens can be recognized by the host immune response, requiring immunosuppressive regimens for suppression.[18]
  - *Autologous* (patient's own stem cells). Autologous transplant requires extraction of the patient's stem cells, which are frozen in storage, while the patient is prepared with partial or complete bone marrow ablation with high-dose chemotherapy and/or whole body radiation therapy. Stored stem cells are infused to faciliatate cell production in the bone marrow.
- Slightly more autologous than allogeneic HSCTs are performed each year in the United States. See Fig. 8.3. In 2009, 9778 autologous and 7012 allogeneic transplants were performed (see Fig. 8.4), most for MM, lymphomas, and some leukemias. In 2009, among patients ≤20 years old, 1815 allogeneic transplants were done, mostly for ALL, AML, AA, and other nonmalignant diseases, and 787 allogeneic transplants for Hodgkin's disease and other cancers.[19]

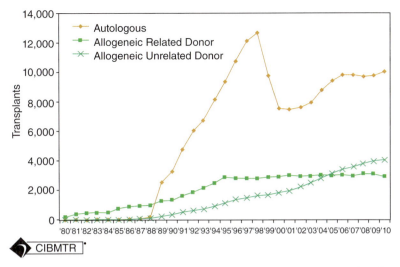

Figure 8.3 Hematopoeitic Stem Cell Transplants in the U.S., 1980–2010. Reprinted with permission of the Center for International Blood and Marrow Transplant Research. Pasquini MC, Wang Z. Current use and outcome of hematopoietic stem cell transplantation: CIBMTR Summary Slides, 2011. Available at: http://www.cibmtr.org.

Figure 8.4 Indications for Hematopoetic Stem Cell Transplants in the U.S., 2009. NHL, non-Hodgkin's lymphoma; AML, acute myelogenous leukemia; HD, Hodgkin's disease; ALL, acute lymphocytic leukemia; MDS/MPD, myelodysplastic syndrome/myeloproliferative diseases; CML, chronic myelogenous leukemia. Reprinted with permission of the Center for International Blood and Marrow Transplant Research. Pasquini MC, Wang Z. Current use and outcome of hematopoietic stem cell transplantation: CIBMTR Summary Slides, 2011. Available at: http://www.cibmtr.org.

- Prior to transplantation, a conditioning regimen of myeloablative chemotherapy is given to eradicate malignant cells, and in allogeneic transplantation, to induce immune suppression that permits donor stem cell engraftment.
- Post-HSCT patients are generally on long-term immunosuppressant therapy:
  - Corticosteroids and cyclosporine have been the traditional modality of long-term immunosuppression in posttransplant patients.
  - Other commonly utilized immunosuppressant medications include mycophenolate mofetil, tacrolimus, sirolumus, methotrexate, thalidomide, and rituximab.
  - The use of immunosuppressants has been linked to several oral side effects including viral infections, fungal infections, erythema, mucositis, and xerostomia.
  - Solid tumors and hematological malignancies may develop several years post-HSCT.
  - The most common oral malignancy is squamous cell carcinoma, necessitating active monitoring of the oral cavity in transplant patients.
  - There is also a higher incidence of NHL's in posttransplant patients.
- Allogeneic HSCT recipients are at risk for graft-versus-host disease (GVHD). See Chapter 12.
- For many of these patients, GVHD is a chronic, ongoing phenomenon.[20]
- Up to 70% of post-allogeneic HSCT patients exhibit some form of manifestation of GVHD.

III. Dental Management

Evaluation

Leukemia

An assessment of the patient's health status can be made by pertinent questions asked during a thorough history including questioning for recurrent fevers, spontaneous bleeding, recurring infection, unplanned weight loss, weakness, and fatigue. Prompt referral to the primary physician is warranted should a dentist suspect a patient being in leukemic state.

Anemia

Based on oral symptoms, a dentist may be the first health-care professional able to identify patients whose anemic status may be yet undiagnosed.

Lymphoma

Dental specialists may aid in identification and diagnosis of lymphoma. Management of the

---

Key questions to ask the patient with leukemia

- What kind of leukemia do you have? When were you diagnosed?
- Are you currently on or planning to begin chemotherapy? How often do you receive your chemotherapy? When was your last chemotherapy session?
- Do you have side effects like oral mucositis? Have your blood counts (white cells and platelets) gotten critically low?
- Are you in remission? Is a bone marrow or stem cell transplant planned for you?

Hematological Disease

? Key questions to ask the leukemia patient's physician

- What is the patient's complete blood count, including absolute neutrophil count and platelet count?
- Does the patient have a central venous catheter?
- What is the schedule of treatments so safe dental treatment can be planned around treatment?
- If myelosuppression is a side effect, how severe has the neutropenia and thrombocytopenia been? When after chemotherapy did this occur? What other toxic side effects has the patient experienced?
- Is the patient with an acute dental/periodontal abscess better managed with systemic (oral or intravenous) antibiotics until blood counts recover rather than undergoing a surgical procedure today?

? Key questions to ask the patient with anemia

- What kind of anemia do you have? When were you diagnosed?
- What treatments have you received?

? Key questions to ask the anemic patient's physician

- What is the severity level of the patient's anemia?
- What treatments are planned for the patient? Does the patient receive blood transfusions?

? Key questions to ask the patient with lymphoma

- What kind of lymphoma do you have/have you had? When were you diagnosed?
- What treatment will/did you receive? Radiation therapy? Chemotherapy? Bone marrow or stem cell transplant? When was this or will this be happening?

Key questions to ask the lymphoma patient's physician

- Is the patient going to receive chemotherapy? [If so ask questions under leukemia]
- Is the patient going to receive or has the patient received radiation therapy? If so, to what dose and are/were the salivary glands included in the field?
- When does the patient need to begin radiation therapy?
- What dose of radiation will/did the mandible and/or maxilla receive?

Key questions to ask the patient with multiple myeloma

- When was your multiple myeloma diagnosed?
- What treatment are you receiving? Chemotherapy? Steroids? Are you now or have you ever taken an injection of a bisphosphonate drug such as Zometa® or Aredia® to help prevent bone lesions? If so when did you start taking this medication?

Key questions to ask the multiple myeloma patient's physician

- What treatment has been done and is planned for the patient?
- Is the patient on a bisphosphonate, and if so, do you recommend a medication holiday for any needed dental surgery?

symptoms accompanying lymphoma is often related to the oncologist's overall medical management.

MM

Dental specialists may aid in the identification and diagnosis of MM. An assessment of the patient's health status can be made by pertinent questions asked during a thorough history including questioning for recurrent fevers, spontaneous bleeding, recurring infection, unplanned weight loss, weakness, bone pain, and fatigue. MM may also present with initial complains of paresthesia in the orofacial region secondary to myelomatous involvement of facial and jaw bones. Prompt referral to the primary physician is warranted.

Dental Treatment Modifications

Leukemias, Lymphoma, and MM

Dental treatment for patients with leukemia, lymphoma, or MM can be divided into three phases:

Prior to Chemotherapy, Radiotherapy, or HSCT: The dentist must identify sources of *existing or potential* infection such as periapical and periodontal abscesses or potential infections such as asymptomatic periapical pathology, severely mobile teeth, or teeth with vertical bone defects. Patients with partially erupted 3rd molars and those with histories of pericoronitis are also of particular concern. The oncologist should be consulted prior to scheduling treatment. Oral surgery should be completed ideally 10–14 days before myelosuppressive chemotherapy or conditioning for HSCT.[21] Dental prophylaxis, periodontal scaling and root planning, and oral hygiene instructions should be accomplished prior to medical therapy provided the patient's leukemic status, as determined with the oncologist, can withstand such therapy. If xerostomia is anticipated, in office fluoride treatment should be given, with initiation of a daily prescription fluoride regimen. Use of intravenous bisphosphonate drugs in MM predisposes patients to bisphosphonate-related osteonecrosis of the jaws (BRONJ), making dental evaluation and dental surgical care prior to bisphosphonate use important for BRONJ prevention.

During Chemotherapy, Radiotherapy, or HSCT Conditioning Therapy: The patient may exhibit oral symptoms such as recurring fungal and viral infections, which require appropriate antifungal and antiviral medications. Therapy-induced oral mucositis may be managed by palliative agents such as viscous lidocaine, anesthetic mouth rinses, and the use of oral moisturizing agents. Recombinant human keratinocyte growth factor has shown promising results in alleviating oral mucositis secondary to cancer chemotherapy and radiotherapy.[22] Conditioning regimens for HSCT can create severe oral complications. HSCT recipients with mucositis or undergoing conditioning therapy should be under routine dental surveillance and should maintain safe oral hygiene by performing oral rinses four to six times/day with sterile water, normal saline, or sodium bicarbonate solution and brush teeth at least two times a day with a soft toothbrush and floss daily if this can be done atraumatically and the patient's blood counts are adequate to withstand this activity.[21]

As dental treatments such as extractions, endodontics, and aggressive periodontal therapy may increase the risk of uncontrolled bleeding and infection, these treatments are often postponed until after the patient is medically stable. A leukemic patient is medically stable when there is a remission of blast cells in bone marrow and peripheral blood, with an overall improvement in health status and a return to normal blood counts. Oral lesions and more specifically gingival bleeding, edema, and erythema may be a sign of relapse of the patient's leukemic status.

After Chemotherapy, Radiotherapy, or HSCT: In a patient who is in remission of leukemia, routine dental procedures may be performed by cautiously monitoring the patient's health status by consultation with the oncologist. While stable, individuals in remission may need periodic intervention to manage xerostomia, complications of GVHD (if allogeneic HSCT has been performed), and recurring oral infections. The dentist will be required to play an active role in managing these chronic oral conditions. Dental professionals may be called upon to monitor, diagnose, and manage BRONJ in MM patients undergoing bisphosphonate therapy. Management of BRONJ may range from antibacterial rinses, long-term antibiotic therapy to surgical debridement of affected areas.[23]

Prophylactic and preventive dentistry should be pursued with diligence in patients while stable. Any oral lesion should be thoroughly evaluated if noted by the patient. Patients treated with bisphosphonates should be counseled on the risks of BRONJ. Patients with residual xerostomia from radiation to the salivary glands should have periodic and frequent oral hygiene visits, home care, use of fluoride supplements and prompt therapy for early signs of dental decay are highly encouraged. Post-HSCT patients on chronic immunosuppressive medications should be reminded that any oral lesion noted by the patient should be thoroughly evaluated. Elective dental care should be delayed 1 year after HSCT.

Anemia

Dental treatment of significantly anemic patients is best performed after consultation with their primary physician. The use of systemic medications in these patients needs to be carefully considered. Adequate hemostasis during invasive procedures is essential. Primary wound closure should be performed when possible to avoid additional blood loss. Preventive dentistry should involve dental prophylaxis and reinforcement of dental hygiene.

Oral Lesion Diagnosis and Management

Leukemias

Leukemias are accompanied by several identifying phenomena, which may occur in the oral cavity[1-3] including the following:

Petechiae: Petechiae are small erythematous macules seen on the skin and mucosa about

Figure 8.5 Mucosal ulcer in a leukemic patient. Photo courtesy of Eric T. Stoopler.

Figure 8.6 Gingival erythema and enlargement in a leukemic patient.

1–2 mm in size, which occur due to minor capillary hemorrhages.

Mucosal Ulcers: Intraoral ulceration in leukemic patients may commonly be a consequence of severe neutropenia. In some cases, multiple neutropenic ulcers may abound the entire oral cavity. See Fig. 8.5.

Gingival Enlargement: Gingival enlargement may be an early oral manifestation in some subtypes of AML (subtypes M4 and M5) and less commonly in ALL. See Fig. 8.6.

Gingival Bleeding and Severe Periodontitis: Spontaneous gingival bleeding and aggressive periodontal disease in absence of appreciable local etiological factors may be a sign of leukemia.

Fungal Infections: Pseudomembranous candidiasis is a common finding in immunocompromised patients, including leukemic patients. Deep fungal infections such as aspergillosis and mucormycosis are less common oral deep fungal infections but can be seen in patients who have persistent immunodeficiency related to leukemia treatment.

Viral Infections: Herpes simplex virus (HSV) infection is the most common viral infection in leukemic patients and can manifest as ulcerative lesions on any oral mucosal surface. See Fig. 8.7. Less common are Cytomegalovirus (CMV) infections, which may be found as one or more necrotic ulcers in patients with persistent immune deficiency.

Anesthesia/Paresthesia: Anesthesia or paresthesia of various branches of the trigeminal nerve (including the inferior alveolar or mental nerves) secondary to aggregation of leukemic infiltrate (an infiltration of leukemic cells) along these nerves may be observed in leukemic patients.[24]

Treatment of oral lesions in leukemic patients should be focused on the overall oncological management of the underlying disease state of the affected individual, if oral manifestations are a direct consequence of the systemic disease. Referral to specialists versed in oral mucosal lesions in medically complex patients is recommended to manage oral lesions associated with leukemia.

Symptoms such as gingival enlargement, gingival bleeding, paresthesia, mucosal ulcers, and petechiae occasionally may resolve when the patient's leukemia has been effectively controlled. The diagnosis of oral infections and their appropriate treatment will often be managed by the oral health-care provider. Antifungal therapy includes topical and systemic use of nystatin, clotrimazole, fluconazole, and, in deep fungal infections, voriconazole or amphotericin B. Antiviral therapy includes acyclovir, valacyclovir, and famciclovir for HSV and ganciclovir and foscarnet for CMV and occasionally for resistant HSV infections. Antiviral and antifungal medications can have significant side effects and pose the potential for drug interactions.

Palliative management of oral ulcers may include use of magic mouthwash or viscous lidocaine as local anesthetic agents. Mouth-moistening agents for cancer therapy-induced xerostomia may also be beneficial for the patient.

Anemia

Oral lesions may include the following:

1. Pallor: Along with pallor of skin, anemic patients may exhibit pallor on the oral mucosa especially on the floor of the mouth.
2. Petechiae: Petechiae are pinpoint erythematous spots on oral mucosa, as a consequence of microhemorrhages under the skin. See Fig. 8.8.
3. Mucosal ulcers: Vitamin B_{12}-deficiency and iron-deficiency anemia may be accompanied by oral mucosal ulcers.
4. Gingival hyperplasia and bleeding may occur in patients with AA. See Fig. 8.9.

Figure 8.7 Intraoral herpetic infection in a leukemic patient.

Figure 8.8 Petechiae and mucosal pallor in a 36-year-old white male with aplastic anemia. (Severe thrombocytopenia [platelet count: 10,000/mm^3], anemia [hemoglobin: 8.5 g/dL], and leukopenia [white blood cell count: 1000 cells/μL]).

Figure 8.9 Gingival inflammation/hyperplasia and candidiasis due to leukopenia in a patient with aplastic anemia.

5. Jaundice: Hemolysis in patients with hemolytic anemia leads to hyperbilirubinemia.
6. Glossodynia: Burning sensation inside the mouth, especially the tongue is observed in iron-deficiency anemia.
7. Atrophic tongue: Depapillation of the dorsal tongue may be a sign of iron-deficiency anemia.
8. Chipmunk facies in individuals with thalassemia major: Bimaxillary protrusion and alveolar enlargement contribute to the chipmunk facies appearance of thalassemia

Figure 8.10 Periapical film showing stair step appearance of alveolar bone due to compensatory marrow expansion in a patient with SCA.

major. Alveolar ridge enlargement occurs due to compensatory expansion of the bone marrow.
9. Alveolar bone in patients with SCA exhibits a step ladder pattern radiographically. See Fig. 8.10.
10. Generalized radiolucency of the mandible due to marrow hyperplasia in SCA. See Fig. 8.11.

Management of oral lesions involves identifying and correcting, if possible, the type of anemia through active medical intervention. Supportive dental care may include use of chlorhexidine mouthwash or palliative rinses in exposed mucosal surfaces.

Lymphoma

Hodgkin's lymphoma has not been associated with specific oral lesions. However, NHL can present with significant oral manifestations[2,12] such as the following:

1. Intraoral lymphatic involvement: Waldeyer's tonsillar ring along the soft palate and oropharynx is the most common intraoral site of lymphoma, followed by salivary glands and mandible. However, intraoral lymphomas have been reported on the palate, gingiva, buccal sulcus, alveolar ridge, and floor of the mouth. See Fig. 8.12.

Figure 8.11 Panoramic radiograph of a 28-year-old African-American with sickle cell anemia, history of acute chest syndrome and stroke, on chronic exchange transfusions. Note generalized radiolucency and large trabeculations in mandible.

Figure 8.12 Intraoral non-Hodgkin's lymphoma in a patient with HIV infection.

Figure 8.13 Radiation caries in patient with salivary gland deficit from head and neck radiation for non-Hodgkin's lymphoma.

2. Petechiae
3. Mucosal ulcers
4. Fungal infections
5. Viral infections
6. Oral paresthesia

Patients with a history of radiation therapy for a head and neck lymphoma may exhibit xerostomia, propensity to oral fungal infections, and radiation-induced dental caries. See Fig. 8.13.

MM

Plasmocytomas, which are solitary neoplastic proliferations of plasma cells in the bone and soft tissues, may occur within the maxillofacial bone complex or intraoral soft tissues. See Fig. 8.14. MM may also present with amyloid protein deposition of the tongue, causing tongue enlargement, which can result in malocclusion.[7]

MM commonly involves the jaw bones and can present with pain and paresthesia of the maxillofacial bones. It may cause intraoral signs such as tooth loss, or mobility. MM has a distinct radiographic appearance in the maxillofacial bones as single or multiple noncorticated irregular "punched-out" radiolucencies.[7] See Fig. 8.15.

GVHD

Oral lesions associated with GVHD[20] include mucosal lesions, benign soft tissue growths, xerostomia, superficial mucoceles, erythema, fibrosis, and scarring of the oral mucosa. Treatment modalities for oral mucosal lesions associated with GVHD involves topical and intralesional corticosteroids and other immunosuppressants such as topical tacrolimus. Xerostomia may be managed by hydration measures, use of saliva substitutes and coating agents, and with prescription of secretory stimulants such as pilocarpine and cevimeline. Trauma from sharp tooth cusps and restorations aggravated by xerostomia may produce inflammation, and the dentist may be required to eliminate sources of friction by smoothening and polishing sharp teeth and restorations. Palliative support for managing oral discomfort may be attained by prescribing viscous lidocaine or magic mouthwash. Refer to Chapter 12 for more information.

Risks of Dental Care

Hemostasis

Leukemia, Lymphoma, and AA

Patients should be told that persistent bleeding after minor dental procedures needs to be evaluated. Platelet count should be available prior to invasive dental treatment in patients with leukemia or who are receiving chemotherapy. Platelet counts below 50,000 often will require platelet transfusion to support surgical hemostasis.

Figure 8.14 Left mandible plasmacytoma in a 58-year-old African-American female with multiple myeloma.

Figure 8.15 Panoramic radiograph of a 47-year-old African-American male with late-stage IIIB multiple myeloma. Note punched-out radiolucencies of the mandible representing lytic bone lesions of the disease.

Susceptibility to Infection

Leukemia and Lymphoma

Uncontrolled infection and poor wound healing is a risk associated with aggressive dental procedures including extractions, endodontic therapy, deep scaling, and periodontal surgery when the patient's blood counts are low or unstable. Based on oncological input, some patients may require antibiotic prophylaxis prior to invasive dental therapy.

Anemia

- Antibiotic prophylaxis *may* be indicated prior to aggressive dental procedures in poorly controlled SCA to prevent risk of potential infection. In patients with SCA, odontogenic infections should be treated vigorously with appropriate antibiotics and antimicrobial mouth rinses to avoid infection precipitating a crisis.[5]
- AA patients will require consultation with a physician prior to treatment and possible antibiotic prophylaxis or platelet support for those with severe neutropenia or thrombocytopenia, respectively.[6]

MM

- A relapse in the patient's primary hematological malignancy may cause increased numbers of immature blast cells in the bone marrow, which may be the cause of uncontrolled infection following dental procedures.

Drug Actions/Interactions

Anemia

- Consider use of dental anesthesia without epinephrine in poorly controlled anemia. There is no contraindication for use of local anesthetic with vasoconstrictor in patients with SCA.[5] Controversy remains because the use of epinephrine is believed by some to cause vascular occlusion and hence impede circulation.
- Avoid medications that can precipitate hemolysis in hemolytic anemias. These medications include sulfonamides, aspirin, chloramphenicol, dapsone, penicillin, streptomycin, and isoniazid, among others.
- Avoid hypoxia when using nitrous oxide sedation in SCA by assuring adequate flow rate, not less than 50% supplemental oxygen and adequate duration of 100% oxygen delivery at the end of the analgesia delivery session.[5]
- Avoid the use of salicylates for pain management in SCA because the acid effect of salicylates can trigger an oxidative crisis—combination of acetaminophen and a narcotic (codeine, oxycodone, or hydrocodone) is a better alternative.[5]
- Use caution when prescribing respiratory depressants such as barbiturates and strong narcotics due to poor oxygen transfer in anemic individuals.

MM

An oral side effect as a result of MM therapy including the use of bisphosphonates is BRONJ.[23] Clinically, BRONJ lesions are of exposed necrotic bone surrounded by inflamed soft tissue. Radiographically, erosion of the bone may be visible when BRONJ is advanced. See Fig. 8.16. See Table 19.5 for management of BRONJ.

Patient's Ability to Tolerate Dental Care

Lymphoma

History of radiotherapy could have an impact on wound or bone healing from extractions and dental surgery; however, radiation doses for lymphoma are typically in the 45–50 Gy range, compared with the higher risk doses of 60–70 Gy used for squamous cell carcinomas of the oral cavity.

Figure 8.16 Bisphosphonate osteonecrosis (BRONJ) of the mandible in a 50-year-old with refractory IgA kappa multiple myeloma treated with monthly zolendronic acid who presented with a large necrotic area of posterior right mandible. Biopsy showed severe osteonecrosis with focal acute osteomyelitis and abundant microorganisms consistent with *Actinomyces* species. All teeth had been removed 5 years ago.

IV. Recommended Readings and Cited References

Recommended Readings

NIDCR. *Dental Provider's Oncology Pocket Guide*. Available at: http://www.nidcr.nih.gov/OralHealth/Topics/CancerTreatment/ReferenceGuideforOncologyPatients.htm. Accessed December 2011.

Cited References

1. DeRossi SS, Garfunkel A, Greenberg MS. Chapter 16. Hematological diseases. In: Burket's Oral Medicine: Diagnosis and Treatment, 10th ed. Greenberg MS, Glick M, eds. 2003, pp. 429–53. B.C. Decker, Inc., Hamilton, Ontario, Canada.
2. Little JW, Falace DA, Miller CS, Rhodus NL. Chapter 24. Disorders of white blood cells. In: Dental Management of the Medically Compromised Patient, 7th ed. 2008, pp. 373–95. Mosby, St. Louis, MO.
3. Burke VP, Startzell JM. The leukemias. Oral Maxillofac Surg Clin North Am 2008;20(4):597–608.
4. Weiss G, Goodnough LT. Anemia of chronic disease. N Engl J Med 2005;352(10):1011–23.
5. Da Fonseca M, Oueis HS, Casamassimo PS. Sickle cell anemia: a review for the pediatric dentist. Pediatr Dent 2007;29(2):159–69.
6. Valdez IH, Patton LL. Aplastic anemia: current concepts and dental management. Spec Care Dentist 1990;10(6):185–9.
7. Stoopler ET, Vogl DT, Stadtmauer EA. Medical management update: multiple myeloma. Oral Surg Oral Med Oral Pathol Oral Radiol Endod 2007;103(5):599–60.
8. Koo HH. Philadelphia chromosome positive acute lymphoblastic leukemia in childhood. Korean J Pediatr 2011;54(3):106–10.
9. Leukemia and Lymphoma Society. *Disease Information and Support*. Available at: http://www.lls.org/#/diseaseinformation/leukemia/. Accessed December 11, 2011.
10. DeRossi SS, Raghavendra S. Anemia. Oral Surg Oral Med Oral Pathol Oral Radiol Endod 2003;95(2):131–41.
11. Little JW, Falace DA, Miller CS, Rhodus NL. Chapter 23. Disorders of red blood cells. In: Dental Management of the Medically Compromised Patient, 7th ed. 2008, pp. 362–72. Mosby, St. Louis, MO.
12. Mawardi H, Cutler C, Treister N. Medical management update: non-Hodgkin lymphoma. Oral Surg Oral Med Oral Pathol Oral Radiol Endod 2009;107(1):e19–33.

13. Lanzkron S, Strouse JJ, Wilson R, Beach MC, Haywood C, Park HS, et al. Systematic review: hydroxyurea for the treatment of adults with sickle cell disease. Ann Intern Med 2008;148(12): 939–55.
14. Ezzat AA, Ibrahim EM, El Weshi AN, Khafaga YM, AlJurf M, Martin JM, et al. Localized non-Hodgkin's lymphoma of Waldeyer's ring: clinical features, management, and prognosis of 130 adult patients. Head Neck 2001;23(7): 547–58.
15. American Academy of Pediatric Dentistry. *Common Laboratory Values*. Available at: http://www.aapd.org/media/policies_guidelines/rs_labvalues.pdf. Accessed December 2011.
16. Elin RJ. Appendix: reference intervals and laboratory values. In: Goldman's Cecil Medicine, 24th ed. Goldman L, Schafer AI, eds. 2012, pp. 2558–69. Saunders Elsevier, Inc., Philadelphia.
17. Terpos E, Sezer O, Croucher PI, García-Sanz R, Boccadoro M, San Miguel J, et al. The use of bisphosphonates in multiple myeloma: recommendations of an expert panel on behalf of the European Myeloma Network. Ann Oncol 2009; 20(8):1303–17.
18. Epstein JB, Raber-Durlacher JE, Wilkins A, Chavarria MG, Myint H. Advances in hematologic stem cell transplant: an update for oral health care providers. Oral Surg Oral Med Oral Pathol Oral Radiol Endod 2009;107(3):301–12.
19. Pasquini MC, Wang Z. *Current use and outcome of hematopoietic stem cell transplantation: CIBMTR Summary Slides*. 2011. Available at: http://www.cibmtr.org.
20. Imanguli MM, Alevizos I, Brown R, Pavletic SZ, Atkinson JC. Oral graft-versus-host disease. Oral Dis 2008;14(5):396–412.
21. Centers for Disease Control and Prevention. Guidelines for preventing opportunistic infections among hematopoietic stem cell transplant recipients: recommendations of the CDC, Infectious Disease Society of America, and the American Society of Blood and Marrow Transplantation. MMWR Recomm Rep 2000; 49(No. RR-10):1–128.
22. Weigelt C, Haas R, Kobbe G. Pharmacokinetic evaluation of palifermin for mucosal protection from chemotherapy and radiation. Expert Opin Drug Metab Toxicol 2011;7(4):505–15.
23. Migliorati CA, Casiglia J, Epstein J, Jacobsen PL, Siegel MA, Woo SB. Managing the care of patients with bisphosphonate-associated osteonecrosis: an American Academy of Oral Medicine position paper. J Am Dent Assoc 2005;136(12):1658–68.
24. Sasaki M, Yamazaki H, Aoki T, Ota Y, Sekiya R, Kaneko A. Bilateral numb chin syndrome leading to a diagnosis of Burkitt's cell acute lymphocytic leukemia: a case report and literature review. Oral Surg Oral Med Oral Pathol Oral Radiol Endod 2011;111(3):e11–6.

Bleeding Disorders

Dena J. Fischer DDS, MSD, MS
Joel B. Epstein DMD, MSD, FRCD (C), FDS RCS (Edin)

I. Background

Description of Disease/Condition

Bleeding disorders are conditions of varying severity that affect normal hemostasis, resulting in prolonged or excessive bleeding. These disorders may be congenital or acquired and cause quantitative and/or qualitative abnormalities in blood elements (i.e., vascular endothelial cells, platelets, coagulation proteins). Specific conditions are defined by deficiencies or abnormalities of blood components (see Table 9.1).

Pathogenesis/Etiology

Hemostasis is the process of blood clot formation and can be divided into four phases: (1) vasoconstriction, (2) platelet plug formation, (3) blood coagulation, and (4) fibrinolysis. Immediately following tissue injury, damaged blood vessels constrict, which temporarily decreases blood flow and pressure within the vessel. Vasoconstriction is followed by mechanical blockage of the injury by a platelet plug. Platelets become activated and adhere to damaged endothelium to form a loose platelet plug. These steps initiate a series of reactions known as the coagulation cascade. These enzymatic reactions involving 13 coagulation factors end in the formation of a fibrin clot that stabilizes the platelet plug. Eventually, as the damaged vessel repairs itself, the clot is degraded proteolytically through a process called fibrinolysis.

Bleeding or bruising that is spontaneous or excessive after injury may be caused by abnormal platelet number/function or vascular integrity and/or defects in coagulation or fibrinolysis. Most bleeding disorders are caused by quantitative or qualitative abnormalities of platelets or coagulation proteins.

Platelet Disorders

Quantitative platelet defects can result from decreased production of platelets caused by bone marrow dysfunction, increased splenic sequestration, or increased consumption of

The ADA Practical Guide to Patients with Medical Conditions, First Edition. Edited by Lauren L. Patton.
© 2012 American Dental Association. Published 2012 by John Wiley & Sons, Inc.

Table 9.1. Definitions of Bleeding Disorders

Platelet disorders	
Thrombocytopenia	Decreased number of functioning platelets caused by decreased platelet production or accelerated platelet destruction/removal
Immune thrombocypenic purpura (ITP)	An autoimmune disorder causing platelet destruction due to the presence of antibodies against the patient's own platelets
Drug-induced platelet disorders	Drugs may reversibly or irreversibly cause inhibition of platelet function.
Coagulation disorders	
von Willebrand disease	An autosomal dominant hereditary bleeding disorder caused by a deficient or defective plasma von Willebrand factor (vWF)
Hemophilia A	An X-linked genetic disorder resulting in deficient or defective clotting Factor VIII
Hemophilia B	An X-linked genetic disorder resulting in deficient or defective clotting Factor IX
Disseminated intravascular coagulation (DIC)	An acquired coagulation disorder characterized by uncontrolled thrombin activation and release, resulting in severe thrombosis that may be fatal
Drug-induced coagulation disorders	Drugs may prevent synthesis of coagulation cascade factors and have the potential to result in prolonged bleeding.

platelets in acquired medical conditions (i.e., immune thrombocytopenic purpura [ITP]). ITP is characterized by the development of antibodies to one's own platelets. Thrombocytopenia can also develop from dysfunctional platelet activity, which may be due to medications or acquired medical conditions (i.e., hematological malignancies, bone marrow disorders, end-stage renal disease). There are also a number of rare inherited qualitative platelet disorders that can result in symptoms from mild bleeding to severe mucocutaneous hemorrhage. Examples include Glanzmann thrombasthenia, Bernard–Soulier syndrome, and platelet storage pool defects.[1]

Coagulation Disorders

Coagulation disorders may be congenital or acquired. Congenital coagulation disorders are uncommon and are characterized by the presence of a single abnormality that can account for the entire clinical picture. von Willebrand disease (vWD) is an autosomal dominant condition that results from the deficiency of von Willebrand factor (vWF) associated with Factor VIII, which varies in severity and type. Many individuals with vWD remain undiagnosed until exposed to trauma or surgery. Hemophilias are sex-linked recessive disorders that result in a deficiency of Factor VIII (in hemophilia A) or Factor IX (in hemophilia B). Although almost all hemophiliac patients are male, it is possible for females who are usually carriers to be affected. Patients with hemophilia A or B often present with similar clinical presentations.

The clinical severity of hemophilia is typically inversely proportional to the measured level of factor coagulant activity (e.g., Factor VIII level). Factor levels are genetically determined and do not vary with time. Severe disease occurs at factor level of less than 1% of normal, moderate at 1–5%, and mild disease above 6%. Normal coagulation factor levels range from 60% to 150%. Approximately 60% of all cases of hemophilia A are severe, while 20–45% of hemophilia B cases are severe. Inhibitors or alloantibodies to Factor VIII and Factor IX develop in 10–30% of patients with severe hemophilia due to genetic and environmental exposures. Factor VIII inhibitor levels are assessed with the Bethesda inhibitor assay (BIA) where the number of Bethesda units (BUs) reflects the inhibitor level, and the amnestic response of the inhibitor to factor concentration replacement therapy reflects the response type. A high-titer, high-responder-type inhibitor patient is the most difficult to manage with factor replacement products because normal replacement products are rapidly inactivated by the inhibitor becoming ineffective.

Acquired coagulation disorders are more common than congenital disorders and are more complex in their pathogenesis. Disseminated intravascular coagulation (DIC) is a condition in which massive activation of the clotting cascade gives rise to uncontrolled thrombin formation, resulting in thrombosis and further activation of the clotting cascade, causing further coagulopathy and bleeding. This may be a manifestation of underlying leukemia, other cancer, obstetric complications, massive tissue injury, or infections, and requires urgent management. Patients with severe liver disease are susceptible to hemorrhage because many of the proteins involved in the coagulation cascade are synthesized in the liver, particularly Factors II (thrombin), VII, IX, and X. Decreased levels of such factors are observed in patients with severe liver disease. In addition, there is reduced clearance of activated clotting factors by the liver. Furthermore, moderate thrombocytopenia is common, resulting from decreased platelet production and increased platelet destruction by hypersplenism.

Drug-Induced Disorders

Certain drugs can cause acquired platelet disorders. One of the most common drugs is aspirin, which irreversibly binds to the enzyme cyclooxygenase, causing blockage of thromboxane and prostaglandin synthesis, thereby preventing platelet release and aggregation for the life of the platelet (approximately 9 days). Other nonsteroidal anti-inflammatory drugs (NSAIDs) also inhibit cyclooxygenase, but the inhibition is reversible. Dipyridamole (Persantine® or combined with aspirin in the drug Aggrenox®) is a thromboxane synthase inhibitor that blocks platelet aggregation. Platelet adenosine diphosphate (ADP) receptor agonists, such as toclopidine (Ticlid®), clopidogrel (Plavix®), and prasurgel (Effient®), are prescribed for the prevention of thromboembolic disease and atherosclerotic events. These antiplatelet agents inhibit platelet aggregation by interfering with platelet ADP binding and are irreversible inhibitors of platelet function. It generally takes 5–7 days after discontinuation of irreversible platelet inhibitors for platelets to return to their baseline function.

Drug-induced coagulation disorders are most commonly caused by the coumarin anticoagulants such as warfarin (Coumadin®), which is prescribed to prevent venous thrombosis and systemic embolism in susceptible patients. Coumadin® acts as a vitamin K antimetabolite, interfering with the synthesis of Factors VII, IX, and X as well as prothrombin. The primary effect of Coumadin® is in the common pathway due to inadequate amounts of prothrombin. In addition, heparin and low-molecular-weight heparins (LMWHs) are fast-acting anticoagulant drugs that bind antithrombin III, which inhibit thrombin and other coagulation factors, resulting in the inhibition of fibrin formation. Fondaparinux (Arixtra®) is an injectable Factor Xa inhibitor used similarly to the LMWH drugs. Newly available oral direct thrombin (Factor IIa) inhibitor dabigatran (Pradaxa®) and Factor Xa inhibitor rivaroxaban (Xarelto®) are used to prevent stroke in patients with atrial fibrillation and venous thromboembolism in patients who have recently undergone total knee or hip replacement. They do not require laboratory monitoring, have less associated bleeding complications than Coumadin®, and have half-lives of 14–17 hours (dabigatran) and 5–13 hours (rivaroxiban), compared with 2.5 days for warfarin.[2]

Epidemiology

There are numerous etiologies of platelet and coagulation abnormalities. More common congenital and acquired conditions are the following:

- *ITP*: Estimated incidence of 50–100 new cases per year, equally distributed between children and adults. ITP is more prevalent in young women.
- *vWD*: The most common inherited bleeding disorder in the United States with a prevalence estimated to be 1.3% of the general population.[3]
- *Hemophilia A*: Hemophilia A accounts for approximately 80% of hemophilia cases in the United States, affecting approximately 1 in 5000 male births.
- *Hemophilia B*: Hemophilia B accounts for approximately 13% of hemophilia cases in the United States, affecting approximately 1 in 35,000 male births.
- *Coumarin Therapy-Induced Anticoagulation Disorder*: Coumadin® is prescribed to approximately 1 million individuals in the United States each year.

Coordination of Care between Dentist and Physician

- The first step in assessing the risk for bleeding is obtaining a comprehensive medical and medication history. A bleeding disorder may be suspected when a patient complains of excessive bruising or bleeding that may be secondary to known trauma or bruising at sites with no recollection of trauma. Oral signs include gingival oozing (see Figs. 9.1 and 9.2), petechiae, and ecchymoses. In patients who are considered to be at risk for

Figure 9.1 Spontaneous gingival oozing in a patient with severe thrombocytopenia.

Figure 9.2 Spontaneous gingival oozing in a patient with leukemia and severe thrombocytopenia.

bleeding, appropriate laboratory tests should be performed and interpreted to evaluate the potential for bleeding complications. If warranted, prophylactic measures should be taken prior to performing dental care.
- Dental procedures that involve any type of soft or hard tissue damage can potentially cause bleeding. Patients with a diagnosed bleeding disorder require management in coordination with a medical provider prior to performing any dental procedure that has the potential to cause bleeding. Oral soft tissue lesions, including petechiae, ecchymoses, and hematomas, are frequently encountered in patients with clinically significant bleeding disorders.
- Depending on the underlying disorder and its severity, measures may have to be taken prior to, during, and following dental procedures. Consultation with a physician or specialist physician including hematologist or cardiologist is recommended in more complicated cases. In some circumstances, treatment may be best provided in a hospital setting, where pre- and/or posttreatment infusions and/or emergency management can be more easily coordinated.

 II. Medical Management

Identification

Bleeding disorders vary in severity and etiology. Many patients with congenital and/or severe bleeding disorders may be aware of their underlying condition. However, patients with newly acquired disease may be unaware of their disorder. Furthermore, patients on antiplatelet or anticoagulant medications that may contribute to abnormal bleeding tendencies may not be aware of their increased risk for bleeding. Bleeding symptoms differ based on the origin of the hemostatic disorder, and clinical presentation can assist in establishing the diagnosis. See Table 9.2.

Table 9.2. Clinical Bleeding Symptoms Differ Based on Nature of Hemostatic Disorder

Clinical Findings	Platelet and Vascular Disorders	Coagulation Disorders
Petechiae	Characteristic	Rare
Ecchymoses	Characteristic, usually small and multiple	Common, often large and solitary
Deep dissecting hematomas	Rare	Characteristic
Hemarthroses	Rare	Characteristic
Delayed surgical bleeding	Rare	Common
Bleeding from superficial cuts and scratches	Persistent, often profuse	Minimal

Medical History

A thorough medical and medication history is critical prior to performing dental care on a patient to assess risk for bleeding. Furthermore, patients diagnosed with bleeding disorders prior to 1985 may have received contaminated blood transfusions and may be at risk for blood-transmitted infectious diseases, such as HIV/AIDS, hepatitis B, and hepatitis C. Affirmative responses to confidential medical history questions in the following areas will alert the dentist to the possible need for further inquiry:

- hemophilia, vWD, or other congenital coagulation disorders;
- bruises easily;
- epistaxis (frequent nosebleeds);
- prolonged bleeding after trauma/surgery including dental procedures;
- history of multiple blood transfusions;
- blood malignancies or dyscrasias;
- current or recently terminated cancer treatment;
- advanced liver disease/hepatitis;

- end-stage renal disease receiving hemodialysis (heparin is administered during dialysis treatment);
- current use of antiplatelet or anticoagulant medications such as aspirin, Coumadin®, ADP inhibitors, LMWH therapy, direct thrombin or Factor Xa inhibitors;
- medical conditions for which one may be on prophylactic antiplatelet or anticoagulant therapy:
  - atrial fibrillation,
  - prosthetic heart valve,
  - history of deep vein thrombosis (DVT),
  - post-myocardial infarction,
  - history of cerebrovascular accident (CVA).

Physical Examination

The physical examination may contribute to identification of orofacial conditions that may be caused by a primary bleeding disorder.
Examples include:

- petechiae (more common with thrombocytopenia/platelet disorders);
- ecchymoses and purpura (more common with thrombocytopenia/platelet disorders);
- hematoma (more common with coagulation disorders);
- spontaneous gingival bleeding (see Figs. 1.11, 9.1, and 9.2).

A bleeding disorder may also occur secondary to an acquired medical condition. Examples include the following:

- *Hematological Malignancies*: These may present with nonspecific mouth ulcerations, gingival hyperplasia (see also Chapter 8).
- *Cancer Treatment*: Cancer chemotherapy may result in depletion of functioning platelets (see also Chapter 13).
- *Advanced Liver Disease*: Many of the proteins involved in coagulation are synthesized in the liver. Patients with advanced disease may experience deficiencies in coagulation proteins (see also Chapter 6).
- *End-Stage Renal Disease*: Patients receiving dialysis treatment may experience qualitative platelet abnormalities due to uremia. Furthermore, heparin is often administered with dialysis treatment, thereby placing patients at risk of bleeding on the day of dialysis treatment (see also Chapter 5).

Laboratory Testing

Common laboratory tests are ordered and can contribute to the diagnosis. The most common laboratory screening would consist of a platelet count, prothrombin time (PT)/international normalized ratio (INR), and activated partial thromboplastin time (aPTT). See Table 9.3. There are more specific tests such as assays for quantity of specific coagulation factors or factor activity. Relative levels of common laboratory test values in various conditions are shown in Table 9.4.

Platelet Tests

Platelet Count

- While there is a large variation among the general population, an individual's count tends to remain within a certain range.
- Platelet replacement therapy for surgical procedures may be warranted at a platelet count <50,000 cells/mL.
- Maintenance platelet replacement therapy may be warranted at a platelet count <10,000–20,000 cells/mL.

Ivy Bleeding Time

- The skin is incised and observed for primary hemostasis in a standardized manner.
- A prolonged bleeding time in patients with a platelet count higher than 100,000 cells/mL suggests impaired platelet function.
- This test is a poor indicator of mucosal and oral-surgery-induced bleeding and is therefore of limited clinical utility.[4]

Table 9.3. Common Laboratory Tests Used to Assess Hemostasis

Laboratory Test	Normal Range	What It Measures
Platelet count	150,00–400,00 cells/mL	Platelet quantity
Ivy bleeding time (BT)	<6 minutes	Platelet function (quantity and quality)
PFA-100	Closure time <193 seconds	Quantitative and qualitative measurement of platelet adhesion, activation, and aggregation
Prothrombin time (PT)	11–14 seconds	Factors II (prothrombin), V, VII, and X, and fibrinogen
International normalized ratio (INR)	1.0	
Activated partial thromboplastin time (aPTT)	27–38 seconds	Factors II, V, VIII, IX, X, XI, and XII
Thrombin time (TT)	9–13 seconds	Abnormalities in the conversion of fibrinogen to fibrin

PFA-100, platelet function analyzer 100.

Table 9.4. Relative Levels of Common Laboratory Screening Test Results for Hemostatic Disorders

Condition	Platelet Count	Bleeding Time/PFA-100	PT/INR	aPTT	TT
Aspirin therapy	↓ or ↔	↑	↔	↔	↔
Coumarin therapy	↔	↔	↑↑	↑	↔
Heparin therapy	↔	↔	↔	↑↑	↑
Hemophilia A or B	↔	↔	↔	↑↑	↔
Thrombocytopenia	↓↓	↑↑	↔	↔	↔
Severe liver disease	↓	↑	↑↑	↑↑	↑↑
Renal hemodialysis	↓	↔	↔	↑	↔
Leukemia	↓	↑	↔	↔	↔
Vessel wall defect	↔	↑	↔	↔	↔
Fibrinogenolysis	↔	↔	↑	↑	↑↑
DIC	↓↓	↑↑	↑↑	↑↑	↑↑

↑, mild increase; ↑↑, moderate to marked increase; ↓, mild decrease; ↓↓, moderate to marked decrease; ↔, normal level; PFA-100, platelet function analyzer 100; PT, prothrombin time; INR, international normalized ratio; aPTT, activated partial thromboplastin time; TT, thrombin time; DIC, disseminated intravascular coagulation.

Platelet Function Analyzer 100 (PFA-100)

- A prolonged closure time in patients with a platelet count higher than 100,000 cells/mL suggests impaired platelet function.

Liver Function Tests

Some patients with advanced liver disease may present with both quantitative and qualitative platelet disorders in addition to clotting defects. Liver function tests may provide additional information regarding the risk of bleeding. Any dental treatment performed on patients with advanced liver disease should be done in coordination with a physician. See Chapter 6.

Coagulation Tests

PT/INR

- PT measures factors of the extrinsic coagulation pathway. A prolonged PT indicates a deficiency or defect.
- It is reported as the INR, which standardizes PT results across laboratories.
- The INR is elevated in patients taking Coumadin®. Depending on the specific clinical indication for therapy, patients on warfarin are typically maintained between 2.0 and 3.0.
- Indications for anticoagulant therapy include treatment and long-term prophylaxis for DVT as well as prevention for complications associated with prosthetic heart valves, atrial fibrillation, CVA, and post-myocardial infarction. Patients with recurrent DVT and prosthetic heart valves may be maintained at levels up to 3.5.

aPTT

- aPTT measures the factors in the intrinsic and common coagulation pathways. A prolonged aPTT indicates a deficiency or defect.
- This may be utilized to monitor the effects of heparin therapy but not LMWHs.
- This can be used to assess bleeding risk in hemophiliacs since this test includes Factors VIII and IX.

Thrombin Time (TT)

- TT can be prolonged because of hypofibrinogenemia, abnormal fibrinogen (dysfibrinogen), or the presence of inhibitors (fibrin degradation products) that interfere with fibrin polymerization.

Medical Treatment

Platelet Disorders

Treatment of thrombocytopenia is typically directed toward identifying the cause. Prednisone therapy, splenectomy, and intravenous gammaglobulin are possible treatment options. Platelet transfusions may be warranted with very low platelet counts (<10,000 cells/mL).

Coagulation Disorders

Transfusions of specific coagulation factors (e.g., monoclonal or recombinant Factor VIII, IX, or VIIa), cryoprecipitate (containing Factor VIII, fibrinogen, vWF, and Factor XIII), or fresh frozen plasma (containing all coagulation factors in normal concentrations, especially Factors V and VIII) may be required to replace deficiencies of specific blood products when trauma occurs or surgery is planned. Some hemophiliacs with repetitive joint bleeding will be educated to self-administer factor concentrates (called home therapy) and will be placed on twice or thrice weekly factor concentrate prophylactic infusions at 25–40 units/kg to maintain trough factor levels of 3–5% and help preserve joint function so as to avoid the need for total joint replacements.

Desmopressin (1-deamino-8-D-arginine vasopressin [DDAVP]), available for parenteral use (0.3 µg/kg intravenously over 15–20 minutes) or as Stimate® nasal spray (one 150 µg spray in each nostril), may correct or prevent bleeding episodes by release of vWF from blood vessel endothelial stores in patients with mild–moderate hemophilia, some types of vWD, uremic bleeding, and cirrhosis.[5–7] DDAVP creates transient two- to fourfold increases in Factor VIII and vWD levels. With vWD, the therapeutic goal is to correct deficiencies in vWF activity to >50% of normal, and this can often be accomplished with DDAVP administration.

In hemophiliacs, factor replacement therapy is required to control hemostasis. Replacement guidelines strive to obtain plasma levels at 25–30% factor activity for minor bleeds, while treatment or prevention of severe bleeds, including major dental surgery, requires a level of 50–100% activity.[7] Hemophiliacs with inhibitors to factor replacement therapy may not respond or will only minimally respond to factor replacement therapy. In such circumstances, alternative factor replacement therapies may circumvent the inhibitor. For example, recombinant activated Factor VII has been found to be safe and efficacious in 70–85% of bleeding episodes in hemophilia A and B patients with inhibitors.[8] Inhibitors tend to occur in more severely affected patients, who tend to receive the greatest number of factor concentrates.[9] With all bleeding disorders, the use of adjunctive antifibrinolytic agents such as ε-aminocaproic acid (EACA) or tranexamic acid may also be warranted.

Drug-Induced Disorders

The goals of medical management with antiplatelet or anticoagulant medications are prophylaxis and management of thromboembolic disease. Correction of excess anticoagulation with Coumadin® is with use of vitamin K injections, which is slow, or more urgently with transfusion of fresh frozen plasma. Correction of overdosage of parenteral heparin occurs immediately with parenteral use of protamine sulfate. Aspirin and the platelet ADP receptor antagonists have no antidote for correction.

III. Dental Management

Evaluation

In a patient suspected of having a bleeding disorder, it is necessary to ask specific questions about their experiences with bleeding and bruising. A history of surgical procedures, tooth extractions, or significant injury without abnormal bleeding is good evidence against the presence of a congenital hemorrhagic disorder.

Furthermore, when assessing appropriate dental management for the patient with a bleeding disorder, the dental provider should consider the types of dental treatment required, potential for hemorrhage while undergoing dental therapy, presence of local factors that increase the potential for hemorrhage, necessity for block anesthesia, and number of anticipated visits to complete the dental treatment. These considerations should be discussed with the medical consultant. Dental procedures that involve soft or hard tissue damage can potentially cause bleeding. The highest risk procedures include dentoalveolar surgery, especially multiple extractions, and surgical periodontal procedures. Lower risk procedures in which excessive bleeding is rarely encountered, even in those with severe hemophilia, include rubber dam clamp placement and use of retraction cord.

Dental Treatment Modifications

With these key questions answered and appropriate modifications taken, patients with congenital or acquired bleeding disorders can safely receive dental care. The timing or extent of the planned treatment may need to be modified after consultation with a physician and consideration of the severity of the bleeding disorder.

Key questions to ask the patient

- Has a physician ever diagnosed you with a bleeding disorder? Do you recall the diagnosis? What is the name of the physician managing treatment for this condition?
- What type of clinical bleeding tendencies do you have? Have you had any dental surgical procedures and problems with bleeding?
- How often do you get bruises? What size are the bruises? Do you remember trauma prior to bruising?
- Have blood transfusions been necessary after surgery or trauma?
- If teeth have been extracted previously, were return visits required for packing or suturing? Was medical intervention (i.e., transfusion) required?
- When bleeding occurs, is it superficial (i.e., mucosal and/or gingival bleeding, recurrent epistaxis [nosebleeds], ecchymoses) or deep (i.e., hematomas, hemarthrosis)? *Superficial bleeding is suggestive of platelet disorders, while deep-tissue bleeding may indicate clotting factor deficiencies.*
- What prescribed and over-the-counter medications do you take? What is the dose and schedule of medication intake? Do you take aspirin or medications that contain aspirin? What is the name of the physician who prescribes your anticoagulant/antiplatelet medication(s)? How frequently are you monitored for appropriate dosage and effects of these medications?

Key questions to ask the physician

- What is the patient's coagulation disorder and the level of severity?
- What are the laboratory values associated with the patient's bleeding disorder?
- What is the reason for the anticoagulant/antiplatelet therapy? How stable is the therapy and the patient's INR if on Coumadin®?
- May the patient temporarily discontinue the anticoagulant/antiplatelet therapy prior to dental surgery? *The nature and extent of the invasive dental procedure should be explained to the physician.* If discontinuing anticoagulant/antiplatelet therapy is recommended, how many days prior to and following the surgical procedure may the patient discontinue the medication?
- If the patient has severe hemophilia, is the patient on weekly factor replacement therapy or home therapy (self-treats)? If so, what schedule and what replacement level are achieved? Have you directed the patient about required factor replacement levels prior to dental procedures? Do you recommend factor replacement therapy prior to specific dental procedures (block anesthesia, scaling and root planning, dental extractions) or recommend referral and/or admission to the hospital for dental surgery?

Platelet Disorders

Platelet transfusions are effective for some indications and may be warranted in thrombocytopenia patients with platelet counts <50,000 cells/mL prior to surgical procedures.

Coagulation Disorders

In hemophiliacs, dental treatment may be best performed in a hospital setting by a dentist who is experienced in the treatment of hemophiliacs.[10] The dentist should work in close coordination with the patient's hematologist and should be familiar with the type and severity of disease. Before dental treatment, factor replacement is administered to raise the level to 25–30% for inferior alveolar block anesthesia and at least 50% for dental extractions. Topical hemostatic and local antifibrinolytic agents such as topical thrombin (converts fibrinogen to fibrin), EACA (25% Amicar® syrup), and tranexamic acid (trans-p-aminomethyl-cyclohexane carboxylic acid [AMCA] available only in Europe as 4.8% oral mouthwash; as Cyclokapron® tablet and injection form in the United States) may contribute to hemostasis. Deciduous teeth should not be removed prior to natural exfoliation.

Often in preparation for dental extractions in patients with severe hemophilia A, hematologists will recommend correction to 50–100% Factor VIII levels preoperatively by infusion of 50–100 IU/dL; intraoperative use of hemostatic agents such as Gelfoam®, Avitene®, Surgicel®, or Instat® and suturing; and postoperative use of Amicar® syrup as a 25 mg/kg swish and spit every 8 hours for 7 days.[11,12] Caution to avoid traumatizing surgical sites with hard food substances is important. Hemophiliacs trained in home therapy can be directed by their physician to self-infuse a specific dose of a selected factor concentrate product in preparation for dental treatment as shown in Fig. 9.3.

With vWD, the therapeutic goal is to correct deficiencies in vWF activity to >50% of normal.

Figure 9.3 Self-infusion of Factor VIII concentrate by a patient prior to dental extraction.

Management is determined by the type and severity of vWD. DDAVP is generally sufficient for most patients; however, certain types of vWD may require Factor VIII replacement therapy or platelet transfusions. The use of adjunctive antifibrinolytic agents may also be warranted.

Drug-Induced Disorders

The dentist and physician should jointly decide the appropriate management strategy for a patient receiving coumarin therapy, taking into account the extent of dental treatment required, potential for hemorrhage, and potential complications of discontinuing the anticoagulant therapy. Figures 9.4 and 9.5 provide guidelines and pathways for determining safe dental management for patients on Coumadin®.

A PT/INR should be taken on a patient taking Coumadin® within 24 hours of the scheduled dental procedure. There is evidence that minor oral surgical procedures can be safely performed on a patient with an INR below 3.5.[13–16] For extensive dental treatment such as full-mouth extraction, treatment modifications include dividing the planned procedures into numerous appointments or, after consultation with the patient's physician, making a decision to withhold Coumadin® for 2–3 days or substituting heparin or LMWH

Dental Procedure	Suboptimal INR Range		Normal Target INR Range			Out of Range
	<1.5	1.5 to < 2.0	2.0 to < 2.5	2.0 to 3.0	> 3.0 to 3.5	> 3.5
				Mechanical Prosthetic Heart Valves		
			Atrial Fibrillation; Venous Thrombosis; Pulmonary or Systemic Embolism; Acute MI			
Examination, radiographs, impressions, orthodontics						
Simple restorative dentistry, supragingival prohylaxis						
Complex restorative dentistry, scaling & root planing, endodontics					Probably safe	
Simple extraction, curettage, gingivoplasty, biopsy				Local measures§	Local measures§	
Multiple extractions, single bony impaction extraction			Local measures§	Local measures§	Local measures§	
Gingivectomy, minor periodontal flap surgery, apicoectomy, single implant placement	Probably safe	Probably safe	Probably safe			
Full mouth or full arch extractions	Probably safe	Local measures§				
Extensive flap surgery, extraction of multiple bony impactions, multiple implant placement	Probably safe					

INR= International Normalized Ratio; MI= Myocardial Infarction. Green indicates that it is safe to proceed in a routine manner (local factors such an periodontitis/gingival inflammation can increase severity of bleeding; the clinician should consider all factors when making a risk assessment). Yellow, use caution, but in many instances the procedure can be safely performed with judicious use of local measures. Red, procedures not advised at current INR level; refer to physician for Coumadin® adjustment.

§ Increased need for use of local measures such as sutures, oxidized cellulose, microfibrillar collagen hemostat, topical thrombin and/or epsilon aminocaproic acid or tranexamic acid. (Herman WW, Konzelman Jr JL, Sutley SH. Current perspectives on dental patients receiving coumarin anticoagulant therapy. JADA 1997:128(3):327-35. Copyright © 1997 American Dental Association. All rights reserved. Adapted 2011 with permission of the American Dental Association.)

Figure 9.4 Safety of outpatient dental procedures for patients on Coumadin®.

(referred to as bridging therapy), performing the surgery, then resuming anticoagulation with Coumadin. If intravenous heparin is used, the procedure should be performed in a hospital setting to facilitate administration of heparin and obtaining bloodwork expeditiously. With LMWHs, after careful coordination with the patient's cardiologist, individuals may undergo oral/dental surgical procedures in an outpatient setting. Subcutaneously delivered LMWHs (enoxaparin [Lovenox®], dalteparin [Fragmin®], and ardeparin [Normiflo®]) permit outpatient treatment of thromboembolic conditions that previously required inpatient hospitalization for unfractionated intravenous heparin administration. For patients placed on a bridging regimen, the Coumadin® is generally discontinued 4–5 days prior to surgery and generally starting 3 days before surgery daily or twice daily LMWH is instituted. The morning of the planned dental surgery, the subcutaneous LMWH is not given to the patient, and the INR is confirmed to be at an adequate level to maintain hemostasis. Surgery is performed, the patient is placed back on the LMWH and coumarin therapy resumed after the procedure on the day of surgery, and the LMWH is discontinued when adequate anticoagulation (INR ≥ 2.0) is achieved with Coumadin®. Physician monitoring of the INR is required during bridging therapy.[17] A typical bridging patient instruction sheet is seen in Fig. 9.6.

Figure 9.5 Algorithm for nonurgent dental care of patients receiving coumarin therapy.

BRIDGING (Substitution) THERAPY: Pre- and Postdental Surgery. Coumadin® taken every evening and Low-Molecular-Weight Heparin (LMWH) taken once daily.									
Coumadin®	PM last dose	none	none	none	PM ___mg	PM ___mg	PM ___mg	PM ___mg	PM ___mg
LMWH #	none	none	AM	AM	none	AM	AM	AM	AM
Labs					AM-INR				AM-INR§
Days	−4	−3	−2	−1	0 (day of surgery)	1	2	3	4

\# Low-molecular-weight heparin, e.g., enoxaparin at 1.5 mg/kg once daily
* Restart Coumadin® at your previous dose, § If adequate this is last day for LMWH dose.

Figure 9.6 Bridging therapy.

For the patient taking dabigatran (Pradaxa®) or rivaroxaban (Xarelto®), preparation for dental treatment may not require any modification of anticoagulant status; however, if the planned dental surgery is expected to cause significant postoperative hemorrhage, consultation with a physician is recommended. Currently, discontinuation of the drug for 24 hours is sufficient to restore normal hemostasis.

Patients with acquired drug-induced functional platelet defects caused by aspirin, NSAIDs, and ADP receptor inhibitors can have minor invasive dental procedures performed without altering the medication dosage.[18,19] Continuation of the drug can prevent the risk of cardiovascular or other medical complications, and any excessive bleeding can be controlled by local hemostatic measures, such as sutures and absorbable collagen hemostatic products, except in the case of leukemic patients with neutropenia where placement of foreign materials can act as nidus of infection.

Oral Lesion Diagnosis and Management

Petechiae

Petechiae are small red extravasation lesions that occur secondary to trauma and are more common in the presence of thrombocytopenias. See Figs. 1.7 and 1.8.

Ecchymoses

Ecchymoses are larger extravasation lesions, often bright red in color. See Figs. 1.8 and 9.7.

Hematomas

Hematomas are exophytic lesions that range in color from brown to red and are composed of clotted blood. See Fig. 1.10. These deep lesions may present in patients with congenital or acquired coagulation disorders secondary to trauma. A hematoma developing in a joint space is called a hemarthrosis.

Figure 9.7 Ecchymosis after prophylaxis treatment in a thrombocytopenic patient with acute leukemia. Note the red extravasation lesion.

 ## Risks of Dental Care

Hemostasis

The potential exists for postoperative bleeding complications resulting from dental treatment in patients with congenital or acquired platelet or coagulation disorders. Patients with known or suspected bleeding disorders should undergo assessment of their hemostatic function prior to dental treatment that may involve soft or hard tissue trauma. Pre- and postoperative therapy such as discontinuing antiplatelet or anticoagulant medication, infusion of platelets or clotting factor concentrates, and/or adjunctive local hemostatic measures may be warranted in consultation with the patient's physician to support invasive dental procedures. Local measures can be utilized to control hemorrhage, including mechanical procedures (i.e., sutures, pressure), absorbable collagen products (i.e., Gelfoam®, Surgicel®), and chemical agents (i.e., topical thrombin, tranexamic acid mouthwash, EACA syrup [Amicar®]). Abnormal clot formation is a risk as shown in Fig. 9.8.

Figure 9.8 Patient with severe hemophilia A, 4 days post-extraction impacted #32 with a "liver" clot which has a liver-like texture and appearance and extrudes from the socket, bleeding easily. It may bleed easily and requires removal by curettage for continued healing, possibly with presurgical factor concentrates, local hemostatics, and Amicar® use. The "liver clot," extruding on to cover some of the occlusal surface of tooth #31, is due to venous bleeding with prolonged oozing and is rich in hemoglobin.

Drug Actions/Interactions

The anticoagulation effect of coumarin therapy can be substantially increased by antibiotic (e.g., metronidazole, penicillin, erythromycin, cephalosporins, tetracycline) or antifungal (e.g., fluconazole) therapy. If antibiotics are employed prior to or as part of treatment, periodic monitoring of INR is recommended. Coumadin® potency can also be decreased with medications such as barbiturates, ascorbic acid, and dicloxacillin.

Patients with congenital or acquired coagulation disorders should not be prescribed aspirin or NSAIDs because of their increased bleeding potential.

Recognition of Potential Medical Emergencies

In hemophiliacs, deep-tissue bleeding (hematoma formation), hemarthrosis, and hematuria can be life threatening and are the common forms of clinical bleeding. Bleeding of the mouth, tongue, or neck that impairs the airway, as well as retroperitoneal hemorrhage or intracranial hemorrhage, may cause acute threats to life. An inferior alveolar nerve block in a hemophiliac in which the artery is nicked can induce life-threatening hematoma formation.

Special Considerations

Heparin

Heparin acts as an antithromboplastin, preventing the enzymatic conversion of prothrombin to thrombin. It is administered intravenously and has a brief duration of action (4 hours). Heparin is commonly used during renal dialysis treatment. Consequently, dentists should not treat patients requiring hemodialysis on the day of therapy due to the increased potential for bleeding with heparin.

Uremia

Uremia is a consequence of renal failure that results in the retention of nitrogenous waste products that are normally excreted into the urine. This condition produces functional abnormalities of platelets. In patients with end-stage renal disease, the dentist should work closely with the nephrologist in assessing platelet function prior to performing invasive dental procedures.

Alcohol

Alcohol can sometimes impair platelet function, with an effect that is proportional to the degree of alcohol ingestion.

IV. Recommended Readings and Cited References

Recommended Readings

Bacci C, Maglione M, Favero L, Perini A, Di Lenarda R, Berengo M, et al. Management of dental extraction in patients undergoing anticoagulant treatment. Results from a large, multicentre, prospective, case-control study. Thromb Haemost 2010;104(5): 972–5.

Douketis JD, Berger PB, Dunn AS, Jaffer AK, Spyropoulos AC, Becker RC, et al. The perioperative management of antithrombotic therapy: American College of Chest Physicians Evidence-Based Clinical Practice Guidelines (8th Edition). Chest 2008;133(6 Suppl.):299S–339S.

Garcia D, Libby E, Crowther MA. The new oral anticoagulants. Blood 2010;115(1):15–20.

Jeske AH, Suchko GD. Lack of a scientific basis for routine discontinuation of oral anticoagulation therapy before dental treatment. J Am Dent Assoc 2003;134(11):1492–7.

Nematullah A, Alabousi A, Blanas N, Douketis JD, Sutherland SE. Dental surgery for patients on anticoagulant therapy with warfarin: a systematic review and meta-analysis. J Can Dent Assoc 2009;75(1):41. Available at: http://www.cda-adc.ca/jcda/vol-75/issue-1/41.pdf.

Perry DJ, Noakes TJ, Helliwell PS; British Dental Society. Guidelines for the management of patients on oral anticoagulants requiring dental surgery. Br Dent J 2007;203(7):389–93.

Cited References

1. Simon D, Kunicki T, Nugent D. Platelet function defects. Haemophilia 2008;14(6):1240–9.
2. Gomez-Moreno G, Sguilar-Salvatierra A, Martin-Piedra MA, Guardia J, Calvo-Guairda JL, Cagrera M, et al. Dabigatran and rivaroxaban, new oral anticoagulants, new approaches in dentistry. J Clin Exp Dent 2010;2(1):e1–5. Available at: http://www.medicinaoral.com/odo/volumenes/v2i1/jcedv2i1p1.pdf.
3. Favaloro EJ. Von Willebrand disease: local diagnosis and management of a globally distributed bleeding disorder. Semin Thromb Hemost 2011; 37(5):440–55.
4. Brennan MT, Shariff G, Kent ML, Fox PC, Lockhart PB. Relationship between bleeding time test and postextraction bleeding in a healthy control population. Oral Surg Oral Med Oral Pathol Oral Radiol Endod 2002;94(4): 439–43.
5. Stanca CM, Montazem AH, Lawal A, Zhang JX, Schiano TD. Intranasal desmopressin versus blood transfusion in cirrhotic patients with coagulopathy undergoing dental extraction: a randomized controlled trial. J Oral Maxillofac Surg 2010;68(1):138–43.
6. Mannucci PM, Remuzzi G, Pusineri F, Lombardi R, Valsecchi C, Mecca G, et al. Deamino-8-D-arginine vasopressin shortens the bleeding time in uremia. N Engl J Med 1983;308(1):8–12.
7. Nichols WL, Hultin MB, James AH, Manco-Johnson MJ, Montgomery RR, Ortel TL, et al. von Willebrand disease (VWD): evidence-based diagnosis and management guidelines, the National Heart, Lung, and Blood Institute (NHLBI) Expert Panel report (USA). Haemophilia 2008;14(2): 171–232.
8. Hedner U, Glazer S, Falch J. Recombinant activated factor VII in the treatment of bleeding episodes in patients with inherited and acquired bleeding disorders. Transfus Med Rev 1993;7(2): 78–83.
9. Yee TT, Pasi KJ, Lilley PA, Lee CA. Factor VIII inhibitors in haemophiliacs: a single-center experience over 34 years, 1964–1997. Br J Haematol 1999;104(4):909–14.
10. Brewer AK, Roebuck EM, Donachie M, Hazard A, Gordon K, Fung D, et al. The dental management of adult patients with haemophilia and other congenital bleeding disorders. Haemophilia 2003;9(6):673–7.
11. Brewer A, Correa ME. Guidelines for Dental Treatment of Patients with Inherited Bleeding Disorders. 2006. No. 40. World Federation of Hemophilia, Montreal, Quebec, Canada. Available at: http://www.wfh.org/2/docs/Publications/Dental_Care/TOH-40_Dental_treatment.pdf. Accessed December 11, 2011.
12. Zanon E, Martinelli F, Bacci C, Zerbinati P, Girolami A. Proposal of a standard approach to dental extraction in haemophilia patients. A case-control study with good results. Haemophilia 2000;6(5):533–6.
13. Herman WW, Konzelman JL Jr., Sutley SH. Current perspectives on dental patients receiving coumarin anticoagulant therapy. J Am Dent Assoc 1997;128(3):327–35.
14. Menendez-Jandula B, Souto JC, Oliver A, Montserrat I, Quintana M, Gich I, et al. Comparing self-management of oral anticoagulant therapy with clinic management: a randomized trial. Ann Intern Med 2005;142(1):1–10.

15. Lockhart PB, Gibson J, Pond SH, Leitch J. Dental management considerations for the patient with an acquired coagulopathy. Part 1: coagulopathies from systemic disease. Br Dent J 2003;195(8): 439–45.
16. Hirsh J, Fuster V, Ansell J, Halperin JL. American Heart Association/American College of Cardiology Foundation. American Heart Association/American College of Cardiology Foundation guide to warfarin therapy. Circulation 2003;107 (12):1692–711.
17. Douketis JD, Johnson JA, Turpie AG. Low-molecular-weight heparin as bridging anticoagulation during interruption of warfarin: assessment of a standardized periprocedural anticoagulation regimen. Arch Intern Med 2004;164(12):1319–26.
18. Brennan MT, Valerin MA, Noll JL, Napeñas JJ, Kent ML, Fox PC, et al. Aspirin use and postoperative bleeding from dental extractions. J Dent Res 2008;87(8):40–4.
19. Napenas JJ, Hong CH, Brennan MT, Furney SL, Fox PC, Lockhart PB. The frequency of bleeding complications after invasive dental treatment in patients receiving single and dual antiplatelet therapy. J Am Dent Assoc 2009;140(6):690–5.

Autoimmune and Connective Tissue Diseases

Scott S. De Rossi DMD
Katharine N. Ciarrocca DMD, MSEd

I. Background

Conditions commonly referred to as connective tissue diseases and/or autoimmune diseases include systemic lupus erythematosus (SLE), rheumatoid arthritis (RA), primary biliary cirrhosis (PBC), fibromyalgia (FM), the various sclerosing syndromes such as progressive systemic sclerosis (PSS) or scleroderma, and Sjögren's syndrome (SS). Collectively, these disorders affect a significant portion of the United States population, where patients can often appear to be in good health, but whose medical illness may adversely affect their oral cavity or the provision of dental care.

Description of Disease/Condition
SLE

SLE is a chronic, inflammatory autoimmune disorder of unknown etiology that affects many organ systems. Autoantibodies and immune complexes set off an array of immunological reactions, resulting in activation of the complement system, leading to vasculitis, fibrosis, and tissue necrosis. The clinical course of SLE is defined by periods of remission and exacerbation.

RA

RA is an autoimmune disease manifesting as a chronic systemic inflammatory disorder. The disease has a wide clinical spectrum with considerable variability in joint and extra-articular manifestations.

PBC

PBC is a chronic and progressive cholestasic disease of the liver. The major pathology of this disease is a destruction of the small-to-medium bile ducts, which leads to progressive cholestasis, liver dysfunction, and ultimately end-stage liver disease.

FM

FM is a syndrome of persistent widespread pain, stiffness, fatigue, disrupted sleep, and cognitive difficulties, often accompanied by multiple other unexplained symptoms, anxiety

The ADA Practical Guide to Patients with Medical Conditions, First Edition. Edited by Lauren L. Patton.
© 2012 American Dental Association. Published 2012 by John Wiley & Sons, Inc.

and/or depression, and functional impairment of activities of daily living.

PSS (Scleroderma)

PSS, or scleroderma, is a disease characterized by skin induration and thickening accompanied by various degrees of tissue fibrosis and chronic inflammatory infiltration in numerous visceral organs, prominent fibroproliferative vasculopathy, and humoral and cellular immune alterations.

SS

SS is a chronic, autoimmune, inflammatory disorder characterized by lymphocytic infiltration of the exocrine glands in multiple sites, most commonly the lacrimal and salivary glands. It can occur alone (primary SS) or in conjunction with another autoimmune rheumatic disease (secondary SS).

Pathogenesis/Etiology

SLE

SLE is the prototype systemic autoimmune disease, as virtually all components of the immune system contribute to the characteristic autoimmunity and tissue pathology. The etiopathogenesis of lupus comprises genetic contributions, environmental triggers, and stochastic events.[1] Autoantibodies and their antigens, cytokines, and chemokines amplify immune system activation and generate tissue damage. Autoantibody production occurs years prior to the development of clinical signs and symptoms of SLE.[2]

RA

Although the cause of RA is unknown, genetic, environmental, hormonal, immunological, and infectious factors may play significant roles.[3] An external trigger (e.g., infection, trauma) elicits an autoimmune reaction, leading to synovial hypertrophy and chronic joint inflammation along with the potential for extra-articular manifestations in genetically susceptible individuals. Synovial cell hyperplasia and endothelial cell activation are early events in the pathological process that progresses to uncontrolled inflammation and consequent cartilage and bone destruction.

PBC

PBC is characterized by a T-lymphocyte-mediated assault on small intralobular bile ducts. A constant attack on the bile duct epithelial cells leads to their gradual destruction and eventual disappearance. The sustained loss of intralobular bile ducts causes the signs and symptoms of cholestasis, and eventually results in cirrhosis and liver failure.[4]

FM

FM is currently understood to be a disorder of central pain processing or a syndrome of central sensitivity. Although the pathogenesis of FM is not completely understood, research shows biochemical, metabolic, and immunoregulatory abnormalities.[5]

PSS (Scleroderma)

The exact etiology of PSS is unclear; however, the following pathogenic mechanisms are always present: endothelial cell injury, fibroblast activation, and cellular and humoral immunological derangement. Vascular dysfunction is one of the earliest alterations of systemic sclerosis and may represent the initiating event in its pathogenesis.[6]

SS

The etiology of SS is not well understood. The presence of activated salivary gland epithelial cells expressing major histocompatibility complex (MHC) class II molecules and the identification of inherited susceptibility markers suggest that environmental or endogenous antigens trigger a self-perpetuating inflammatory response in susceptible individuals. In addition, the continuing presence of active interferon pathways in SS suggests ongoing activation of the innate immune system.[7]

Epidemiology

SLE

- An estimated 161,000–322,000 women are currently afflicted with SLE in the United States, with 1 in 1000 white and 1 in 250 black women affected.[8]
- Ninety percent are young to middle-aged women.
- The 10-year survival rate is >90%, with 20-year survival rates near 80%.

RA

- An estimated 1.3 million adults have RA.[8]
- Annual worldwide incidence of RA is approximately three cases per 10,000 population, and the prevalence rate is approximately 1%, increasing with age and peaking at age 35–50 years.
- RA affects all populations, although the disease is much more prevalent in some groups (e.g., 5–6% in some Native American groups) and much less prevalent in others (e.g., black persons from the Caribbean region).
- Women are affected by RA approximately three times more often than men, but sex differences diminish in older age groups suggesting a hormonal component.

PBC

- The incidence of PBC has been estimated as 4.5 cases for women and 0.7 cases for men (2.7 cases overall) per 100,000 population.[4]
- Women account for 75–90% of patients.
- Men develop similar symptoms and clinical course of disease, but they appear to be at higher risk for developing hepatocellular carcinoma.
- Onset of PBC usually occurs in persons aged 30–65 years.

FM

- It is estimated that 5 million U.S. adults are afflicted with FM.[9]
- FM exhibits no race predilection but shows a drastic female predominance with a female-to-male ratio of approximately 9:1.
- FM can occur in individuals of all ages.

PSS (Scleroderma)

- An estimated 49,000 U.S. adults have PSS.[8]
- Incidence and prevalence of PSS are estimated at 19 and 240 cases per million population, respectively.
- Peak onset occurs in individuals aged 30–50 years.
- The risk of systemic sclerosis is four to nine times higher in women than in men.

SS

- Primary SS affects 0.4–3.1 million U.S. adults.[8]
- SS affects 0.1–4% of the population.
- The female-to-male ratio of SS is 9:1.
- SS can affect individuals of any age but is most common in elderly people.
- Onset typically occurs in the 4th–5th decade of life.

Coordination of Care between Dentist and Physician

Rheumatological diseases are chronic and often difficult to diagnose. A careful examination of the face, temporomandibular joints, and oral cavity for evidence of oral mucosal dryness or lupus-like oral lesions can assist in the diagnostic process for many of these diseases. Salivary measurements and minor salivary gland biopsies from the labial mucosa can contribute to the diagnosis of SS. The relationship between SS and lymphoma underscores the importance of the oral health-care provider aiding in the diagnosis and monitoring of these patients. Among patients with SS, the incidence of non-Hodgkin's lymphoma is 4.3% (18.9 times higher than in the general population), with a median age at diagnosis of 58 years. The mean time to the development of non-Hodgkin's lymphoma after the onset of SS is 7.5 years. In addition, patients with major joint dysfunction who undergo total joint replacement will require consideration for antibiotic prophylaxis (AP). While this is controversial, a decision whether to use prophylactic antibiotics should be coordinated between dentist and physician/orthopedic surgeon on an individualized basis.

II. Medical Management

Identification

SLE

The manifestations of SLE exhibit no typical pattern of presentation. Small-vessel vasculitis, resulting from immune-complex deposition leads to renal, cardiac, hematological, mucocutaneous, and central nervous system (CNS) destruction. In addition, polyserositis (inflammation of the serous membranes) results in joint, peritoneal, and pleuropericardial symptoms. Diagnosis is made by a combination of laboratory tests and clinical manifestations including 4 of 11 criteria.[10,11]

Raynaud's phenomenon can occur in a variety of rheumatological diseases as shown in Fig. 10.1.

RA

The hallmark feature of this condition is persistent symmetric polyarthritis (synovitis) that affects the hands (see Fig. 10.2) and feet, although any joint lined by a synovial membrane may be involved. The criterion for an RA diagnosis uses a score-based algorithm based on four areas: joint involvement, serology test results, acute-phase reactant test results, and patient self-reporting of signs/symptom duration. A score of 6 of 10 or greater must be met

---

American College of Rheumatology Criteria for the Diagnosis of Systemic Lupus Erythematosus

A diagnosis of SLE can be made with reasonable probability if 4 of the 11 criteria are met, serially or simultaneously, during a period of observation. Serology is used to support a diagnosis.

Arthritis
Serositis (pleuritis or pericarditis)
Malar rash
Discoid rash
Photosensitivity
Oral ulcers
Renal disease (proteinuria or cellular casts)
Neurological disease (psychosis or seizures)
Hematological disease (hemolytic anemia, thrombocytopenia, leukopenia, or lymphopenia)
Immunological manifestations (anti-Sm nuclear antigen, anti-native DNA, false-positive antiphospholipid antibodies)
Antinuclear antibodies

Adapted from Tan et al.[10] and Hochberg.[11]

Figure 10.1 Patient's hand with Raynaud's syndrome. Note purple tone to fingertips of cyanotic phase.

Figure 10.2 Hands of a 43-year-old with rheumatoid arthritis showing small joint synovitis. DIP, distal interphalangeal joint; PIP, proximal interphalangeal joint; MCP, metacarpophalangeal joint; IP, interphalangeal joint.

for a classification of definitive RA applied to patients with synovitis in at least one joint that cannot be better explained by an alternative diagnosis.[12] Patients with a score that falls below 6/10 may be reassessed over time. Progression of RA is shown in Table 10.1.

PBC

Many people with PBC have no symptoms of the disease when they are initially diagnosed. Routine blood tests for an evaluation for other conditions lead to diagnosis in 25% of patients.

FM

Patients with FM may meet criteria for three or more central sensitivity syndromes. Most patients do not appear chronically ill, although they may look fatigued or agitated.

PSS (Scleroderma)

Some types of scleroderma affect only the skin, while others affect the whole body.

- *Localized scleroderma* usually affects only the skin on the hands and face. It develops

Table 10.1. Progression of Rheumatoid Arthritis

Stage 1 (early)	No destructive changes observed upon radiographic examination; radiographic evidence of osteoporosis is possible
Stage 2 (moderate)	Radiographic evidence of periarticular osteoporosis, with or without slight subchondral bone destruction; slight cartilage destruction is possible; joint mobility is possibly limited, but no joint deformities are observed; adjacent muscle atrophy is present; extra-articular soft-tissue lesions (e.g., nodules, tenosynovitis) are possible
Stage 3 (severe)	Radiographic evidence of cartilage and bone destruction in addition to periarticular osteoporosis; joint deformity (e.g., subluxation, ulnar deviation, hyperextension) without fibrous or bony ankylosis; muscle atrophy is extensive; extra-articular soft-tissue lesions (e.g., nodules, tenosynovitis) are possible
Stage 4 (terminal)	Presence of fibrous or bony ankylosis, along with criteria of stage 3

> **Criteria for rheumatoid arthritis diagnosis**
>
> 1. Confirmed presence of synovitis (swelling) in at least 1 joint
> 2. Absence of alternative diagnosis that better explains the synovitis
> 3. Achievement of a total score of 6 or greater out of 10 points in the 4 domains (sum of point scores in Category A–D)
>   A. Joint involvement
>   　　1 large joint (i.e., shoulders, elbows, hips, knees, ankles) = 0 point
>   　　2–10 large joints = 1 point
>   　　1–3 small joints (with or without involvement of large joints) (i.e., metacarpophalangeal, proximal interphalangeal, 2nd–5th metatarsophalangeal, thumb interphalangeal, and wrist joints) = 2 points
>   　　4–10 small joints (with or without involvement of large joints) = 3 points
>   　　>10 joints (at least 1 small joint, plus any combination of large and additional small joints or joints such as temporomandibular, acromioclavicular, sternoclavicular) = 5 points
>   B. Serology (at least 1 serology test result is needed for classification)
>   　　Negative RF *and* negative ACPA = 0 point
>   　　Low-positive RF *or* low-positive ACPA = 2 points
>   　　High-positive RF *or* high-positive ACPA = 3 points
>   C. Acute-phase reactants (at least 1 test result is needed for classification)
>   　　Normal CRP *and* normal ESR = 0 point
>   　　Abnormal CRP *or* abnormal ESR = 1 point
>   D. Duration of symptoms
>   　　<6 weeks = 0 point
>   　　≥6 weeks = 1 point
>
> Key: ACPA, anticitrullinated protein antibody; RF, rheumatoid factor; CRP, C-reactive protein; ESR, erythrocyte sedimentation rate.
> Adapted from Aletaha D, Neogi T, Silman AJ, Funovits J, Felson DT, Bingham CO 3rd, et al. 2010 Rheumatoid Arthritis Classification Criteria. An American College of Rheumatology/European League Against Rheumatism Collaborative Initiative. Arthritis Rheum 2010;62(9):2569–81.

slowly, and rarely, if ever, spreads throughout the body or causes serious complications.

- *Systemic scleroderma* may affect large areas of skin and organs such as the heart, lungs, or kidneys. There are two main types of systemic scleroderma: (1) limited disease or CREST syndrome = calcinosis, Raynaud's syndrome, esophageal dysmotility, sclerodactyly (see Fig. 10.3), telangiectasia; or (2) diffuse disease.

Figure 10.3 Sclerodactyly in a patient with scleroderma.

SS

The clinical presentation of SS may vary. The onset is insidious. It usually starts in women aged 40–60 years, but it also can affect men and children. The first symptoms in primary SS can be easily overlooked or misinterpreted, and diagnosis can be delayed for as long as several years.

Medical History and Physical Exam

SLE

Medical history and physical assessment reveals the diversity of this multisystem disease that can have phases of stability and exacerbations, called lupus flares.

- *Renal Disease*: Localization of immune complexes in the kidney is the precipitating factor in the development of lupus nephritis and can lead to a rapidly progressing glomerulonephritis or a less aggressive form of renal disease resulting from cumulative, chronic tissue injury during previous flares of SLE. Ultimately, cell proliferation, inflammation, necrosis, and fibrosis result in significant impairment of renal function.
- *Cardiac Disease*: Cardiac manifestations include pericarditis, pericardial effusion, myocardial infarction, and valvular disease. The most common of all cardiac lesions in these patients is a nonbacterial verrucous valvular lesion, known as Libman–Sacks endocarditis.
- *Hematological Disease*: Anemia, leukopenia, and thrombocytopenia are significant complications of SLE and/or its treatment. Anemia in these patients is most commonly associated with hemodialysis therapy, while leukopenia results from the immunosuppressive therapies. Thrombocytopenia occurs in up to 25% of patients, with extreme thrombocytopenia (<20,000 platelets per cubic millimeter) occurring in 5–10% of these patients.[13]
- *Mucocutaneous Disease*: The cutaneous manifestations of SLE include photosensitive rashes, alopecia (hair loss), periungual telangiectasias (involving the nail folds), and livedo reticularis (purplish networking discoloration of skin). The malar or "butterfly rash," which affects fewer than half of patients, and the discoid rash are the two most characteristic rashes of SLE (see Fig. 1.4).
- *Oral Conditions*: Over 75% of SLE patients have oral complaints including ulcerations, xerostomia, and burning mouth. Ulcerations, erythema, and/or keratosis, commonly affecting the vermilion, gingiva, buccal mucosa, and palate found in patients with SLE may be confused with lichen planus.
- *Musculoskeletal Conditions*: Arthralgia with "morning stiffness" is the most common initial manifestation of SLE, and over 75% of patients develop a true arthritis that is symmetric, nonerosive, and usually involves the hands, wrists, and knees. Involvement of the temporomandibular joint has been documented in up to 60% of SLE patients.
- *Neuropsychiatric Disease*: Diffuse and focal cerebral dysfunction including psychosis, seizures, cerebrovascular accidents, and peripheral sensorimotor neuropathies account for greater than 60% of neuropsychiatric manifestations.

RA

Affected joints show inflammation with swelling, tenderness, warmth, and decreased range of motion (ROM). Atrophy of the interosseous muscles of the hands is a typical early finding. Joint and tendon destruction may lead to deformities such as ulnar deviation, boutonniere and swan-neck deformities, hammer toes, and, occasionally, joint ankylosis. Common joint physical findings include stiffness, tenderness, pain on motion, swelling, deformity, and limitation of motion.

Extra-articular manifestations include:

- rheumatoid nodules;
- peripheral neuropathy (affects nerves, most often those in the hands and feet, and can result in tingling, numbness, or burning);

- anemia;
- scleritis (inflammation of the blood vessels in the eye that can result in corneal damage, scleromalacia, and, in severe cases of nodular scleritis, perforation);
- infections (patients with RA have a higher risk for infections; immunosuppressive drugs further increase that risk);
- osteoporosis (more common than average in postmenopausal women with RA; the hip is particularly affected; risk for osteoporosis appears to be higher than average in men with the disease who are older than 60);
- heart disease (RA can affect blood vessels and increase the risk for coronary ischemic heart disease);
- SS;
- lymphoma and other cancers (RA-associated immune system alterations may play a role).

PBC

Fatigue is the first reported symptom, with 10% experiencing severe pruritus of unknown cause. Right upper quadrant discomfort occurs in 8–17% of patients.[14] Physical examination findings depend on the stage of the disease. In the early stages, examination findings are normal. As the disease progresses, the following may be found:

- hepatomegaly;
- hyperpigmentation;
- splenomegaly;
- jaundice;
- Sicca syndrome (xerophthalmia, xerostomia);
- signs of advanced liver disease are spider nevi, palmar erythema, ascites, temporal and proximal muscle wasting, and peripheral edema.

FM

Patients may complain of chronic widespread pain lasting more than 3 months, fatigue, poor sleep, stiffness, cognitive difficulties, multiple somatic symptoms, anxiety, and/or depression.

Figure 10.4 Location of the nine paired tender points that make up the 1990 American College of Rheumatology criteria for fibromyalgia. Source: NIAMS. Available at: http://www.niams.nih.gov/HealthInfo/Fibromyalgia/default.asp.

Except for painful tender (or trigger) points and, perhaps, signs of deconditioning, physical examination findings are normal in patients with FM. The tender-point examination should be performed first during the physical examination, because a number of factors may influence the sensitivity of the tender points during the examination. Pain, not just tenderness, is present at multiple FM tender points (see Fig. 10.4).[15]

PSS (Scleroderma)

Skin symptoms of scleroderma may include:

- fingers or toes that turn blue or white in response to hot and cold temperatures;

- hair loss;
- skin hardness;
- skin that is abnormally dark or light;
- skin thickening, stiffness, and tightness of fingers, hands, and forearm;
- small white lumps beneath the skin, sometimes oozing a white substance that looks like toothpaste;
- sores (ulcers) on the fingertips or toes;
- tight and mask-like skin on the face (see Fig. 1.5).

Bone and muscle symptoms may include:

- joint pain;
- numbness and pain in the feet;
- pain, stiffness, and swelling of fingers and joints.

Breathing problems may result from scarring in the lungs and can include:

- dry cough;
- shortness of breath.

Digestive tract problems may include:

- constipation/diarrhea;
- difficulty swallowing;
- esophageal reflux or heartburn.

Figure 10.5 Bilateral parotid gland selling in a patient with Sjögren's syndrome.

SS

Most individuals with SS present with Sicca symptoms, such as xerophthalmia (dry eyes), xerostomia (dry mouth), and parotid gland enlargement (see Fig. 10.5).[16] In addition, numerous extraglandular features may develop, such as arthralgia, arthritis, Raynaud's phenomenon, myalgia, pulmonary disease, gastrointestinal disease, leukopenia, anemia, lymphadenopathy, neuropathy, vasculitis, renal tubular acidosis, and lymphoma.

Patients may describe the effects of dry mouth in the following ways:

- inability to eat dry food (e.g., crackers) because it sticks to the roof the mouth;
- tongue sticking to the roof of the mouth;
- putting a glass of water on the bed stand to drink at night (and resulting nocturia);
- difficulty speaking for long periods of time or the development of hoarseness;
- higher incidence of dental caries and periodontal disease;
- altered sense of taste;
- difficulty wearing dentures;
- development of oral candidiasis with angular cheilitis, which can cause mouth pain.

Laboratory Testing

SLE

SLE is characterized by the production of numerous different autoantibodies, including antinuclear antibodies (ANAs), anti-native DNA, rheumatoid factor (RF), anti-SM, anti-Ro, and anti-La, many of which produce specific laboratory and clinical abnormalities. However, these autoantibodies can also be seen in a number of connective tissue diseases and are summarized in Table 10.2. Diagnosis is made by a combination of laboratory tests and clinical manifestations.[17]

Revised International Classification Criteria for Sjögren's Syndrome

I. Ocular symptoms: a positive response to at least one of the following questions:
   1. Have you had daily, persistent, troublesome dry eyes for more than 3 months?
   2. Do you have a recurrent sensation of sand or gravel in the eyes?
   3. Do you use tear substitutes more than three times a day?
II. Oral symptoms: a positive response to at least one of the following questions:
   1. Have you had a daily feeling of dry mouth for more than 3 months?
   2. Have you had recurrently or persistently swollen salivary glands as an adult?
   3. Do you frequently drink liquids to aid in swallowing dry food?
III. Ocular signs—that is, objective evidence of ocular involvement defined as a positive result for at least one of the following two tests:
   1. Schirmer's I test, performed without anaesthesia (<5 mm in 5 minutes)
   2. Rose bengal score or other ocular dye score (>4 according to van Bijsterveld's scoring system)
IV. Histopathology: in minor salivary glands (obtained through normal-appearing mucosa) focal lymphocytic sialoadenitis, evaluated by an expert histopathologist, with a focus score >1, defined as a number of lymphocytic foci (which are adjacent to normal-appearing mucous acini and contain more than 50 lymphocytes) per 4 mm^2 of glandular tissue.
V. Salivary gland involvement: objective evidence of salivary gland involvement defined by a positive result for at least one of the following diagnostic tests:
   1. Unstimulated whole salivary flow (<1.5 mL in 15 minutes)
   2. Parotid sialography showing the presence of diffuse sialectasias (punctate, cavitary, or destructive pattern), without evidence of obstruction in the major ducts.
   3. Salivary scintigraphy showing delayed uptake, reduced concentration, and/or delayed excretion of tracer.
VI. Autoantibodies: presence in the serum of the following autoantibodies:
   1. Antibodies to Ro (SSA) or La (SSB) antigens, or both

Revised rules for classification

For primary Sjögren's syndrome (SS)
- In patients without any potentially associated disease, primary SS may be defined as follows:
  - The presence of any four of the six items is indicative of primary SS, as long as either item IV (Histopathology) or VI (Serology) is positive.
  - The presence of any three of the four objective criteria items (i.e., items III, IV, V, VI).
  - The classification tree procedure represents a valid alternative method for classification, although it should be more properly used in clinical–epidemiological survey.

For secondary SS
- In patients with a potentially associated disease (for instance, another well-defined connective tissue disease), the presence of item I or item II plus any two from among items III, IV, and V may be considered as indicative of secondary SS.

Exclusion criteria
- Past head and neck radiation treatment
- Hepatitis C infection
- Acquired immunodeficiency disease (AIDS)
- Preexisting lymphoma
- Sarcoidosis
- Graft-versus-host disease
- Use of anticholinergic drugs (since a time shorter than fourfold the half-life of the drug)

Source: Vitali et al.[16]

Table 10.2. Percentage of Autoantibodies Associated with Specific Connective Tissue Diseases

Autoantibody Type	Autoimmune Disease			
	Systemic Lupus Erythematosus	Rheumatoid Arthritis	Sjögren's Syndrome	Diffuse Scleroderma
ANA	95–100	30–60	95	80–95
Anti-native DNA	60	0–5	0	0
Rheumatoid factor	20	72–85	75	25–33
Anti-Sm	10–25	0	0	0
Anti-Ro	15–20	0–5	60–70	0
Anti-La	5–20	0–2	60–70	0

ANA, antinuclear antibodies; anti-Sm, antibody to Smith antigen; anti-Ro, antibody to Ro antigen (SS-A); anti-La, antibody to La antigen (SS-B).

RA

ANAs are elevated in 30–60% of patients, while RF is seen in up to 85% of patients with RA (see Table 10.2). Progressive, radiographic changes, including juxta-articular demineralization, joint space narrowing, and the development of joint erosions are diagnostic criteria for RA.

PBC

- The hallmark of this disease is the presence of antimitochondrial antibodies (AMAs) in the sera.
- Significant elevations of the alkaline phosphatase (ALP), γ-glutamyl transpeptidase (GGTP), and immunoglobulin levels (mainly immunoglobulin M [IgM]) are usually the most prominent findings in liver function tests
- An elevation of the aminotransferases alanine aminotransferase (ALT) and aspartate aminotransferase (AST) can be identified in most patients with PBC.
- Lipid levels and cholesterol levels may be increased, with an increased high-density lipoprotein (HDL) fraction.
- Increased erythrocyte sedimentation rate (ESR).
- As the disease progresses to cirrhosis, an elevated bilirubin level, a prolonged prothrombin time, and a decreased albumin level can be found.

FM

There are no characteristic laboratory test findings in FM.

PSS (Scleroderma)

- ANAs are present in about 80–95% of affected patients, usually with a speckled or centromere pattern. A nucleolar pattern, although less common, is more specific for systemic sclerosis.
- Anticentromere antibodies are present in about 45–50% of patients with limited disease and are rare in patients with diffuse disease.

SS

Clinical and laboratory testing used to help confirm a diagnosis of SS, and which are reliable data to classify SS, include the following:

- objective measurement of saliva secretion to confirm salivary gland hypofunction;

- objective measurement of tear secretion to confirm lacrimal gland hypofunction;
- salivary gland biopsy for scoring of the chronic inflammation, usually taken from the lower labial mucosa;
- autoantibody testing, to reveal the presence of serum autoantibodies to SS-associated antigen-A (anti-SS-A or anti-Ro) or -B (anti-SS-B or anti-La).

Medical Treatment

SLE

An organ-specific approach is used to manage SLE by rheumatologists. Long-term corticosteroids are the principal treatment modality for the management. High doses are usually reserved for significant renal and CNS disease. Small to moderate doses are used to treat the serositis and inflammatory arthritis. Aspirin, hydroxychloroquine, and prednisone remain the only U.S. Food and Drug Administration (FDA)-approved drugs for SLE.[18]

RA

- The objectives of RA therapies include the reduction of inflammation and pain, the preservation of function, and the prevention of deformity.
- Nonpharmacological measures include physical therapy, orthotic devices, and occasionally surgery.
- Medication-based therapies comprise several classes of drugs, including nonsteroidal anti-inflammatory drugs (NSAIDs), disease-modifying antirheumatic drugs (DMARDs), immunosuppressants, biological response modifiers, and corticosteroids.[19]

PBC

- Ursodeoxycholic acid (UDCA) is the major medication used to slow the progression of the disease.
- Immunosuppressive agents such as methotrexate, cyclosporine, corticosteroids, and colchicine inhibit immune reactions that mediate the progression of the disease.
- Liver transplantation appears to be the only lifesaving procedure.

FM

The overall approach for chronic pain in FM involves a multifaceted treatment plan that incorporates various adjuvant medicines, aerobic exercise, and psychological and behavioral approaches to reduce distress and promote self-efficacy and self-management (e.g., relaxation training, activity pacing, visual imagery, distraction). Opioids, hypnotics, anxiolytics, and certain skeletal-muscle relaxants may be used with caution because of the potential for abuse.

PSS (Scleroderma)

- Primary drug treatment aims at inhibiting tissue fibrosis and vascular and immune system alterations, although the FDA has not approved any therapies for PSS.
- Skin thickening can be treated with numerous experimental drugs or interventions (D-penicillamine, interferon-gamma, mycophenolate mofetil, cyclophosphamide, photopheresis, allogeneic bone marrow transplantation).
- Specific symptoms and signs are treated with targeted medical management specific for pruritis, Raynaud's, arthralgias, gastrointestinal symptoms, and so on. Prednisone, immunosuppressants, and chelating agents remain the treatments of choice.

SS

Goals for management of patients with SS involve oral health management and multidisciplinary care as shown in Table 10.3.

Table 10.3. Five Goals of Management for Patients with Sjögren's Syndrome

Alleviating symptoms	Diet and habit modifications Frequent and regular sips of water Avoidance of dry, hard, sticky, acidic foods Avoidance of excess caffeine and alcohol Salivary substitutes and lubricants: rinses, gels, sprays Toothpastes Use of bedside humidifier during sleeping hours
Instituting preventive measures	Increased frequency of oral/dental evaluation and recall maintenance—every 3 months Daily use of highly fluoridated dentifrice Topical fluoride application at home and in office (solution, gel, foam, or varnish); topical: over the counter (0.05% sodium fluoride); prescription (1.0% sodium fluoride, 0.4% stannous fluoride)
Treating oral conditions	Dental caries: Restorative therapy, topical fluoride Oral candidiasis: clotrimazole troches: 10 mg dissolved orally four to five times daily for 10 days; nystatin/triamcinolone ointment for angular cheilitis: apply topically four times daily; systemic therapy for immunocompromised patients; denture antifungal treatment: soaking of denture for 30 minutes daily in chlorhexidine or 1% sodium hypochlorite Bacterial infections: systemic antibiotics for 7–10 days, chlorhexidine 0.12%: rinse, swish, and spit 10 mL twice daily Ill- or poor-fitting prostheses: denture adjustment, hard and soft reline, use of denture adhesives, implant-borne prostheses
Improving salivary function (if possible)	Sugar-free, xylitol-containing mints, candies, and gum Sialogogues: pilocarpine: 5–10 mg orally three times daily; cevimeline: 30 mg orally three times daily

Managing underlying systemic conditions	Multidisciplinary management with other health-care providers:
	   Endocrinology
	   Rheumatology
	   Internal medicine
	   Hematology/oncology
	   Radiation oncology
	   Nephrology/transplant medicine

III. Dental Management

Evaluation

Patients with known autoimmune and connective tissue disease should have a focused interview with the dentist.

SS

In evaluation of patients with SS, the patient interview (see Dry Mouth Questionnaire) and clinical assessment can reveal signs that a patient's salivary flow rate is decreased.[20] For example:

- Does the mucosa appear dry?
- Does the mirror stick to the mucosa?

Key questions to ask the patient

When were you diagnosed?
Is your mouth dry?

Additional disease-specific questions:
For the patient with SLE
    Is your disease stable? If not, then when was your last flare?
    Do you have kidney disease?
For the patient with RA
    Have you had any joint surgeries? And if so what procedure and when?
    Do you have movement difficulties? When during the day is your mobility at its best?
For the patient with PBC
    What is the health status of your liver?
    Do you bleed excessively?
For the patient with scleroderma
    Is your disease stable? If not, then when was your last flare?
    Do you have mobility limitations?
For the patient with fibromyalgia
    Have you been having headaches or temporomandibular joint pain?
For the patient with a total joint replacement
    Which joint was replaced? When was this?
    Was that the first time the joint was replaced or did it need to be redone?
    How stable is your current joint prosthesis?

Key questions to ask the physician

How stable is the patient's rheumatological condition?
Do you feel the patient (on high-dose steroids) is adrenal suppressed and would require steroid supplementation for dental surgical procedures?
Are you planning any pulse steroid or immunosuppressant therapy in the near future for the patient?

Additional disease-specific questions:
For the patient with SLE
    How advanced is the patient's SLE? Does the patient have lupus nephritis? Does the patient have cardiac disease?
    What is the patient's most recent complete blood count (CBC) and prothrombin time (PT)/INR?
For the patient with PBC
    What is the patient's most recent CBC and PT/INR?
For the patient with a total joint replacement
    Is the prosthetic joint stable?
    Has the patient ever had a prosthetic joint infection?
    Do you feel antibiotic prophylaxis is necessary prior to dental procedures (all, just surgical?) for this patient? What antibiotic regimen do you suggest?

> **Dry Mouth Questionnaire**
>
> 1. Does the amount of saliva in your mouth seem to be too little, too much, or you don't notice it?
> 2. Do you have any difficulties swallowing?
> 3. Does your mouth feel dry when eating a meal?
> 4. Do you sip liquids to aid in swallowing dry food?
>
> Reference: Fox et al.[20]

- Is there a lack of pooled saliva in the floor of mouth?
- Is there difficulty in expressing saliva from the major gland ducts?
- Is it clear and of good consistency?
- Is there an increase in caries in unusual areas (e.g., mandibular incisors)?

In addition, milking the parotid glands to inspect the consistency and amount of saliva is important.

Dental Treatment Modifications

SLE

General guidelines for treatment of patients with SLE and other connective tissue disorders with systemic involvement are shown in Table 10.4.

RA

- Patients with secondary SS will often require intensified oral hygiene instruction, dietary instruction and modifications, home/professional fluoride therapy, antimicrobial mouth rinses, more frequent recall/radiographs, and aggressive treatment of dental disease.[21]
- Patient education and physical comfort in the dental chair should be important considerations for the dental practitioner. Altering the position of the dental chair, allowing the patient to rest periodically, shifting positions or use of pillows, and scheduling shorter appointments can be used to improve patient comfort in the dental setting.
- Home care can present a serious challenge to patients with reduced manual dexterity. Floss holders, irrigating devices, electric toothbrushes, and modifications to traditional toothbrushes may be helpful (see Fig. 18.3 for toothbrush modifications).
- Patients with RA may demonstrate some temporomandibular joint involvement during the course of their disease. Narrowed joint spaces, flattened condyles, erosions, subchondral sclerosis, cysts, and osteoporosis can be seen radiographically.
- An increased incidence of advanced periodontal disease has been seen in patients with long-standing RA. It does not appear that inadequate oral hygiene due to functional impairment is a primary factor in RA-associated periodontal disease.
- Xerostomia affects greater than 40% of patients with RA, making the patient more susceptible to caries, periodontal changes, and candidiasis.

PBC

Liver disorders are important to the dentist due to a potential bleeding tendency, intolerance to drugs (general anesthetics, benzodiazepines), and the underlying causes for the liver dysfunction. A thorough history will usually alert the clinician to potential problems. Preoperative blood testing to include serum bilirubin,

Table 10.4. General Guidelines for Dentists Treating Patients with Connective Tissue Disease

Before dental care
- Consultation with the patient's physician/rheumatologist to assess extent of connective tissue-related end-organ disease and current therapies (as secondary conditions can themselves affect provision of care—e.g., end-stage renal disease and myocardial infarction)
- Obtain a baseline complete blood count with differential
- Consider routine chemistry panel in patients with lupus nephritis or PSS-related renal impairment
- Postpone elective care during SLE exacerbation or during pulse therapy
- Assess potential for adrenal suppression and use replacement therapy when appropriate
- Prescribe prophylactic antibiotics when indicated to minimize the risk of endocarditis and prosthetic joint infection
- Consider preoperative antibiotics for patients on immunosuppressive therapy and low absolute neutrophil count
- Use stress-reducing measures when appropriate:
    - Consider sedative premedication
    - Schedule short, morning appointments
    - Pain and anxiety control
- Be prepared for medical emergencies in the dental clinic:
    - Adrenal suppression
    - Cardiovascular status
    - Impaired hemostasis

During dental care
- Assess oral mucosal disease and TMJ involvement and treat as appropriate
- Assess xerostomia and provide treatment when appropriate
- Assess facial muscular pain and dysfunction in polymyositis
- Use sutures and adjunctive hemostatic agents when indicated
- Use stress-reducing measures when appropriate

After dental care
- Use appropriate dosing intervals of medications for patients with renal insufficiency/hemodialysis
- Use caution when prescribing NSAIDs/aspirin in SLE patients as they may precipitate a flare and consider dose adjustments for RA patients on NSAID regimens
- Consider oral suspension medications for scleroderma patients with reflux and esophageal involvement
- Consider postoperative antibiotics for patients on immunosuppressive therapy
- Evaluate for TMJ dysfunction and consider serial imaging studies
- Schedule frequent recall maintenance (every 3–4 months)

NSAIDs, nonsteroidal anti-inflammatory drugs; SLE, systemic lupus erythematosus; RA, rheumatoid arthritis; PSS, progressive systemic sclerosis; TMJ, temporomandibular joint.

albumin, AST, ALT, GGTP, ALP, CBC with differential, and prothrombin time/international normalized ratio (PT/INR) may be indicated. See also Chapter 6.

FM

Provision of dental care for patients with FM usually requires little, if any, modification. Major clinical considerations for FM patients include comorbid temporomandibular disorder (TMD) and possible drug interactions.[22]

- If TMD is present in patients with FM, it is advisable to minimize jaw fatigue during dental treatment.
- Avoid prolonged periods of jaw opening, if possible.

- Allow frequent breaks during prolonged dental treatment for jaw rest.
- Provide jaw support during treatment by using a bite block, mouth prop, and hand support, if necessary.
- There may be an increased risk of caries secondary to medication-induced xerostomia.

PSS (Scleroderma)

- One of the most challenging aspects for dental practitioners of treating patients with scleroderma is the physical limitations caused by narrowing of the oral aperture and rigidity of the tongue.[23] The inability to access posterior dentition in order to accomplish oral hygiene and dental treatment during progression of the disease may necessitate treatment plan modification (see Table 10.5).
- The dentist should instruct patients in jaw physical therapy in an effort to maintain the masticatory function.
- For patients with the diffuse form of the disease, dentists must consider the extent of visceral disease as that may affect the provision of dental care.
- Patients with xerostomia will require supplemental fluoride therapy and frequent recall maintenance.

SS

- Preventive measures are critical in the overall management of a patient with reduced saliva.
- Increased frequency of oral and dental evaluation and recall maintenance every 2–3 months is imperative.
- Nutritional counseling recommending a low-carbohydrate diet is also needed.
- In addition, topical fluoride application, at home or in the dental office, with solutions, gels, foams, or varnishes, is important in preventing dental caries.
- The identification and management of other oral conditions such as candidiasis, bacterial infections, and ill-fitting prostheses are important.

Table 10.5. Orofacial Findings in Progressive Systemic Sclerosis and Their Management

Orofacial Findings	Management
Sicca syndrome	Cevimeline, pilocarpine, salivary substitutes
Periodontitis	Hygiene education, scaling and root planning, biannual maintenance sequences, antibiotic therapy
Plaque and/or anticoagulant-induced gingival hemorrhage	Hygiene education, scaling and root planing procedures, antifibrinolytic mouth rinses
Caries	Conservative dentistry, dental prophylaxis with fluoride treatment
Mandibular bone resorption	No treatment, simple follow-up
Severe MIO (<30 mm)	3 months of elongation exercises
Edentulation	Fractionated in case of severe MIO; partial, complete removable dentures, dental implants
Perioral "whistle" lines	Pulsed CO_2 laser

MIO, maximal interincisal opening.
Adapted from Alantar et al.[23]

Total Joint Replacement

An estimated 600,000 joint prostheses are placed in the United States each year. About 12,000 (2%) of those become infected, resulting in a cost of about $30,000 per occurrence. Most prosthetic joint infections occur within 3 months after surgery and are termed "early infections." Those occurring later than 3 months after surgery are called "late prosthetic joint infections" (LPJIs).

Prosthetic joints are infected in one of four ways:

- contamination at the time of surgery;
- spread from an adjacent area;
- hematogenous spread;
- reactivation of an infection from a previous joint infection.

Early recommendations called for antibiotic prophylaxis (AP) for all patients with prosthetic joints before dental procedures. Some of the emphasis came from studies in which a huge ($>1 \times 10^9$) inoculum of *Staphylococcus aureus* was injected into rabbits, and from case reports that claimed a relationship, often in spite of a late onset of infection (>6 months after the procedure). A survey conducted in 2000 suggests that the majority of orthopedic surgeons favor prophylaxis, in spite of the lack of scientific evidence.[24]

In 1997, with input from members of the Infectious Diseases Society of America (IDSA), the American Dental Association (ADA) and American Academy of Orthopedic Surgeons (AAOS) published an advisory statement regarding the dental treatment of patients with prosthetic joints and a revised statement in 2003.[25] AP was not recommended for patients with pins, plates, or screws, or for otherwise healthy patients with total joint replacements.

Patients at greater risk due to specific medical conditions should be considered candidates for prophylaxis. These include patients whose prostheses were less than 2 years old or those who had "high-risk" conditions such as:

- inflammatory arthropathies (RA, SLE);
- drug-induced or radiation-induced immunosuppression;
- previous joint infection;
- malnourishment;
- hemophilia;
- human immunodeficiency virus infection;
- insulin-dependent diabetes;
- malignancy.

In February 2009, without collaborative involvement with organized dentistry or nonorthopedic physician specialties, the AAOS published what it labeled an "Information Statement" entitled "Antibiotic Prophylaxis for Bacteremia in Patients with Joint Replacements." Given the potential adverse outcomes and cost of treating an infected joint replacement, the AAOS recommended that clinicians consider AP for all total joint replacement patients prior to any invasive procedure that may cause bacteremia. There was no clear explanation or scientific basis for this change in position. The risk/benefit and cost/effectiveness ratios fail to justify the administration of routine AP.

If one were to follow the information statement of the AAOS authors, the following four assumptions all would have to be true for a clinician to believe the actions are in the patient's best interest:

- Bacteremia from oral flora arising from dental procedures causes LPJIs.
- There is a temporal relationship between dental procedures and LPJIs.
- AP prevents bacteremia resulting from dental procedures and subsequent LPJIs.
- One cannot compare late LPJIs and infective endocarditis because of differing anatomy, blood supply, microorganisms, and mechanisms of infection.

Analysis of reported cases of LPJIs demonstrates that joint infections rarely are caused by bacterial species common to the mouth. There is no credible evidence to link LPJIs with dental procedures.[26]

Issuance of future joint society consensus recommendations is under discussion. In the interim, dentists must use their clinical judgment.

Three Choices for the Clinician[27]

- Inform patients who have prosthetic joints about the lack of scientific evidence to support AP in their situation and the potential for a drug reaction to AP so that patients can make informed decisions. The problem with this approach is that patients may become confused by the conflicting information.
- Base clinical decisions entirely on the 2003 consensus statement and other literature published since then. The problem with this approach is potential medicolegal jeopardy if they do not contact the orthopedist for recommendations and then follow them.
- Contact the patient's orthopedic surgeon, briefly discuss or outline in a letter the current dilemma, and suggest that they both follow the 2003 guidelines until a new joint consensus statement is approved. If the orthopedist elects to follow the 2009 AAOS information statement and recommends AP for a patient who would not receive AP according to the 2003 guidelines, then the dentist should ask the orthopedist to write the prescription for antibiotics.

Oral Lesion Diagnosis and Management

SLE

- *Oral Lesions*: Most of the oral lesions of SLE are caused by vasculitis and appear as ulceration or mucosal inflammation. Oral ulcerations are often transient and occur during acute SLE exacerbations and regress without intervention. Lip lesions commonly appear with a central atrophic area surrounded by a keratinized white border with small radiating striae (see Fig. 10.6). These manifestations of SLE may be the initial sign of the disease. The diagnosis of these lesions is accomplished by routine biopsy or direct immunofluorescence staining.
- *Xerostomia*: Some oral conditions of SLE may directly result from salivary gland dysfunction. Xerostomia can increase the occurrence of dental caries, periodontal disease, and candidiasis.

PBC

Oral complications may be associated with liver failure or xerostomia.

Advanced Liver Disease

- Gingival bleeding
- Petechiae and ecchymosis
- Jaundice of skin and mucosa
- Lichen planus

Secondary SS

- Parotitis (45–90% of patients with PBC can exhibit evidence of sialoadenitis)
- Dental attrition/erosion
- Xerostomia
- Glossitis
- Angular cheilitis
- Candidiasis

PSS (Scleroderma)

- Severe microstomia (see Fig. 10.7), limitation in mouth opening, and submucosal fibrosis represent major limitations to dental care.
- Salivary production may be decreased and pooling of saliva may be absent. Oropharyngeal

Figure 10.6 Cutaneous and oral lesions associated with systemic lupus erythematosus (SLE). (a) Lesion on labial commissure. (b) Tongue lesion. (c,d) Buccal mucosa oral ulcers of SLE.

and esophageal cancers are more common in persons with diffuse systemic sclerosis.
- There may be radiographic abnormalities like periodontal ligament space widening (33% of cases) or osteolytic lesions (7%).
- Increased risk of caries secondary to medication-induced xerostomia and difficulty with oral hygiene.

SS

The clinical complications of hyposalivation and xerostomia include (see Fig. 10.8):

Figure 10.7 Microstomia in PSS.

Figure 10.8 Clinical complications of xerostomia in Sjögren's syndrome. (a) Dry pebbly appearance of tongue; (b) dry, slick tongue and angular cheilitis; (c) rampant dental caries; (d) cuspal dental caries.

- mucosal abnormalities;
- dental caries;
- periodontal disease;
- halitosis;
- candidiasis;
- difficulty with mastication, swallowing, and speaking.

 Risks of Dental Care

Hemostasis

SLE

- Prior to performing dental surgery, consultation with the physician for understanding of recent platelet count is advised. No elective surgical procedures should be performed in patients with a platelet count <50,000 cells/mm^3.
- The use of primary closure and adjunctive hemostatic measures is recommended for thrombocytopenic patients. Microfibrillar collagen (Avitene®, Collaplug®) and oxidized regenerated cellulose (Gelfoam®, Surgicel®) may be helpful.
- The use of platelet inhibiting NSAIDs or salicylates for postoperative pain management should be avoided.

RA

- Analgesics with potential to inhibit platelet aggregation are commonly used. However, postsurgical bleeding is rare and can be managed with local measures.

PBC

- Patients may have the tendency for excessive bleeding due to liver dysfunction.

Susceptibility to Infection

SLE, RA, and PBC

- A preoperative complete blood count can aid the dentist in screening for leukopenia.
- There may be increased potential for infection secondary to medication-induced immune suppression.
- Consider antibiotic coverage for patients who have been on long-term, high-dose, daily corticosteroid therapy or other immune suppressants and patients with an absolute neutrophil count <500–1000 cells/mm^3.

Drug Actions/Interactions

Commonly used drugs for connective tissue disease and their toxicities are shown in Table 10.6.

SLE

- Use appropriate dosing intervals of medications for SLE patients who have renal insufficiency or are receiving hemodialysis.
- Use caution when prescribing NSAIDs or aspirin.

RA

- Prior to prescribing additional NSAIDs during dental care, practitioners must assess the patient's current regimen to avoid toxic levels, renal impairment, or exacerbation of peptic ulcer disease.
- Adrenal insufficiency is a potential problem with long-term corticosteroid use.

PBC

- PBC may lead to unpredictable hepatic metabolism of medications.
- Patients on long-term corticosteroids may be adrenally suppressed.

FM

- Use caution when using local anesthetic containing vasoconstrictors for patients taking amitriptyline or venlafaxine, as it may precipitate a hypertensive crisis.
- Use caution when prescribing the following:
  - Opioid analgesics for patients taking tricyclic antidepressants, as they may increase overall patient sedation.
  - Macrolide antibiotics, chiefly erythromycin and clarithromycin, as they may interact with the cytochrome P-450 enzyme system and increase therapeutic levels of other medications.
  - NSAIDs for patients taking selective serotonin reuptake inhibitors, as they may increase risk for prolonged bleeding.

Patient's Ability to Tolerate Dental Care

SLE

- Elective dental care should be deferred if patient is in a lupus flare.

RA and PBC

- Replacement therapy prior to certain dental procedures for adrenally suppressed individuals may be indicated to prevent cardiovascular collapse.
  - Long-lasting local anesthetics, postoperative pain medications, and sedative premedication should be considered for these patients.

Table 10.6. Drug Toxicities of Medications Used to Treat Connective Tissue Diseases

Drug	Disease	Toxicity
Azathioprine	RA	Stomatitis, nausea, vomiting, hepatotoxicity, pancytopenia, rash, arthralgia
Calcium channel antagonists	Raynaud's phenomenon	Gingival overgrowth, rash, dizziness, headache, congestive heart failure
Corticosteroids	RA, SLE	Candidiasis, hypertension, osteoporosis, cataracts, peptic ulcers, psychosis, delayed wound healing
Cyclophosphamide	SLE, PSS	Stomatitis, cardiotoxicity, myelosuppression, hepatotoxicity, pulmonary fibrosis, neoplasms, thrombocytopenia
Cyclosporine		Renal impairment, hypertension, gingival overgrowth
D-penicillamine	RA, PSS	Rash, stomatitis, dysgeusia, proteinuria, myelosuppression, infrequent but serious autoimmune disease
Danazol	Thrombocytopenia in SLE	Stomatitis, acneiform rash, cholestatic jaundice, anxiety
Gold, oral	RA	Same as injectable but less frequent, diarrhea
Gold salts, injectable	RA	Rash, stomatitis, myelosuppression, proteinuria thrombocytopenia
Hydroxychloroquine sulfate	RA, SLE	Mucosal discoloration, lichenoid reaction, convulsions, retinal and corneal changes, leukopenia, thrombocytopenia, nausea, vomiting
Methotrexate	RA, SLE	GI symptoms, stomatitis, rash, alopecia, infrequent myelosuppression, hepatotoxicity, rare pulmonary toxicity
Mycophenolate mofetil	RA, SLE	Hyper- or hypotension, peripheral edema, chest pain, tachycardia, headache, insomnia, fever, dizziness, anxiety, rash, nausea, vomiting, abdominal pain, diarrhea or constipation, anorexia, dyspepsia, leukopenia, anemia, thrombocytopenia, leukocytosis, ascites, paresthesia, tremor, weakness, abnormal liver or kidney function, dyspnea, cough, sinusitis, pleural effusion, bacterial, candidal and herpetic infections
NSAIDs	RA	GI symptoms including indigestion, ulceration, hemorrhage, small-bowel ulceration; stomatitis, renal, neurological, pulmonary, hepatic, hematological, dermatological, displacement of protein-bound drugs
Omeprazole	Reflux in PSS	Xerostomia, mucosal atrophy, dysgeusia, diarrhea, abdominal pain, proteinuria, hematuria, pancytopenia
Sulfasalazine	RA	Stomatitis, Stevens–Johnson syndrome, hepatitis, convulsions, leukopenia, thrombocytopenia, toxic nephrosis, myocarditis

RA, rheumatoid arthritis; SLE, systemic lupus erythematosus; PSS, progressive systemic sclerosis; GI, gastrointestinal; NSAIDs, nonsteroidal anti-inflammatory drugs.

FM

- Dependent on jaw pain as well as how well the patient is feeling that day.

PSS (Scleroderma)

- Replacement therapy prior to certain dental procedures for adrenally suppressed individuals may be indicated to prevent cardiovascular collapse.
  - Long-lasting local anesthetics, postoperative pain medications, and sedative premedication should be considered for these patients.
- Avoid prolonged periods of jaw opening, if possible.
- Allow frequent breaks during prolonged dental treatment for jaw rest.
- Provide jaw support during treatment by using a bite block, mouth prop, and hand support, if necessary.

Recognition of Potential Medical Emergencies

SLE, RA, and PBC

- *Recognition*: As the mainstay of treatment of autoimmune connective tissue diseases is systemic corticosteroids, dentists must be aware of the potential for adrenal crisis.
- *Management Protocol*: If the patient shows signs/symptoms of adrenal crisis (vomiting, abdominal pain, low blood pressure, syncope, hypoglycemia, confusion), immediate emergency medical treatment is necessary.

IV. Recommended Readings and Cited References

Recommended Readings

American College of Rheumatology. *Clinical support*. 2011. Available at: http://www.rheumatology.org/practice/clinical/

Napenas JJ, Lockhart PB, Epstein JB. Comment on the 2009 American Academy of Orthopaedic Surgeons' information statement on antibiotic prophylaxis for bacteremia in patients with joint replacements. J Can Dent Assoc 2009;75(6):447–9.

Cited References

1. Rahman A, Isenberg DA. Systemic lupus erythematosus. N Engl J Med 2008;358(9):929–39.
2. Cooper GS, Dooley MA, Treadwell EL, St Clair EW, Parks CG, Gilkeson GS. Hormonal, environmental, and infectious risk factors for developing systemic lupus erythematosus. Arthritis Rheum 1998;41(10):1714–24.
3. Barton A, Worthington J. Genetic susceptibility to rheumatoid arthritis: an emerging picture. Arthritis Rheum 2009;61(10):1441–6.
4. Mayo MJ. Natural history of primary biliary cirrhosis. Clin Liver Dis 2008;12(2):277–88.
5. Yunus MB. Fibromyalgia and overlapping disorders: the unifying concept of central sensitivity syndromes. Semin Arthritis Rheum 2007;36(6):339–56.
6. Arnett FC. Is scleroderma an autoantibody mediated disease? Curr Opin Rheumatol 2006;18(6):579–81.
7. Price EJ, Venables PJ. The etiopathogenesis of Sjögren's syndrome. Semin Arthritis Rheum 1995;25(2):117–33.
8. Helmick CG, Felson DT, Lawrence RC, Gabriel S, Hirsch R, Kwoh CK, et al. Estimates of the prevalence of arthritis and other rheumatic conditions in the United States. Part I. Arthritis Rheum 2008;58(1):15–25.
9. Lawrence RC, Felson DT, Helmick CG, Arnold LM, Choi H, Deyo RA, et al. Estimates of the prevalence of arthritis and other rheumatic conditions in the United States. Part II. Arthritis Rheum 2008;58(1):26–35.
10. Tan EM, Cohen AS, Fries JF, Masi AT, McShane DJ, Rothfield NF, et al. The 1982 revised criteria for the classification of systemic lupus erythematosus. Arthritis Rheum 1982;25(11):1271–7.
11. Hochberg MC. Updating the American College of Rheumatology revised criteria for the classification of systemic lupus erythematosus. Arthritis Rheum 1997;40(9):1725.
12. Aletaha D, Neogi T, Silman AJ, Funovits J, Felson DT, Bingham CO 3rd. 2010 Rheumatoid Arthritis

Classification Criteria: an American College of Rheumatology/European League against Rheumatism collaborative initiative. Ann Rheum Dis 2010;69(9):1580–8.
13. De Rossi SS, Glick M. Lupus erythematosus: considerations for dentistry. J Am Dent Assoc 1998;129:333–9.
14. Solis Herruzo JA, Solis Munoz P, Munoz Yague T. The pathogenesis of primary biliary cirrhosis. Rev Esp Enferm Dig 2009;101(6):413–23.
15. Wolfe F, Smythe HA, Yunus MB, Bennett RM, Bombardier C, Goldenberg DL, et al. The American College of Rheumatology 1990 criteria for the classification of fibromyalgia: report of the Multicenter Criteria Committee. Arthritis Rheum 1990;33(2):160–72.
16. Vitali C, Bombardieri S, Jonsson R, Moutsopoulos HM, Alexander EL, Carsons SE, et al. Classification criteria for Sjögren's syndrome: a revised version of the European criteria proposed by the American-European Consensus Group. Ann Rheum Dis 2002;61(6):554–8.
17. D'Cruz DP, Khamashta MA, Hughes GR. Systemic lupus erythematosus. Lancet 2007;369(9561):587–96.
18. Appel GB, Contreras G, Dooley MA, Ginzler EM, Isenberg D, Jayne D, et al. Mycophenolate mofetil versus cyclophosphamide for induction treatment of lupus nephritis. J Am Soc Nephrol 2009;20(5):1103–12.
19. Saag KG, Teng GG, Patkar NM, Anuntiyo J, Finney C, Curtis JR. American College of Rheumatology 2008 recommendations for the use of nonbiologic and biologic disease-modifying antirheumatic drugs in rheumatoid arthritis. Arthritis Rheum 2008;59(6):762–84.
20. Fox PC, Busch KA, Baum BJ. Subjective reports of xerostomia and objective measures of salivary gland performance. J Am Dent Assoc 1987;115(4):581–4.
21. Treister N, Glick M. Rheumatoid arthritis: a review and suggested dental care considerations. J Am Dent Assoc 1999;130(5):689–98.
22. Balasubramaniam R, Laudenbach JM, Stoopler ET. Fibromyalgia: an update for oral health care providers. Oral Surg Oral Med Oral Pathol Oral Radiol Endod 2007;104(5):589–602.
23. Alantar A, Cabane J, Hachulla E, Princ G, Ginisty D, Hassin M, et al. Recommendations for the care of oral involvement in patients with systemic sclerosis. Arthritis Care Res 2011;63(8):1126–33.
24. Lockhart PB, Brennan MT, Fox PC, Norton HJ, Jernigan DB, Strausbaugh LJ. Decision-making on the use of antimicrobial prophylaxis for dental procedures: a survey of infectious disease consultants and review. Clin Infect Dis 2002;34(12):1621–26.
25. American Dental Association, American Academy of Orthopaedic Surgeons. Antibiotic prophylaxis for dental patients with total joint replacements. J Am Dent Assoc 2003;134(7):895–9.
26. Berbari EF, Osmon DR, Carr A, Hanssen AD, Baddour LM, Greene D, et al. Dental procedures as risk factors for prosthetic hip or knee infection: a hospital-based prospective case-control study. Clin Infect Dis 2010;50(1):8–16.
27. Little JW, Jacobson JJ, Lockhart PB. The dental treatment of patients with joint replacements: a position paper from the American Academy of Oral Medicine. J Am Dent Assoc 2010;141(6):667–71.

HIV/AIDS and Related Conditions

Lauren L. Patton DDS

I. Background and Rationale

Description of Disease

Human immunodeficiency virus (HIV) is the etiological agent for acquired immune deficiency syndrome (AIDS). HIV is a retrovirus in the *Lentivirus* group.

Definition

The 2008 Centers for Disease Control and Prevention (CDC) definition of HIV and AIDS for public surveillance[1] is based on the laboratory evidence of HIV-1 or HIV-2 infection, the CD4 cell count, and the presence of AIDS-defining conditions outlined in the 1993 case definition.[2] See Table 11.1. Patients with laboratory-confirmed HIV infection may be in one of four HIV infection stages: Stage 1, 2, 3/AIDS, or unknown.

Pathogenesis/Etiology

Once transmission of HIV occurs, the retrovirus enters human cells, particularly the CD4+ (T-helper) lymphocytes in the peripheral blood and undergoes replication. Additional HIV virus is created and returned to the circulation, ultimately destroying the lymphocyte in the process. CD4+ lymphocyte depletion results in compromise of the host cell-mediated immune response.

Primary or acute infection and seroconversion usually occur without the display of any signs or symptoms; however, a small number of patients may experience a viral syndrome similar to the flu. In the next 6 months, HIV-specific antibody responses can be detected by standard HIV antibody tests. During the clinically latent or asymptomatic period of months to years, viral replication continues but the patient experiences few or no symptoms of HIV disease. Without medical intervention,

> **AIDS-defining conditions:**
>
> - Candidiasis of bronchi, trachea, or lungs
> - Candidiasis, esophageal
> - Cervical cancer, invasive
> - Coccidioidomycosis, disseminated or extrapulmonary
> - Cryptococcosis, extrapulmonary
> - Cryptosporidiosis, chronic intestinal (greater than 1 month's duration)
> - *Cytomegalovirus* disease (other than liver, spleen, or nodes)
> - *Cytomegalovirus* retinitis (with loss of vision)
> - Encephalopathy, HIV related
> - Herpes simplex: chronic ulcer(s) (greater than 1 month's duration), or bronchitis, pneumonitis, or esophagitis
> - Histoplasmosis, disseminated or extrapulmonary
> - Isosporiasis, chronic intestinal (greater than 1 month's duration)
> - Kaposi's sarcoma
> - Lymphoma, Burkitt's (or equivalent term)
> - Lymphoma, immunoblastic (or equivalent term)
> - Lymphoma, primary, of the brain
> - *Mycobacterium avium* complex or *Mycobacterium kansasii*, disseminated or extrapulmonary
> - *Mycobacterium tuberculosis*, any site (pulmonary or extrapulmonary)
> - *Mycobacterium*, other species or unidentified species, disseminated or extrapulmonary
> - *Pneumocystis carinii* pneumonia
> - Pneumonia, recurrent
> - Progressive multifocal leukoencephalopathy
> - *Salmonella* septicemia, recurrent
> - Toxoplasmosis of the brain
> - Wasting syndrome due to HIV

eventually viral replication overcomes the host immune response and CD4+ counts begin a progressive decline. The immune system deteriorates, and patients become increasingly susceptible to opportunistic infections such as oral candidiasis and the most common AIDS-defining condition, *Pneumocystis carinii* pneumonia (PCP). Death may ensue in 2–3 years following diagnosis with an AIDS-defining illness if medical care is not accessed or effective at halting disease progression.

Epidemiology

In June 1981, five previously healthy young men in Los Angeles, CA, with PCP, two of whom had died, were the first cases of HIV/AIDS reported in the world. Thirty years after this, the U.S. CDC reported that there are an estimated 33.3 million people living with HIV infection worldwide at the end of 2009[3]:

- Prevalence: Estimated U.S. persons living with HIV infection at the end of June 2008 = 1,178,350, of which 21% are undiagnosed and unaware of their HIV infection.[4]
- Incidence: Estimated new infections in the United States each year = 56,300 people.
- Gender: Of persons living with HIV/AIDS at year end 2008, 72% were adolescent and adult men, 26% were adolescent and adult women, and 2% were children under age 13 years.
- Age: All ages are affected, but the most common age group for new HIV cases (15%) is 20–24 years.
- Race/ethnicity: New HIV cases are in African-Americans (52%), whites (28%), Hispanics (17%), and others (3%). African-American men and women are estimated to have an incidence rate seven times higher than for whites.
- Risk behavior: Transmission risks of new HIV cases diagnosed in 2009 are reported as male-to-male sexual contact (MSM) (57%), high-risk heterosexual contact (31%), injection drug use (IDU) (9%), and MSM and IDU (3%).[4]
- Perinatal HIV transmission, for example, from mother to child during pregnancy, labor and delivery, and breast-feeding, has declined dramatically to less than 2% of births from HIV-infected mothers, as a result of maternal HIV testing and use of antiretroviral therapy (ART) during pregnancy and labor and delivery, and avoidance of breast-feeding.

Table 11.1. The 2008 Surveillance Case Definition for HIV Infection among Adults and Adolescents (Aged ≥13 Years), United States, 2008[1]

Stage	Laboratory Evidence	Clinical Evidence
Stage 1	Laboratory confirmation of HIV infection *and* CD4+ T-lymphocyte count of ≥500 cells/µL or CD4+ T-lymphocyte percentage of ≥29	None required (but no AIDS-defining conditions)
Stage 2	Laboratory confirmation of HIV infection *and* CD4+ T-lymphocyte count of 200–499 cells/µL or CD4+ T-lymphocyte percentage of 14–28	None required (but no AIDS-defining conditions)
Stage 3 (AIDS)	Laboratory confirmation of HIV infection *and* CD4+ T-lymphocyte count of <200 cells/µL or CD4+ T-lymphocyte percentage of <14	*or* documentation of an AIDS-defining condition (with laboratory confirmation of HIV infection)[b]
Stage unknown[a]	Laboratory confirmation of HIV infection *and* no information on CD4+ T-lymphocyte count or percentage	*and* no information on the presence of AIDS-defining conditions

Laboratory confirmation of HIV infection from either (1) positive result from an HIV antibody screening test (e.g., reactive enzyme immunoassay [EIA]) confirmed by a positive result from a supplemental HIV antibody test (e.g., Western blot or indirect immunofluorescence assay test) or (2) positive result or report of a detectable quantity (i.e., within the established limits of the laboratory test) from any of the following HIV virological (i.e., non-antibody) tests: HIV nucleic acid (DNA or RNA) detection test (e.g., polymerase chain reaction [PCR]); HIV p24 antigen test, including neutralization assay; HIV isolation (viral culture).
[a] Every effort should be made to report CD4+ T-lymphocyte counts or percentages and the presence of AIDS-defining conditions at the time of diagnosis.
[b] Documentation of an AIDS-defining condition supersedes a CD4+ T-lymphocyte count of ≥200 cells/µL and a CD4+ T-lymphocyte percentage of total lymphocytes of ≥14. Definitive diagnostic methods for these conditions are available in Appendix C of the 1993 revised HIV classification system and the expanded AIDS case definition and from the National Notifiable Diseases Surveillance System.

Coordination of Care between Dentist and Physician

- Primary medical care guidelines for persons initiating HIV care[5] state that the review of systems should include questioning about common HIV-related oral conditions including thrush or oral ulceration and the physical examination should include a careful examination of the oropharynx for evidence of candidiasis, oral hairy leukoplakia, mucosal Kaposi's sarcoma, aphthous ulceration, and periodontal disease.
- For optimal preventive oral health care, the physician should recommend dental consultation once HIV infection has been diagnosed and sought promptly when orofacial manifestations of HIV or acute dental disease develops since an oral infection can become life threatening in the severely immune compromised patient. Oral health care should be planned with consideration of the patient's medical status.
- The dentist's oral screening exam and/or use of a rapid oral-based point-of-care HIV antibody test in the dental office may help to identify new HIV infections and facilitate patient access to medical care. Whenever the dental practitioner identifies HIV-associated oral lesions in a patient of unknown HIV status, the dentist should discuss the possibility of HIV infection with the patient. Applicable state law should be consulted regarding confidentiality and other obligations.

II. Medical Management

Identification

While many HIV-infected patients will be aware of their serostatus, some will be unknown to the dentist because they are asymptomatic, have no physical signs and are unaware that they are seropositive, or withhold that information. A history of AIDS or HIV seropositivity may be supplied by the patient, or HIV infection may be suspected on the basis of the medical history or physical examination.

Medical History

Affirmative responses to confidential medical and social history questions in the following areas will alert the dentist to the possible need for further inquiry:

- AIDS or HIV infection;
- recurring infections (i.e., oral, tuberculosis [TB], pulmonary, gastrointestinal, sexually transmitted diseases);
- history of IDU;
- blood transfusions (1979–1985);
- hemophilia;
- malignancies (e.g., Kaposi's sarcoma and non-Hodgkin's lymphoma) known to be associated with HIV infection;
- symptoms associated with HIV infection such as night sweats, prolonged diarrhea, unexplained weight loss, and fever;
- history of viral hepatitis.

Further inquiry might include questions concerning the following:

- Unsafe sexual practices known to be associated with HIV transmission especially in high-risk populations (e.g., prostitutes, men who have sex with men, IDUs, hemophiliacs) or having multiple sexual partners.
- Association with persons who have certain infectious diseases (i.e., viral hepatitis, AIDS, TB, sexually transmitted diseases). If the response is affirmative, there must be follow-up questions to ascertain if the contact was such that HIV could have been transmitted.
- Rejection as a blood donor.

Physical Examination

The physical examination is important in identifying and monitoring orofacial conditions that may be associated with HIV infection.[6]

Examples include:

- candidiasis;
- hairy leukoplakia;
- oral warts;
- linear gingival erythema;
- ulcerative necrotizing gingivitis and periodontitis;
- prolonged, extensive, and/or frequently occurring herpes simplex infections;
- more severe and prolonged recurrent aphthous ulcers;
- salivary gland enlargement;
- Kaposi's sarcoma;
- cervical lymphadenopathy.

If the history or physical examination suggests the possibility of undiagnosed HIV infection, the provider should coordinate care with the primary care physician for a complete medical evaluation and laboratory testing.

Laboratory Testing
HIV Antibody Tests

HIV testing and referral are recommended for patients whose medical history or oral examination reveals the possibility of HIV infection. Early HIV detection and access to HIV medical care and ART can improve the quality and prolong the life span of the patient, as well as help to prevent future virus transmission.

> HIV testing should be done only in conformity with state laws regarding the legality and confidentiality of such testing. The medical, social, and legal implications of an HIV antibody test are extensive, and therefore, pre- and posttest patient counseling may be required. The practitioner ordering the test must assure that any necessary written informed consent is given, that precounseling is done before the test is taken if required by state law, that state reporting and contact tracing laws, if any, are followed and that further counseling and referral are available at the same time that the test results are disclosed to the patient.

To aid in HIV prevention efforts, the CDC revised its guidance to make HIV antibody testing routine in all health-care settings under general consent for medical care, unless the patient declines (opt-out screening), with pre-vention counseling no longer required[7]:

- Enzyme-linked immunosorbent assay (ELISA) and enzyme immunoassay (EIA). They are 99% sensitive but generate a number of false positives. They are used for rapid antibody screening tests and as the first test in the conventional test sequence.
- The more specific Western blot assay is used for confirmation.
- It is important to remember that seroconversion (positive HIV antibody test) may not occur for up to 6 months following exposure and infection.

Several HIV test technologies have been approved by the U.S. Food and Drug Administration that vary by fluid tested (whole blood, serum, plasma, oral fluids, and urine) and time required to run the test (conventional vs. rapid tests). Testing options facilitate access to testing and increase acceptability of testing.

The OraQuick ADVANCE® Rapid HIV-1/2 antibody test (OraSure Technologies, Inc., Bethlehem, PA) is a way to measure HIV-antibody response in oral mucosal exudate in 20 minutes and can be used in the dental office. See Fig. 11.1.

CD4+ Lymphocyte Counts

Normal range: 600–1600 cells/μL of blood; median: 1000 cells/μL:

- This is the most widely available marker of immune system competence in the patient with HIV/AIDS.[8]
- It is an excellent predictor of pending risk of HIV-associated opportunistic infection, disease progression, and survival in clinical trials and cohort studies.
- This guides the prophylactic use of antimicrobial medications to prevent the appearance of HIV opportunistic infections.
- Initial immune suppression (CD4 < 500 cells/μL) signals the first appearance of systemic and oral opportunistic infections.
- Severe immune suppression (CD4 < 200 cells/μL) predisposes patients to life-threatening infections (e.g., toxoplasmosis and cryptococcosis).
- CD4+ counts may be obtained every 6–12 months or more frequently if a patient is altering the ART regimen or has new clinical signs or symptoms.

HIV Viral Load

Dynamic range <40 to >750,000 copies/mL:

- This is the most widely available marker of viral replication in the HIV-positive individual.[8]
- It is most commonly assessed by a reverse transcriptase-initiated polymerase chain reaction (RT-PCR) technique to determine the number of copies of HIV ribonucleic acid (RNA) in the peripheral blood.

Figure 11.1 (a) Test swab; (b) test results. OraQuick ADVANCE Rapid HIV-1/2 antibody test (OraSure Technologies, Inc.).

- It is an excellent predictor of pending risk of CD4+ cell decline over a 3- to 4-month period and thus, HIV-associated opportunistic infections.
- This guides the selection and modification of ART regimens with achieving and maintaining an undetectable viral load (e.g., HIV RNA < 40 copies/μL) as the goal.
- It is obtained at baseline prior to initiating ART, 4 weeks after treatment initiation or regimen change, and reassessed every 3–4 months (or whenever a CD4+ cell count is obtained).

Hematology

In patients who are HIV positive, routine hematological tests are often assessed, which include

- total white blood cell count;
- differential white blood cell count, including absolute neutrophil count (ANC);
- hematocrit and hemoglobin;
- platelet count.

While all values may be suppressed, particularly in advanced AIDS, it is rare that the values are suppressed to critical levels that would require medical management or transfusion prior to dental surgical procedures.[9] When this is the case, the patient is likely to report thrombocytopenia or severe neutropenia on the health history.

Medical Treatment

The goals of medical treatment are to decrease the viral load, increase the patient's immune competence, and treat or prevent opportunistic infections. ART currently includes the following five drug classes:

- nucleoside/nucleotide reverse transcriptase inhibitors (NRTIs);
- non-nucleoside reverse transcriptase inhibitors (NNRTIs);
- protease inhibitors (PIs);
- entry inhibitors (chemokine coreceptor antagonists or fusion inhibitors);
- integrase inhibitors.

Currently, a standard ART regimen does not exist, and therefore, a regimen consists of a combination of drugs from different classes typically referred to as highly active antiretroviral therapy (HAART).[10] The parameters used to develop a regimen for individual patients include viral load levels and CD4+ count, and drugs are selected in combination to interfere with multiple stages of HIV replication. In an effort to identify antiretroviral drug-resistant HIV strains and to assist in drug selection, genotyping and phenotyping may be performed.

III. Dental Management

Evaluation

The HIV-infected patient should have a comprehensive dental evaluation that includes a complete radiographic examination. Particular attention should be given to detecting the presence of orofacial manifestations associated with HIV infection. The examination should be done with consideration of the patient's immunological and hematological status and general medical condition.

Dental Treatment Modifications

With these key questions answered and appropriate modifications taken, HIV-infected patients can safely receive dental care. The patient's "chief complaint" should be addressed promptly with infection eliminated and preventive habits established. Maintaining gingival and periodontal health may help to prevent the rapid forms of periodontal destruction that may occur with

Key questions to ask the patient

- What medications are you currently taking?
- When were you last tested for CD4+ count and viral load? Do you know the results?
- When were you last tested for TB and what was the result? If positive, did you take preventive medications and for how long?
- Do you have any drug allergies, for example, itching, swelling, or breathing problems, after taking medicines?
- Have you had or do you have hepatitis B or C or liver cirrhosis?
- Have you had any bleeding problems?
- Has your physician ever told you that you had endocarditis?
- Do you currently smoke, drink alcohol, or use recreational drugs?
- Do you have a prosthetic joint?
- Are there any other medical problems for which you are currently being evaluated or treated, for example, hypertension, diabetes, or coronary artery disease?

Key questions to ask the physician

- What medications is the patient taking and do you feel the patient is adherent to the recommended drug regimen?
- What is the latest CD4+ count and viral load and have they been stable or rising or declining over time?
- What is the patient's current TB screening status/result?
- What is the most recent complete blood count (CBC) with differential, platelet count and additional coagulation studies if they have been done?
- Has the patient been assessed for HBV or HCV infection? If so, what was the result?
- Does the patient have a cardiac valvular prosthesis or a history of endocarditis that requires antibiotic prophylaxis?
- Does the patient have a prosthetic joint for which you recommend antibiotic prophylaxis?
- Are there any other medical concerns about the patient that you would like to share?

immune suppression. Appropriate emergency treatment should be rendered and pain relieved in all stages of the disease.

The majority of HIV-infected patients will be medically healthy, thus requiring little or no modification of dental treatment. With advanced HIV disease, timing or extent of the dental treatment plan may need to be modified according to the immunological and hematological status and general medical condition of the patient. Fatigue during prolonged procedures may be experienced by patients with significant anemia. The frequency of follow-up dental appointments should be arranged on an individualized basis in order to closely monitor oral health.

Coinfections of Concern to Dentistry

TB (See also Chapter 3)

TB is spread by airborne transmission, particularly in closed spaces, of *Mycobacterium tuberculosis*. People coinfected with HIV and TB have a substantially increased risk of developing active TB compared with the 5% early and 5% late risk for immune-competent persons without HIV infection. Longer courses of therapy and prophylaxis are recommended for HIV-infected patients with TB.

All HIV-infected persons should be given a tuberculin skin test.[11] The Mantoux skin test should be repeated annually along with anergy testing, using control allergens such as tetanus or *Candida*, because anergy is more common in individuals with reduced CD4 counts.

The dental team should be alert to possible signs and symptoms of TB including general symptoms of fatigue, malaise, weight loss, fever, and night sweats as well as pulmonary symptoms of prolonged coughing or coughing up blood. Referral to a physician for evaluation and needed treatment prior to elective dental care is recommended. Patients should not receive elective dental care until they are noninfectious. A definitive noncontagious status can be confirmed by three consecutive negative sputum cultures for acid-fast bacilli. Emergent dental care should be provided in a facility that has the capacity for airborne infection isolation and has a respiratory protection program in place.

Hepatitis B (HBV)/Hepatitis C (HCV) Virus Infection (See also Chapter 6)

Due to similar routes of transmission, there is an increased prevalence of HBV/HCV infection among those with HIV, with HCV found in approximately one-third of all HIV-infected people in the United States.[12] HBV or HCV infection may impact the course and management of HIV disease by increasing the risk of ART-induced hepatotoxicity. HIV coinfection is associated with higher HCV viral loads and a more rapid progression of HCV-related liver disease, which leads to an increased risk of cirrhosis.

Viral hepatitis that is sufficiently severe to result in liver dysfunction, will lead to altered drug metabolism and coagulopathies. Patients with significant liver disease may require additional coagulation laboratory tests such as the prothrombin time/international normalized ratio (PT/INR) and partial thromboplastin time (PTT) to assess function of the liver-dependent coagulation Factors II, VII, IX, and X, and liver function tests to gauge the ability of the liver to metabolize drugs.

Oral Lesion Diagnosis and Management

A number of oral lesions have been associated with HIV disease.[6,13] Suggested drug treatment regimens for several common or severe oral conditions are presented in Table 11.2. Oral

Table 11.2. Treatment of Oral Manifestations of HIV

Oral Manifestation	Medication: Unit Dose/Formulation	Prescribing Information
Oral candidiasis	Nystatin (Mycostatin®)	
	100,000 u/mL oral suspension	2–5 mL QID, rinse × 2 minutes and swallow for 10–14 days
	200,000 u pastille	1–2 pastilles dissolved slowly 4–5 × day for 10–14 days
	Clotrimazole (Mycelex®)	
	10 mg troche	Dissolve 1 troche in the mouth 5 × day for 10–14 days
	Ketoconazole (Nizoral®)	
	200 mg tablets	2 tablets stat, then 1 tablet QD with meal for 10–14 days
	Fluconazole (Diflucan®)	
	100 mg tablets	2 tablets stat, then 1 tablet QD for 10–14 days
	Itraconazole (Sporanox®)	
	100 mg capsules	2 capsules after meals QD for 10–14 days
	Miconazole (Oravig™)	
	50 mg buccal tablet	1 tablet applied to canine fossa QD for 14 days
Angular chelitis	Nystatin-triamcinolone acetonide (Mycolog II®) ointment	
	2% ketoconazole cream	Apply to affected areas after meals and QHS as needed
	1% clotrimazole ointment	
	2% miconazole ointment	

(Continued)

Table 11.2. (*Continued*)

Oral Manifestation	Medication: Unit Dose/Formulation	Prescribing Information

Recurrent herpes simplex virus infection	Acyclovir (Zovirax®)
	  200 mg tablet
	Valacyclovir (Valtrex®)
	  500 mg caplet
		1–3 tablets 5 × day for 10 days
		
		2 caplets TID for 10 days

Herpes zoster (shingles)	Acyclovir (Zovirax®)
	  800 mg tablet
	Valacyclovir (Valtrex®)
	  500 mg caplet
	Famciclovir (Famvir®)
	  125 mg tablet
		1 tablet 5 × day for 10 days
		
		2 caplets TID for 10 days
		
		4 tablets TID for 10 days

Linear gingival erythema	Chlorhexidine (Peridex®, Periogard®) 0.12% oral rinse	½ ounce BID rinse × 30 seconds and spit for 14 days

Necrotizing ulcerative periodontitis	Chlorhexidine (Peridex®, Periogard®)
	  0.12% oral rinse
	
	Metronidazole (Flagyl®)
	  250–500 mg tablet
	Clindamycin (Cleocin®)
	  150 mg capsule
	Amoxicillin/clavulanate (Augmentin®)
	  250–500 mg capsule
		½ ounce BID rinse × 30 seconds and spit for 14 days
		
		1 tablet QID for 7 days
		
		1 capsule QID for 7 days
		
		1 capsule TID for 7 days

Major aphthous ulcers	Fluocinonide (Lidex®)
	  0.05% ointment mixed 50–50 with Orabase®
	Clobetasol proprionate (Temovate®)
	  0.05% ointment mixed 50–50 with Orabase®
	Triamcinalone acetonide (Kenalog®)
	  3 mg/mL intralesional injection
	Dexamethasone (Decadron®)
	  Elixir 0.5 mg/5 mL
	
	Prednisone (Deltasone®)
	  20 mg tablet
	Thalidomide (Thalomid®)
	  100 mg tablet
		Apply coat to ulcer QID for 7–14 days
		
		Apply coat to ulcer QID for 7–14 days
		
		1.3-mL injection every third day for 12 days
		
		5-mL oral rinse and spit 3–4 × day OR 15-mL oral rinse and swallow QID for 7 days
		
		1 tablet TID for 7 days
		
		2 tablet BID for 5 days, then 2 tablet QD for 9 days

u, unit; mg, milligram; mL, milliliter; QD, once daily; QHS, at bedtime; BID, twice daily; TID, three times daily; QID, four times daily.

Figure 11.2 Pseudomembraneous candidiasis of the (a) buccal mucosa, (b) palate and (c) ventral tongue.

candidiasis is the most frequently occurring oral manifestation of HIV. It indicates an increased risk of HIV disease progression and is associated with reduced CD4+ counts. Oral hairy leukoplakia is considered the second most common oral lesion among HIV-seropositive adults. Prevalence of oral lesions associated with HIV varies across study population, with most HIV-infected adults having oral candidiasis and/or hairy leukoplakia at some point during the course of disease progression. Among HIV-infected children, oral candidiasis, aphthous stomatitis, parotid gland enlargement, and linear gingival erythema may occur. The use of HAART has improved the immune competence of individuals with HIV and thus decreased the prevalence of most oral mucosal diseases.

Candidiasis

Candidiasis in HIV-infected patients typically presents as one of three forms: (1) the white, removable, curd-like plaques of pseudomembranous candidiasis (commonly referred to as "thrush") as shown in Fig. 11.2; (2) the red atropic areas of erythematous candidiasis, as shown in Fig. 11.3; or (3) the radiating fissures from the corners of the mouth characteristic of angular cheilitis. Combinations of these may also be seen in a patient at a given time. Oral candidiasis may place the significantly immune-suppressed patient at increased risk for the

Figure 11.3 Erythematous candidiasis of the palate.

AIDS defining condition of esophageal candidiasis that presents with the additional symptoms of pain on swallowing and occasional substernal chest pain.

Management of candidiasis typically involves topical treatment with either clotrimazole oral troches or nystatin formulations until CD4+ counts fall below 150–200 cells/μL. For systemic antifungal treatment or prevention of frequent recurrences, fluconazole is the most often prescribed and clinically effective drug. Itraconazole may be an effective alternative among patients with severe immune suppression and oral candidiasis resistant to fluconazole. Candidal infections should be treated for 10–14 days, and therapy should be continued

Figure 11.4 Oral hairy leukoplakia of the left tongue.

Figure 11.5 Nodular Kaposi's sarcoma of the palate.

for 2–3 days after the disappearance of clinical signs. Tobacco smoking may exacerbate candidal recurrences and tobacco cessation efforts should be encouraged.

Hairy Leukoplakia

Oral hairy leukoplakia, typically characterized by asymptomatic, white, vertically corrugated, hyperkeratotic patches on the lateral border of the tongue as shown in Fig. 11.4, almost always indicates HIV seropositivity. It may be an important finding as it is a marker of immune suppression, higher viral load, and HIV disease progression. Caused by the Epstein–Barr virus, it naturally undergoes periods of exacerbation and remission, and treatment of the viral source is rarely needed. Because hairy leukoplakia may be superinfected with *Candida* and can resemble candidiasis, a trial of antifungal therapy may be helpful if symptoms of burning are reported. Epidemiologically, it is more common among MSM.

Kaposi's Sarcoma

Kaposi's sarcoma appears as red, bluish, or purplish macular or nodular lesions that do not blanche with compression, most often occurring on the palate or gingiva, as shown in Fig. 11.5. The lesions are frequently asymptomatic until they enlarge or ulcerate. This indolent, vascular, mucocutaneous neoplasm may erode alveolar bone causing tooth mobility. Human herpesvirus-8 (Kaposi's sarcoma-associated herpesvirus) has been identified as the etiological agent. Kaposi's sarcoma is seen almost exclusively among MSM and has dramatically decreased in occurrence in the last 10 years. In an HIV-positive patient, Kaposi's sarcoma establishes a diagnosis of AIDS. Biopsy of a suspicious lesion may be indicated to confirm a clinical impression and help plan therapy for the lesion. The patient's physician should be made aware of biopsy results.

Treatment depends on the location, size, severity of symptoms, and number of lesions present. Low-dose radiation therapy, surgical excision, and intralesional injection with vinblastine or sodium tetradecyl sulfate have been used for palliative treatment for painful advanced lesions that may interfere with normal function.

Oral Warts (Condyloma Acuminatum)

Oral warts are caused by the human papillomavirus (HPV) and may be sexually transmitted.

Figure 11.6 Oral wart on (a) the tongue and (b) lower lip.

When they occur in the mouth, they are often present on other mucocutaneous surfaces. Oral warts vary in appearance from white- to pink-colored papules to nodules with a smooth, raised, papillary or cauliflower-like surface as shown in Fig. 11.6. Evaluation for removal is recommended when they interfere with function or are of esthetic concern. All forms of treatment result in a high recurrence or reinfection rate. Surgical removal, topical application of 25% podophyllin solution in a tincture of benzoin, 0.5% podophyllotoxin, or interferon injections may be used.

HIV-Associated Periodontal Diseases

Linear gingival erythema presents as a fiery red gingival margin, with absence of significant accumulation of plaque.

Necrotizing ulcerative gingivitis presents as rapid localized destruction of the gingiva and is characterized by punched out interdental papillae as shown in Fig. 11.7. Affected patients are usually refractory to conventional therapy and may have mild pain and occasional bleeding.

Necrotizing ulcerative periodontitis resembles in some respects, acute necrotizing ulcerative gingivitis (ANUG) superimposed on rapidly

Figure 11.7 Necrotizing ulcerative gingivitis (maxillary arch) and necrotizing ulcerative periodontitis (mandibular arch).

progressive periodontitis. However, in contrast to ANUG, these patients complain of spontaneous bleeding and severe, deep-seated pain, which is not readily relieved by analgesics. These atypical rapidly progressive periodontal infections should be treated as soon as possible utilizing tissue debridement, thorough scaling and root planing (when indicated), in combination with 0.12% chlorhexidine gluconate rinses or povidone iodine solution and

Figure 11.8 Herpes simplex virus infection (herpes labialis) at labial commissure.

antibiotics for acute episodes. A vigorous home care regimen with the usual oral hygiene approaches, including 0.12% chlorhexidine rinses, is recommended. Once the acute phase is under control, the patient should be followed at 1- to 2-month intervals with treatment interventions as needed.

Herpes Simplex Virus Infection

Herpes may present as orofacial vesicles and/ or ulcerations. As shown in Fig. 11.8, these round or irregular, shallow, small (<3–4 mm) painful ulcers may enlarge, become confluent and extensive, and have prolonged courses. Diagnosis can be aided by cytological examination or confirmed by viral culture in the vesicular phase. Rapid institution of antiviral therapy for recurrent herpes infections will reduce lesion severity.

Varicella Zoster Virus Infection

Zoster, commonly referred to as shingles, is caused by reactivation of latent *Varicella zoster* virus with immune compromise. It presents in a distinctly unilateral distribution as painful, itching vesicles that coalesce to form ulcers. This distribution follows one or more branches of the trigeminal nerve. While self-limiting in 10–14 days, treatment with an antiviral medication may be indicated to reduce the symptoms and duration of the lesions. In the absence of specific contraindications, consideration should be given to prescribing short-term, high-dose corticosteroid prophylaxis for postherpetic neuropathy. Adequate hydration, nutrition, and management of fever and pain are important. An ophthalmologist should evaluate patients with involvement of the ophthalmic division of the trigeminal nerve.

Recurrent Aphthous Ulcerations

HIV-positive patients may exhibit painful, intraoral, slow healing ulcers that may recur. Multifaceted approaches including hematology laboratory assessment, culture and sensitivity, cytology, and biopsy often do not produce a definitive etiological source such as herpes simplex, cytomegalovirus, severe neutropenia, or TB. Major aphthous ulcers as shown in Fig. 11.9, which may be over 6 mm in diameter, are more common with severe immune suppression.

Accessible ulcers, if few in number, may first be treated with an application of a topical steroid ointment or cream. If the ulcers are numerous and/or inaccessible, dexamethasone elixir may be swished or gargled and expectorated three to four times a day. If none of the above is effective, systemic treatment with prednisone or thalidomide may be helpful. Drug interactions, side effects, and adrenal suppression must be considered, and consultation with the patient's physician is recommended.

Xerostomia

Benign lymphoepithelial lesions of the salivary glands may occur and result in glandular enlargement and xerostomia. Use of saliva substitutes may reduce patient discomfort, especially before and during meals and at bedtime. Caffeine and alcohol should be avoided.

Figure 11.9 Major aphthous ulcers of (a) the tongue and (b) upper labial mucosa.

Chewing sugarless gum may be helpful in the removal of food debris and may stimulate salivary flow. Use of cholinergic medications may be considered. If specific medications are identified as the probable cause of the xerostomia, the dentist may discuss with the prescribing physician the possible alteration of drug, dose, or schedule to improve patient comfort and oral health. Utilization of topical fluorides may be needed for control of dental caries.

Bacterial Infections

Unusual bacterial infections sometimes occur in the oral cavity of HIV-infected patients. Treatment of these infections should be based on culture and sensitivity testing. Because of the possibility of drug resistance and interference with other medications the patient may be taking, treatment of unusual organisms or infections refractory to first-line antibiotics should be coordinated with the patient's physician.

 Risks of Dental Care

Hemostasis

The potential exists for postoperative bleeding complications resulting from dental treatment in patients with altered hemostasis. Patients with diagnosed coagulopathies such as hemophilia, other inherited coagulation disorders, liver dysfunction, or thrombocytopenia may be at increased risk. These patients should have their hemostatic function assessed, with coagulation studies, prior to invasive dental treatment. Pre- and postoperative therapy such as infusion of clotting factor concentrates, fresh frozen plasma, platelet transfusions, or other medical interventions may be needed to support oral surgical procedures.

Although up to 20% of HIV-seropositive patients demonstrate a reduction in the number of circulating platelets, it is rare that this reduction would be clinically significant for dental treatment.[9] Elective dental treatment should not be performed if the platelet count is <50,000 cells/μL.

Susceptibility to Infection

Several studies and a systematic review report no significant increase in dental treatment complications in HIV-positive patients compared with HIV-negative patients. When dental extractions result in complications, they are the typical complications and are mild and readily amenable to outpatient management.[14,15]

> **Antibiotic prophylaxis for dental treatment for HIV-infected patients**
>
> With the exception of known indications for antibiotic prophylaxis (e.g., past history of endocarditis or a prosthetic heart valve* and possibly with prosthetic joints†), antibiotic prophylaxis before dental treatment is not indicated solely because of the patient's HIV positivity. The decision to use prophylactic antibiotics depends on the concomitant medical conditions, the procedure to be performed, and the patient's degree of neutropenia (absolute neutrophil count below 500 cells/mm^3). If prophylactic antibiotics are used, consultation with the patient's physician is advisable since overgrowth of resistant microorganisms may present a significant problem.
>
> * The American Heart Association recommends antibiotic prophylaxis for the following patients:
> - prosthetic cardiac valve or prosthetic material used for cardiac valve repair;
> - previous infective endocarditis;
> - congenital heart disease (CHD) including (1) unrepaired cyanotic CHD, including palliative shunts and conduits; (2) completely repaired congenital heart defect with prosthetic material or device, whether placed by surgery or catheter intervention, during the first 6 months after the procedure; or (3) repaired CHD with residual defects at the site or adjacent to the site of a prosthetic patch, or prosthetic device (which inhibit endothelialization);
> - cardiac transplantation recipients who develop cardiac valvulopathy.
>
> † The American Dental Association and American Academy of Orthopedic Surgeons recommend consideration of antibiotic prophylaxis for patients with total joint replacements who have HIV comorbidity.

Drug Actions/Interactions

A number of drugs used to treat HIV infection or its complications have potential interactions with drugs prescribed by dentists. See Table 11.3. Before administering any medication, the dentist should check for possible interactions with medications the patient is taking. In addition, ART and some drugs used to treat opportunistic infections have adverse reactions that may have an impact on the oral cavity. These adverse reactions include oral ulcerations, erythema multiforme, cushingoid facies, parotid lipomatosis, perioral paresthesias, taste alterations, xerostomia, stomatitis, and bone marrow suppression. Of particular note, patients with HIV disease may also be prescribed antidepressants, with resultant drug-induced xerostomia placing them at increased risk of dental caries and mucosal candidal infection.

Many of the PIs and the NNRTIs interfere with cytochrome P450 CYP3A drug-metabolizing enzymes in the liver, consequently altering the metabolism of benzodiazepines that are frequently used in conscious sedation techniques and creating precautions for use of macrolide antibiotics.

Individuals who are currently using cocaine or crack cocaine should not receive dental treatment within 6 hours of last drug use since during this time, they are at increased risk of myocardial ischemia and cardiac arrhythmias. Use of epinephrine-containing local anesthetics following cocaine administration is not recommended because cocaine potentiates the response of sympathetically innervated organs to epinephrine, which could result in a hypertensive crisis, myocardial infarction, or cerebral vascular accident.

Patient's Ability to Tolerate Dental Care

In general, patients with HIV/AIDS are able to tolerate outpatient dental care well and are at

Table 11.3. Antiretriviral Drugs and Interactions/Precautions for Drug Prescribing in Dentistry[a] and Drug Toxicities of Concern for Dental Practice (Resource: Lexi-Comp Online, Accessed December 26, 2011)

Antiretroviral Drugs Brand Name (Generic)[a]	Interactions and Precautions for Drug Prescribing in Dental Practice	Drug Toxicities of Concern for Dental Practice
Nucleoside/nucleotide reverse transcriptase inhibitors (NRTIs)		
Combivir® zidovudine + lamivudine	See Retrovir®	See Retrovir® and Epivir®
Emtriva® emtricitabine	n/a	Hyperpigmentation
Epivir® lamivudine (3TC)	n/a	Neutropenia, thrombocytopenia
Epzicom® abacavir + lamivudine	n/a	See Epivir® and Ziagen®
Retrovir® zidovudine (AZT)	Coadministration with clarithromycin enhances myelosuppressive effect and decreases zidovudine concentration; fluconazole may decrease the metabolism of zidovudine	Anemia, neutropenia, oral mucosal pigmentation, taste perversion, dysphagia, oral ulcers
Trizavir® abacavir + zidovudine + lamivudine	See Retrovir®	See Retrovir®, Epivir®, and Ziagen®
Truvada® tenofovir DF + emtricitabine	See Viread®	See Emtriva® and Viread®
Videx® didanosine (ddI)	Nonenteric coated didanosine may decrease the absorption of azole antifungals	Xerostomia, peripheral neuropathy
Viread® tenofovir (TNF)	Avoid acyclovir and valacyclovir that decrease excretion of tenofovir	n/a
Zerit® stavudine (d4T)	n/a	Peripheral neuropathy, exacerbates bone marrow suppression
Ziagen® abacavir (ABC)	n/a	Oral ulceration, erythema multiforme, paresthesias
Protease inhibitors		
Agenerase® amprenavir (APV)	*Benzodiazepine precaution, azole antifungal precaution, macrolide antibiotic precaution,* avoid dexamethasone that decreases amprenavir effect, avoid metronidazole with amprenavir oral solution at risk of propylene glycol toxicity	n/a

(Continued)

Table 11.3. (*Continued*)

Antiretroviral Drugs Brand Name (Generic)[a]	Interactions and Precautions for Drug Prescribing in Dental Practice	Drug Toxicities of Concern for Dental Practice
Aptivus® tipranavir (TPV)	*Benzodiazepine precaution, azole antifungal precaution, macrolide antibiotic precaution*	Increased bleeding in hemophiliacs, may impair platelet aggregation and increase bleeding risk
Crixivan® indinavir (IDV)	*Benzodiazepine precaution, azole antifungal precaution, macrolide antibiotic precaution, may increase concentration of fentanyl*	Increased bleedng in hemophiliacs, anemia
Invirase® saquinavir (SQV)	*Benzodiazepine precaution, azole antifungal precaution, macrolide antibiotic precaution*	Increased bleedng in hemophiliacs, taste alteration, oral ulceration, dysphagia, neutropenia, thrombocytopenia, anemia
Kaletra® lopinavir + ritonavir (LPV/RTV)	See Norvir® and *benzodiazepine precaution*; increases levels of clarithromycin, ketoconazole, and itraconazole; decreases level of voriconazole; diminishes therapeutic effect of tramadol; metronidazole may interact with alcohol in Kaletra® oral solution	See Norvir® and increased bleeding in hemophiliacs, neutropenia, ulcerative stomatitis, xerostomia, facial edema
Lexiva® fosamprenavir (FPV)	*Benzodiazepine precaution, azole antifungal precaution, macrolide antibiotic precaution, may enhance the toxic effect of meperidine*	Increased bleeding in hemophiliacs, cushingoid appearance, erythema multiforme, neutropenia, hemolytic anemia
Norvir® ritonavir (RTV)	*Benzodiazepine precaution*; avoid meperidine, propoxyphene, piroxicam; ketoconazole increases ritonavir levels; clarithromycin and erythromycin reduce ritonavir levels; ritonavir may increase levels of prednisone; metronidazole may enhance adverse effects of ritonavir	Increased bleeding in hemophiliacs, may cause cushingoid appearance, paresthesias, taste perversion, parotid lipomatosis
Reyataz® atazanavir (ATV)	*Benzodiazepine precaution, azole antifungal precaution, macrolide antibiotic precaution*, increases serum concentration of fentanyl, may enhance the toxic effect of meperidine	Increased bleeding in hemophiliacs, may cause cushingoid appearance, erythema multiforme, neutropenia, anemia, thrombocytopenia

Table 11.3. (Continued)

Antiretroviral Drugs Brand Name (Generic)[a]	Interactions and Precautions for Drug Prescribing in Dental Practice	Drug Toxicities of Concern for Dental Practice
Prezista® darunavir (DRV)	*Benzodiazepine precaution, azole antifungal precaution, macrolide antibiotic precaution,* darunavir may increase the serum concentration of topical lidocaine, may enhance the toxic effect of meperidine	Increased bleeding in hemophiliacs, may cause cushingoid appearance, erythema multiforme, oral lesions, facial edema, osteonecrosis, pancytopenia, paresthesias, xerostomia
Viracept® nelfinavir (NFV)	*Benzodiazepine precaution, azole antifungal precaution, macrolide antibiotic precaution,* increases the serum concentration of fentanyl, may enhance the toxic effect of meperidine	Increased bleeding in hemophiliacs, may cause cushingoid appearance, neutropenia, thrombocytopenia, anemia, paresthesias, mouth ulcers
Non-nucleoside reverse transcriptase inhibitors (NNRTIs)		
Complera™ rilpivirine + tenofovir DF + emtricitabine	See Truvada® and Edurant™	See Truvada® and Edurant™
Edurant™ rilpivirine	Avoid dexamethasone that decreases rilipivirine effect and decrease dexamethasone effect; concomitant use with ketoconazole, fluconazole, or itraconazole reduces azole concentration and elevates rilpivirine concentration; avoid erythromycin and clarithromycin	n/a
Intelence® etravirine	May decrease serum concentration of itraconazole and ketoconazole, may increase serum concentration of voriconazole, decreases serum concentration of clarithromycin	May cause cushingoid appearance, erythema multiforme, anemia, paresthesias, stomatitis, xerostomia
Rescriptor® delavirdine	May increase serum concentration of fentanyl, may diminish therapeutic effect of tramadol	May cause cushingoid appearance, erythema multiforme, anemia, thrombocytopenia, pancytopenia, mouth ulcers, gum hemorrhage

(Continued)

Table 11.3. *(Continued)*

Antiretroviral Drugs Brand Name (Generic)[a]	Interactions and Precautions for Drug Prescribing in Dental Practice	Drug Toxicities of Concern for Dental Practice
Sustiva® efavirenz	*Benzodiazepine precaution*, may increase serum concentration of fentanyl, decreased concentration of itraconazole and voriconazole, voriconazole may increase efavirenz concentration	May cause cushingoid appearance, abnormal taste, erythema multiforme, paresthesias, neutropenia
Viramune® nevirapine	Decreased concentration of voriconazole, voriconazole may increase nevirapine concentration	Oral ulceration, erythema multiforme
Entry inhibitors		
Fuzeon® enfuviritide (ENF, T-20)	n/a	Neutropenia, thrombocytopenia, xerostomia, taste disturbance
Selzentry® maraviroc	Avoid ketoconazole, itraconazole, clarithromycin	Neutropenia, anemia, herpes exacerbation, stomatitis, osteonecrosis
Integrase inhibitor		
Isentress® raltegravir	n/a	Neutropenia, thrombocytopenia, facial wasting

[a] This list is constantly changing with new medications and new drug interactions and toxicities reported. The dentist should consult with a contemporary electronic drug interaction program, pharmacist, or the treating physician before prescribing drugs. *Benzodiazepine precaution*, avoid midazolam, triazolam, diazepam, and/or alprazolam: at risk for increased and prolonged sedation and respiratory depression; *azole antifungal precaution*, concomitant administration with azole antifungals increases levels of both drugs; *macrolide antibiotic precaution*, concomitant administration with macrolide antibiotics (erythromycin, azithromycin, and/or clarithromycin) increases serum concentration of both drugs and decreases antibiotic effectiveness; n/a, not applicable.

no greater risk of medical emergencies in the dental office than individuals without HIV/AIDS.

Special Considerations

Infection Control

Patients with HIV/AIDS can be managed in traditional dental settings using the infection control measures recommended by the CDC.[16]

Occupational Exposures to HIV

All health-care facilities should have a written blood-borne pathogen policy that includes management of exposures. As shown in Table 11.4, the U.S. Public Health Service has published updated recommendations for the management of health-care personnel occupational exposures to blood and other body fluids that might contain HBV, HCV, or HIV[17] and for postexposure prophylaxis (PEP).[18] Dental care personnel who sustain an exposure incident (defined as specific

Table 11.4. Management of Occupational Blood Exposures[11]

Provide immediate care to the exposure site	Wash wounds and skin with soap and water Flush mucous membranes with water
Reporting of exposure	Access to medical provider for testing Access to postexposure protocol Documentation for workers' compensation or disability claims
Determine risk associated with exposure by:	Type of fluid (e.g., blood, visibly bloody fluid, other potentially infectious fluid or tissue, and concentrated virus) Type of exposure (i.e., percutaneous injury, mucous membrane or nonintact skin exposure, and bites resulting in blood exposure)
Evaluate exposure source	Assess the risk of infection using available information Test known sources for HBsAg, anti-HCV, and HIV antibody (consider using rapid testing) For unknown sources, assess risk of exposure to HBV, HCV, or HIV infection Do not test discarded needles or syringes for virus contamination
Evaluate exposed person	Assess immune status for HBV infection (i.e., by history of HBV vaccination and vaccine response)
Give PEP for exposures posing risk of infection transmission.	HBV—If source patient HBsAg+ or unknown, check HBsAb status of exposed. If exposed is unvaccinated or nonresponder (<10 mIU/mL): HBIGx1 and initiate hepatitis B (HB) vaccination. HCV—PEP not recommended HIV—PEP recommendations depend on HIV disease severity of source patient and severity of occupational injury. Initiate PEP as soon as possible, preferably within hours of exposure. Offer pregnancy testing to all women of childbearing age not known to be pregnant. Seek expert consultation if viral resistance is suspected. Administer PEP for 4 weeks if tolerated.
Perform follow-up testing and provide counseling.	Advise exposed persons to seek medical evaluation for any acute illness occurring during follow-up.
HBV exposures	Perform follow-up HBsAb testing in persons who receive HBV vaccine. Test for anti-HBs 1–2 months after last dose of vaccine. HBsAb response to vaccine cannot be ascertained if HBIG was received in the previous 3–4 months.
HCV exposures	Perform baseline and follow-up testing for anti-HCV and ALT 4–6 months after exposure. Perform HCV RNA at 4–6 weeks if earlier diagnosis of HCV infection is desired. Confirm repeatedly reactive anti-HCV EIAs with supplemental tests.
HIV exposures	Perform HIV antibody testing for at least 6 months postexposure (e.g., at baseline, 6 weeks, 3 months, and 6 months). Perform HIV antibody testing if illness compatible with an acute retroviral syndrome occurs. Advise exposed person to use precautions to prevent secondary transmission during the follow-up period. Evaluate exposed person taking PEP within 72 hours after exposure to monitor for drug toxicity for at least 2 weeks.

ALT, alanine amino-transferase; EIAs, enzyme immunoassays; HBIG, hepatitis B immunoglobulin; HBsAg, hepatitis B surface antigen; HBsAb, hepatitis B surface antibody; HBV, hepatitis B virus; HIV, human immunodeficiency virus; anti-HCV, hepatitis C antibody; HCV RNA, hepatitis C virus ribonucleic acid (HCV viral load); PEP, postexposure prophylaxis.

eye, mouth, other mucous membrane, nonintact skin, or parenteral contact with blood or other potentially infectious materials that results from the performance of an employee's duties) should immediately consult a physician for follow-up evaluation and possible HIV PEP with antiretroviral medications. The question of HBV and HCV exposure should also be addressed. Dental health-care workers should be vaccinated against HBV.

It is primarily through contact with blood that the dentist or dental personnel could be at risk for becoming infected coincidental to providing dental treatment. Such risk is, however, extremely low. The average risk of HIV transmission after a percutaneous exposure to HIV-infected blood has been estimated to be approximately 0.3% (95% confidence interval [CI] = 0.2–0.5%) (this represents 3/1000 HIV-contaminated sharps injuries) and after a mucous membrane exposure, approximately 0.09% (95% CI = 0.006–0.5%).[16,17] While saliva itself has not been shown to be a vehicle of HIV transmission, saliva in dentistry is considered to be contaminated with blood and is a potentially infectious material. For comparison purposes, the risks of seroconversion from HBV- and HCV-contaminated percutaneous injuries are 23–37% and 1.8%, respectively.[16,17]

None of the 57 U.S. health-care workers who have voluntarily reported to the CDC with documented HIV seroconversion temporally associated with an occupational HIV exposure were dental care providers.[19] Fortunately, the quantity of blood exposure and depth of injury in dental settings is usually limited.

Epidemiological and laboratory studies suggest that several factors might affect the risk of HIV transmission after an occupational exposure[19,20]:

- exposure to a larger quantity of blood from the source person as indicated by a device visibly contaminated with the patient's blood;
- a procedure that involved a needle being placed directly in a vein or artery, or a deep injury;
- a source patient had terminal illness possibly reflecting either the higher plasma viral load with advanced AIDS or other viral characteristics such as the presence of syncytia-inducing strains of HIV in long-term HIV disease.

In a sentinel case-control study of health-care workers, HIV seroconversion was decreased fivefold with the use of 28 days of zidovudine PEP.[20] The CDC guidelines for the management of occupational exposures to HIV and recommendations for PEP, consider the infection status of the source patient, the volume of exposure, and ART drug toxicities.[17,18] Adverse symptoms, such as nausea and diarrhea, are common with PEP; however, side effects can often be managed by prescribing antimotility or antiemetic agents. For most HIV exposures that warrant PEP, a basic 4-week, two-drug (there are several options) regimen is recommended. A three-drug regimen may be recommended for HIV exposures that pose an increased risk of transmission (based on the infection status of the source and the type of exposure). Occupational exposures should be considered urgent medical concerns.

Patient Education

HIV-infected patients should be told about the necessity of dental treatment, with particular emphasis on the possibility of acceleration of oral disease if they are immune compromised. Patients or their caregivers may be taught to perform periodic orofacial examinations and be encouraged to contact the dentist whenever signs and/or symptoms of HIV-associated oral diseases occur.

While no case of HIV transmission through casual contact has been documented, patients should be advised not to share blood-contaminated devices such as toothbrushes.

Ethics and Professional Conduct

Advisory Opinions 1.B.2 Confidentiality of Patient Records and 4.A.1. Patients with

> **ADA principles of ethics and code of professional conduct**
>
> **Section 1. Principle: Patient Autonomy ("self-governance")**
> **Advisory Opinion 1.B.2. Confidentiality of Patient Records.**
>
> The dominant theme in Code Section I-B is the protection of the confidentiality of a patient's records. The statement in this section that relevant information in the records should be released to another dental practitioner assumes that the dentist requesting the information is the patient's present dentist. There may be circumstances where the former dentist has an ethical obligation to inform the present dentist of certain facts. Code Section 1.B. assumes that the dentist releasing relevant information is acting in accordance with applicable law. Dentists should be aware that the laws of the various jurisdictions in the U.S. are not uniform, and some confidentiality laws appear to prohibit the transfer of pertinent information, such as HIV seropositivity. Absent certain knowledge that the laws of the dentist's jurisdiction permit the forwarding of this information, a dentist should obtain the patient's written permission before forwarding health records which contain information of a sensitive nature, such as HIV seropositivity, chemical dependency or sexual preference. If it is necessary for a treating dentist to consult with another dentist or physician with respect to the patient, and the circumstances do not permit the patient to remain anonymous, the treating dentist should seek the permission of the patient prior to the release of data from the patient's records to the consulting practitioner. If the patient refuses, the treating dentist should then contemplate obtaining legal advice regarding the termination of the dentist-patient relationship.
>
> **Section 4. Principle: Justice**
> **Advisory Opinion 4.A.1. Patients with Bloodborne Pathogens.**
>
> A dentist has the general obligation to provide care to those in need. A decision not to provide treatment to an individual because the individual is infected with HIV, HBV, HCV or another bloodborne pathogen, based solely on that fact, is unethical. Decisions with regard to the type of dental treatment provided or referrals made or suggested should be made on the same basis as they are made with other patients. As is the case with all patients, the individual dentist should determine if he or she has the need of another's skills, knowledge, equipment or experience. The dentist should also determine, after consultation with the patient's physician, if appropriate, if the patient's health status would be significantly compromised by the provision of dental treatment.

Bloodborne Pathogens from *ADA Principles of Ethics and Code of Professional Conduct* provide ethical guidance.

IV. Recommended Readings and Cited References

Recommended Readings

Kaplan JE, Benson C, Holmes KH, Brooks JT, Pau A, Masur H, et al. Guidelines for prevention and treatment of opportunistic infections in HIV-infected adults and adolescents recommendations from CDC, the National Institutes of Health, and the HIV Medicine Association of the Infectious Diseases Society of America. MMWR Recomm Rep 2009;58(RR-4):1–207.

The National Clinician's Post-Exposure Prophylaxis Hotline. 2010. The Regents of the University of California. PEPline. Available at: http://www.ucsf.edu/hivcntr/Hotlines/PEPline

Shiboski CH, Patton LL, Webster-Cyriaque JY, Greenspan D, Traboulsi RS, Ghannoum M, et al. The Oral HIV/AIDS Research Alliance: updated case definitions of oral disease endpoints. J Oral Pathol Med 2009;38(6):481–8.

Cited References

1. Schneider E, Whitmore S, Glynn KM, Dominguez K, Mitsch A, McKenna MT, et al. Revised surveillance

case definitions for HIV infection among adults, adolescents, and children aged <18 months and for HIV infection and AIDS among children aged 18 months to <13 years—United States, 2008. MMWR Recomm Rep 2008;57(RR-10): 1–8. Available at: http://www.cdc.gov/mmwr/preview/mmwrhtml/rr5710a1.htm. Accessed December 26, 2011.
2. Centers for Disease Control. 1993 revised classification system for HIV infection and expanded surveillance case definition among adolescents and adults. MMWR Recomm Rep 1992;41(RR-17): 1–19.
3. Center for Disease Control and Prevention. Thirty years of HIV—1981–2001. MMWR Morb Mortal Wkly Rep 2011;60(21):689.
4. Centers for Disease Control and Prevention. HIV Surveillance Report. 2009; vol. 21. Available at: http://www.cdc.gov/hiv/surveillance/resources/reports/2009report/index.htm. Accessed December 26, 2011.
5. Aberg JA, Gallant JE, Anderson J, Oleske JM, Libman H, Currier JS, et al. Primary care guidelines for the management of persons infected with human immunodeficiency virus: recommendations of the HIV Medicine Association of the Infectious Diseases Society of America. Clin Infect Dis 2004;39(5):609–29.
6. EC-Clearinghouse on Oral Problems Related to HIV Infection, WHO Collaborating Centre on Oral Manifestations of the Immunodeficiency Virus. Classification and diagnostic criteria for oral lesions in HIV infection. J Oral Pathol Med 1993;22(7):289–91.
7. Branson BM, Handsfield HH, Lampe MA, Janssen RS, Taylor AW, Lyss SB, et al. Revised recommendations for HIV testing of adults, adolescents and pregnant women in health-care settings. MMWR Recomm Rep 2006;55(RR-14): 1–17.
8. Patton LL, Shugars DC. Immunologic and viral markers of HIV-1 disease progression: implications for dentistry. J Am Dent Assoc 1999; 130(9):1313–22.
9. Patton LL. Hematologic abnormalities among HIV-infected patients: associations of significance for dentistry. Oral Surg Oral Med Oral Pathol Oral Radiol Endod 1999;(5)88:561–7.
10. Panel on Antiretroviral Guidelines for Adults and Adolescents. Guidelines for the use of antiretroviral agents in HIV-1-infected adults and adolescents. Department of Health and Human Services. October 14, 2011; pp. 1–167. Available at: http://www.aidsinfo.nih.gov/ContentFiles/AdultandAdolescentGL.pdf. Accessed December 26, 2011.
11. Centers for Disease Control. Tuberculosis and human immunodeficiency virus infection: recommendations of the Advisory Committee for the Elimination of Tuberculosis (ACET). MMWR Morb Mortal Wkly Rep 1989;38:236–8, 243–50.
12. Sulkowski MS, Mast EE, Seeff LB, Thomas DL. Hepatitis C virus infection as an opportunistic disease in persons infected with human immunodeficiency virus. Clin Infect Dis 2000;30(Suppl. 1):S77–84.
13. Baccaglini L, Atkinson JC, Patton LL, Glick M, Ficarra G, Peterson DE. Management of oral lesions in HIV-positive patients. Oral Surg Oral Med Oral Pathol Oral Radiol Endod 2007;103(Suppl. 1):S50.e1–S50.e23.
14. Bonito AJ, Patton LL, Shugars DA, Lohr KN, Nelson JP, Bader JD, et al. Management of Dental Patients Who Are HIV-Positive. Evidence Report/Technology Assessment No. 37. AHRQ Publication No. 01-E042. 2002. Agency for Healthcare Research and Quality, Rockville, MD. Available at: http://www.ncbi.nlm.nih.gov/books/NBK33702/. Accessed December 26, 2011.
15. Patton LL, Shugars DA, Bonito AJ. A systematic review of complication risks for HIV-positive patients receiving invasive dental treatments. J Am Dent Assoc 2002;133(2):195–203.
16. Kohn WG, Collins AS, Cleveland JL, Harte JA, Eklund KJ, Malvitz DM et al. Guidelines for infection control in dental healthcare settings—2003. MMWR Recomm Rep 2003;52 (RR-17):1–61.
17. Centers for Disease Control and Prevention. Updated U.S. Public Health Service guidelines for the management of occupational exposures to HBV, HCV, and HIV and recommendations for postexposure prophylaxis. MMWR Recomm Rep 2001;50(RR-11):1–52.
18. Panlilio AL, Cardo DM, Grohskopf LA, Heneine W, Ross CS; U.S. Public Health Service. Updated U.S. Public Health Service guidelines for the management of occupational exposures to HIV

and recommendations for postexposure prophylaxis. MMWR Recomm Rep 2005;54(RR-09): 1–17.
19. Do AN, Ciesielski CA, Metler RP, Hammett TA, Li J, Fleming PL. Occupationally acquired human immunodeficiency virus (HIV) infection: national case surveillance data during 20 years of the HIV epidemic in the United States. Infect Control Hosp Epidemiol 2003;24(2):86–96.
20. Cardo DM, Culver DH, Ciesielski CA, Srivastava PU, Marcus R, Abiteboul D, et al. A case-control study of HIV seroconversion in health care workers after percutaneous exposure. N Engl J Med 1997;337(21):1485–90.

Immunological and Mucocutaneous Disease

Bassam A. Issa BDS
Michael T. Brennan DDS, MHS

I. Background

The immune system helps protect the body against foreign agents. In the case of autoimmune diseases, the immune system attacks healthy cells in the body. The conditions discussed in this chapter are considered to be of immune origin, although other etiological agents may be identified in the future. The interactions of the immune system contribute to the magnitude of the disease process. When the immune system is triggered, a cascade of humoral and cellular immune responses is initiated. In many of these diseases, antibodies against normal epithelium are found in the circulation.

Description of Diseases/ Conditions and Management

Allergy and Allergic Reactions

Allergic reactions are immune responses mediated by immunoglobulin E (IgE). These inflammatory reactions occur after repeated contact with an external antigen (*allergen*) in previously sensitized individuals. Some patients are more prone to severe and recurring reactions than others.

Contact Stomatitis

Hypersensitivity to allergens is common within the oral cavity. Allergens creating reaction of the oral mucosa include:

- foods;
- dental materials, flavoring, and other chemicals in toothpaste and mouthwashes;
- medications.

Clinical Features of Contact Stomatitis

- Oral mucosal erythema and edema.
- Gingiva with generalized uniform redness.
- Buccal mucosa might become puffy and dark red.
- Lips appear swollen, erythematous, and subject to chronic ulcerations.

The ADA Practical Guide to Patients with Medical Conditions, First Edition. Edited by Lauren L. Patton.
© 2012 American Dental Association. Published 2012 by John Wiley & Sons, Inc.

> **Classification of hypersensitivity reactions**
>
> Type I: Anaphylactic
> Type II: Cytotoxic
> Type III: Immune complex mediated
> Type IV: Cell mediated or delayed

Figure 12.1 Contact stomatitis of the maxilla due to a denture allergy.

The patient usually complains of a burning sensation and sensitivity or irritation to hot, cold, alcohol, and spicy food. An allergy to denture base material occurs when the acrylic has been incompletely cured. See Fig. 12.1.

Angioedema

Angioedema is a clinical presentation of a group of allergic conditions with different etiological pathways. Angioedema usually develops as a regional, painless swelling of the lips, cheek, or tongue. It is of a great concern when the posterior anatomical structures are involved, because the airway becomes subject to compromise. Upon cessation of contact with the allergen, the swelling subsides usually within 24–48 hours. The two forms of angioedema are acquired and hereditary:

- Acquired angioedema is the most common form and is usually the result of a recent ingestion of a medication such as penicillin, nonsteroidal anti-inflammatory drugs (NSAIDs), or angiotensin-converting enzyme (ACE) inhibitors (e.g., lisinopril).
- Hereditary angioedema is a rare form of the disease, inherited as an autosomal dominant trait. In these patients, the swelling develops after mild trauma to the area.

Orofacial Granulomatosis (OFG)

OFG is an uncommon immunologically mediated disorder characterized by persistent or recurrent soft tissue enlargement, ulceration, and a variety of other orofacial features. The chronic inflammation of OFG is often characterized by the presence of granulomas in the subepithelial tissues. Risk factors include genetics, food allergy, dental material allergy, microbial etiology, and immunological etiology.

Graft-versus-Host Disease (GVHD)

GVHD occurs mainly in recipients of allogeneic hematopoietic stem cell transplantation (HSCT) for treatment of hematological diseases. See Chapter 8. Antigenic differences between the donor and the host will lead to graft rejection unless the donor cells in the graft are given advantage over host cells. Such advantage is achieved through suppression of the host immune cells by chemotherapy with or without irradiation in order to deplete the host immune system and allow successful engraftment of donor stem cells.

Clinical Features of GVHD

Both acute (aGVHD) and chronic (cGVHD) phases of this complication develop often involving multiple organs. The phases occur after different times following transplant; however, consensus criteria define each by their clinical characteristic and pathological features rather than chronologically[1]:

- aGVHD occurs within 100 days of HSCT, but can persist beyond that time or recur. It has a relatively uniform clinical picture, classically manifested by erythematous rash, diarrhea, and/or liver involvement; generally occurs early posttransplant; and is the major cause of early mortality.
- cGVHD typically occurs beyond day 100 posttransplant and can affect almost every major organ but most commonly involves skin, oral, vaginal, and conjunctival mucosa; salivary and lacrimal glands; and the liver. Approximately 40–70% of engrafted patients surviving the initial transplant will eventually develop cGVHD, which can persist for long periods of time and require long-term management from multiple disciplines.[2]

Figure 12.2 Reticular pattern of the soft palate and uvula associated with chronic graft-versus-host disease (GVHD) in a child post-bone marrow transplant.

Risk Factors

- Prior diagnosis of aGVHD is the risk factor associated most consistently with subsequent cGVHD.
- Increasing donor and recipient age.
- Increasing (T cell) dose in the graft.
- Female donor and male recipient combination.
- Unrelated donors.
- Total body irradiation.

Clinical Similarity to Autoimmunity

In many cases, the manifestations of aGVHD and cGVHD resemble both clinically and histologically autoimmune disorders such as lichen planus (LP), Sjögren's syndrome, and systemic lupus erythematosus[1,3]:

- **Oral Findings in aGVHD**
  Mucosal erythema, ulcerations, and painful desquamative oral lesions occur often in patients undergoing immunosuppression for HSCT. However, a true clinical case definition of oral acute GVHD is lacking as several factors contribute to oral lesion development during the first few weeks following transplant.

- **Oral Findings in cGVHD**
  Classic features of oral cGVHD include lichenoid changes (see Fig. 12.2), ulcerations, salivary gland dysfunction, restricted oral opening, mucoceles, and rarely squamous cell carcinoma.

Treatment of GVHD

Multiple factors must be considered when treating a patient with oral GVHD. The clinician may need to try various treatments and possibly treatment combinations to manage oral GVHD symptoms. Pharmacotherapy for oral GVHD may be systemic, topical, or injectable. The two systemic immunosuppressive drugs used most commonly are cyclosporine and corticosteroids, either alone or in combination. Other systemic agents are also used.

Topical corticosteroids such as clobetasol or fluocinonide may be used for local management for oral cGVHD.

Vesiculobullous Conditions

Vesiculobullous diseases are a group of severe, potentially life-threatening diseases, characterized by blisters and erosions of skin and/or mucous membranes. In these conditions, autoantibodies are formed that will impact different components of the mucous membrane or skin. Based on histopathological, immunological, and clinical criteria, autoimmune bullous diseases are classified into two major groups associated with autoantibodies to desmosomal (pemphigus group) or hemidesmosomal proteins (subepidermal blistering diseases, e.g., pemphigoid diseases and epidermolysis bullosa acquisita [EBA]).

Pemphigus Group and Pemphigus Vulgaris (PV)

Pemphigus is a group of rare, potentially life-threatening autoimmune mucocutaneous diseases that are characterized by blistering that affects stratified squamous epithelium and results in cutaneous or mucosal blistering, or both. It affects less than 0.5 patients/100,000 population/year,[4] and there are several variants. PV is the main variant and the one that usually affects the mouth. The remaining of the discussion relates to PV.

Etiology and Pathogenesis of PV

- Most cases are idiopathic; isolated cases have an identifiable trigger such as diet or drugs (ACE inhibitors, NSAIDs, and some antibiotics).
- A significant number of cases show a strong genetic, as well as ethnic relationship, primarily within the Ashkenazi Jews and those of the Mediterranean descent.[5]
- The pathological process is mediated by autoantibodies that target the extracellular adhesion components, which in case of oral PV is mainly desmoglein 3.[6]

Clinical Features of PV

- The oral mucosa is usually affected at an early stage in PV.
- Blisters, which eventually lead to chronic erosions and ulcers, are seen mainly on the buccal mucosa, palate, ventral surface of the tongue, and lips. See Fig. 12.3.

Figure 12.3 Area of ulceration on the lower labial mucosa seen in a patient with pemphigus vulgaris.

- Advanced stages consist of severe desquamative or erosive gingivitis.
- Oral lesions are almost invariably followed by lesions on the skin.
- PV may be occasionally associated with other autoimmune disorders, particularly rheumatoid arthritis, lupus erythematosus, or Sjögren's syndrome.

Diagnosis of PV

- In patients with PV and active blistering, firm sliding pressure separates normal-looking epithelium (Nikolsky sign), but this is neither sensitive nor specific.
- Biopsy of the perilesional tissue with histological examination and immunostaining is crucial.
- Assay of serum antibody titers by indirect immunofluorescence may also help guide prognosis and treatment.

Treatment of PV

Treatment is initially aimed at bringing the disease under control rapidly until it is possible to reduce it gradually. Treatment is invariably with systemic corticosteroids; other treatments include cyclosporine, dapsone, tacrolimus, rituximab, and intravenous immunoglobulins in steroid-resistant PV.

Mucous Membrane Pemphigoid (MMP)

MMP is a chronic autoimmune subepithelial blistering disease. MMP can be localized or extensive and can affect both mucosal and cutaneous surfaces.[7]

Epidemiology of MMP

- Found in 2–5 per 100,000 population a year.
- Occurs twice as often in women as men.
- Primarily affects middle-aged and older adults. However, children may also be affected.

Pathogenesis of MMP

In MMP, autoantibodies attack antigen sites in the molecules connecting the epithelium to the connective tissue and prevent the linkage of molecules in the hemidesmosomes. The major antigens involved in oral MMP are believed to be BP180 and laminin 5.

Clinical Features of MMP

- MMP may arise at any mucosal site, most commonly the oral and conjunctival mucosa.
- Eighty-five percent of cases will have oral involvement without concomitant skin involvement, and it may be the only site of disease.
- Lesions usually involve the gingival, palatal, and buccal mucosa, and less over the tongue and lips.
- The gingival presentation is typically painful erythematous and tender erosions with desquamation, either spontaneously or with very minimal physical trauma, such as with toothbrushing. Often, there is an inability to maintain oral care with consequent heavy accumulation of plaque and an additional inflammatory burden from this source. Small vesicles may be observed that rupture easily, but in comparison to those of PV, are long lasting and well defined. See Fig. 12.4.
- Over time, there may be scarring at the sites of repeated vesiculobullous lesion development and healing, mainly over the posterior soft palate.

Figure 12.4 Erosive gingival lesion in a patient with mucous membrane pemphigoid.

Treatment of MMP

Management of MMP depends on the severity of the disease. Widespread disease involving the eye, throat, or skin requires the expertise of a medical specialist:

- Patients with oral lesions may be treated with topical or intralesional corticosteroids.
- Desquamative gingivitis is often managed with topical steroids in a soft occlusal splint.
- Patients with more severe symptoms may require systemic corticosteroids, dapsone, tacrolimus, or other steroid sparing drugs.
- Excellent oral hygiene to reduce the plaque is recommended.

EBA

Epidermolysis bullosa (EB) constitutes a group of diverse inherited skin conditions characterized by blistering of the cutaneous and mucous membranes. EB is classified into three major types according to the level of tissue separation within the cutaneous basement membrane zone: EB simplex, EB dystrophic, and EB junctional.[8] The other acquired type of EB is EBA, which is a cutaneous subepidermal autoimmune blistering disease that results from autoantibodies directed against collagen VII, a major component of anchoring fibrils. The remaining of the discussion relates to EBA.

Epidemiology of EBA

- EBA is a rare disease with a prevalence of approximately 0.2/million population.[9]
- There is no sex or racial predilection known.

Clinical Features of EBA

- EBA is characterized by the appearance of skin fragility and noninflammatory tense, subepidermal vesicles, and bullae that heal with scarring and milia (keratin-filled cysts).
- Lesions are usually on the upper extremities, but they may appear on any mucocutaneous surface.

Diagnosis of EBA

EBA cannot be diagnosed only by clinical findings; biopsy and immunofluorescence studies are necessary.

Treatment of EBA

Symptomatic therapy is the mainstay of the clinical management. Cases of EBA treated with cyclosporine, colchicine, photochemotherapy, and intravenous immunoglobulins found favorable responses with each treatment.[10]

Erythema Multiforme (EM)

EM is a reactive mucocutaneous disorder in a disease spectrum that is comprised of a group of acute self-limiting skin reactions, which are occasionally chronic and recurrent. Classified within this group are erythema minor (EMm), erythema major (EMM), Steven–Johnson syndrome (SJS), and toxic epidermal necrolysis (TEN).[11,12]

Etiology of EM

- EMm and EMM are often associated with a preceding herpes simplex virus (HSV) infection.

Common precipitating factors of erythema multiforme

Infections	Gastrointestinal
Herpes simplex	Crohn's disease
Mycoplasma pneumonia	Ulcerative colitis
Histoplasmosis	

Drugs	Others
Penicillin	Malignancies
Fluoroquinolones	Vaccinations
Phenytoin	
Carbamazepine	
Cephalosporins	
Digitalis	
Ibuprofen	
Naproxen	

- Typical EM lesions develop 10–14 days following the clinical manifestations of HSV infection.
- A significant immunogenetic element is also associated with the pathogenesis.
- Aside from HSV infection, a wide range of other viral, bacterial, and fungal infections has been implicated in triggering EM.
- SJS and TEN are mainly associated with drugs as risk factors (antibiotics and analgesics).

EMm

EMm is characterized clinically by cutaneous disease. Skin lesions consist of typical target (*bull's-eye*) lesions that are less than 3 cm in diameter round shape with a well-defined border that are usually present on the extensor surfaces of the extremities. The cutaneous lesions of EMm involve less than 10% of the body surface area. Nikolsky's sign is negative. Lesions last for 1–3 weeks and heal without scarring. Some patients will experience prodromal systemic symptoms such as fever and chills.

- Mucous membrane involvement in EMm is uncommon, but when present, it is usually limited to the oral cavity.

Figure 12.5 Erosive-type lesions of the lower lip seen in a patient with erythema multiforme.

- The oral lesions initially manifest with edema, erythema, and erythematous macules of the lips and buccal mucosa, followed by the development of multiple vesicles and bullae that quickly rupture and result in a pseudomembrane. See Fig. 12.5.
- The lips tend to become swollen and show bloody encrustations.

EMM

EMM spans a wide range of clinical presentations that include mucocutaneous involvement, ranging from severe EMm to mild SJS. The cutaneous involvement is usually less than 10% of body surface area, but generally more severe than EMm. Affected patients have symmetrically typical cutaneous target lesions and/or atypical and raised target lesions that heal within 1–6 weeks.[13]

- The oral mucosa is the most commonly involved mucosal surface. In EMM, oral lesions are larger than that of EMm with ulceration of all oral mucosal surfaces.
- Lesions start as erythematous macules that form vesicles. The vesicles tend to rupture and leave areas of erosions. The oral lesions usually heal without scarring.
- Affected patients may have trismus and dysphagia.

- Cervical lymphadenopathy may also be present.

SJS

SJS is a disorder characterized by sudden onset erosions of the mucous membranes (predominantly the oral mucosa and conjunctivae) together with blistering of the skin. Some still consider EMM and SJS to be the same disease. The skin lesions are atypical flat target lesions and macules rather than classic target lesions, and more widespread. Nikolsky's sign is positive.

- The buccal mucosa, palate, and vermillion border are the most commonly affected sites. Mucosal blisters rapidly form and rupture to leave irregular hemorrhagic erosions with grayish white pseudomembranes.
- The oral lesions are painful, causing dysphagia, breathing difficulties, and hypersalivation.
- The mucocutaneous lesions last for 2–6 weeks and about one-third of affected individuals have prodromal symptoms that include fever, headache, pharyngitis, and arthralgia.
- Additionally, there is a risk of scarring of mucosal lesions, unlike EMm and EMM.
- Although most cases are thought to be caused by medications, infections may also trigger SJS. Mortality rate is 10%.

TEN

TEN is clinically characterized by poorly defined erythematous macules, and by epidermal detachment that ranges from 10% to 30% of the body surface. TEN can clinically resemble second-degree superficial burns. The onset of the skin lesions (after taking the suspected causative agent) is 1–16 days. TEN usually develops suddenly and often has a poor prognosis with a mortality rate of 30–40%:

- The oral lesions resemble those of SJS.

Diagnosis of TEN

- Because the histopathological and immunopathological features are nonspecific, the diagnosis is often based on clinical presentation and the exclusion of other vesiculobullous disorders.
- The detection of intralesional HSV-DNA may be useful tests to differentiate herpes-associated EM from drug-associated EM and SJS.

Treatment of TEN

If the oral mucosa is affected, mouthwashes containing local anesthetics may help in relieving painful oral symptoms. High-potency topical steroids and short courses of systemic prednisone have been reported to be very effective in controlling lesions of EMm of non-HSV etiology. In patients with HSV-associated EMm, antiviral therapy, such as acyclovir 400 mg twice daily, has been reported to be of clinical benefit, particularly preventing recurrences. Treatment of widespread cutaneous and mucosal lesions in EMM, SJS, and TEN often necessitates a multidisciplinary systemic management.

Aphthous Stomatitis (AS)

AS represents the most common oral ulcerative condition.

Epidemiology of AS

The prevalence of AS is estimated at 1.03%.[14] Among adults, AS is more common in women, whites, nonsmokers, and people under the age of 40 years and of high socioeconomic status.[15]

Etiology and Pathogenesis of AS

The precise etiology remains unclear. Immune mechanisms appear to play an important role. A positive family history is seen in one-third of patients. Cell-mediated immunity and formation of immune complexes may also play a role

> **Aphthous stomatitis-like ulcers associated with systemic diseases**
>
> Behçet's disease
> Inflammatory bowel disease (Crohn's disease, ulcerative colitis)
> HIV
> Marshall syndrome
> Mouth and Genital Ulcers with Inflamed Cartilage (MAGIC) syndrome
> Sweet syndrome
> Reiter syndrome

in AS development. In addition, a B-lymphocyte-mediated mechanism has been implicated.

A number of nonimmunological contributing factors have been identified in AS. However, there is no strong evidence to support the causative role of these factors. These include:

- hematinic deficiencies: B_{12}, iron, and folic acid;
- microbial elements;
- environmental or behavioral factors: oral trauma, stress, or smoking cessation;
- sensitivity to food such as tomatoes, chocolates, nuts, and dairy products;
- hormonal changes related to the menstrual cycle;
- chemical compounds (sodium lauryl sulfate);
- medications (beta-blockers, nicorandil, ACE inhibitors).

Clinical Presentation of AS

- Well-demarcated, oval or round recurrent oral ulcers with a white or yellow pseudomembrane and a surrounding erythematous halo. See Fig. 12.6.
- Lesions may appear initially as red macules, but quickly form the classic ulcer.
- Most ulcers develop on freely movable non-keratinized oral mucosa. They are sometimes mistaken for HSV infection. Recurrent HSV ulcers are typically seen on nonmovable, keratinized mucosa.

Figure 12.6 Ulceration of the upper labial mucosa in a patient with recurrent aphthous stomatitis.

- AS ulcers are painful, and in severe cases, they can be disabling.
- Although sometimes prodromal symptoms such as burning sensation or focal erythema may be present, these are usually ignored by most patients until the painful ulcer develops.[14]

Classification of AS Ulcers

Ulcers are usually classified based on their size, duration, and the presence or absence of scarring after healing into minor, major, and herpetiform ulcers:

- *Minor aphthae (Mikulicz aphthae)* represent the most common variety accounting for 80–85% of AS. These ulcers are less than 1.0 cm in diameter. During an exacerbation, a single lesion or multiple concurrent lesions may appear. Each lesion lasts for 10–14 days and heals spontaneously without scarring. These ulcers are found on the nonkeratinized and movable mucosa.
- *Major aphthae (Sutton's disease)* comprise about 10–15% of cases. The onset is usually at puberty, and chronic recurrence may persist for many years.[16] These ulcers are greater than 1 cm in diameter, deeper, more painful, and may take up to 6 weeks to heal. Scarring is common. AS may compromise the patient's nutritional status.
- *Herpetiform aphthous ulcers* are the least common type. They present as crops of 1- to 3-mm ulcers that heal within 10–14 days without scarring. They may appear anywhere in the oral cavity and are commonly mistaken for HSV infection. They generally have a later age of onset than either major or minor AS.[17]

Diagnostic Tests for AS

To investigate the potential role of nutritional deficiencies, a panel of blood tests that include a complete blood count, iron, folate, and vitamin B_{12} is recommended. Additional diagnostic tests may include Tzank smear; viral, bacterial, and fungal cultures; and colonoscopy.

Treatment of AS

The diagnosis, clinical presentation, severity of AS, and the presence or absence of extraoral lesions is important to determine the selection of treatment. Educating patients about the benign nature of AS and the importance of stress reduction and elimination of trauma is advised. Patients are encouraged to avoid foods that may trigger or prolong the eruption of new aphthae.

Topical corticosteroid agents such as triamcinolone acetonide with Orabase®, fluocinonide 0.05%, or clobetasol propionate 0.05% are the first choice of treatment for minor and herpetiform aphthae. Systemic treatment in severe cases may be necessary. A variety of medications have shown to be effective each with potential adverse effects. Oral prednisone, colchicine, dapsone, pentoxifylline, and thalidomide are some examples.

Behçet's Disease (BD)

BD is a systemic vasculitis characterized by recurrent oral and genital ulcers, cutaneous lesions, ocular, gastrointestinal, and neurological manifestations. It was recognized as a syndrome by Dr. Hulushi Behçet, a Turkish physician, in 1937.

Epidemiology of BD

BD is prevalent along the Silk Road, an ancient trading route between the Mediterranean and East Asia. The prevalence is highest in Turkey (420 per 100,000 population), and less than 1 per 100,000 in the United Kingdom and the United States.[18]

Etiology and Pathogenesis of BD

The etiology of BD is unknown, but the most widely accepted theory is that an environmental, hemostatic, or immunological stimulus elicits an abnormal immune response in a genetically susceptible host.

Diagnosis of BD

BD is a clinical diagnosis without any specific laboratory test. The International Study Group for BD proposed the criteria for the diagnosis of the condition in 1990.[19]

Clinical Features of BD

Mucocutaneous features are the most common presenting symptoms of the disease, while eye, vascular, and neurological elements are the most serious:

- Oral ulcers manifest as aphthous ulcers. See Fig. 12.7.
- Genital ulcers.

> **International Study Group Diagnostic Criteria for Behçet's Disease, 1990**
>
> Recurrent oral ulceration *plus two of the following*:
> - recurrent genital ulceration
> - eye lesions
> - skin lesions
> - positive pathergy test

- Cutaneous lesions: papulopustular lesions, acneform lesions, and erythema nodosum.
- Ocular disease: usually bilateral, common, and severe in men, and can vary from a gritty sensation and blurring of vision to severe pain and blindness.
- Musculoskeletal: arthralgia or arthritis.
- Cardiovascular: superficial thrombophlebitis, deep venous thrombosis, arterial obstruction, and aneurysms.
- Gastrointestinal: mucosal ulcers, abdominal pain, and diarrhea.
- Central nervous system: acute or subacute brainstem syndrome, and headaches.

Treatment and Prognosis of BD

The goal of the treatment is to prevent irreversible organ damage. Management is tailored to the type and severity of symptoms, and to the sex and age of the patient. Young or male patients usually have more severe manifestations. Mucocutaneous disease is usually treated with topical agents, particularly topical corticosteroids. However, when attacks are frequent or severe, systemic therapy with colchicine, pentoxifylline and dapsone may be useful. In refractory cases, thalidomide, azathioprine, tumor necrosis factor antagonists may be necessary.[20]

Figure 12.7 Areas of ulcerations involving the palate in a 16-year-old male with Behçet's disease.

Lichen Planus (LP)

LP is a chronic autoimmune systemic disease that commonly involves the mucosa of the oral cavity, but can involve other sites, including the skin, the vaginal mucosa, the nails, and the scalp (resulting in alopecia). The reported prevalence rates of oral LP vary from 0.5% to 2.2% of the population. The typical age of presentation is between 30 and 60 years, and it is more common in women.[21]

Etiology/Pathogenesis of LP

- Despite recent advances in understanding the immunopathogenesis of oral LP, the initial triggers of lesion formation and the essential pathogenic pathways are unknown.
- Allergic reactions, stress or anxiety, and viral infections especially hepatitis C infection have a controversial role.

Clinical Features of LP

LP commonly affects the oral mucosa, usually in the absence of skin lesions. Mucosal lesions are multiple and almost always have a bilateral distribution. They commonly take the form of white papules that gradually enlarge and coalesce to form either a reticular or a plaque-like pattern. A characteristic feature is the presence of white lines (*Wickham's striae*) radiating from the papules. In the reticular form, there is a lace-like network of raised white lines. See Fig. 12.8. The plaque-like form resembles leukoplakia. In some patients, the lesions are erythematous or ulcerated. These different forms may coexist in the same patient. The gingiva are commonly the site of erythematous/erosive LP.

There are lesions that resemble LP both clinically and histopathologically. Usually, these lesions are referred to as "lichenoid" lesions:

- Oral lichenoid contact lesions result from an allergic contact stomatitis. They are seen in direct topographic relationship to dental restorative materials, most commonly amalgam, or other contacted agents (e.g., cinnamon).
- Oral lichenoid drug reactions more commonly occur as a temporal association with taking certain medications, for example, ACE inhibitors and NSAIDs.
- Oral lichenoid lesions may develop as part of GVHD.

Figure 12.8 White reticular pattern with an ulcerated center on the right buccal mucosa in a patient with lichen planus.

Diagnosis of LP

- The clinical features alone may be sufficiently diagnostic, especially when presenting with a reticular pattern.
- The need for a biopsy for histological confirmation of the diagnosis is not definitive.

Treatment and Prognosis of LP

The elimination of precipitating factors is an important step in symptom management. Minimizing mechanical trauma from a sharp cusp, or chemical trauma from acidic, spicy, or strongly flavored foods and beverages should be encouraged and can lead to symptomatic improvement. The accumulation of bacterial plaque may also exacerbate the condition. The use of alternative oral hygiene measures including the use of alcohol-free chlorhexidine gluconate mouth rinses may be helpful.

Small and asymptomatic areas of reticular or plaque-type LP may not require treatment. Four main classes of medical interventions are used with various results. These include corticosteroids, retinoids, calcineurin inhibitors, and ultraviolet phototherapy.

There is an ongoing controversy as to whether oral LP is associated with an increased risk of malignant transformation. The annual malignant transformation rate is 0.2–0.5%. Patients should be encouraged to discontinue habits that are likely to increase the risk of malignant transformations. Long-term monitoring is recommended.

II. Recommended Readings and Cited References

Recommended Readings

American Academy of Oral Medicine. Patient Information Sheets. Available at: http://www.aaom.com/patients/. Accessed March 17, 2012.

Neville BN, Damm DD, Allen CM, Bouquot JE. Oral and Maxillofacial Pathology, 3rd ed. 2009. Saunders Elsevier, St. Louis, MO.

Sapp JP, Eversole LR, Wysocki GP. Contemporary Oral and Maxillofacial Pathology, 2nd ed. 2004. Mosby Elsevier, St. Louis, MO.

Sciubba JJ. Autoimmune oral mucosal diseases: clinical, etiologic, diagnostic, and treatment considerations. Dent Clin North Am 2011;55(1):89–103.

Siegel MA, Silverman S Jr., Sollecito TP. Clinician's Guide. Treatment of Common Oral Conditions, 7th ed. 2009. American Academy of Oral Medicine, Edmonds, WA.

Cited References

1. Filipovich AH, Weisdorf D, Pavletic S, Socie G, Wingard JR, Lee SJ, et al. National Institute of Health consensus development project on criteria for clinical trials in chronic graft-versus-host disease: I. Diagnosis and staging working group report. Biol Blood Marrow Transplant 2005;11(12): 945–56.
2. Fraser CJ, Bhatia S, Ness K, Carter A, Francisco L, Arora M, et al. Impact of chronic graft-versus-host disease on the health status of hematopoietic cell transplantation survivors: a report from the Bone Marrow Transplant Survivor Study. Blood 2006;108(8):2867–73.
3. Baird K, Pavletic SZ. Chronic graft versus host disease. Curr Opin Hematol 2006;13(6):426–35.
4. Bystryn JC, Rudolph JL. Pemphigus. Lancet 2005;366(9479):61–73.
5. Kricheli D, David M, Frusic-Zlotkin M, Goldsmith D, Rabinov M, Sulkes J, et al. The distribution of pemphigus vulagaris-IgG subclasses and their reactivity with desmoglein 3 and 1 in pemphigus patients and their first degree relatives. Br J Dermatol 2000;143(2):337–42.
6. Scully C, Challacombe SJ. Pemphigus vulgaris: update on etiopathogenesis, oral manifestations, and management. Crit Rev Oral Biol Med 2002; 13(5):397–408.
7. Darling MR, Daley T. Blistering mucocutaneous diseases of the oral mucosa—a review: part 1. Mucous membrane pemphigoid. J Can Dent Assoc 2005;71(11):851–4.
8. Sawamura D, Nakano H, Matsuzaki Y. Overview of epidermolysis bullosa. J Dermatol 2010;37(3): 214–9.
9. Bernard P, Vaillant L, Labeille B, Bedane C, Arbeille B, Denoeux JP, et al. Incidence and distribution of subepidermal autoimmune bullous skin disease in three French regions. Bullous Diseases French Study Group. Arch Dermatol 1995;131(1):48–52.
10. Engineer L, Ahmed AR. Emerging treatment for epidermolysis bullosa aquisita. J Am Acad Dermatol 2001;44(5):818–28.
11. Al-Johani KA, Fedele S, Porter S. Erythema multiforme and related disorders. Oral Surg Oral Med Oral Pathol Oral Radiol Endod 2007;103(5): 642–54.
12. Katz J, Livneh A, Shemer J, Danon YL, Peretz B. Herpes simplex-associated erythema multiforme (HAEM): a clinical therapeutic dilemma. Pediatr Dent 1999;21(6):359–62.
13. Ayangco L, Rogers RS. Oral manifestations of erythema multiforme. Dermatol Clin 2003;21(1): 195–205.
14. Chattopadhyay A, Shetty KV. Recurrent aphthous stomatitis. Otolaryngol Clin North Am 2011;44(1):79–88.

15. Scully C. Clinical practice. Aphthous ulceration. N Engl J Med 2006;355(2):165–72.
16. Scully C, Porter S. Recurrent aphthous stomatitis: current concepts of etiology, pathogenesis and management. J Oral Pathol Med 1989;18(1):21–7.
17. Femiano F, Lanza A, Buonaiuto C, Gombos F, Nunziata M, Piccolo S, et al. Guidelines for diagnosis and management of aphthous stomatitis. Pediatr Infect Dis J 2007;26(8):728–32.
18. Sakane T, Takeno M, Suzuki N, Inaba G. Behcet's disease. N Engl J Med 1999;341(17):1284–91.
19. International Study Group for Behcet's Disease. Criteria for diagnosis of Behcet's disease. Lancet 1990;355(8697):1078–80.
20. Yazici Y, Yurdakul S, Yazici H. Behçet's syndrome. Curr Rheumatol Rep 2010;12(6):429–35.
21. Al-Hashimi I, Schifter M, Lockhart PB, Wray D, Brennan M, Migliorati CA, et al. Oral lichen planus and oral lichenoid lesions: diagnostic and therapeutic considerations. Oral Surg Oral Med Oral Pathol Oral Radiol Endod 2007;103(Suppl.):S25.e1–12.

Head and Neck Cancer

Steven M. Roser DMD, MD, FACS
Steven R. Nelson DDS, MS
Srinivasa Ramachandra MD, BDS, FDS RCS (Eng)

I. Background

Description of Disease/Condition

Head and neck cancers vary by histopathology and location in this region, yet 90% arise from the lining mucosa of the oral cavity and pharynx, also referred to as the upper aerodigestive tract.

This chapter emphasizes the "mucosal" or epithelial-derived squamous cell carcinoma (SCC). The majority of non-epithelial-derived tumors in the head and neck region are lymphomas (non-Hodgkin's and Hodgkin's lymphomas) (see Chapter 8 "Hematological Diseases"). The biology of head and neck SCC (HNSCC) differs from other cancers of the thyroid, skin, brain, eye, and manifestations of lymphomas in the head and neck.

Pathogenesis/Etiology

Risk Factors

Tobacco, alcohol use, ultraviolet light, viral infection, radiation, genetic factors, malnourishment, diet, and chemical exposures to betel quid and areca nut are established risk factors for head and neck cancers, with tobacco and alcohol use causing more than 80% worldwide, including the United States (see also Chapter 16, "Substance Use Disorders").

Tobacco

Tobacco use in any form can cause head and neck tumors, with risk increasing in proportion to the duration and intensity of usage. Patients with head and neck cancer who continue tobacco use carry a high risk for a second primary tumor in the region.

- Cigarette smokers have a cancer incidence six to eight times higher than nonsmokers.
- Cigar, pipe, filtered cigarette, and "beedi" or "bidi" smoking have a dose–response relationship to oral, pharyngeal, and laryngeal cancers.
- Smokeless tobacco, chewing tobacco, and snuff use results in an increased risk of invasive tumors arising from premalignant

> **Anatomic glossary of head and neck**
>
> - **Nasal**—the nasal cavity and paranasal sinuses, including the sphenoid, frontal, ethmoid, and maxillary sinus
> - **Oral cavity**—lips, buccal mucosa, gingiva, anterior two-thirds of the tongue, floor of the mouth, retromolar trigone, and hard palate
> - **Pharynx**—a long tubular structure from behind the nose to the region of voice box and esophagus divided into nasopharynx, oropharynx, and hypopharynx
> - **Nasopharynx**—upper third of pharynx posterior to nasal and superior to oropharynx up to the skull base containing the eustachian tubal apertures in lateral walls
> - **Oropharynx**—base of the tongue, soft palate, uvula, tonsillar area, and posterior pharyngeal wall
> - **Hypopharynx**—the lower third of the pharynx, between the oropharynx and esophagus, including the areas around the upper part of the voice box (pyriform sinuses, post cricoid area of the posterior larynx, and larynx)
> - **Larynx**—the voice box is a short passageway formed by the cartilage just below the pharynx in the neck and includes the epiglottis, which prevents food from entering the air passages
> - **Lymph nodes**—located in the neck, lymph nodes can have cancer spread to them from tumors in the head and neck areas and other regions.
> - **Major salivary glands**—parotid glands, submandibular glands, and sublingual glands. The mouth, lips, palate, and tongue contain multiple minor salivary glands.

lesions of the oral and oropharyngeal mucosa.
- Cancer incidence also has a positive correlation with exposure to the polycyclic aromatic hydrocarbons, nitrosamines, and aromatic amines, along with many other carcinogens, found in tobacco smoke.[1]
- Second-hand tobacco smoke is an environmental hazard, creating risk of head and neck cancers in nonsmokers.
- Cancer risk decreases after 5 years of smoking cessation, and risk is comparable with nonsmokers after 20 years of abstinence.

Alcohol

- Alcohol has been identified as a carcinogenic agent in many cohort studies.[2] However, the exact mechanism of carcinogenesis is not well known. Alcohol may promote carcinogenesis by acting as a solvent, that is, enhancing the penetration of carcinogens in oral tissues, or it may act as a cofactor along with tobacco.
- All types of alcohol have been associated with increased risk.
- Certain genetic predispositions and polymorphisms are enhanced by alcohol intake.[3]

Human Papillomavirus (HPV)

- HPV is a sexually transmitted virus; oncogenic types 16 and 18 have been found to have a causal role in a subgroup of head and neck invasive tumors of the oropharynx and oral cavity.
- Sites most commonly related to HPV infection are the base of the tongue and tonsils.

HPV-associated head and neck cancers have a different risk profile from non-HPV-associated head and neck tumors—that is, patients are usually young, nonusers of tobacco and alcohol; possess a distinct molecular profile; have a better outcome after complete treatment; and have a lower incidence of second cancers.

> **Common head and neck cancers by location**
>
> **Nasal cavity, vestibule, and paranasal malignancies**
> *Epithelial tumors*: squamous cell carcinoma, sinonasal undifferentiated carcinoma, olfactory neuroblastoma (esthesioneuroblastoma)
> *Nonepithelial tumors*: mucosal melanoma, osteosarcoma, chondrosarcomas, synovial sarcomas, rhabdomyosarcoma, fibrosarcoma
>
> **Nasopharyngeal malignancies**
> Squamous cell carcinoma, lymphomas, nasopharyngeal carcinoma (keratinizing, nonkeratinizing, and undifferentiated types), fibrosarcoma
>
> **Oral cavity**
> *Epithelial*: squamous cell carcinoma, verrucous carcinoma
> *Nonepithelial*: striated muscle rhabdomyosarcoma, angiosarcoma/Kaposi
>
> **Oropharynx**
> Squamous cell carcinoma, lymphoepithelialomas, lymphomas
>
> **Hypopharynx**
> Squamous cell carcinoma
>
> **Larynx**
> *Epithelial*: squamous cell carcinoma, verrucous carcinoma
> *Nonepithelial*: adult rhabdomyosarcoma
>
> **Thyroid malignancies and parathyroid malignancies**
> Papillary carcinoma, follicular carcinoma, medullary thyroid carcinoma, anaplastic thyroid carcinoma
>
> **Salivary gland malignancies**
> Mucoepidermoid carcinoma, adenoid cystic carcinoma, acinic cell carcinoma, adenocarcinoma, squamous cell carcinoma
>
> **Skin**
> Squamous cell carcinoma, basal cell carcinoma, melanomas, angiosarcoma
>
> **Facial bones**
> Osteosarcoma of the mandible, synovial sarcoma

Betel Quid

- Betel quid is a mixture of areca nut, slaked lime, and spices rolled in betel leaf. Gutkha and pan masala are variants with tobacco.
- Chewing this mixture is a strong risk factor for cancer of the oral cavity and oropharynx in Southeast Asia and immigrants from this region to the United States.
- Oral submucous fibrosis, a premalignant lesion, is also a result of areca consumption.

Ultraviolet Light

- Exposure among outdoor workers is associated with a very high incidence of lip cancers, with SCC most commonly occurring on the lower lip. See Fig. 13.1.

Epstein-Barr Virus (EBV)

- EBV causes nasopharyngeal carcinoma.

Diet

- A diet rich in fruits, vitamin A, zinc, carotene, and tocopherol is protective from HNSCC.

Figure 13.1 Squamous cell carcinoma of the lower lip in a 61-year-old white male with a history of cigarette smoking. Courtesy of Dr. Bert Wood.

- Nitrite-rich preserved meat consumption increases risk for nasopharyngeal carcinomas.

Other Factors

Also suggested as risks for HNSCC are: heredity; environmental and occupational exposure to formaldehyde, asbestos, wood dust, and industrial pollutants like polycyclic aromatic hydrocarbons[4]; radiation exposure from environmental, medical, or occupational reasons; and immunosuppressant medications used after transplant surgery.

Pathogenesis/Progression

The majority of HNSCCs develop from premalignant lesions such as leukoplakia and erythroplakia, which present with histological findings of dysplasia; however, not all dysplastic lesions progress to carcinoma (see Chapter 16, "Substance Use Disorders"). Current research indicates that the development of cancer is driven by an accumulation of genetic and epigenetic changes within a clonal population of cells.[5]

Epidemiology

Incidence

- Head and neck cancer is the fifth most common cancer worldwide.
- In the United States, approximately 40,000–50,000 people are diagnosed with head and neck cancer each year.[6]

According to the Surveillance Epidemiology and End Results (SEER) data in the United States, there is a marked difference in incidence, tumor site, and outcome between sexes, socio-economic status, and race after standardization for age.

Sex: Male-to-female ratios are 2:1 to 3:1, more strongly male dominated for larynx cancers than tumors of the oral cavity and pharynx.

Race: African-American men have a higher incidence per 100,000 people, are diagnosed at later stages, and have poorer 5-year survival compared with whites in the United States.

Age: Incidence of head and neck cancer also increases with age, wherein the majority prevalence occurs between 50 and 70 years. Although HPV-positive head and neck cancer has been noted in younger individuals, the mean age of laryngeal SCC has a peak incidence at 70 years and pharyngeal SCC incidence increases from teens to peak at the age of 80 years.

Incidence Trends: The U.S. SEER registries for 1973–2004 revealed that the incidence of oral SCC increased in the sites potentially linked to HPV infection, with an annual percentage change at +0.80%, whereas it decreased in the sites unrelated to HPV infection.[7]

Mortality

- In the United States, approximately 10,000–11,000 people die from head and neck cancers annually.[6]

- In the United States, the mortality from oral cavity and oropharynx cancer decreased from 5.1 to 3.8 per 100,000 people in men and from 2 to 1.4 per 100,000 people in women, age adjusted, 1992–2007.
- Worldwide disparities in time of detection, care, and tumor characteristics result in immense differences in mortality. Mortality rates in western Europe and the United States are lower when compared with central and eastern Europe.

Coordination of Care between Dentist and Physician

Therapeutic interventions and prognosis differ widely depending on the stage at diagnosis, location and histology of the tumor. Coordination of care is important before, during, and after cancer therapy due to the extent, nature, severity, and duration of complications of therapy in the head and neck region that can impact esthetics, speaking, mastication, deglutition, overall nutrition, comfort, and quality of life.

> **Signs and symptoms of head and neck cancer presentation**
>
> - "Sore" in the mouth that bleeds and fails to heal
> - White or red patch in the mouth, which cannot be dislodged
> - Lump in the tongue, inner cheek of the mouth (buccal mucosa), floor of the mouth
> - Difficulty swallowing or pain while swallowing
> - Hoarseness or change in voice, difficulty in speech
> - Reduced mouth opening, nonarticular pathology
> - Blood in sputum
> - Mobile or dislodged tooth without any trauma or significant gum disease
> - Nasal fullness with bleeding
> - Development of double vision (diplopia)
> - Sensation loss or radiating pain
> - Neck lumps
> - Swelling on the upper or lower jaw or under the lower jaw
> - Earache or reduced hearing
> - Tearing of eyes (epiphora)
> - Fracture of jaws without trauma

II. Medical Management

Identification

Head and neck cancers can be asymptomatic until they are quite advanced. They present with insidious symptoms. Expeditious diagnosis and treatment has an impact on cancer outcomes.

Visual screening is a simple method for early detection of oral lesions. An American Dental Association Council on Scientific Affairs Expert Panel on Screening for Oral SSCs provided evidence-based clinical recommendations.[8] The panel emphasized that screening for oral cancer is one component of a thorough hard-tissue and soft-tissue examination that follows patient history and risk assessment and that both benefits and limitations result from screening, with limited evidence that screening impacts oral cancer mortality rates. See Table 13.1.

Adjunctive Screening Tests

Aids to oral, oropharyngeal cancer, and precancerous lesion screening are not widely used due to the lack of randomized controlled trials or large-scale studies that are sufficiently sensitive and specific in comparison to the gold standard of biopsy results to demonstrate effectiveness and general lack of assessment in populations seen in general dental practices.[9] Another disadvantage is their inability to differentiate cancer from precancerous lesions.[12]

1. *Toluidine blue (tolonium chloride)* is currently not approved as a stand-alone test by the

Table 13.1. Recommendations of the American Dental Association Council on Scientific Affairs Expert Panel on Screening for Oral Squamous Cell Carcinomas, Based on Evidence (April 2009)

Topic	Recommendation
Screening during routine examinations[a]	The panel suggests that clinicians remain alert for signs of potentially malignant lesions or early-stage cancers in all patients while performing routine visual and tactile examinations, particularly for patients who use tobacco or who are heavy[b] consumers of alcohol.
Follow-up for seemingly innocuous lesions	For seemingly innocuous lesions, the panel suggests that clinicians follow up in 7–14 days to confirm persistence after removing any possible cause to reduce the potential for false-positive screening results.
Follow-up for lesions that raise suspicion of cancer and those that are persistent	For lesions that raise suspicion of cancer or for lesions that persist after removal of a possible cause, the panel suggests that clinicians communicate the potential benefits and risks of early diagnosis. Considerations include the following: • that even suspicious lesions identified during the course of a routine visual and tactile examination may represent false positives. • that clinical confirmation (a second opinion) can be sought from a dental or medical care provider with advanced training and experience in diagnosis of oral mucosal disease so as to reduce the potential for a false-positive or false-negative oral cancer screening result. • that a malignancy or nonmalignancy can be confirmed only via microscopic examination that requires a surgical biopsy. • that a decision to pursue a biopsy to confirm the presence or absence of a malignancy should be made in the context of informed consent.
Use of lesion assessment devices	Although transepithelial cytology has validity in identifying disaggregated dysplastic cells, the panel suggests surgical biopsy for definitive diagnosis.

[a] There is insufficient evidence that use of commercial devices for lesion detection that are based on autofluorescence or tissue reflectance enhance visual detection of potentially malignant lesions beyond a conventional visual and tactile examination. *Source*: Patton et al.[9]
[b] Heavy alcohol consumption is defined as follows: for men, consumption of an average of more than two drinks per day; for women, consumption of an average of more than one drink per day. *Sources*: Pelucchi et al.[10] and Centers for Disease Control and Prevention.[11]
Source: Adapted from Rethman et al.[8]

U.S. Food and Drug Administration (FDA), but widely used sporadically worldwide. It is either applied on suspicious lesions or used as a mouth rinse and spit to stain early oral SCC and high-grade dysplasia. There is confusion over inclusion of equivocal staining lesions as positive or negative.[12]

2. *Transepithelial oral cytology* (Oral CDx® Brush Test®, OralCDx Laboratories, Inc., Suffern, NY). It has been studied with a design not to brush test low-suspicion lesions based on clinical features. Brush cytology does not provide a definitive diagnosis like scalpel biopsy diagnosis. When an abnormal result is reported, a surgical biopsy has to be performed.

3. *Tissue reflectance or chemiluminescence* (reflective tissue fluorescence)—(ViziLite® Plus with TBlue®, Zila, Inc., Fort Collins, CO; Microlux™, AdDent, Inc., Danbury, CT; Orascoptic DK™, Orascoptic, A Kerr Co., Middleton, WI). It is a direct visual exam

using a blue light after application of a 1% acetic acid solution wash to remove oral debris and allow visualization after cellular dehydration. Under blue-white illumination, normal epithelium appears blue and abnormal tissue appears distinctly white. This aceto-white area can be marked with tolonium chloride for biopsy (ViziLite Plus® with TBlue®).

4. *Narrow-emission tissue autofluorescence* (VELscope® Vx, LED Dental, Burnaby, BC, Canada). This is fluorescence imaging, which uses a blue excitation light. Normal oral mucosa emits a pale green autofluorescence when seen through a filter. In contrast, abnormal or suspicious tissue appears dark. However, proper filtration is critical and large sample studies are lacking.

5. *Multispectral technology* (autofluorescence and tissue reflectance) (Identafi® 3000, Tirmira, Houston, TX). This uses autofluorescence and reflectance multispectral technology. Violet light fails to absorb in abnormal tissue and fails to admit very low blue fluorescence, appearing dark brown or black. Amber light is absorbed by hemoglobin in blood and is used to delineate vasculature with tissue reflectance.

6. *HPV screening* (OraRisk® HPV test, OralDNA® Labs, Quest Diagnostics, Madison, NJ). This test analyzes a saline mouth rinse sample using DNA amplification by polymerase chain reaction (PCR) assay for the presence of HPV infection.

Medical History/Physical Examination

A detailed patient history of symptoms, risk factors, environmental or occupational exposures including tobacco and alcohol use, medical and surgical history, and family history is obtained and recorded prior to physical examination.

Components of the physical examination for the head and neck cancer patient include the following:

- *Inspection* of the skin and scalp for nodules, ulcers, and pigmented areas.
- *Neurological exam* of all cranial nerves for sensory and motor function of the eye, face, jaws, ears, swallowing, shoulder, and tongue.
- *Extraoral examination* for lymph nodes, nodules or masses, thyroid size and mobility, symmetry, consistency, and tenderness. Any decrease in jaw opening, loss of sensation, motor function, swallowing difficulty, or bony architecture changes and lip consistency are noted. Areas around the ears are examined for tenderness, nodularity, and asymmetry. Malignant lymph node enlargements tend to be nonpainful and nontender to palpation, hard and indurated on palpation, and fixed to underlying muscle and tissues compared with inflammatory and infectious lymph nodes that may be painful, tender, and rubbery to palpation and mobile in all directions. Typical head and neck lymphatic drainage patterns can give an indication of possible location of tumors. See Fig. 13.2.
- *Intraoral examination with bimanual palpation* of cheeks, tongue, and floor of the mouth. A mouth mirror-assisted exam is made of all regions of the mouth, tonsillar area, and hard and soft palate.
- *Indirect laryngoscopy* is carried out with a mirror to visualize tongue base, nasopharynx, epiglottis, and true and false vocal cords with surrounding wall mucosa.
- *Nasal flexible endoscopy* involves applying a local anesthetic spray, and then using a flexible endoscopy for visualization of nasal cavity, nasopharynx, soft palate movement, pooling of secretions, ulcerations, erythema, and papillary projections. Asymmetry is recorded.
- *Triple endoscopy examination under anesthesia.* Head and neck tumors may be synchronous with primary SCC in the esophagus, lower airway, and the lungs. Thus, laryngoscope, bronchoscope, and esophagoscope examinations may be used to visualize and allow

LEVEL AND NODAL GROUPS	CANCER SITES of LYMPHATIC SPREAD
I--Submental and submandibular nodes	Lip; anterior tongue; floor of mouth; gingiva; buccal mucosa
II--Upper jugulodigastric group	Oral cavity; pharynx; larynx
III--Middle jugular nodes	Nasopharynx; oropharynx; oral cavity; hypopharynx; larynx
IV--Inferior jugular nodes	Hypopharynx; subglottic larynx; esophagus
V-- Posterior triangle group	
VI--Anterior compartment group	

Figure 13.2 Neck node levels and head and neck cancer lymphatic drainage patterns.

biopsy under anesthesia, particularly when the primary tumor location is unknown and metastatic neck nodes are the presenting sign.

Laboratory Testing

There are no mandated laboratory tests in the diagnosis of an HNSCC. However, cancer patients undergoing chemotherapy may require a complete blood count with white cell differential; basic metabolic, renal and liver function, and nutrition status markers; and possibly immunological studies for viruses and tumor markers.

Diagnostic Imaging

- *Panoramic dental X-rays* are very useful as initial follow-up imaging of oral cavity lesions with good detail of hard-tissue architecture and involvement.
- *Plain chest X-rays* in two perpendicular exposures are performed to review any primary tumors or cancer spread to the lungs from the HNSCC.
- *Computed tomography (CT) scan* may be the most valuable diagnostic image, as it offers good detail of tumor size and character, and identifies occult primary and any lymph node spread. It can delineate bony erosion and involvement. CT scans with good resolution are used in reconstruction planning after tumor resection surgery. CT scans are also used to monitor any recurrence and progression of disease.
- *Magnetic resonance imaging (MRI)* provides details of tumor size, character, and bony extension of the tumor if marrow space is involved. MRI is more sensitive than CT in

delineation of soft-tissue details and soft-tissue extent of the tumor. MRI can also identify tumor from sinus secretions, neural spread, and intracranial extent. However, the gain in sensitivity of detail is lost in specificity in comparison to CT scan. Motion artifact is a particular problem in hypopharynx and larynx. Nasopharynx and oropharynx imaging is superior with gadolinium contrast-enhanced MRI.
- *Positron emission technology (PET) scan* is used for the identification of metastasis, tumor recurrence, and aggressive malignant processes. It is less sensitive in occult primary tumor identification. It works on the principle of increased tracer uptake in highly metabolic tumor sites.

Biopsy

Biopsy of the tumor or suspicious lesion can be performed with a scalpel blade, a cutting ring punch, forceps, and needles. Specimens are sent to the laboratory for microscopic, immunological, and special staining.

Fine Needle Aspiration (FNA)

This is a method of obtaining specimens from tumors and masses in the head and neck area, including thyroid nodules. A needle is passed through the overlying skin or mucosa, allowing suction to be applied at the outer end of the needle while multiple passes are made collecting a sample for histological analysis.

Histological Tumor Grading

Histopathological evaluation of tumor cells and architecture from the biopsy or final tumor specimen is conducted to determine the amount of abnormal differentiation from its original structure in order to establish the histological grade. Cancer cells undergoing hyperplasia will have lack of differentiation. Poorly differentiated tumors are considered high-grade tumors, are more aggressive, and have worse prognosis. In contract, well-differentiated tumors are considered low-grade tumors, are less aggressive, and have better prognosis.

Staging

Staging is based on the American Joint Committee for Cancer (AJCC) TNM classification system for tumor extent. Three main parameters, tumor size (T), tumor cell spread to draining lymph nodes (N), and tumor cell spread to distant parts of the body as metastasis (M), are assessed clinically, by imaging, and then pathologically. Designation of "x" is for unknown, unable to be assessed, status of tumor.

- For the oral cavity and oropharynx:
  T0 = no evidence of primary;
  T1 = tumor ≤2 cm diameter;
  T2 = tumor 2–4 cm;
  T3 = tumor >4 cm;
  T4 = any size tumor but invades adjacent structures.
  N0 = no nodes;
  N1 = one node <3 cm same side as primary;

Key considerations before biopsy
- Differential diagnosis by clinical evaluation prior to biopsy
- Clear path in mind of further referral, if necessary, before biopsy
- If imaging is indicated, consider chronology of biopsy contributing to any artifact
- Optimal technique to get the best representative sample
- Knowledge of investigations needed on the specimen obtained

Prognosis	Stage	T	N	M
Better	0	Tis	N0	M0
	I	T1	N0	M0
	II	T2	N0	M0
	III	T3	N0	M0
		T1,T2,T3	N1	M0
	IVA	T4	N0,N1	M0
		any T	N2	M0
	IVB	any T	N3	M0
Poorer	IVC	any T	any N	M1

Example:
T1N1M0 – primary tumor is 2 cm or less at its largest diameter with metastasis to a single same sided regional lymph node which is not larger than 3 cm at its largest dimension.

Figure 13.3 Head and neck cancer TNM stage grouping.

N2a = one node of 3–6 cm same side as primary;
N2b = multiple nodes all <6 cm on same side as primary;
N2c = one or more nodes, none >6 cm on both sides or opposite side of primary;
N3 = lymph node >6 cm.
M0 = no distant metastases;
M1 = distant metastases present.

- Each head and neck cancer type has its own AJCC staging classification system, which helps in treatment planning and prognosis evaluation.
- T, N, and M are combined in an overall stage assignment. See Figs. 13.3 and 13.4.

Figure 13.4 Neck lymphadenopathy in a 63-year-old white male with T3N2c SCC of left posterior pharynx and tonsil.

Prognosis

- Cancers of the oral cavity and oropharynx have a relatively poor prognosis. Their 5-year survival rate is approximately 50–60%, with early presentation (lower stage) resulting in a better prognosis.
- Well-differentiated tumors have a better prognosis than poorly differentiated tumors.
- Tumor invasion out of the lymph node capsule, perineural infiltration, and local and regional recurrences have poor survival outcomes and need concurrent or multiple modalities of treatment.

Medical Treatment

The three commonly used modalities to treat head and neck cancer are surgical excision, radiation therapy, and chemotherapy, either as single therapy or in combination. The anatomical location of the tumor, stage, size, involvement of adjacent normal structures, patient medical condition, and the expertise available are all taken into account to determine which modality or combination of treatments is recommended.

Treatment of Specific Tumor Sites

Lip Tumors

- SCC predominates on the lower lip and basal cell cancer on the upper lip. This is among the most common cancers of the oral region.
- It is primarily treated with surgery in early stages with tumor-free margins (4–6 mm) at the edges of resection.
- Radiation is reserved for patient preference and tumors unsuitable for resection.
- Younger patients have poor prognosis. There is good cure rate if there is no extension to neck lymph nodes and no nerve involvement.
- A neck clearance of lymph nodes is carried out if the lesion is of high risk and advanced stage. The neck dissection includes both sides if the tumor is in the midline.

SCC of Oral Cavity (Tongue, Floor of the Mouth, Other Oral Mucosa)

- Stage I or II tumors are treated with surgical resection with wide clear margin (at least 0.5 cm) free of tumor or definitive radiotherapy for 6–7 weeks with 60–70 gray (Gy) and have similar survival outcome. Surgery has less associated morbidity and is usually preferred. A limited (supraomohyoid) neck dissection is also carried out on the side of the tumor. There is debate about the utility of neck dissection if there is limited depth of invasion and no lymph nodal spread.
- Many floor of the mouth cancers present after deep invasion into the tongue, muscles of the floor of the mouth, and the adjacent bone. See Fig. 13.5.
- Most tongue cancers occur on the lateral border of the oral tongue (anterior two-thirds) and are able to be diagnosed at an early stage. See Fig. 13.6.
- Stage III and IV tumors are managed with combination of surgery and radiation therapy.
- Invasion of the mandible may require composite resection. If a large segment is

Figure 13.5 T2N2b moderately differentiated, invasive SCC of the floor of the mouth in a 62-year-old African-American female.

Figure 13.6 T3N0 moderately differentiated SCC of the right oral tongue in a 25-year-old white male.

removed, then subsequent reconstruction by bone and soft tissue harvested from another part of the body may be required, along with the use of metal plates or bars for retention.

Cancer of the Oropharynx

- Tumors in this region have poor surgical access.
- HPV association is a favorable prognostic cancer, especially for oropharyngeal tumors with good response to adjuvant chemotherapy and radiation.[13]
- Transoral laser surgery and transoral robotic surgery (TORS) are the latest technology-assisted surgical approaches with wide uptake.

Cancer of the Hypopharynx and Larynx

- The hypopharynx has 8–10% of HNSCCs.
- Cancers in this region can cause vocal cord fixation, injure nerves, and spread into the esophagus.
- Difficulty swallowing, pain, pooling of saliva, subsequent weight loss, and malnutrition are common associated problems.
- Surgical treatment of the larynx includes open and transoral laser approaches.
- Organ preservation with chemoradiation improves outcomes, which is a significant consideration.

Cancer of the Nasopharynx

- Primary therapy for nasopharyngeal cancer is chemoradiation.
- Radiation is delivered through the muscles of mastication and can result in radiation fibrosis and significant trismus.
- Surgical resection in this region has high morbidity and does not improve survival outcomes.

Salivary Gland Cancers

- Seventy percent arise in parotid glands, contributing about 1% of HNSCCs. Yet, only about 25% of all parotid gland tumors are malignant.
- The history of previous radiation is a significant risk factor for salivary tumors.
- Mucoepidermoid carcinoma is the most common salivary gland cancer among adults and children, with higher incidence in the parotid gland.
- Adenoid cystic carcinoma is more common among the submandibular, sublingual, and minor salivary glands.
- Polymorphous low-grade adenocarcinoma is the most common on the palate.
- Presentation of salivary tumors can be asymptomatic, painless swellings or painful, slow growing, bleeding masses, with voice change and nasal obstructive symptoms. It can be nodular, solid, or cystic. On rare occasion, it causes facial palsy and intraoral asymmetry.
- Surgery is based on tumor size, relationship to the facial nerve, and degree of invasion into surrounding tissues.
- Radiotherapy is indicated in advanced-stage disease and when there are adverse prognostic factors, including perineural and vascular invasion, close or positive margins, and histological high grade.

Treatment Modalities

Surgical Resection and Maxillofacial Defects

- Tumor surgery and resection of the mandible or maxilla, tongue, larynx, and hard palate can lead to deficiencies of form and function.
- Rehabilitation methods to reconstruct defects of surgical resection attempt to restore critical functions of breathing, swallowing, speech, secretion control, and restoration of esthetics to improve quality of life.
- Reconstructive options include vascular free flaps harvested from other body parts,

bone grafts, prosthetic material, splints, and obturators.
- There is an increased efficiency in virtual treatment planning using computer-aided reconstruction techniques for reconstructing surgical defects with autologous grafts and vascular composite flaps. See Fig. 13.7.

Radiation Therapy

- Common indications for radiation are advanced tumor stage with positive lymph nodes, nerve invasion, spread through blood vessels and lymphatic channels, extra capsular spread, and increased tumor thickness.

Figure 13.7 Virtual surgery planning for resection of the left mandible due to invasion by retromolar trigone SCC. (a) 3D reconstruction of the mandible. (b) Replacement by patient's left fibula from the CT scan of the patient's left lower extremity. (c) Transparency of fibula reconstruction over native mandible. (d) Case planning with reconstruction plate.

- Conventional external-beam radiation therapy is a 5-days-per-week course of a daily dose of 1.5–2 Gy per fraction for a total dose of 62–70 Gy. Fractioning of the dose delivered, boost protocols, and accelerated fractionation are better techniques to deliver radiation.
- Radiation-planning techniques and delivery have improved efficacy and reduced morbidity. Radiation therapy is focused to the desired field by various techniques, including three-dimensional conformal treatment planning with intensity modulated radiotherapy (IMRT) and image-guided radiotherapy (IGRT).

IMRT works by constantly reshaping the field and intensity of the beam based on the position of the tumor in relation to the dynamic radiation source. It creates a differential between normal and cancerous tissue, helping to avoid dosage to healthy tissue. The result is fewer functional side effects, reduced additional radiation to adjacent structures, and lessened morbidity than the patient might have with standard radiotherapy. It is often used in "parotid sparing" protocols, where the side with the primary tumor receives 70 Gy and the opposite side receives 50 Gy in an attempt to negotiate the radiation beams so as to avoid higher doses to the parotid gland.

In *proton beam therapy (IMPT)*, protons are used to minimize the morbidity from radiation and minimize the dose to adjacent critical structures, such as the salivary glands, eyes, and thyroid tissue. There are increased treatment costs but better tumor control by focused higher dosage delivery.

Implant brachytherapy involves the local application of cesium-131 or iridium-192 in radiation delivery catheters by surgical approach (interstitial or intracavitary) to areas of the tongue and oral cavity tumors. It has significant side effects and cost that are barriers to use.

Amifostine is an organic thiophosphate, cytoprotective free radical-scavenging agent given intravenously 15 minutes prior to radiation therapy to protect from the harmful effects of cisplatin and radiation, including xerostomia. Tolerance, cost, and adverse effects are barriers to wider utilization.

Chemotherapy

Chemotherapy for HNSCC is used primarily for organ preservation in advanced disease and may be used for palliative treatment. Three approaches are as follows:

1. *Neoadjuvant Therapy or Induction Chemotherapy*: Chemotherapy is administered before locoregional surgery or radiotherapy.
2. *Adjuvant Therapy*: Chemotherapy and radiotherapy are simultaneously administered after surgery in high-risk patients reducing metastatic burden.
3. *Concurrent Chemoradiation for Organ Preservation*: Simultaneous chemotherapy and radiotherapy are a definitive and curative treatment for instances in laryngeal tumors. Radiation is used with cisplatin and 5-fluoruracil for the additive (or supra-additive) radiosensitizing effect of chemotherapy on the effectiveness of the radiation treatment.

The types of chemotherapy agents are:

- alkylating agents—cisplatin;
- antibiotics—derivatives of antimicrobial compounds from *Streptomyces*-like doxorubicin, bleomycin, and mitomycin;
- antimetabolites—methotrexate and 5-fluorouracil;
- alkaloids—vincristine and vinblastine;
- taxanes—paclitaxel and docetaxel.

Nonspecific toxic effects of chemotherapy include a maculopapular rash, neutropenia, preponderance to bleed with platelet dysfunction, hand–foot syndrome, and facial erythema including flushing, gingival bleeding, mucosal hemorrhages, alopecia, stomatitis, and xerostomia.

III. Dental Management

Evaluation

An understanding of where the patient is in the course of diagnosis and treatment and the type of therapy used is critical to treatment planning.

Dental Treatment Modifications

Patients Receiving Chemotherapy

Dental Management prior to Chemotherapy

- Prechemotherapy dental examination to eliminate oral sources of bacteremia and reduce severity of complications.
- A preventive dental treatment plan should be instituted.
- Extraction of unsalvageable teeth should be completed at least 7 days prior to onset of chemotherapy.

Dental Management during Chemotherapy

- Good oral hygiene must be maintained.
- The patient should use an extra-soft nylon bristle toothbrush to reduce risk for trauma (or soft bristles rinsed under hot water to soften them).
- Electric and/or ultrasonic toothbrushes may be used, if used atraumatically. An appropriate flossing technique and 0.12% chlorhexidine mouth rinse may be useful adjuncts for plaque and gingivitis control.
- If the gingival tissue bleeds easily or the neutrophil count is critically low, brushing should be discontinued and the teeth cleansed with moist gauze pads.
- Commercial mouth rinses may dry the tissue and may need to be avoided.
- Removable prostheses should not be worn while sleeping, or at any time if they cause tissue irritation. Denture adhesives should also be avoided, and denture soaking solutions must be changed daily.
- Only the minimally necessary dental interventions should be provided to control acute

Key questions to ask the patient

If prior to treatment:
- What type of cancer do you have? Where is it located? Have you previously been treated for head and neck cancer?
- What cancer treatments are planned? Who is on your cancer team (surgical oncologist, radiation oncologist, medical oncologist)? When will your treatment start?
- What has your cancer doctor told you to expect for side effects of your treatment?

If posttreatment:
- Where was your primary tumor? Do you know the cancer stage? Were neck nodes involved?
- What treatments for your cancer did you receive? What parts of your head and neck were radiated and what was the highest dose you received? What type of surgery did you have? Did you receive chemotherapy?
- Have you experienced any adverse consequences from your prior cancer therapy?

> **Key questions to ask the physician**
>
> **If prior to treatment:**
> - What are the tumor location, type, and stage? When was it first diagnosed? Is this the first head and neck cancer in this patient?
> - What treatments are planned?
> - If *radiation therapy* is planned:
>   - What is the planned field of radiation?
>   - What will be the dose in gray (Gy) of the radiation to the alveolar bone of maxilla and mandible? Parotid and submandibular/sublingual glands? Muscles of mastication?
>   - Will parotid sparing IMRT be used? Will any other radioprotective aids such as amifostine be used? What level of salivary gland deficit is expected?
>   - When will the treatment begin and what is the planned schedule?
> - If *surgical resection* is planned:
>   - What surgery is planned? Will the patient require a surgical stent or surgical oburator? Will the patient require postsurgical maxillofacial rehabilitation?
>   - Will access for the patient to perform oral hygiene and/or dentist to restore or remove teeth in the future be compromised?
> - If *chemotherapy* is planned:
>   - What is the schedule for the chemotherapy?
>   - Do you anticipate any bone marrow suppression? If so, will this be severe?
>   - Do you anticipate any oral mucositis as a side effect?
>
> **If posttreatment:**
> - Where was the primary tumor? What was the histopathology and stage?
> - What treatments were received? When was treatment given? Were attempts made to preserve salivary gland function?
> - What areas of the mandible and maxilla were involved to what dose of radiation? Can you please be as specific as possible about radiation dose to the tooth area locations: for example, right side, left side, maxilla only, mandible only, both maxilla and mandible, wisdom teeth only, all molars, premolars, up to canine, including in all teeth.

dental problems occurring during active phases of myelosuppression. Review of the hematological profile and consultation with the physician are critical for optimal timing of dental intervention. The most optimal time for dental treatment would be the week prior to the next dose of chemotherapy for the patient receiving chemotherapy on a monthly cycle.

- When there is an emergent dental problem and significant deficiencies are noted in the blood cell count (absolute neutrophil count less than $500/mm^3$ and platelet count less than $50,000/mm^3$), transfusion of blood components and broad-spectrum parenteral antibiotic prophylaxis should be considered before dental treatment.
- If the patient is scheduled to receive blood component transfusions as part of the supportive regimen, the emergent dental problem can usually be palliated and definitive dental treatment scheduled immediately following the blood transfusion.

Dental Management following Chemotherapy

- Definitive dental care may be provided for patients after chemotherapy is completed.

Patients Receiving Radiation Therapy to the Head and Neck

Dental Management prior to Radiation Therapy

Points of discussion with the cancer team:

- Urgency of completion of dental care needs.
- Allowable delay in cancer treatment for dental care management, without affecting cancer treatment efficacy.
- Planned field and total dosage of radiation therapy, specifically including the salivary glands and tooth-bearing alveolus.
- Use of radiation implants (brachytherapy), which is locally more destructive than external beam therapy.
- Planned use of any radioprotective techniques or drugs for preserving salivary function.

Discussion with patient:

- The patient's resources, ability, and commitment to lifelong aggressive preventive measures including meticulous oral hygiene, daily fluoride applications, and frequent follow-up dental maintenance visits.

Oral/dental evaluation and treatment planning:

- All hopeless and questionable teeth (i.e., teeth with advanced periodontitis or impacted, nonessential, or nonrestorable teeth), root fragments, and other bone pathology within the field of radiation should be removed prior to radiation, particularly in the posterior mandible and if alveolus is to receive a total dose >50 Gy.
- Extractions including alveoloplasty with tension-free primary tissue closure and any other dental or preprosthetic surgery should be performed to allow 14–21 days of healing, if possible.

Treatment and maintenance of salvageable teeth:

- Prophylaxis and home care instructions should be provided. Include analysis and modification of diet to eliminate cariogenic foods.
- High-priority restorations and elimination of sites of irritation should be accomplished.
- Orthodontic bands within the field of radiation should be removed.
- Dentures should be left out as much as possible during radiation therapy and should be cleaned daily, and denture adhesives should not be used.
- To prevent demineralization of tooth structure, daily 5000 ppm fluoride toothpaste or 1.1% neutral sodium fluoride gel as brush on or in custom gel-applicator trays should be used once daily for 5 minutes.
- Supplemental use of remineralizing products such as Recaldent™ (amorphous calcium phosphate) in Prospec™ MI Paste/MI Paste Plus™ (GC America Inc., Alsip, IL) may be considered.

Dental Management during Radiation Therapy

- Restorative treatment may be provided in the first 2 weeks before mucositis becomes severe.
- Denture use will depend on severity of mucositis and fit of prostheses.
- Mucositis and candidiasis may require management.

- Oral hygiene, daily fluoride use, and nutritional maintenance are important.
- Trismus prevention is recommended if muscles of mastication are in the field.

Dental Management after Radiation Therapy

- Recall visits every 3–6 months to evaluate for recurrence and side effects of radiation.
- Further caries prevention by fluoride varnish use.
- Prompt detection and restoration of dental caries.
- Assessment of oral hygiene and preventive maintenance regimen compliance with daily prescription-strength fluoride use.
- Determination of the feasibility and timing of prosthetic reconstruction. Traumatic pressure on thin dry alveolar and palatal mucosa should be avoided to prevent the development of ulcerations. Endosseous implants in radiated bone appear to have a higher initial failure rate,[14,15] but once integrated, survival is not reduced compared with implants in nonradiated bone.[16]
- If dental surgery is required, the dentist must consult with the radiation oncologist to determine the total radiation dose in gray to the bone that is involved in the planned surgery to help determine risk of nonhealing and development of osteoradionecrosis (ORN). The total radiation dose in gray to the alveolus in the area of the planned surgery is the most important factor in post-radiation dental treatment planning.

Oral Lesion Diagnosis and Management

Side Effects/Consequences of Head and Neck Radiation Therapy and/or Chemotherapy

Supportive care evidence-based treatment guidelines have been developed by the Multinational Association of Supportive Care in Cancer.[17] Complications can be generally classified as:

- acute or early transient, occurring only during therapy;
- chronic or late continuing or beginning, sometimes months to years, after completion of treatment.

- *Mucositis*
  - *Timing (acute)*: The most common, almost universal, acute oral effect of cancer therapy. It presents around 1–2 weeks into radiotherapy and 7 days after chemotherapy onset and subsides around the same period after completion of therapy. See Fig. 13.8. It can be severe in 90% of oral and pharyngeal cancer patients receiving radiation therapy and 65% of those treated for larynx or hypopharynx cancer.[18]
  - *Clinical presentation*: Mucosa is painful, atrophic, ulcerative, and denuded with destruction of the epithelial surface. It appears to be worse near metal restorations.
  - *Treatment*: Maintain good oral hygiene with regular mouth rinsing with bland rinses of saline and baking soda and brushing with a soft brush. Topical pain relief with 2% viscous lidocaine or benzydamine (where available); diphenhydramine elixir alone or mixed 50% with Maalox® or Kaopectate®; dyclonine HCL throat lozenges; Gelclair® (Helsinn Healthcare S.A., Lugano, Switzerland); Caphosol® (EUSAPharma (USA), Inc., Langhorne, PA); MuGard™ (Access Pharmaceuticals, Dallas, TX); or systemically with analgesics from nonsteroidal anti-inflammatory to combination narcotic agents.
  - *Prevention*: No effective preventative available for radiation mucositis; cryotherapy (sucking ice chips) during 5-fluoruracil, etidronate, and high-dose melphalan chemotherapy may be of some

Figure 13.8 (a,b) Mucositis of the palate and dorsum of the tongue of a patient on day 6 of combined chemoradiation therapy in a 41-year-old white female.

benefit. Patients receiving high-dose chemotherapy and total body irradiation for autologous stem-cell transplantation may benefit from keratinocyte growth factor-1 (palifermin) for 3 days prior to conditioning treatment and for 3 days posttransplantation for the prevention of oral mucositis.[19]

- **Fungal and Viral Infections**
  - *Timing (acute and chronic)*: Candida and herpetic infections occur in radiation patients and those undergoing preparation for hematopoetic stem-cell transplants.
  - *Clinical presentation*: These are due to changes in microbial load of oral mucosa and skin.
  - *Treatment*: Acyclovir or valaciclovir for herpes simplex virus.[20] Gastrointestinal tract absorbed drugs, like fluconazole or ketoconazole or a higher dose of clotrimazole, may be beneficial for the treatment of oral candidiasis.[21]
  - *Prevention*: Acyclovir or valaciclovir for herpes simplex virus.[20]

- **Hypogeusia/Dysgeusia**
  - *Timing (acute and chronic)*: Radiation doses greater than 60 Gy may lead to permanent loss of taste.
  - *Clinical presentation*: Loss of taste sensation possibly related to factors like reduced salivary flow, taste chemoreceptor destruction, and mucositis.
  - *Treatment*: None.
  - *Prevention*: None.

- **Salivary Gland Dysfunction and Xerostomia**
  - *Timing (chronic)*: A radiation dose as low as 25 Gy can cause salivary gland degeneration.
  - *Clinical presentation*: Serous glands degenerate faster than mucous glands causing acidic and thicker flow. This change causes difference in taste, speech, deglutition, mastication, antimicrobial presence, and remineralization. Mucosal dryness leads to inability to wear prostheses and thus to poor nutrition. See Fig. 13.9.
  - *Treatment*: Sipping water, over-the-counter saliva substitutes containing carboxymethylcellulose with added mucopolysaccharide or glycerate polymer gel base, saliva stimulants (sugarless preferably xylitol-containing mints or sour candy or gum), mouth rinse of ¼ teaspoon of glycerine in 8 oz of water, or prescription sialogogues: pilocarpine or cevimeline. Carbonated, acidic, alcohol-based products including

Figure 13.9 (a,b) Dry palatal and floor of the mouth mucosa 1.5 years post-72 Gy for SCC of the left tonsil and neck in a 61-year-old white male. Patient received hyperbaric oxygen for the exposed bone.

Figure 13.10 Radiation caries: (a) radiation caries 2 years after receiving 70 Gy for nasopharyngeal carcinoma; (b) radiation caries after radiation for SCC of the supraglottic larynx in a 39-year-old black female.

mouthwashes should be avoided. Coat lips with petrolatum ointment. Humidify sleeping area.[22]
- *Prevention*: Parotid gland sparing radiation techniques; possibly amifostine or pilocarpine during radiation therapy.[22]

- **Dental Caries**
  - *Timing (chronic)*: Related to radiation-induced salivary gland deficits.
  - *Clinical presentation*: Radiation or rampant caries progressing quickly in anatomical areas of teeth normally immune to caries. Cusp tip and circumferential cervical areas including canines are caries susceptible. See Fig. 13.10.
  - *Treatment*: Rapid restoration with amalgam, fluoride-releasing resin-modified glass ionomer restorative material, composite resins for anterior esthetic areas only, or full-coverage crowns.[23]
  - *Prevention*: Professionally applied and daily prescription strength topical fluoride treatments, mouth rinses, remineralizing agents, xylitol-containing products, and restricted sugar-containing foods help to prevent accelerated caries.

- *Trismus*
  - *Timing (chronic)*: Related to radiation fibrosis of the muscles of mastication.
  - *Clinical presentation*: Tonic contraction of masticatory muscles, temporomandibular joint contractions, and mucosal degeneration can cause limitation of mouth opening.
  - *Treatment*: Physiotherapy exercises with appliances as simple as taped tongue depressors are useful along with analgesic, anti-inflammatory medications.
  - *Prevention*: By performing mouth opening exercises in 20 maximal opening without pain cycles thrice daily. This can be accomplished by opening against gentle pressure generated by placing the hand against the midline mandible or with use of a handheld unit such as the TheraBite® Jaw Rehabilitation System™ (Craniomandibular Rehab, Inc., Denver, CO). Vertical dimension has to be maintained by daily exercises during radiation therapy.[24]

- *Osteoradionecrosis (ORN)*
  - *Timing (chronic)*: Related to hypoxic, hypocellular, hypovascular changes in alveolar bone that may undergo necrosis spontaneously or induced by infection or trauma (surgery). This happens months to years after radiation therapy and is dose related. There is about a 3% risk in the field of radiation regardless of whether teeth are removed before or after radiation.[25] Risk is higher in the posterior arch, mandible, and if doses to bone exceed 60 Gy or involve brachytherapy near the surgical site. Etiopathogenesis proposed is free radical formation, endothelial dysfunction, inflammation, and microvascular thrombosis leading to bone and tissue necrosis.
  - *Clinical presentation*: Bone within the field becomes devitalized, and mucosal or cutaneous dehiscence exposes underlying devascularized bone. See Fig. 13.11.
  - *Treatment*: Local debridement of sequestrated bone, resection with nonvascular bone reconstruction, microvascular composite flap reconstruction, and hyperbaric oxygen therapy are treatment options. Medical treatments proposed are pentoxifylline and tocopherol. Free tissue transfer has the best outcome. Hyperbaric

Figure 13.11 Osteoradionecrosis (ORN): (a) ORN of the right mandible of the patient in Fig. 13.10b; (b) ORN of the right mandible in an 87-year-old black female with history of 65 Gy to SCC right mandible 22 years earlier.

oxygen therapy is used with resection to treat ORN.
- *Prevention*: Local trauma to periodontal tissues, like extractions, are inciting factors for ORN. Mandibular surgery in the radiation field and continued tobacco smoking are identified as high risk. Preradiation extractions of only the diseased dentition has better prognosis than postradiation exposure. Hyperbaric oxygen therapy at 20 presurgical and 10–20 postsurgical treatments may be given adjunctively; however, ORN preventive effectiveness is controversial.[25]

- **Dental and Facial Skeletal Delay**
  - *Timing (chronic)*: Tumoricidal doses of radiation to growing child facial regions.
  - *Clinical presentation*: Underdevelopment of the growing facial bones; arrested growth; modified tooth eruption patterns; irregularities in enamel and dentin of the developing dentition.
  - *Treatment*: Growth and development monitoring, and orthodontic and restorative dentistry.
  - *Prevention*: None.

- **Speech and Swallowing**
  - *Timing (acute and chronic)*: Surgical and nonsurgical (organ preservation chemoradiation) interventions.
  - *Clinical presentation*: Speech and swallowing problems.
  - *Treatment*: May require maxillary obturators, speech and swallowing therapy, or permanent gastrostomy tube for feeding.
  - *Prevention*: None.

- **Nutritional Status**
  - *Timing (acute and chronic)*: Related to surgery, radiation therapy, and/or chemotherapy.
  - *Clinical presentation*: Poor healing, immune compromise, development of fistulas. Poor nutrition is an independent negative prognostic sign.
  - *Treatment/prevention*: High protein, high moisture content nutritional supplements are often required. Gastrostomy or tube feeding into the stomach and intestine is used as primary nutrition or supplementation.[26]

 Risks of Dental Care

Hemostasis

Thrombocytopenia, and increased bleeding risk, may result from some myelosuppressive chemotherapy protocols. Myelosuppression occurs in 25–30% of people taking cisplatin.

Susceptibility to Infection

Neutropenia may result from some myelosuppressive chemotherapy protocols making patients prone to bacterial infections. When mucositis and severe neutropenia are present, oral bacteria may seed oral ulcers and cause septicemia.

Xerostomia may predispose to oral candidiasis.

Drug Actions/Interactions

Chemotherapy drugs may be myelosuppressive or locally cytotoxic to mucosa.

Patient's Ability to Tolerate Dental Care

Tolerance of dental care is dependent on local cytotoxic effects of chemotherapy and radiation therapy to the oral mucosa. Patients will not be comfortable receiving dental care while mucositis is present.

IV. Recommended Readings and Cited References

Recommended Readings/ Resources

American Cancer Society. Available at: http://www.cancer.org.

National Institute of Dental and Craniofacial Research. *Cancer treatment and oral health.* Available at: http://www.nidcr.nih.gov/OralHealth/Topics/CancerTreatment/.

Oral Cancer Foundation. Available at: http://www.oralcancerfoundation.org.

Oral Health in Cancer Therapy—A Guide for Health Care Professionals, 3rd ed. Rankin KV, Jones DL, Redding SW, eds. 2008. Texas Dental Oncology Education Program. Available at: http://www.doep.org/. Accessed November 25, 2011.

Surveillance, Epidemiology, and End Results (SEER) Program. Available at: http://seer.cancer.gov/index.html.

Cited References

1. Hecht SS. Tobacco smoke carcinogens and lung cancer. J Natl Cancer Inst 1999;91(14):1194–210.
2. Cancela Mde C, Ramadas K, Fayette JM, Thomas G, Muwonge R, Chapuis F, et al. Alcohol intake and oral cavity cancer risk among men in a prospective study in Kerala, India. Community Dent Oral Epidemiol 2009;37(4):342–9.
3. Druesne-Pecollo N, Tehard B, Mallet Y, Gerber M, Norat T, Hercberg S, et al. Alcohol and genetic polymorphisms: effect on risk of alcohol-related cancer. Lancet Oncol 2009;10(2):173–80.
4. Gustavsson P, Jakobsson R, Johansson H, Lewin F, Norell S, Rutkvist LE. Occupational exposures and squamous cell carcinoma of the oral cavity, pharynx, larynx, and oesophagus: a case-control study in Sweden. Occup Environ Med 1998;55(6):393–400.
5. Lingen MW, Pinto A, Mendes RA, Franchini R, Czerninski R, Tilakaratne WM, et al. Genetics/epigenetics of oral premalignancy: current status and future research. Oral Dis 2011;17(Suppl. 1):7–22.
6. Siegel R, Ward E, Brawley O, Jemal A. Cancer statistics, 2011: the impact of eliminating socioeconomic and racial disparities on premature cancer deaths. CA Cancer J Clin 2011;61(4):212–36.
7. Chaturvedi AK, Engels EA, Anderson WF, Gillison ML. Incidence trends for human papillomavirus-related and -unrelated oral squamous cell carcinomas in the United States. J Clin Oncol 2008;26(4):612–9.
8. Rethman MP, Carpenter W, Cohen EE, Epstein J, Evans CA, Flaitz CM, et al. Evidence-based clinical recommendations regarding screening for oral squamous cell carcinomas. J Am Dent Assoc 2010;141(5):509–20.
9. Patton LL, Epstein JB, Kerr AR. Adjunctive techniques for oral cancer examination and lesion diagnosis: a systematic review of the literature. J Am Dent Assoc 2008;139(7):896–905.
10. Pelucchi C, Gallus S, Garavello W, Bosetti C, La Vecchia C. Cancer risk associated with alcohol and tobacco use: focus on upper aero-digestive tract and liver. Alcohol Res Health 2006;29(3):193–8.
11. Centers for Disease Control and Prevention. Alcohol: Frequently Asked Questions. 2008. Centers for Disease Control and Prevention, Atlanta, GA. Available at: www.cdc.gov/alcohol/faqs.htm#10. Accessed March 10, 2010.
12. Lingen MW, Kalmar JR, Karrison T, Speight PM. Critical evaluation of diagnostic aids for the detection of oral cancer. Oral Oncol 2008;44(1):10–22.
13. Fakhry C, Westra WH, Li S, Cmelak A, Ridge JA, Pinto H, et al. Improved survival of patients with human papillomavirus-positive head and neck squamous cell carcinoma in a prospective clinical trial. J Natl Cancer Inst 2008;100(4):261–69.
14. Coulthard P, Patel S, Grusovin GM, Worthington HV, Esposito M. Hyperbaric oxygen therapy for irradiated patients who require dental implants: a Cochrane review of randomised clinical trials. Eur J Oral Implantol 2008;1(2):105–10.
15. Ihde S, Kopp S, Gundlach K, Konstantinovi_ UNDEFINED VS. Effects of radiation therapy on craniofacial and dental implants: a review of the literature. Oral Surg Oral Med Oral Pathol Oral Radiol Endod 2009;107(1):56–65.
16. Linsen SS, Martini M, Stark H. Long-term results of endosteal implants following radical oral cancer surgery with and without adjuvant radiation therapy. Clin Implant Dent Relat Res 2009;October 16 [epub ahead of print].
17. Peterson DE, Bensadoun RJ, Lalla RV, McGuire DB. Supportive care treatment guidelines: value, limitations, and opportunities. Semin Oncol 2011;38(3):367–73.
18. Sonis ST. Oral mucositis. Anticancer Drugs 2011;22(7):607–12.
19. Keefe DM, Schubert MM, Elting LS, Sonis ST, Epstein JB, Raber-Durlacher JE, et al. Updated clinical practice guidelines for the prevention

and treatment of mucositis. Cancer 2007;109(5): 820–31.
20. Glenny AM, Fernandez Mauleffinch LM, Pavitt S, Walsh T. Interventions for the prevention and treatment of herpes simplex virus in patients being treated for cancer. Cochrane Database Syst Rev 2009;(1):CD006706.
21. Worthington HV, Clarkson JE, Khalid T, Meyer S, McCabe M. Interventions for treating oral candidiasis for patients with cancer receiving treatment. Cochrane Database Syst Rev 2010;(7): CD001972.
22. Shiboski CH, Hodgson TA, Ship JA, Schiødt M. Management of salivary hypofunction during and after radiotherapy. Oral Surg Oral Med Oral Pathol Oral Radiol Endod 2007;103:S66.e1–19.
23. Pendrys DG. Resin-modified glass-ionomer cement (RM-GIC) may provide greater caries preventive effect compared with composite resin, but high-quality studies are needed. J Evid Based Dent Pract 2011;11(4):180–2.
24. Bensadoun RJ, Riesenbeck D, Lockhart PB, Elting LS, Spijkervet FK, Brennan MT, et al. A systematic review of trismus induced by cancer therapies in head and neck cancer patients. Support Care Cancer 2010;18(8):1033–8.
25. Wahl MJ. Osteoradionecrosis prevention myths. Int J Radiat Oncol Biol Phys 2006;64(3):661–9.
26. Ravasco P, Monteiro-Grillo I, Marques Vidal P, Camilo ME. Impact of nutrition on outcome: a prospective randomized controlled trial in patients with head and neck cancer undergoing radiotherapy. Head Neck 2005;27(8):659–68.

Neurological Disorders

Robert G. Henry DMD, MPH

I. Background

Description of Diseases/Conditions

Because the nervous system comprises the brain, spinal cord, and spinal and peripheral nerves, functional capacity and life itself may be lost when disease or damage occurs. Neurological diseases/conditions can be classified in 12 major categories as described in the International Classification for Diseases (ICD)-10, Chapter 6: Diseases of the Nervous System.[1] This chapter will review the most common and representative neurological disorders that dentists are likely to see in dental practice with the exception of the Alzheimer's disease (AD) and other dementias, which will be discussed in Chapter 18.

Parkinson's Disease (PD)

In 1817, James Parkinson, an English surgeon described a condition he termed "the shaking palsy," with tremor at rest, rigidity, and bradykinesia (slowness of movement), today referred to as PD. PD is a progressive neurodegenerative condition of neurons that produce dopamine, primarily located in the substantia nigra. It is the second most common neurodegenerative condition after AD.

Multiple Sclerosis (MS)

MS, the most common autoimmune disease of the central nervous system (CNS), is a complex neurological condition. The pathological hallmark of MS is the plaque, which is an area of demyelination along an axon, limited to the white matter of the CNS and randomly located in more than one area of the brain or spinal cord.

Cerebrovascular Accident (CVA) or Stroke

A CVA is a serious and often fatal neurological event occurring when the blood supply to a part of the brain is suddenly interrupted, resulting in necrosis, or "infarction," of the affected tissue. If the blockage of the artery is temporary and blood flow is quickly restored, the brain may recover quickly. It can also cause mild to

The ADA Practical Guide to Patients with Medical Conditions, First Edition. Edited by Lauren L. Patton.
© 2012 American Dental Association. Published 2012 by John Wiley & Sons, Inc.

severe disabilities, and possibly death hours, days, or weeks after the initial stroke event. Death varies based on age and type of stroke:

- 80% after an intracerebral hemorrhage;
- 50% after a subarachnoid hemorrhage;
- 30% from an ischemia from thromboembolism.

Stroke is the leading cause of serious, long-term disability in the United States. Approximately 50% who survive the acute period (first 6 months) are alive 7 years later.

Of stroke survivors,

- 10% recover with no impairment;
- 50–70% regain functional independence but will have a mild residual disability;
- 15–30% are permanently disabled;
- 20% require institutional care (help with daily tasks such as bathing and dressing).[2]

Amyotrophic Lateral Sclerosis (ALS)

The most common disease of motor neuron diseases, ALS, also known as Lou Gehrig's disease, after the famous baseball player who acquired this disease in the 1930s in the prime of his career at age 36, involves progressive dysfunction of the nerves from the spinal cord and brain controlling voluntary muscle movement.

Traumatic Brain Injury (TBI)

Brain injury (BI) is defined as damage to the brain caused by a *primary insult* such as trauma or a *secondary insult* such as metabolic and physiological events that occur after the primary damage.

Epilepsy (and Other Seizure Disorders)

The term "epilepsy" refers to a group of disorders characterized by chronic, recurrent, paroxysmal seizure activity; altered consciousness; or involuntary movements caused by abnormal and spontaneous electrical activity in the brain. Seizures may be accompanied with motor manifestations (convulsive) or may occur with other changes in neurological function (sensory, cognitive, and emotional). Symptoms are produced by excessive temporary neuronal discharges, which result from intracranial or extracranial causes. Epilepsy can occur as a result of trauma or be a developmental condition.

Epileptic seizures are divided into two major classes: partial, subdivided into simple and complex, and generalized based on clinical and electroencephalographic (EEG) features.[3]

Partial Seizures

Simple Partial or Focal Seizures

- Occur in 75–80% of epileptics.
- Characterized by neuronal discharge from a recognized cortical locus that is not associated with loss of consciousness.
- Signs include episodes of altered sensation, cognitive function, or loss of motor activity.
- Known as "auras" if they precede a complex or secondarily generalized seizure.
- Symptoms vary, depending on the brain region involved and can have motor signs (movement of a body part), sensory signs (visual or olfactory changes), psychic signs (fear, anxiety, hallucinations), or autonomic signs (dizziness, tachycardia, sweating).[4]

Complex Partial Seizures

- Originate in the frontal and/or temporal lobes.
- Result in impaired consciousness with altered behavior, sensation, or motor activity that can last from 30 seconds to 2 minutes.
- The motor activity often consists of repetitive automatic movements of the face or limbs.

Generalized Seizures

Generalized seizures begin with a widespread, excessive discharge involving most or all of the brain at the same time. They are divided into several types, including the following:

Tonic–Clonic Seizures

- Clinical signs of generalized tonic–clonic convulsions (grand mal seizure) are classic and followed in order.
  - *Aura* (a brief sensory alteration) consists of auditory, gustatory, olfactory, hallucinations, slurring of speech, frequent blinking, irritability, and/or mood changes.
  - Sudden loss of consciousness, with an "epileptic cry" caused by air being forced out by the contraction of the diaphragm through a partially closed glottis.
  - *Tonic phase* (lasting <1 minute) happens when body contracts producing muscular rigidity; person may become cyanotic, tachycardic, and hypertensive.
  - *Clonic phase* (lasting seconds to several minutes) is characterized by forceful jerking of the head, trunk, and extremities. Loss of bladder control is common, and patients may bite their tongues, cheeks, or lips.
  - *Postictal phase* is characterized by a slow return to consciousness, headache, disorientation, muscle soreness, and sleepiness.

Status Epilepticus

- A tonic–clonic seizure lasting >5 minutes without a recovery period and is a serious medical emergency.
- Caused by abrupt withdrawal of an anticonvulsant medication or an abused substance (cocaine, amphetamines).
- Possible airway obstruction and aspiration, which can lead to severe hypoxemia, acidosis, permanent BI or death.
- Supplemental oxygen followed by parenteral administration of a benzodiazepine should be administered after initiation of the emergency response system.

Absence or Petit Mal Seizures

- Seconds of unconsciousness without an absence of body tone.
- Signs include appearance of daydreaming, rapid blinking of the eyelids, minor movements of the hands, and/or subtle facial twitching without generalized muscular activity.

Myoclonic Seizures

- A brief jerk or series of jerks that may involve a small part of the body, such as a single finger, hand, or foot, or may involve both sides of the body simultaneously, most often the shoulders or upper arms.
- They are generally of short duration (minutes) and have no postictal phase.

Atonic Seizures or Drop Seizures

- Sudden loss of muscle tone occurs throughout most or all of the body, which may include head nodding or limb dropping, or the patient collapsing to the ground.

Clonic Seizures (of Focal Epilepsy)

- Rhythmic, jerking movements of body parts, such as the arms or legs, with impaired consciousness.

Tonic Seizures

- Stiffening of the body or limb; can result in falling if the person is standing with risk of traumatic injury to the head, and oral and dental structures.
- Last up to 20 seconds and are followed by a postictal state.[4]

Epidemiology

Epidemiologic aspects of the selected conditions are listed in Table 14.1.

Table 14.1. Epidemiology of Selected Neurological Disorders in the United States

Condition	Prevalence	Incidence	Gender	Age	Race/Ethnicity
Parkinson's disease (PD)	1 million (1 in 300)	50,000 new cases/year (three- to fourfold increase expected)	More common in men than women	1% <50 years 2.5% >70 years	No racial predilection
Multiple sclerosis (MS)	380,000 people (1 per 850)	Incidence has been increasing	Affects women two times as often as men	Affects young adults age 15–50 years old	Higher in temperate regions and less along equator
Cerebrovascular accidents (CVAs)	4.7 million (survivors); 3rd most common cause of death	Over 700,000 new cases a year (averages one stroke/minute)	Increased incidence in young men and old women	Onset age 20–40 years 28% <65 years 50% >75 years	Increased incidence in racial/ethnic minorities
Amyotrophic lateral sclerosis (ALS) (Lou Gehrig's)	30,000 cases of ALS in the United States	More than 5000 people/year	Affects men more than women	Generally diagnosed after age 55 years	No preference
Traumatic brain injuries (TBIs)	More than 75,000 deaths from TBI/year (400 per 100,000 disabled survivors)	More than 1.7 million TBIs every year	Young men ages 16–24 account for nearly 50% of all motor vehicle accidents	Infants (shaken baby syndrome) and older adults from falls; two-thirds of TBI occur in persons <36, with vehicular accidents accounting for 50%	No preference
Epilepsy	3 million	About 200,000 new cases/year; 0.5% overall; 10% of the U.S. population will have a seizure in a lifetime	No gender prevalence	Increased incidence with age; as many as 1% of children under 20, 3% of those who are 75+	Higher among racial minorities than among Caucasians

Pathogenesis/Etiology

PD

The cause of PD is unknown, although several factors are associated with PD including viral infections, genetic mutations, stroke, brain tumor, and head injuries that damage specific cells affected by the dopamine in the brain. Certain environmental factors increase the risk of developing PD including exposure to manganese (such as miners or welders), mercury, carbon disulfide, certain agricultural herbicides, and certain drugs (contaminated heroin, neuroleptics such as phenothiazines and butyrophenones).

MS

The etiology of MS is unknown; however, it is widely believed that the disease is triggered by an infectious agent that causes autoimmune-mediated inflammation leading to demyelination and axonal injury. The area of demyelination initially disrupts the conduction of a nerve impulse, but with recovery, conduction is slowed and the refractory period is prolonged. Conduction along these segments is sensitive to temperature changes and may fail if the temperature rises. Affected areas of the brain may range in size from 1 mm to several centimeters in diameter. Demyelination from inflammation, most often of the optic nerve, brain stem, and cervical spinal cord, results in tissue destruction, swelling, and breakdown of the blood–brain barrier.[5] A genetic component may exist, as the risk of a first-degree relative developing MS is two to four times that of the general population.

CVA or Stroke

There are two main causes of stroke:

- Ischemic (87% of all strokes): arterial blockage in the brain.
  - *Thrombus*—occlusion of a cerebral artery by a blood clot formed on the arterial wall obstructing blood flow.
  - *Embolus*—having the clot break off from the arterial wall and travelling through the bloodstream until it cannot pass through, thus obstructing blood flow distal to the embolus resulting in infarction.
  - Primary risk factors: atherosclerosis and cardiac pathology such as a previous myocardial infarction and atrial fibrillation.
- Hemorrhagic (13% of all strokes): bleeding into the brain due to arterial rupture.
  - *Intracerebral* (10%)—bleeding into the brain.
  - *Subarachnoid* (3%)—bleeding into the space between the brain and inner lining of the skull.
  - Primary risk factor: hypertension.

There are known risk factors for stroke, some modifiable (smoking, lack of exercise, physical inactivity, obesity) and others immutable (older age, people of color, male gender, family history). Other confounding risks, subject to medical management, include diabetes, hypertension, congestive heart failure, prior stroke, high cholesterol, atrial fibrillation, carotid stenosis, and possibly periodontitis due to the effect of inflammatory products (C-reactive protein, interleukins, etc.) on systemic vasculature.[6-8] Medications such as estrogens, pseudoephedrine and phenylephrine can also be risk factors for strokes by creating a hypercoagulable state or by increasing blood pressure. Having multiple risk factors greatly increases the risk of stroke.

A *transient ischemic attack* (TIA) is defined as a stroke that lasts less than 24 hours and has no residual effects. While most TIAs last less than 10 minutes, up to one-third of patients will have noticeable changes on brain imaging studies that indicate injury to the brain.

The type of deficit that occurs from a stroke is directly dependent on the size and location of the infarct or hemorrhage. If many small strokes occur in the brain, a person can develop a condition called *multi-infarct dementia (MID)*. People with MID may have a wide variety of symptoms including mental deterioration with memory loss (dementia), walking problems, facial muscle problems such as difficulty talking and opening the eyelids, and weakness or numbness in one or more body areas.[6]

ALS

ALS is characterized by degeneration of the cells in both the upper and lower motor neurons of the spinal cord and cerebral cortex. Degeneration of descending pathways leads to weakness and spasticity of the muscles in the limbs, and eventually progresses to muscle atrophy and death from respiratory failure within 3–5 years in about 50% of patients. The cause of ALS is unknown, but a genetic abnormality is currently the focus of researchers.

TBIs

The causes of head injury include falls, assaults, motor vehicle accidents, shaken baby syndrome, and sports concussions. With severe head injury, brain damage occurs because of the direct trauma to the brain resulting in disruption of the brain, shearing of axons, and intracerebral hemorrhage. Injuries occur at the site of trauma, and also the opposite side of injury, called a contre-coup injury. Contre-coup injuries result from acceleration/deceleration forces moving the brain within the skull. Secondary insults can occur due to brain edema, which causes intracranial pressure to rise and lead to cerebral herniation or hypoperfusion causing brain cells to die. Extradural hematomas, resulting from middle meningeal artery bleeding into the extradural space can cause rapid deterioration following an apparently good recovery from a head injury.

Epilepsy (and Other Seizure Disorders)

Epilepsy may occur when there are

- disruptions to the normal connections between nerve cells in the brain;
- imbalances of natural chemicals or neurotransmitters that are important to the signalling among nerve cells;
- changes in the membranes of nerve cells that alter their normal sensitivity.[9]

Some of these disruptions, imbalances, and changes may develop early in life and may be related to early exposures and events. Others may be acquired later.

Conditions and events that may lead to epilepsy are:

- unknown cause (cryptogenic) or idiopathic (syndrome-like)—these account for two-thirds of seizures;
- oxygen deprivation (e.g., during childbirth);
- brain infections (e.g., meningitis, encephalitis, cysticercosis, or brain abscess);
- TBI or head injury;
- stroke (resulting from a block or rupture of a blood vessel in the brain);
- other neurological diseases (e.g., AD);
- brain tumors;
- certain genetic disorders.

Beyond epilepsy, there are a number of medical conditions such as having a high fever, low blood sugar, alcohol or drug withdrawal, and immediately following a brain concussion, that can cause seizures. For people who experience a seizure under such circumstances, without a history of seizures at other times, there is only the need to treat the underlying medical condition that caused the seizure.

Seizures in epilepsy can be evoked by specific stimuli. Approximately 1 of 15 patients reports that seizures occurred after exposure to flickering lights, monotonous sounds, music, or a loud noise. Syncope as occurring in the dental setting and low oxygen to the brain, are also known to trigger seizures.

Coordination of Care between Dentist and Physician

A detailed health history will help to determine the stability of the specific disorder and the frequency or nature of medical care received. For example, how long an epileptic patient has been seizure free, should indicate that he or she is under good control. Similarly, the medical history will include medications used to treat the neurological condition, and dentists should know their actions, interactions (if any) to dental medications and local anesthetics used, and side effects or adverse reactions to expect (such as xerostomia).

There are a number of neurological conditions that may occur for the first time in a dental office as a result of a dental procedure or increase in stress (stroke, seizure in epilepsy, Bell's palsy). Other neurological conditions can mimic dental problems such as trigeminal neuralgia (TN) and toothache. Because of these potential interrelationships, dentists must be alert to oral signs and symptoms that may indicate undiagnosed or emergently occurring neurological conditions.

A dental consultation should be routine as many of the medications used in managing neurological conditions have adverse and detrimental oral side effects such as dry mouth and gingival overgrowth that require dental management. Medical providers may identify drooling in late-stage PD patients and request dental intervention. Similarly, stroke patients may need modified preventive oral care regimens to accommodate to functional disabilities.

Invasive or oral surgical dental interventions should be planned with the input of the medical team or, in most cases, the neurologist. For some conditions, such as stroke, elective dental care should be deferred until risk factors (such as underlying hypertension) are under control. For other conditions, such as ALS, MS, epilepsy, and PD, dental care should be coordinated with the time of day that the person's movements or symptoms are best managed.

II. Medical Management

Parkinson's Disease (PD)

Identification, Medical History, and Physical Exam Findings

The classical features of PD are known by the acronym TRAP:

- *Tremor*: trembling or shaking of one hand at rest that looks like a person is rolling a pill. Generally the first sign, occurring in 70% of untreated patients.
- *Rigidity*: difficulty writing due to stiff muscles.
- *Akinesia* (impaired movement) or bradykinesia: altered gait characterized by loss of arm swing, shorter steps, difficulty starting or stopping, and slowness.
- *Postural instability*: stooped posture.

In late disease, there may be cognitive impairment of memory and concentration, global dementia, mood disturbances, insomnia, and fatigue. The frequency of dementia is controversial but may occur in as many as 25% of PD patients. There is no specific laboratory test for PD.

Medical Treatment

There is no standard medical treatment for PD. Listed in Table 14.2 are the six classes of drugs commonly used to treat the patient's symptoms once they cause lifestyle problems such as

Table 14.2. Medications Used in the Management of Parkinson's Disease (PD)[a]

Drug Classes	Examples/Drugs	Drug Effect	Adverse Effect	Dental Concerns
Dopamine precursor	Levodopa (L-dopa) Carbidopa/levodopa *Sinemet CR®*	Drug precursor that is metabolized into dopamine in the brain	Dyskinesia, fatigue, headache, anxiety, confusion, insomnia, orthostatic hypotension	When uncontrolled movements occur, sedation may be needed to treat; caution when getting up from dental chair; L-dopa—dry mouth
Dopamine agonists	Bromocriptine *Parlodel®* Pramipexole *Mirapex®* Ropinirole HCl *Requip®*	Mimics the action of dopamine	Psychosis (hallucinations, delusions), orthostatic hypotension, nausea dyskinesia	Caution when getting up from dental chair; Mirapex® interacts with erythromycin
Dopamine-releasing agent	Amantadine *Symmetrel®*	Enhances dopamine transmission	Anticholinergic effects: sedation, urinary retention, peripheral edema, nausea, constipation, confusion	Dry mouth, nausea, sedation, caution when leaving dental chair
Monoamine oxidase B inhibitor	Selegiline *Eldepryl®* *Zelapar®*	Prevents metabolism of dopamine in the brain	Dizziness, orthostatic hypotension, nausea	Caution when leaving dental chair. No adverse problems with using epinephrine or levonordefrin
Cathchol-O-methyl-transferase (COMT) inhibitors	Tolcapone *Tasmar®* Entacapone *Comtan®*	Used with levodopa to prevent breakdown in intestine, allowing more levodopa to reach the brain	Dyskinesia, psychosis, orthostatic hypotension, nausea, diarrhea, abnormal taste	Caution with use of vasoconstrictors; monitor vital signs and limit dose to two carpules containing 1:100,000 epinephrine or less; aspirate injections
Anticholinergic	Trihexyphenidyl HCL *Artane®* Benztropine mesylate *Cogentin®*	Blocks the effect of acetylcholine (another brain neurotransmitter) to rebalance its levels with dopamine	Sedation, urinary retention, dry mouth	Dry mouth

[a] Modified from Little, Falace, Miller, and Rhodus, 2008. Table of Drugs Used in the Management of PD. pp. 477–478.
CR, controlled release; HCl, hydrochloride.

slowness or imbalance (falls). Dopaminergic drugs are reserved for advanced PD because their activity lessens with long-term treatment and their use can result in long-term complications including psychosis. Other therapies include protein-restricted diet, exercise to maintain muscle tone, neurosurgery including deep brain stimulation and thalamotomy (removing the thalamus) or pallidotomy (removing the globus pallidus), and transplantation of fetal embryonic cells.[10]

Multiple Sclerosis (MS)

Identification, Medical History, Physical Exam, and Laboratory Testing

Common presenting symptoms include the following[5]:

- *Disturbance in visual function*: distortion of the central vision; impairment of color perception; pain on eye movement; nystagmus; double vision; vision loss.
- *Sensory symptoms*: Feeling "numb"; cold, pins, and needles; swelling or "tightness" in the arms, legs, or trunk.
- *Motor weakness*: Affecting the legs which produces paraplegia; may have marked spasticity, incoordination, difficulty walking, loss of balance and vertigo; bowel and bladder incontinence; spastic paresis of skeletal muscles causing imprecise speech or tremor in speaking.
- *Fatigue*: Prominent, increases in the afternoon.

There are two main patterns of disease as seen in Fig. 14.1:

- *Relapsing remitting (90% of all patients)*: clear relapses followed by recovery; frequency of relapses and duration of remission vary considerably; may go on to produce a secondary progressive form with a progressing increase in disability.

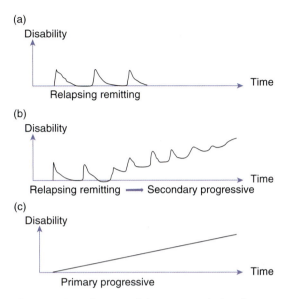

Figure 14.1 Patterns of disease in multiple sclerosis.

- *Primary progressive (10% of all patients)*: deterioration that begins from onset.

MS is diagnosed from the history, clinical exam, cerebral spinal fluid studies, altered sensory evoked potential, and magnetic resonance imaging (MRI) brain scan performed over time.

Medical Treatment

There is no known cure for MS. Multiple treatments are directed toward relief of symptoms.

Medications used to manage the symptoms or prevent relapses of MS are seen in Table 14.3.

Corticosteroids and immunomodulating drugs are mainstays of therapy. Other MS-associated conditions include TN, headache, and optic neuritis.

CVA/Stroke

Identification/Medical History/Physical Exam

A new-onset stroke or TIA requires immediate medical attention to prevent extensive brain

Table 14.3. Medications Used in the Medical Management of Multiple Sclerosis (MS)[a]

Drug Classes	Examples/Drugs	Drug Effect	Adverse Effects	Dental Concerns
Primary drugs				
Corticosteroids	Methylprednisolone	Anti-inflammatory	Immunosuppression/adrenal suppression	Consider adrenal and immune response
Interferon beta-1a Interferon beta-1b	Avonex®, Rebif® Betaseron®	Slows disease progression	Transient flu-like symptoms	None described
Alternatives				
Glatiramer acetate	Copaxone® injection	Reduce rate of clinical relapse	Ulcerative stomatitis, lymphadenopathy, salivary gland enlargement	None described
Mitoxantron	Novantrone® infusion	Arrests cell cycle and used as last resort	Leukopenia, cardiac problems, leukemia, mucositis, stomatitis	
GABA agonist	Baclofen	Antispastic (Manage spasticity)	Sedation	None described
GABA receptor Activators	Benzodiazepines: lorazepam, diazepam			
Modifies calcium Release in muscle	Dantrolene			
Alpha-2 adrenergic agonist	Tizanidine (Zanaflex®)			
Anticholinergics	Ditropan®, Detrol®	Bladder control	Sedation, urinary retention	Dry mouth
Dopamine-releasing agent	Amantadine (Symmetrel®)	Helps to reduce fatigue	Anticholinergic effects: sedation, urinary retention, peripheral edema, nausea, constipation, confusion	Dry mouth, nausea, sedation, caution when leaving dental chair
Antiseizure	Carbamazepine (Tegretol®) Phenytoin (Dilantin®)	Prevents paroxysmal events	Toxic levels may cause confusion	Gingival overgrowth
Antidepressants	Serotonin reuptake inhibitors (Prozac®) Tricyclic antidepressants (Elavil®)	Manage depression occurring in >50% of MS patients	Anticholinergic effects: sedation, urinary retention, peripheral edema, nausea, constipation, confusion	Dry mouth, nausea, sedation, caution when leaving dental chair

[a] Modified from Little, Falace, Miller, Rhodus, 2008, p. 483.
GABA, gamma-aminobutyric acid.

tissue damage. Symptoms of stroke depend on the type and area of brain affected. Signs of ischemic stroke usually occur suddenly, and signs of hemorrhagic stroke usually develop gradually. Classic warning signs include sudden one-sided weakness or numbness in the face, arm, or leg; sudden decrease in the level of consciousness or confusion; trouble speaking, understanding, walking, or seeing in one or both eyes; loss of balance or coordination; severe sudden headache.[5] A patient with a history of stroke may have varying disabilities that compromise the ability to perform normal activities of daily living independently.

Medical Treatment

There are three levels of medical management of the stroke patient:

Prevention: Controlling blood pressure and stopping smoking. Medications that decrease platelet aggregation (aspirin, ticlopidine, and dypyridamole) are used to prevent strokes. Carotid endarterectomy surgery is used when a moderate or severe atherosclerotic blockage in the carotid artery develops.

Early Diagnosis: If a person experiences signs or symptoms of a stroke, early emergency medical service (EMS) transportation to a hospital is critical for computerized tomography (CT) imaging to determine if there has been a TIA or stroke and whether the stroke is hemorraghic or thrombotic. Early diagnosis establishes whether the stroke is due to ischemia from a thromboembolism or from a hemorrhage.

Treatment: Treatment targets preventing further thrombosis or hemorrhage, and thrombolysis with intravenous administration of tissue plasminogen activator (tPA) within 3 hours of ischemic stroke onset. If patients survive, anticoagulants, such as heparin, warfarin, aspirin, platelet receptor agonists (clopidogrel, abciximab, ticlopidine), and Aggrenox® (dipyridamole combined with aspirin), are used to stabilize ischemic strokes and prevent further strokes from thromboembolism. Anticonvulsants may be used to manage seizures that may accompany the postoperative course of stroke.

Recovery and Rehabilitation: Stroke recovery is often divided into two categories:
- *Neurological recovery*: ability of the brain to regain lost abilities; depends on factors including extent and location of brain injury, early treatment, and prestroke health and intellectual status.
- *Functional recovery*: extent of improvement in daily activities such as bathing, dressing, walking, and talking, after neurological recovery ends. A stroke rehabilitation team may include physical, occupational, and speech therapists; nursing; social workers; physicians; and other professionals such as dentists.[6]

Amyotropic Lateral Sclerosis (ALS)

Identification/Medical History/ Physical Exam

Initial symptoms of ALS include muscle cramping, weakness, and atrophy that begin in the small muscles of the hand and forearm. Changes in muscle tone as a result of the progressive deterioration of the motor neurons results in dysphagia, dysarthria, muscle atrophy, and paralysis. Patients retain all sensory and cognitive capabilities, eye movement, and control of the urinary sphincter through the final stages of the disease. Lacking a laboratory test for diagnosing ALS, clinical exam, MRI, and nerve conduction tests can exclude other neuropathies and support the diagnosis but do not confirm it.

Medical Treatment

Treatment is supportive and involves most of the professionals on the medical team; ultimately, gastrostomy tube may be required to support feeding and tracheostomy with ventilator support for respiration. Psychological support for the patient and relatives is important in this relentless, progressive disease. Some drug therapy and other medical interventions have been shown to be useful, including baclofen for spasticity and riluzole, which is a glutamate antagonist that has been shown to improve 18 months of survival by 7% and delay need for tracheostomy.[11]

Traumatic Brain Injury (TBI)

Identification/Medical History/ Physical Exam

TBI can be classified into mild, moderate, and severe categories. The Glasgow Coma Scale is the most commonly used system for classifying TBI severity but is limited in predicting outcomes.[12]

Medical Treatment

Management is aimed at preventing brain damage which depends on the severity of the injury, with loss of consciousness over 5 minutes, altered consciousness, seizures, and skull fracture indicating greater severity and requiring brain CT or MRI assessment. Early management focuses on avoiding hypotension, maintaining oxygenation and avoiding raised intracranial pressure, or reducing it by surgical procedures to evacuate intracranial hematomas and shunt for hydrocephalus.

Once the patient is stable and improving, a rehabilitation team approach works best to manage the sequelae from TBI. There are frequent psychological and behavior difficulties, personality changes, disinhibition, and memory loss. Even after a mild head injury, patients can become anxious, have difficulty concentrating, sleep poorly, and experience posttraumatic stress disorder.

Other symptoms that may develop include problems in cognition, sensory processing, communication, and behavior or mental health. Patients may also experience unilateral or bilateral paresis or paralysis in addition to changes

---

Glasgow Coma Scale (GCS)

Eye opening (E)	Verbal response (V)	Motor response (M)
4 Spontaneously	5 Normal conversation	6 Normal
3 To voice	4 Disoriented conversation	5 Localizes to pain
2 To pain	3 Words, but not coherent	4 Withdraws to pain
1 None	2 No words, only sounds	3 Decorticate posture
	1 None	2 Decerebrate
		1 None

Total GCS = E score + V score + M score (minimum 3; maximum 15)
Score: 13–15 = Mild TBI; 9–12 = Moderate TBI; <8 = Severe TBI

in muscle tone, sensation, bowel and bladder control, edema, and coordination. Depending on the location of the brain damage, the patient may develop contractures, hindering mobility, or respiratory difficulties. The frequency of posttraumatic epilepsy depends on the severity and type of head injury.

Epilepsy (and Other Seizure Disorders)

Identification/Medical Exam and Laboratory Testing

The clinical signs and symptoms of seizures depend on the location of epileptic discharges in the cortex and the extent and pattern of the propagation in the brain.

Diagnosing epilepsy is a multistep process involving the following evaluations:

- seizure activity history, medication review, neurological exam along with supporting blood and clinical laboratory tests to rule out metabolic diseases that can cause seizures;
- EEG is the most valuable diagnostic tool identifying seizure type and predicting the likelihood of recurrence as it records electrical activity of the brain;
- imaging methods such as a CT or MRI and positron emission tomography (PET) scans may identify areas of the brain that produce seizures.

Medical Treatment

- Medications specific for the type of seizure activity, as seen in Table 14.4, to achieve control with minimal side effects.
  - On antiepileptic medications 70% enter remission, becoming seizure free for 5 or more years, while 10% never achieve remission.[13]
- Surgery or pharmacological intervention if an identifiable neoplasm, infection, or metabolic imbalance problem is diagnosed.

- Vagus nerve stimulator for some patients with unsatisfactory seizure control on medications; it delivers short bursts of energy to regions in the brain felt to be responsible for seizures.

III. Dental Management

Evaluation

Although most patients with neurological diseases or conditions will have been clinically diagnosed prior to their dental visit, dentists should be alert to signs and symptoms such as memory deficits, an inability to perform motor or verbal tasks, or personality changes:

- Begin with a careful medical and dental history including a review of medications.
- Communicate in the presence of a family caregiver if the patient has difficulty understanding, or is not capable to give informed consent. The caregiver can verify the history, interpret symptom meaning, ease patient anxiety, and facilitate legal consent.
- For competent, responsive patients, address the patient directly with short, simple phrases, giving only one direction at a time, allowing response time and repeating if needed.
- Nonverbal communication is important and includes exhibiting a relaxed, calm, and confident manner, using direct eye contact, encouraging touch, and demonstrating procedures prior to performing them.

Dental Treatment Modifications

A number of specially adapted preventive products or techniques are very helpful for caregivers to use with patients who have neurological disorders:

- The Collis-Curve™ (Collis Curve, Inc., Brownsville, TX, 1-800-298-4818; http://

Table 14.4. Medications Commonly Used in the Management of Epilepsy[a]

Indication	Medication	Main Side Effects
Primarily partial seizures	Carbamazepine (*Tegretol®*)	Ataxia, dizziness, diplopia, agranulocytosis, thrombocytopenia, liver dysfunction
	Lamotrigine (*Lamictal®*)	Ataxia, dizziness, diplopia, blurred vision, somnolence, headache, nausea, vomiting, rash
Primarily absence seizures	Clonazepam (*Klonopin®*)	Ataxia, drowsiness, general CNS depression, abnormal behavior, palpitations, muscle weakness
	Ethosuximide (*Zarontin®*)	GI upset, liver failure, weight gain, tremors, alopecia
Tonic–clonic seizures	Phenytoin (*Dilantin®*)	Ataxia, confusion, lethargy, gingival overgrowth, blood dyscrasias, skin rash, allergic reaction
	Phenobarbital	Drowsiness, CNS depression, megaloblastic anemia (rare)
	Topiramate (*Topamax®*)	Mood disturbances, confusion, sedation, paresthesias, hyperthermia, acidosis
	Valproic acid (*Depakene®*)	GI upset (indigestion, nausea, and vomiting, cramping, diarrhea, constipation), hypersalivation, anorexia, increased appetite, agranulocytosis, thrombocytopenia
	Divalproex sodium (*Depakote®*)	
Status epilepticus	Midazolam (*Versed®*)	Respiratory depression, decreased blood pressure, nausea, vomiting, diplopia, mood swings

[a] Adapted from Rhodus and Miller, 2008.
GI, gastrointestinal; CNS, central nervous system.

Key questions to ask the patient

- What type of neurological disorder do you have?
- How is your neurological disorder treated?
- What are the signs and symptoms of your neurological disorder?
- What type of stroke did you have? What activities are now difficult for you?
    - Do you have any long-term effects from your stroke?
- How often do you have seizures? When was your last seizure?
    - What brings them on? How long do they last? What happens when you have a seizure? How well controlled is your seizure disorder?
- Do you have any other underlying medical conditions?
- What are the laboratory values associated with your medical conditions?
- Are you on an anticoagulant, or do you have any increased bleeding tendencies?
- What types of medications can you not take?

Key questions to ask the physician

- What is the severity of the patient's neurological disorder?
- Is the patient in remission (controlled disorder) or an active stage of the disorder?
- Does the patient have memory or functional deficits?
- What medications are being prescribed for the patient's neurological disorder?
- Is the patient being treated for other medical conditions?
- What are the patient's most recent laboratory values?
- If the patient has Dilantin®-induced gingival overgrowth, is there a substitute medication that can be tried?

www.colliscurve.com), shown in Fig. 14.2. A specialized toothbrush with three rows of bristles for assisted brushing that, when placed correctly, can clean the lingual, facial, and occlusal surfaces of the teeth at the same time, making it easier for caregivers to use than conventional or electric brushes.

- Open Wide® Disposable Mouth Rest (Specialized Care Co., Inc., Hampton, NH, 1-800-722-7375; http://www.specializedcare.com), shown in Fig. 14.3. A foam mouth prop designed for caregivers to use to keep the mouth open during oral hygiene.
- If a person has trouble gripping, working with occupational therapists to modify a toothbrush with a Velcro® (Velcro USA, Manchester, NH) strap may suffice.

Other conventional preventive products may be helpful for caregivers to maintain oral hygiene and health, including electric toothbrushes, proxabrushes for cleaning between teeth, and fluorides in a patient-tolerable method. Caregivers need to be reminded to

Figure 14.2 Collis-Curve (Collis Curve, Inc.). Note the three rows of bristles.

Figure 14.3 Open Wide (Specialized Care Co., Inc.) disposable mouth rest compared with tongue blade and gauze.

keep their fingers from between the teeth of their patients, due to the danger of being bitten.

PD

Dentists should be able to recognize the main clinical features (TRAP) distinctive for PD. If these are present in an undiagnosed patient, referral to a physician for diagnosis is essential.

For patients diagnosed with PD, dental management concerns include the following:

- Ability of patients to provide daily oral hygiene due to muscle rigidity and tremor. It is important to encourage patients with PD to be as independent as possible in self-care activities, keep the muscles in good shape, and not lose muscle strength. Brushing will take longer and may require adaptive devices.
- Unexpected patient movements in poorly controlled or advanced PD patients that impact the ability to tolerate dental care and may require oral or intravenous sedation.
- Preventing drug interactions from dental/medical medications used in PD management.

MS

Reports of progressive facial pain in a young adult with no dental pathology (simulating TN), visual disturbances, numbness, or muscle weakness, should all alert the dentist of possible undiagnosed MS or other neurological disease and warrant referral to a physician or neurologist. In most cases of patients with MS, because fatigue is often worse in the afternoon, dental appointments should be scheduled in the morning.

Level of dental care depends on disease progression:

- *Initial stage*: (stable and in remission with little motor spasticity and weakness) no modifications are needed and patients can receive routine dental care.
- *Later stages*: patients may need help in transferring from a wheelchair to the dental chair; may require assistance in maintaining routine, daily oral hygiene; if in need of emergency dental care, consultation with the physician is advised.

Stroke/CVA

For stroke patients with residual deficits, treatment plans should be individualized considering the extent of disability and patient and caregiver motivation. All restorations should be placed with ease of cleansability in mind. In addition to recognizing the patient at risk for a stroke (to prevent a stroke or recurrent stroke) and managing a new onset stroke in the office, modifications include the following:

- An appreciation for stroke survivors' deficits and communication styles related to left or right brain injuries. Suggestions for dental professionals working with stroke patients are shown in Tables 14.5 and 14.6.
- Transferring patients and preventing distress during dental treatment.
- Managing oral dysfunctions from stroke and complications from medications, while preventing drug interactions.
- Modifying home care practices, increasing recall visit frequency, providing fluoride supplementation, and supporting the depressed patient.

ALS

As ALS progresses, caregivers will need to take an active role in supporting oral self-care with brushing assistance. Patients may pocket food in the alveolar folds due to weak facial muscles requiring the caregiver to sweep the mouth from back to front to check for retained food after meals.

Table 14.5. Suggestions for Dental Professionals Working with Left-CVA Patients

Left Brain Damage (L-CVA) Findings	Implications
Paralysis to right side Speech and language deficits	Because this patient has trouble communicating, it is easy to *underestimate* his or her abilities, which may be nonverbal. Use simple drawings or write directions to communicate.
Behavior style: slow, cautious, disorganized	Do not rush the patient in doing things.
Memory deficits: auditory	Communicate by eliminating extraneous stimuli; do not raise voice or use "baby talk"; substitute pantomime and demonstration for words; divide tasks into simple steps; give frequent, accurate, and immediate positive feedback; and ask simple and brief questions.
Anxious	Use stress-reduction techniques.

Modified from Stroke Association Org, 2011.

Table 14.6. Suggestions for Dental Professionals Working with Right-CVA Patients

Right Brain Damage (R-CVA) Findings	Implications
Paralysis to left side Spatial and perceptual deficits	Because this patient can speak and write, it is easy to *overestimate* his or her abilities.
Behavior style: quick and impulsive	Do not allow the patient to do things such as transfer by himself unless you are there to watch and help if needed.
Memory deficits: visual including visual field cuts	Move slowly around a patient's head. If moving too quickly into a patient's visual area, the risk of a patient suddenly moving is great.
Cannot monitor self (one-sided neglect)	Most patients will need assistance in brushing the left side of their mouth, as they will not be able to "crossover" to the neglected side; may pouch food on the left side.

Modified from Stroke Association Org, 2011.

TBI

Modifications depend on accommodating to lasting sequelae. In many cases, nitrous oxide and oral or intravenous sedation will help to relax the patient, especially those with post-traumatic stress disorder (see Chapter 15). Oral hygiene concerns remain the same as for other patients with neurological problems, with need for adaptive aids or help from a caregiver.

Epilepsy (and Other Seizure Disorders)

A thorough history should be taken prior to beginning any dental treatment on a patient with a history of epilepsy so as to avoid triggers, to easily recognize and manage seizure events in the dental chair, and to determine if dental injuries have occurred related to seizures. Management recommendations are given in Table 14.7.

Table 14.7. Management of Seizure Risk in the Epileptic Patient

Management Concern	Recommendation

Is there something I need to do to prevent seizure(s) during dental care?	For well-controlled patients: normal care
	Poorly controlled: consult with physician:
	    May require adjustment of anti-seizure medications.
	    Consider treatment with sedation/general anesthesia.

How can I eliminate the precipitating factors for an "aura?"	Careful position of dental light and avoid known precipitating factors. Consider using an extraoral mouthprop (molt).
If a grand mal seizure (status epilepticus) occurs, will I be ready to provide emergency care?	1) Clear area, move bracket and instruments. 2) Place chair in supported supine position. 3) Remove foreign bodies from the person's mouth if possible (but no blind finger sweep). 4) Turn head to sideways to avoid aspiration. 5) Passively restrain to prevent patient from falling out of chair or hitting object. 6) Time the duration of seizure.
Following a seizure in my office, what do I need to do to provide postseizure care?	1) Turn patient's head to side to avoid aspiration. 2) Examine patient for traumatic injuries. 3) Discontinue care and arrange for transport.
If a seizure lasts for more than 5 minutes or my patient becomes cyanotic, in my practice what should I do?	1) Activate emergency rescue system (call 911). 2) Assure patient has an airway and is breathing adequately. 3) If not breathing on his or her own, support airway and give supplemental oxygen. 4) If equipped and trained, give parenteral 10 mg diazepam or 5 mg midazolam.

Adapted from Robbins.[4]

Oral Lesion/Condition Diagnosis and Management

Drooling (PD): Due to the difficulty in swallowing in advanced PD, saliva, which is normally swallowed, spills out of the mouth and causes drooling. This is enhanced by a PD patient's forward posturing and anteriorly flexed head position. Treatment for drooling is difficult and options available include medications (anticholinergics such as glycopyrrolate and benztropine), surgical intervention (transposing of parotid duct),[14] and a newer investigational alternative of injecting botulinum toxin into the excretory glands periodically.[15] All of these methods have limitations, and many patients decide to manage this problem by learning to position their head or having a washcloth or handkerchief at hand.

Dry Mouth (MS, PD, Stroke): Because many of the medications can cause dry mouth (in particular, the anticholinergics, antifatigue agents, and antidepressants), the use of salivary substitutes, salivary stimulants, and fluoride rinses or gels for dentate patients may be indicated.

Trigeminal Neuralgia: TN is 400 times more likely among people with MS than among the general population.[16] Having a high suspicion, identification of a trigger point, and ruling out pain of dental origin should prevent astute dental clinicians from surgically treating apparent tooth-related pain with no other obvious clinical etiology or pathology. Referral to a physician or neurologist for relief of neurological pain from TN by using carbamazepine, clonazepam, amitriptyline, or surgery is recommended.

Dysarthria/Dysphagia (MS, Stroke): Stroke and MS may result in slow, irregular speech with unusual separation of syllables, loss or difficulty in speech, slurred speech, a weak palate, difficulty swallowing, unilateral paralysis of the orofacial muscles, and loss of sensory stimuli of oral tissues. The tongue may be flaccid, with multiple folds, and may deviate on extrusion. Dysphagia is common, and the use of rubber dams to prevent aspiration of materials should be considered whenever possible.[17]

Dilantin®-Induced Gingival Overgrowth (Seizures): Patients taking phenytoin may develop gingival overgrowth related to drug use, dosage, and oral hygiene status. Surgical excision of this excess tissue, with removal of contributing plaque and calculus, is often the only treatment which can be offered. Physicians should be consulted to consider use of alternative antiseizure medication for susceptible patients. See examples in Figs. 14.4 and 14.5.

Figure 14.4 Dilantin®-induced gingival overgrowth.

Figure 14.5 Dilantin®-induced gingival overgrowth is more extensive with poorer oral hygiene.

 ## Risks of Dental Care

Hemostasis

Stroke patients with underlying hypercoagulable conditions will be taking warfarin; a direct thrombin inhibitor, for example, dabigatran (Pradaxa®); or antiplatelet drugs. These patients are at risk of excessive bleeding when performing surgical/invasive dental treatment. If the international normalized ratio (INR) is <3.5, risk is acceptable for undertaking most invasive dental procedures. In cases of INR >3.5, the physician should be consulted to decrease the dose enough to lower the INR to <3.5. In these cases, it is important that the anticoagulant not be discontinued as the risk of a recurrent stroke or myocardial infarction is considered to be greater than that of the risk for bleeding. See Chapter 9.

Seizure disorder patients who take valproic acid, which specifically inhibits the secondary phase of platelet aggregation, or carbamezapine, may develop thrombocytopenia resulting in bleeding complications.[18] In general, antiplatelet agents, such as aspirin, clopidogrel (Plavix®), and dipyridamole, do not lead to significant bleeding problems in oral surgical procedures and do not need to be discontinued. Good surgical technique including gentle technique, removing granulation tissue, and using primary closure and hemostatic agents (Gelfoam®, sutures, topical thrombin) will prevent most postsurgical bleeding episodes.

For stroke patients on anticoagulants or seizure patients on valproic acid, postoperative pain should be managed with acetaminophen-containing products, with or without narcotics.

Susceptibility to Infection

Susceptibility to infection is generally not elevated in patients with neurological disorders with the possible exception of the MS patient chronically using corticosteroids and seizure disorder patients on phenytoin, carbamazepine, or valproic acid that can cause leukopenia.

Drug Actions/Interactions

Drugs for PD often result in xerostomia, nausea, and tardive dyskinesia. Adverse effects of common drugs used in MS are varied. When xerostomia is a significant issue, the patient's physician should be consulted to determine if the amount or type of xerogenic medication can be adjusted. Saliva substitutes and/or salivary stimulants (e.g., xylitol sweetener-containing gum, pilocarpine, bethanechol, cevimeline) can be prescribed.

Patient's Ability to Tolerate Dental Care

Ability to withstand dental treatment is an important consideration for all patients with neurological disorders:

PD: For patients taking antiparkinsonism medications, the dental chair should be inclined slowly and the patient should remain sitting from 3 to 5 minutes before being released. Oral or intravenous sedation is effective in reducing involuntary tremors or dyskinesias for the short time necessary to provide dental treatment but should be used with caution in these patients. Dentists should be aware that many antiparkinsonian drugs can be CNS depressants and prescription sedatives have an additive effect.

MS: Patients in remission are best able to tolerate dental care. For severely disabled adults, intravenous sedation or general anesthesia may be necessary to accomplish the recommended dental treatment. For patients taking corticosteroids, potential adrenal suppression should be considered.

Stroke: The stroke patient's ability to tolerate dental treatment using the American Society of Anesthesiologist (ASA) risk classification is outlined in Table 14.8. In general, ASA III or ASA IV stroke-prone or stroke patients should be seen during midmorning and have appointments that are stress free.

Stroke patients may need assistance transferring to the dental chair. One-person transfers can be done with assisting the patient while standing in front of the patient to prevent falls, using a transfer board for one-person transfers, or with two-person transfers. Two-person wheelchair transfer is shown in Fig. 14.6.

Intraoperative management techniques include:

- monitoring blood pressure prior to and during invasive procedures;
- limiting epinephrine to two to three carpules and avoiding epinephrine impregnated gingival retraction cord;
- practicing good pain control;
- using stress-reduction techniques;
- preventing aspiration through limiting ultrasonic scaling and air–water syringe use,

Table 14.8. ASA Risk According to Stroke Status and Dental Management Recommendations

	Stroke Status	Recommendations
ASA I	No stroke risk factors	No modifications needed
ASA II	One or more stroke risk factors	Refer to physician for medical treatment of risk factors and counsel patient to quit or modify risk factors.
ASA III	History of one or more TIAs or stroke, with or without neurological deficits at least 6 months before dental treatment	Refer for evaluation to medical facility if risk factors not being treated. Manage in dental office according to deficit present.
ASA IV	History of TIA or stroke, with or without neurological deficits, within 6 months of dental treatment	Deferral of dental treatment for at least 6 months due to the fact that TIA/CVA recurrence is highest within the first year. Up to 25% of patients who have a TIA will die within 1 year.

Modified from Malamed, S. *Medical Emergencies in the Dental Office*. 5th ed., 2000.

Figure 14.6 Two-person wheelchair transfer. Wheelchair is prepared by placing close to and parallel to dental chair, locking the wheels and removing the footrests and armrest nearest the dental chair. (Left panel) First clinician stands behind the patient and places his arms under the patient's upper arms and grasps the patient's wrists, with patients arms interlocked across the chest. (Right panel) Second clinician places both hands under the patient's lower thighs and initiates and leads the lift at a prearranged count of 1-2-3. Both clinicians use leg and arm muscles while bending their backs as little as possible and gently lift the patient's torso and legs at the same time. From the National Institutes of Health. Wheelchair Transfer: A Health Care Providers Guide. NIH Publication No. 09-5195. Available at: http://www.nidcr.nih.gov/OralHealth/Topics/DevelopmentalDisabilities/WheelchairTransfer.htm.

using rubber dams for restorative procedures, and obtaining primary closure for extractions.

Most strokes result in paralysis or swallowing problems on the contralateral side (i.e., left-CVA, right hemiplegia). Risk of aspiration increases with the severity of the stroke and is more likely with clear liquids than solids:

- *ALS*: Patients with severe ALS will require short appointments and may have to be transferred from a wheelchair to a dental chair. Because of their severe respiratory problems due to the disease's effect on the muscles that control breathing, deficits in protective airway reflexes develop. A rubber dam for restorative procedures should be used if the patient can breathe through the nose. In order to protect the airway, the dental chair should be placed at 45 degrees, not in a supine position.
- *Epilepsy and Other Seizure Disorders*: Ability to tolerate dental care is enhanced by adequate medical control of seizures and elimination of precipitating factors.

Medical Emergencies

Neurological medical emergencies include seizures and new onset TIA or stroke. For recognition and management of seizures, please see Table 14.7.

TIA/Stroke

Recognition

The health history should reveal possible risk factors for stroke, and appearance of any of the classic warning signs in the dental patient should raise alarm. In addition to traditional risk factors, the finding of calcified carotid artery atheromas (CCAAs) in the region of the carotid bifurcation on a routine panoramic radiograph may indicate an increased risk for stroke, yet systematic reviews have been inconclusive as to significance of the increased risk.[19,20] Until further information is available, a prudent recommendation is to refer the patient with incidental finding of carotid atheromas (usually located near cervical vertebrae 3 and 4 at a 45 degree angle from the angle of the mandible) on panoramic radiographs to the patient's physician for further evaluation.[21]

Management

If a patient were to develop signs and symptoms of a stroke in the dental office, the following sequence should be followed:

1. Terminate the dental procedure.
2. Position the patient in a comfortable position (if conscious, upright, and if unconscious, on back).
3. Assess the patient to determine responsiveness; if unresponsive with no breathing or not normal breathing (only gasping), activate the emergency medical response system (EMS), use the automated external defibrillator, if available, and provide cardiopulmonary resuscitation.
4. Monitor and record vital signs every 5 minutes if the patient is conscious. Blood pressure is generally elevated, whereas the heart rate may be normal or elevated. Summon medical assistance when signs and symptoms indicate a possible stroke, so thrombolytic therapy can be used within the first 3 hours if indicated and residual, neurological deficit is minimized.
5. Most TIA/CVA victims remain conscious and should be allowed to remain seated upright (45 degrees). Do not position the patient supine, as this increases blood flow to the brain, which is potentially dangerous if hypertensive.
6. Oxygen may be administered through a nasal cannula or nasal hood. No CNS depressant should be used as this may affect the patient's condition adversely, or mask neurological signs needed to help diagnose the condition.

7. If neurological signs and symptoms do not resolve when EMS arrives, the victim should be stabilized and transported to a hospital. Loss of consciousness is associated with a poor clinical prognosis in CVA (70–100% initial mortality).

IV. Recommended Readings and Cited References

Recommended Readings

Little JW, Falace DA, Miller CS, Rhodus NL. Chapter 27. Neurologic disorders. In: Dental Management of the Medically Compromised Patient, 7th ed. 2008. Mosby Elsevier, St. Louis, MO.

Malamed SF. Medical Emergencies in the Dental Office, 5th ed. 2000. Mosby, St. Louis, MO.

Cited References

1. World Health Organization. Chapter VI. Diseases of the nervous system. In: International Classification of Diseases (ICD-10). Accessed February 7, 2012. Available at: http://apps.who.int/classifications/icd10/browse/2010/en.
2. Asplund K, Stegmayr B, Peltonen M. Chapter 64. From the twentieth to the twenty-first century: a public health perspective on stroke. In: Cerebrovascular Disease Pathophysiology, Diagnosis, and Management, vol. 2, Ginsberg MD, Bogousslavsky J, eds. 1998. Blackwell Science, Malden, MA.
3. Proposal for revised clinical and electroencephalographic classification of epileptic seizures. The Commission on Classification and Terminology of the International League Against Epilepsy. Epilepsia 1981;22(4):489–501.
4. Robbins MR. Dental management of special needs patients who have epilepsy. Dent Clin North Am 2009;53(2):295–309.
5. Fischer DJ, Epstein JB, Klasser G. Multiple sclerosis: an update for oral health care providers. Oral Surg Oral Med Oral Pathol Oral Radiol Endod 2009;108(3):318–27.
6. Stein J, Silver JK, Frates EP. Risk factors for having a stroke. In: Life after Stroke. The Guide to Recovering Your Health and Preventing Another Stroke. 2006, pp. 3–13, 87–90. Johns Hopkins Press, Baltimore, MD.
7. Henry RG, Smith BJ. Managing older patients who have neurologic disease: Alzheimer's disease and cerebrovascular accident. Dent Clin North Am 2009;53(2):269–94.
8. Kinane D, Bouchard P; Group E of European Workshop on Periodontology. Periodontal diseases and health: consensus report of the Sixth European Workshop on Periodontology. J Clin Periodontol 2008;35(8 Suppl.):333–7.
9. Centers for Disease Control and Prevention. Epilepsy. 2012. Available at: http://www.cdc.gov/Epilepsy/. Accessed March 2012.
10. Hallett M, Litvan I. Evaluation of surgery for Parkinson's disease: a report of the Therapeutics and Technology Assessment Subcommittee of the American Academy of Neurology. The Task Force on Surgery for Parkinson's Disease. Neurology 1999;53(9):1910–21.
11. Fuller G, Manford M. Neurology: An Illustrated Color Text. 2000. Churchill Livingstone, Harcourt Publishers Limited, London, UK.
12. Centers for Disease Control. Glasgow Coma Scale. 2003. Department of Health and Human Services, Centers for Disease Control, Mass Casualties. Available at: http://www.bt.cdc.gov/masscasualties. Accessed October 2011.
13. Epilepsy Foundation. *What is epilepsy?* 2010. Available at: http://epilepsyfoundation.org/aboutepilepsy/whatisepilepsy/statistics.cfm. Accessed October 2011.
14. Hockstein NG, Samadi DS, Gendron K, Handler SD. Sialorrhea: a management challenge. Am Fam Physician 2004;69(11):2628–34.
15. Kalf JG, Smit AM, Bloem BR, Zwarts MJ, Mulleners WM, Munneke M. Botulinum toxin A for drooling in Parkinson's disease: a pilot study to compare submandibular to parotid gland injections. Parkinsonism Relat Disord 2007;13(8):532–4.
16. Maloni HW. Pain in multiple sclerosis: an overview of its nature and management. J Neurosci Nurs 2000;32(3):139–44, 152.
17. Jolly DE, Paulson RB, Paulson GW, Pike JA. Parkinson's disease: a review and recommendations for dental management. Spec Care Dentist 1989;9(3):74–8.
18. Rhodus NL, Miller CS. Chapter 7. Neurologic conditions. In: Clinician's Guide: Medically

Complex Dental Patients, 3rd ed. Rhodus NL, Miller CS, eds. 2009. The American Academy of Oral Medicine. BC Decker Inc., Hamilton, Ontario, Canada.
19. Friedlander AH, Baker JD. Panoramic radiography: an aid in detecting patients at risk of cerebrovascular accident. J Am Dent Assoc 1994;125(12):1598–603.
20. Mupparapu M, Kim IH. Calcified carotid artery atheroma and stroke: a systematic review. J Am Dent Assoc 2007;138(4):483–92.
21. Carter LC, Haller AD, Nadarajah V, Calamel AD, Aquirre A. Use of panoramic radiography among an ambulatory dental population to detect patients at risk of stroke. J Am Dent Assoc 1997;128(7):977–84.

Neurodevelopmental and Psychiatric Disorders

Maureen Munnelly Romer DDS, MPA
Nancy J. Dougherty DMD, MPH

Neurodevelopmental and psychiatric disorders of particular importance to dentistry are discussed in this chapter.

Section 1. Neurodevelopmental Disorders

I. Background

Description of Disorder

Intellectual Disabilities (IDs)/ Mental Retardation

ID is a disability with onset before age 18 years that is characterized by significant limitations both in intellectual functioning and in adaptive behavior, affecting many everyday social and practical skills.[1]

Down Syndrome (DS)

DS (Trisomy 21) is a congenital chromosomal abnormality characterized by systemic anomalies, ID, and a recognizable craniofacial appearance.[2]

Cerebral Palsy (CP)

CP is a general term used to describe a number of neuromuscular disorders that are present at birth or are acquired during infancy. CP affects muscle movement as a result of structural abnormalities or trauma to parts of the brain that control this function.

An International Workshop on the Definition and Classification of Cerebral Palsy, held in 2004, developed the following definition[3]:

> Cerebral palsy (CP) describes a group of disorders of the development of movement and posture, causing activity limitation, that are attributed to non-progressive disturbances that occurred in the developing fetal or infant brain. The motor disorders of CP are often accompanied by disturbances of sensation, cognition, communication, perception, and/or behavior, and/or by a seizure disorder.

The ADA Practical Guide to Patients with Medical Conditions, First Edition. Edited by Lauren L. Patton.
© 2012 American Dental Association. Published 2012 by John Wiley & Sons, Inc.

Autistic Spectrum Disorder (ASD)

ASD includes "classic" autism, Asperger syndrome, and atypical autism or pervasive developmental disorders (PDDs) not otherwise specified. ASDs are characterized by deficits in three major areas[4]:

- social interaction/relatedness;
- verbal/nonverbal communication;
- restricted interests, repetitive/stereotyped behaviors, and resistance to change.

Individuals can present with a wide variety of behavioral characteristics, ranging from mild to very severe involvement. However, these behaviors may change with the acquisition of other developmental skills. Asperger syndrome is a high-functioning form of autism with impaired social interactions, limited repetitive patterns of behavior, and delayed motor milestones and clumsiness. Common comorbidities include mental retardation (intelligence quotient [IQ] <70) in 70% and epilepsy in 25% of cases.[5]

Attention Deficit Hyperactivity Disorder (ADHD)

ADHD is a neurodevelopmental disorder that is characterized by an inability to regulate attention, often with displays of hyperactivity and impulsivity.[4,6,7]

Pathogenesis/Etiology

IDs/Mental Retardation

Genetic disorders are a leading cause of ID. There are over 800 syndromes associated with ID.[8] Intrauterine exposure to toxins (e.g., fetal alcohol syndrome, anticonvulsant medications), intrauterine infections (e.g., cytomegalovirus, rubella, toxoplasmosis), metabolic disorders and neurodegenerative disorders can also cause ID in a child. Other etiologies include perinatal/postnatal conditions such as extreme premature birth, intraventricular hemorrhage, hypoxic–ischemic encephalopathy, traumatic brain injury, and meningitis.

DS

The genetic basis for DS is a mutation resulting in an extra copy of chromosome 21 (seen in 95% of cases). A much smaller number of cases (up to 5%) involve translocation or mosaicism of chromosome 21.

CP

CP may be attributed to structural abnormalities in the brain as well as the central nervous system (CNS) vascular insufficiency resulting in hypoxia to the developing brain. Risk factors for CP include:[9,10]

- intrauterine exposure to toxins or infections,
- preterm birth and low birth weight,
- multiple gestation,
- intrauterine growth retardation,
- maternal thyroid disorders,
- maternal seizure disorder,
- birth asphyxia,
- infections in postnatal period (meningitis, encephalitis),
- intracranial hemorrhage (postnatal),
- kernicterus (postnatal).

ASD

There is no known single cause of autism; etiologies are likely multifactorial. Current research is focusing on factors that could influence the development of the embryonic brain[11]:

- Genetics: High concordance in identical twins and first-degree relatives.
- Environmental and other possible factors:
  - impaired methylation and gene mutations involving metabolism of vitamin D[12];

- maternally derived antibodies, maternal infection, maternal teratogen exposure, heavy metal exposure, and folic acid supplementation[12];
- paternal age at time of conception[13];
- measles, mumps, rubella (MMR) vaccine has been implicated but rejected as a causative factor.[14]

ADHD

A precise etiology for ADHD has not been established. Studies of families with the disorder suggest a strong genetic component, possibly with altered function of neurotransmitters and structural abnormalities in the brain.[6,7]

Epidemiology

IDs/Mental Retardation

- Prevalence of ID is estimated at 1–3% in developed countries.
- Prevalence of severe ID in the United States is estimated at 3–4 per 1000 children and adults, while mild ID is much more common.[15]

Approximately 85% of people with ID are in the mild range with an IQ of 50–70, academically at the level of a sixth grader, and functionally able to live in the community with minimal support.[16] ID itself is not associated with a shortened life span. However, life span may be decreased due to the underlying etiology for the ID. Higher rates of seizure disorders, gastrointestinal complications including feeding dysfunction and gastroesophageal reflux, and respiratory disease are common.

DS

- This occurs in 11.8/10,000 live births in the United States, with a higher rate associated with mothers who are ≥35 years old.[17]
- Approximately 400,000 people with DS currently reside in the United States.[18]

CP

- This is the most common congenital neuromuscular disorder.[19]
- Overall prevalence in developed countries is estimated at 2–3 per 1000 live births, with the rate holding steady for more than 30 years.[10]
- A higher prevalence exists in children born preterm.

Classification

CP can be classified according to the nature of the motor disorder[19]:

- spastic (70–80%),
- dyskinetic (10–15%),
- ataxic (5%).

CP can also be classified topographically, according to which parts of the body are affected:

- quadriplegia (all four extremities, trunk, and oromotor musculature),
- hemiplegia (one side of the body),
- diplegia (legs either solely or more than the arms),
- monoplegia (one limb—very rare).

Patients will often present with a diagnosis encompassing both type and location of disorder, that is, "spastic diplegia."

ASD

- This occurs in between 1 in 80 and 1 in 240, with an average of 1 in 110 children in the United States.[20]
- Boys are four to five times more likely to have an ASD than girls.
- Prevalence has not been linked to social factors such as race, ethnicity, parental education, or socioeconomic status.

ADHD

U.S. prevalence rates of ADHD in school-age children range from 5.6% to 15.9%, with pronounced state-by-state variation, possibly due to differences in diagnostic testing. Boys are almost three times more likely to be diagnosed with ADHD than girls, although it is thought that some of this difference may be attributed to the fact that more boys display hyperactive/impulsive behaviors than girls.[21]

Coordination of Care between Dentist and Physician

Physicians may be the first to notice oral trauma or oral neglect and related infections in patients with neurodevelopmental disorders and should refer the patient to a dental provider for prevention and care. The dentist may require consultation with the physician for patients with complicated medical and behavioral issues.

II. Medical Management

Identification/Medical History/ Physical and Laboratory Examination

IDs/Mental Retardation

Individuals who are considered to be "intellectually disabled" must show deficits not only in cognitive functioning, but also in adaptive functioning (i.e., communication, self-care, home living, and social and interpersonal skills). Cognitive functioning refers to IQ levels, with an IQ below 70 indicating an ID (mean IQ = 100; 70 is 2 standard deviations below the mean).[4]

DS

Systemic anomalies commonly associated with DS include:[2,22]

- congenital cardiac anomalies (40–50% of infants),
- immune deficiencies (T- and B-cell defects, impaired cell, and humoral immune systems),
- overall hypotonicity,
- atlantoaxial instability (12–20%),
- intellectual disability (usually in the range of mild-to-moderate disability),
- increased risk for leukemia,
- increased risk for early-onset Alzheimer's disease.

CP

The clinical picture of CP can vary greatly from mild to severe functional and systemic involvement. In addition to various medical specialists, a team of health-care professionals, including physical, occupational, and speech therapists may be required to optimize the individual's quality of life. Medical complications associated with CP include but are not limited to:[23]

- intellectual disability (seen in 30–50%),
- seizures,
- gastroesophageal reflux,
- dysphagia,
- spinal disorders (scoliosis or kyphosis),
- joint contractures (secondary to spasticity).

ASD

The diagnosis of ASD is behaviorally based. There are no specific genetic, medical, or laboratory tests that are diagnostic for ASD. Deficiency in at least one of the areas of communication, socialization, or restricted behavior must be present before the age of 3. Formal diagnosis requires a two-stage process: developmental screening during "well child" check-ups and if problems are detected, then the child should be referred for the second stage, which is a comprehensive evaluation by a multidisciplinary team.[24]

ADHD

Diagnostic criteria require characteristics to be evident by age 7 and must have had duration of at least 6 months. The disorder is classified into three distinct subtypes[4]:

- predominantly inattentive,
- predominantly hyperactive-impulsive,
- combined type.

Comorbidities include anxiety and depression. Adults with inadequately treated ADHD show a high incidence of illicit drug use, which may indicate an attempt to self-medicate.[7]

Medical Treatment

Auxiliary therapies such as occupational therapy, speech therapy, and parental counseling are also often necessary.[11]

ASD: While there is no U.S. Food and Drug Administration (FDA)-approved treatment for ASD, patients are often on medications to help control hyperactivity, repetitive behaviors, and aggression. Approximately 10% of patients with ASD have an associated genetic disorder (e.g., tuberous sclerosis, Fragile X, Prader–Willi, and Angelman syndromes), which may require additional medical management.[25]

CP: Depending on severity, patients with CP may require antispasmotic and antiseizure medications. They may also need surgery to correct contractures (foot, ankle, hand, wrist, knee, hip, and pelvic) or spinal deformities so as to improve balance, walking, and standing.

ADHD: Treatment consists of behavioral therapy combined with pharmacotherapy. Medications frequently used in the treatment of ADHD[6] are shown in Table 15.1.

III. Dental Management

Evaluation

Important aspects of dental history include ascertainment of legal guardianship status for the patient, assessment of type and adequacy of patient oral hygiene and need for caregiver supportive oral care, past abilities to tolerate dental treatment in the dental office setting, need for anxiety management, sedation or general anesthesia to accomplish treatment, current oral health status, and ability to make improvements in oral health with coaching. The caregiver and legal guardian should be present and participate in interpreting or clarifying the patient's unique communication style or to report on past dental history and challenges with patient communication and cooperation with dental care.

Oral Manifestations

DS

Orofacial features characteristic of individuals with DS, as seen in Fig. 15.1, include:[2,22]

- midface hypoplasia;
- underdeveloped palate with high palatal vault (results in relative Class III malocclusion);
- macroglossia (either true or relative due to small oral cavity) with subsequent strong gag reflex;
- fissured tongue that may protrude and contribute to halitosis (possibly secondary to chronic mouth breathing);
- large thick lips with hypotonia causing mouth drop and the lower lip to protrude;
- dental findings including microdontia, hypodontia, supernumerary teeth, morphological variants, delayed eruption, and maxillary impactions (secondary to underdeveloped palate).

CP

As with medical issues, there is great variation in oral conditions associated with CP. Some of those seen most frequently include:[26,27]

Table 15.1. Oral Side Effects and Interactions of Drugs Used in Neurodevelopmental Disorder (and Some Overlap with Psychiatric and Neurological Disorders)

Drug Generic/Proprietary Names	Class/Indication	Oral Side Effects	Dental Drug Interactions/Precautions
Common drugs to treat autism spectrum disorders (ASDs)			
Fluoxetine Prozac® Sarafem®	Antidepressant (SSRI)/control repetitive behavior in ASD; also treat MDD, OCD, panic attack, ED, ADHD, PTSD, phobias	Dry mouth	None
Sertraline Zoloft®	Antidepressant (SSRI)/control repetitive behavior in ASD; also treat MDD, OCD, PTSD, panic attacks, social anxiety	Dry mouth	Aspirin, NSAIDs, diazepam
Lithium Lithobid®	Antimanic agent/control aggression in ASD, prevent mania in BPD, schizophrenia	Dry mouth, excess saliva, swollen lips, tongue pain, salivary gland enlargement, metallic taste, dysgeusia	NSAIDs, metronidazole
Carbamazepine Tegretol® Carbatrol®	Antiseizure/control aggression in ASD, BPD, seizure disorders	Dry mouth	Acetaminophen, tramadol, alprazolam, lorazepam, doxycycline, erythromycin, clarithromycin, itraconazole, ketoconazole
Valproate/divalproex (valproic acid) Depakene® Depakote®	Antiseizure/control aggression in ASD, mania in BPD, seizure disorders	Bone marrow suppression with thrombocytopenia at high doses, stomatitis, taste perversion, dry mouth	Aspirin, acyclovir, erythromycin, lorazepam
Risperidone Risperdal®	Atypical antipsychotic/control aggression in ASD; also treat schizophrenia, BPD	Dry mouth, hypersalivation, stomatitis	None
Olanzapine Zyprexa®	Atypical antipsychotic/control aggression in ASD; also treat schizophrenia, BPD	Dry mouth	Ciprofloxacin

Common drugs to treat attention deficit hyperactivity disorder (ADHD)

Methylphenidate Ritalin® Concerta®	CNS stimulant/control hyperactivity	Dry mouth	None
Amphetamine and dextroamphetamine Adderall® Dexedrine®	CNS stimulant/control hyperactivity	Dry mouth, dysgeusia	Propoxyphene
Atomoxetine Strattera®	Antidepressant (SNRI), also to treat MDD	Dry mouth	None
Buproprion Wellbutrin® Zyban®	Atypical antidepressant; also for smoking cessation; to treat MDD, seasonal affective disorder	Dry mouth, dysgeusia	Dexamethasone
Imipramine Tofranil®	Antidepressant (tricyclic); also to prevent bedwetting; to treat MDD, ED, panic disorders	Dry mouth, dysgeusia	None

Common antispasmotic drugs to treat cerebral palsy

Baclofen Gablofen® Lioresal®	®Muscle relaxant/antispasmotic	None	None
Dantrolene Dantrium®	Muscle relaxant/antispasmotic	None	None
Botulinum toxin Botox®	Muscle relaxant/antispasmotic	None	None
Cyclobenzaprine Flexeril® Amrix®	Muscle relaxant/antispasmotic	Dry mouth	None

BPD, bipolar disease; CNS, central nervous system; ED, eating disorder; MDD, major depression; NSAIDs, nonsteroidal anti-inflammatory drugs; OCD, obsessive–compulsive disorder; PTSD, posttraumatic stress disorder; SNRI, serotonin–norepinephrine reuptake inhibitor; SSRI, selective serotonin reuptake inhibitor.

Key Questions

Key questions to ask the patient (caregiver) with neurodevelopmental disorders

- What type of disorder does the patient have?
- What type of behaviors/symptoms does the patient have?
- Who is the patient's legal guardian?
- How is oral hygiene accomplished? Does the patient receive assistance? What type, how often, and how well accepted is the assistance? Is there gum bleeding on assisted brushing?
- What attempts have been used to improve oral hygiene and how successful have they been?
- What is the patient's diet and eating habits (sugar content and contact duration with teeth)?
- How has past dental treatment in the dental office setting been managed? Does the patient benefit from tell–show–do or special communication or relaxation/cooperation techniques?
- Does the patient benefit from previsit antianxiety medication use? What dose has been used? Has nitrous oxide/oxygen analgesia been tried? If so, was it successful?
- Do you feel medical stabilization (use of papoose board), conscious sedation, or general anesthesia will be needed to accomplish treatment?
- Has the (nonverbal) patient demonstrated any signs that he or she might be in pain?
- Can the patient indicate he or she is having pain? How is pain demonstrated?

Key questions to ask the physician for the patient with neurodevelopmental disorders

- What has the patient's behavior been like for office procedures such as blood draws and vaccinations?
- If general anesthesia is required, does the patient require other medical procedures that can be done at the same time as the dental care under general anesthesia if done in a hospital setting, for example, gynecological exam and Pap smear, blood draw for laboratory testing, and removal of impacted ear cerumen?

- malocclusions (most frequently Class II, anterior open bite);
- bruxism (more prevalent in individuals with severe intellectual disability);
- persistent sialorrhea (hypersalivation with drooling; seen in individuals with dysphagia);
- extensive calculus deposits (associated with dysphagia, pooling saliva, possible gastrostomy tube feeding).

Dental Treatment Modifications

Traditional behavior management techniques such as tell–show–do are often successful. Direct uncomplicated language should be used, being mindful of the person's biological age and being sure to maintain the person's dignity by not talking "baby talk." It is equally important to address the patient and not just the caregiver or guardian while explaining treatment

Figure 15.1 Young lady with Down syndrome ready for her high school prom.

and options. Issues of guardianship should be determined, and only legal guardians should sign consent if the patient is unable to do so. Treatment planning should be based on the principle of patient-centered care. Plans should start at ideal, and then be adapted or modified after considering the patient's abilities, wants, and needs, as well as his or her ability to tolerate the treatment and maintain restorations.[28]

Oral hygiene and routine preventive care should be emphasized. For patients who cannot reliably swish and spit, chlorhexidine applied to the toothbrush with assisted brushing may be beneficial. Oral hygiene techniques for patients who resist caregiver help may need to be demonstrated to the caregiver. As shown in Fig. 15.2, a useful approach to assisted brushing (after the patient has made an attempt to brush his or her own teeth, if possible) is from behind the patient's head, with the head supported.

Figure 15.2 Positioning for providing oral hygiene for a patient in a wheelchair. From the Practical Oral Care for People with Cerebral Palsy. NIH publication No. 09-5192. Available at: http://www.nidcr.nih.gov/OralHealth/Topics/DevelopmentalDisabilities/PracticalOralCarePeopleCerebralPalsy.htm.

IDs/Mental Retardation

A number of factors can complicate oral health maintenance for individuals with ID. Patients may exhibit oral habits such as bruxism or other self-injurious behaviors, which are seen more frequently in individuals with low cognitive function and sensory impairments.

DS

Individuals with DS are at higher risk than the general public for the development and early onset of periodontal disease.[2,22,29] Rates of periodontal disease have been reported as high as 90–96% in adults[22] and may be due to the compromised immune response and abnormalities in capillary morphology and connective tissue.[29]

Although dental caries incidence in institutionalized children with DS whose diets are closely monitored is low, they maintain caries risk and should receive the same preventive considerations as other children. The deinstitutionalization of individuals with DS and subsequent "normalization" of their diets has led to a caries rate closer to that of the general population.[22]

Risks of Dental Care

Hemostasis and Susceptibility to Infection

DS: Patients are more susceptible to infections due to immune compromise (lymphopenia and defects in neutrophil chemotaxis).[30]

Drug Actions/Interactions

ASD and ADHD: Common medications to treat ASD and ADHD may have interactions and side effects, particularly dry mouth that may require caries-preventive approaches with use of topical fluorides (see Table 15.1).

Patient's Ability to Tolerate Dental Care

It is important from the start to determine each individual's ability to communicate and cooperate.[2,22] Cognition, communication, and behavior should be kept in mind when planning dental treatment. An awareness of each individual's physical and behavioral limitations should guide the oral health professional when providing care. The goal should be to provide optimal oral care while using the least restrictive techniques.

The majority with mild-to-moderate behavioral concerns can be managed within the routine dental setting. For some individuals who have extensive treatment needs or difficult behaviors, it may be necessary to consider sedation or general anesthesia.

DS and CP: The combination of hypotonia and upper airway anomalies may increase risk for adverse events during sedation, factors that should be weighed when planning treatment modalities.

ASD: Patients often present behavioral challenges such as short attention span, rigidity of routines, hyperactivity, easy frustration, tantrums, and echolalia.[31] Standard behavior management techniques such as tell–show–do, and immediate positive and negative reinforcement (paired with firmness, if necessary) can be helpful, but it is important to be flexible in trying different techniques. Modeling, positive reinforcement (praise) after every successful step of procedure with a prize at the end of the visit and the use of clear, short, simple sentences are often useful.[32]

Obtaining a good behavioral history is important as patients may exhibit atypical behaviors. Parent/caregiver should be asked about the patient's idiosyncrasies/stereotypic behaviors, adherence to routines, repetitive motions, attachment to unusual objects, self-injurious behaviors communication level, reactions to noise, reactions to touch (light and deep pressure), and reactions to bright light and previous visits to doctors.

Section 2. Psychiatric Disorders

I. Background

Description of Conditions

Anxiety Disorders

Generalized Anxiety Disorder (GAD)

In GAD, there is an increased sympathetic arousal that results in the physical and emotional symptoms of anxiety and may share symptoms with depression. For a diagnosis of GAD, the worry or physical symptoms must cause clinically significant distress or impairment in social or occupational function.

Obsessive–Compulsive Disorder (OCD)

OCD is a neuropsychiatric disorder characterized by recurrent distressing thoughts (i.e., obsessions) and repetitive behaviors or mental rituals (compulsions). These acts serve to reduce anxiety.[33]

Phobias

Phobia is defined as the presence of the following symptoms: fear that is present and considered out of proportion to the demands of the situation, cannot be reasoned away, and is beyond voluntary control and leads to avoidance of a situation.

Posttraumatic Stress Disorder (PTSD)

PTSD is a chronic psychiatric disorder precipitated by an individual's exposure to some type of terrifying or life-threatening event.[34,35] Hallmarks of PTSD include an individual's reexperiencing the event in such forms as nightmares and flashbacks, avoiding reminders of the event, and persistent hyperarousal.[35]

Mood Disorders

Bipolar Disorder (BPD)

BPD, also known as manic-depressive disorder, is a disorder that causes unusual mood swings from the lows of depression to the highs of euphoria (i.e., mania). Unusual shifts in energy and activity levels are common and the disorder may impede the normal ability to carry out day-to-day tasks. Shifts may occur several times a day or as seldom as a few times a year.[36]

Major Depressive Disorder (MDD)

MDD, or major depression, is characterized by a combination of symptoms that interfere with a person's ability to work, sleep, study, eat, and enjoy once-pleasurable activities. Major depression is disabling and prevents a person from functioning normally.

Psychotic Disorders

Schizophrenia

Schizophrenia is a chronic psychiatric disorder that results in significant psychosocial disability. Symptoms can include hallucinations as well as delusional and disordered thoughts. The diagnosis of schizophrenia is based on a combination of "positive" symptoms (psychotic behaviors not seen in healthy individuals) and "negative" symptoms (disruptions in normal emotions and behaviors). A person with schizophrenia may also display cognitive symptoms such as problems with focus or executive functioning.[37]

Eating Disorders (EDs)

Anorexia Nervosa (AN) and Bulimia Nervosa (BN)

"Eating disorder" is an umbrella term for a group of psychiatric illnesses that manifest in the form of dysfunctional eating patterns. Clinical ED can result in considerable morbidities and mortality.[38] Three major classifications of ED are seen in the Diagnostic and Statistical Manual of Mental Disorders (DSM-IV)[1]:

- *AN* is characterized by an intense fear of gaining weight and an inability to maintain weight at a minimal level (15% below normal).
- *BN* involves recurrent episodes of binge eating, often alternating with purging behaviors including induced vomiting and/or laxative abuse. Weight often remains in the normal range.
- *Eating disorders not otherwise specified* (EDNOS) includes binge-eating disorder and other

dysfunctional eating patterns that do not meet the complete criteria for AN or BN.

Pathogenesis/Etiology
Anxiety Disorders

GAD

GAD typically develops in the decade between the late teens and late twenties, while specific and social phobias exhibit an earlier onset. GAD is a chronic condition and patients may have episodes for 10 years or more.[39] Disrupted modulation of the CNS (both the serotonergic and noradrenergic transmitter systems) has been proposed as a pathophysiological mechanism for anxiety disorders.

OCD

Etiology is not well understood. Theories of pathogenesis include

- genetics;
- serotonin system defects;
- immunological component due to sudden onset of symptoms in children after being infected with group A *Streptococcus*.[40]

Phobias

Phobias usually appear in childhood or adolescence and tend to persist into adulthood. The etiology of specific phobias is not well understood; although there is some evidence that the tendency to develop them may run in families, they are largely innate and do not arise directly from environmental experiences.[41]

PTSD

Not all individuals who are exposed to trauma go on to develop PTSD. Studies suggest the existence of a genetic predisposition that requires a traumatic event to trigger the chronic biological responses seen in PTSD.[34] In PTSD, the negative-feedback system of the hypothalamic–pituitary–adrenal axis appears to have increased sensitivity, which alters the body's response to perceived threats and the ability to cope.[35]

Mood Disorders

BPD

The pathophysiology of BPD is not completely understood. There are clear genetic links with the greatest risk factor for the development of BPD being a family history of the disorder.[42] However, genetics play only one part in the development of BPD, and studies have pointed to defects in mitochondrial energy production as a basis for BPD.[43]

MDD

The pathophysiology of MDD is not well understood but is likely multifactorial. Chronic stress[44] and impaired regulation of serotonin may play a role in the development of MDD. Other factors such as abnormal stress, (e.g., neglect, abandonment, abuse), genetics, and childhood/adolescent life experiences may interact to increase risk.

Psychotic Disorders

Schizophrenia

Schizophrenia has a definite genetic component. The exact biochemical basis for the disease has not been determined, with interest in genetic controls on neurotransmitter function as well as structural abnormalities in brains of people with schizophrenia.[37,45]

EDs

AN and BN

AN and BN are multifactorial in etiology, involving concerns about body weight and shape influenced by cultural and family pressures for thinness, and emotional and personality disorders; genetics and biological factors may also contribute to etiology.

Epidemiology

Anxiety Disorders

GAD

Prevalence in the United States is estimated at 4–7%, 1-year prevalence of 3–5%, and current prevalence of 1.5–3%.[46] GAD is more common among women, unmarried people, racial–ethnic minority groups, and people of low socioeconomic status.[46,47]

OCD

OCD is relatively rare, with a lifetime prevalence of 1.6%. It may appear in adolescence, with over 50% experiencing the onset of symptoms before their mid-20s.[48] OCD is a chronic condition and almost 75% have continuous symptoms, while the remainder may have intermittent symptoms.

Phobias

Phobia is the most common anxiety disorder, with up to 49% of people reporting an unreasonably strong fear and approximately 25% of those people meeting criteria for phobia.[49] An estimated 19.2 million American adults have specific phobias, affecting twice as many women as men.[50]

PTSD

U.S. prevalence of PTSD in men is 3.6%, and 9.7% in women. Higher prevalence rates exist in specific populations such as combat veterans and political refugees.[51] It is unclear if the higher prevalence in women is due to gender differences in response to trauma or if women are subjected to a greater level of trauma during their lifetimes.[35]

Mood Disorders

BPD

The 12-month prevalence rate of BPD is 2.6%.[50] Lifetime prevalence rates decline with age, being 5.9% in 18- to 29-year-olds, 4.5% in 30- to 44-year-olds, 3.5% in 45- to 59-year-olds, and 1.0% in those ≥60 years old. The average age of onset of BPD is 25, and there is a high rate of suicide.[48]

MDD

The 12-month prevalence of MDD is 6.7%.[50] Women are 70% more likely to experience MDD, and Caucasians are 40% more likely than non-Hispanic blacks to have MDD. The average age of onset is 32 years.[48] Rate of heritability of MDD is estimated at 31–42%.[44]

Psychotic Disorders

Schizophrenia

Schizophrenia is estimated to affect 1–1.5% of Americans. Onset is usually in adolescence or early adulthood, typically late teens to mid-20s for men, and late-20s for women.[45]

EDs

AN and BN

Accurate data on prevalence is not available because the majority of individuals with EDs never seek medical or mental health treatment.[52] A recent review posited a prevalence for AN of 0.3% and for BN of 1%. Highest prevalence rates are seen in young white females. The prevalence of EDNOS was estimated at 2.6% in the United States for white women in the 18- to 40-year age group, and as high as 4.5% in black women. Reported incidence rates for males are very low.[52]

Coordination of Care between Dentist and Physician

Oral health-care providers should be aware of clinical findings that may help to identify patients with an ED and to assist them in obtaining a diagnosis and appropriate psychiatric management. Dentists may also detect patients with specific phobias related to aspects of dental care, such as injection needles, the noise of the drill, or the mere physical assessment of oral or dental structures. Psychiatrists may coordinate care with dentists for patients with acute anxiety reaction to dentistry or situational phobias of dental treatment, or where the underlying psychiatric disorders or medications to manage them are being detrimental to oral and general health and require adjustment to support oral health.

 ## II. Medical Management

Identification/Medical History/ Physical and Laboratory Examination

Anxiety Disorders

GAD

GAD is characterized by worry that is:

- diagnosed as excessive and uncontrollable;
- present more days than not in a 6-month period;
- associated with at least three of six symptoms of
  - restlessness,
  - easily fatigued,
  - difficulty concentrating,
  - irritability,
  - muscle tension,
  - sleep disturbance[4];
- worry or physical symptoms must cause clinically significant distress or impairment in social or occupational functioning;
- anxiety is not confined to features of another disorder (i.e., fear of gaining weight as in AN), related to PTSD, developmental disorder, substance abuse, or any other recognized medical condition.

OCD

The diagnostic criteria for OCD include recurrent obsessions or compulsions that are severe enough to be time-consuming, or to cause marked distress or significant impairment. The patient must also recognize the behavior as excessive and unreasonable, the compulsions must not be restricted to another disorder (specific phobia, GAD), and the condition is not a result of physiological effects of a substance or medical condition.[4]

Phobias

The patient must recognize that the fear is excessive and unreasonable and exposure to the phobic stimulus must evoke immediate anxiety. Phobias are *specific* and are cued by the presence or anticipation of a specific object or situation (e.g., flying, heights, animals, injections). In addition, the avoidance, anxious anticipation, or distress in the feared situation(s) interferes significantly with the person's normal routine, occupational or social activities, or relationships, or there is marked distress about having the phobia. The anxiety, panic attacks, or phobic avoidance associated with the specific object or situation are not better accounted for by another mental disorder, such as OCD, PTSD, separation anxiety, social phobia (e.g., avoidance of social situations because of fear of embarrassment, also known as social anxiety disorder), or panic disorder.[4]

PTSD

The symptoms of PTSD can have similarities with those of other anxiety disorders or depression. To be diagnosed with PTSD, a person must have been exposed to a traumatic event, and the symptoms must be present for at least 1 month.[4]

Mood Disorders

BPD

BPD is most often diagnosed during adolescence or early adulthood. The most easily distinguishable feature of BPD is the euphoric and excited mood of mania or irritability lasting throughout at least 1 week. Additional symptoms of mania include inflated self-esteem, decreased need for sleep, increased talkativeness, flight of ideas, distractibility, and increased goal-directed behavior (e.g., psychomotor agitation) and excessive engagement in pleasurable activities that have a high potential for becoming reckless and self-destructive (e.g., spending sprees). This disturbance in mood causes marked impairment in occupational functioning or in usual social activities or relationships with others. Psychological effects of substance abuse, medications, or a medical condition (e.g., hyperthyroidism) must be ruled out.[4]

MDD

Diagnosis of MDD is based on patient interview and a mental status evaluation. Information from family and friends may be helpful, as patients may minimize the symptoms of the disorder. For a diagnosis of MDD:

- At least five of the following symptoms must be present:
  - Insomnia
  - Feelings of worthlessness
  - Fatigue
  - Inability to concentrate
  - Suicidal ideation
  - Psychomotor agitation
  - Loss of appetite
  - Significant weight gain.
- One symptom must also be either loss of interest in activities normally enjoyed or depressed/sad mood.
- Symptoms must persist for a period of more than 2 weeks and should be distinguished from a major depressive episode that is a consequence of grief, chronic substance use, or a transient response to serious medical illness.[4]

No medical tests exist for depression, but laboratory tests may be useful in ruling out medical causes for the symptoms (sleep apnea, vitamin B_{12} deficiency, etc.) and establishing a diagnosis.

Psychotic Disorders

Schizophrenia

To be diagnosed with schizophrenia:[4]

- At least two of the following symptoms must be present during a 1-month period:
  - delusions (e.g., of grandeur, thought control, or persecution);
  - hallucinations (e.g., hearing voices);
  - disorganized speech;
  - grossly disorganized behavior (e.g., frequent crying, bizarre dress) or catatonic behavior;
  - negative symptoms (e.g., blunted affect, disorganized speech, or lack of motivation).
- Occupational or social dysfunction below prior level, including decreased self-care.
- Symptoms present for at least 6 months.

Eating Disorders

AN and BN

Systemic manifestations of ED include:[38]

- cardiac abnormalities, including bradycardia and arrhythmias;
- hypothermia;
- disruption of menstrual cycles (in AN);
- esophagitis (in BN);
- constipation;
- malnutrition;
- osteoporosis;
- psychiatric comorbidities, including depression, anxiety, or OCD.

Medical Treatment

Medications used in psychiatric disorders, their oral side effects, and interactions or precautions in dentistry are shown in Tables 15.1 and 15.2.

Anxiety Disorders

GAD

A combination of medication management with anxiolytics and psychotherapy is advised for GAD. The best outcomes are achieved with involvement of cognitive behavior therapy (CBT), but length of time in treatment and expertise of the therapist can affect outcomes.[53]

OCD

CBT is often an effective treatment for OCD. First-line pharmacological treatment is selective serotonin reuptake inhibitor (SSRI) antidepressants, which may be bolstered by atypical antipsychotics in resistant cases.[54] Pharmacotherapy and CBT reduce the frequency and severity of symptoms; however, full remission is rare.[40]

Phobias

Targeted psychotherapy (desensitization or exposure therapy or CBT) is the first-line treatment for specific phobias, and patients generally respond very well.[55] If the object of the phobia is easy to avoid, however, the patient may never seek treatment. Social phobias may be treated with SSRIs or beta-blockers, in addition to psychotherapy.[55]

PTSD

Treatment for PTSD usually consists of a combination of counseling and pharmacotherapy. The SSRIs are considered first-line drugs for PTSD. Sertraline and paroxetine are the only two that have actually been approved by the FDA for treatment of PTSD. The anticonvulsant, divalproex, is sometimes helpful in alleviating such symptoms as flashbacks, nightmares, impulsiveness, and hyperarousability.[34,35]

Mood Disorders

BDP

The focus of medical management is on a therapeutic alliance between doctor and patient, family and peer support, encouragement of strict adherence to treatment and monitoring and management of symptoms and risk. Maintenance medications approved by the FDA for the treatment of BPD include lithium, lamotrigine, aripiprazole, and olanzapine.[56]

MDD

Treatment is a combination of antidepressant medication, patient education, and psychotherapy. Episodes of major depression among patients with life-altering illnesses complicate treatment and increase risk of suicide.[42] Fortunately, new generations of SSRI antidepressants, the most widely prescribed in the United States, cannot be used to commit suicide and have a lower risk of cardiovascular side effects compared with older classes of antidepressants such as the monoamine oxidase inhibitors and tricyclic antidepressants.[57]

Psychotic Disorders

Schizophrenia

Treatment for schizophrenia consists of pharmacotherapy and psychosocial therapy.[37,45] Medications commonly used to treat schizophrenia include typical antipsychotics and atypical antipsychotics. These medications may cause an array of side effects such as movement disorders (tardive dyskinesia, restless leg syndrome, dystonia), drowsiness and dizziness, blurred vision, and tachycardia.

EDs

AN and BN

Medical management usually involves lengthy psychotherapeutic interventions and nutritional

Table 15.2. Oral Side Effects and Interactions of Drugs used in Psychiatric Disorders

Drug Generic/ Proprietary Names	Class/Indications	Oral Side Effects	Dental Drug Interactions/Precautions
Venlafaxine Effexor®	Antidepressant (SNRI)/major depression; anxiety; panic disorder	Dry mouth	Tramadol, ketoconazole
Aripiprazole Abilify®	Atypical antipsychotic/schizophrenia, BPD	Dry mouth; hypersalivation; involuntary tongue, face, mouth, and jaw movements (tongue sticking out, puffing of cheeks, mouth puckering, chewing movements); trouble swallowing; speech changes	None
Ziparsidone Geodon®	Atypical antipsychotic/schizophrenia	Dry mouth, twitching of face or tongue, difficulty speaking or swallowing	Azithromycin, erythromycin, ketoconazole
Amitriptyline Elavil®	Antidepressant (tricyclic)/MDD, PTSD, chronic pain	Dry mouth, extrapyramidal symptoms, bone marrow suppression, stomatitis, peculiar taste, black tongue, paresthesias	NSAIDs, tramadol, epinephrine-containing local anesthesia
Paroxetine Paxil®	Antidepressant (SSRI)/PTSD, OCD, MDD, GAD, phobias, panic attacks	Dry mouth	Aspirin, NSAIDs, codeine, diazepam, dexamethasone, tramadol, meperidine
Citalopram Celexa®	Antidepressant (SSRI)/OCD, phobias, ED, panic attacks	Dry mouth	NSAIDs, ketoconazole, tramadol
Fluvoxamine Luvox®	Antidepressant (SSRI)/OCD, phobias	Dry mouth	Alprazolam, tramadol, triazolam, diazepam, ketoconazole, NSAIDs
Escitalopram Lexapro®	Antidepressant (SSRI)/OCD, phobias, GAD	Dry mouth	NSAIDs, tramadol
Lamotrigine Lamictal®	Anticonvulsant/mood stabilizer, BPD, seizure disorders, MDD	None	None

(Continued)

Table 15.2. (Continued)

Drug Generic/Proprietary Names	Class/Indications	Oral Side Effects	Dental Drug Interactions/Precautions
Chlorpromazine Thorazine®	Typical antipsychotic/schizophrenia, other psychotic disorders, BPD, severe aggressive behavior in ADHD	Dry mouth	None
Haloperidol Haldol®	Typical antipsychotic/schizophrenia, other psychoses, motor and verbal tics, severe aggressive behavior in ADHD	Dry mouth; hypersalivation; tongue protrusion or fine tongue movement; tardive dyskinesia: uncontrollable rhythmic face, mouth, jaw movements; bone marrow suppression	Erythromycin, narcotics
Perphenazine Trilafon®	Typical antipsychotic/schizophrenia	Dry mouth; hypersalivation; tongue protrusion or fine tongue movement; tardive dyskinesia: uncontrollable rhythmic face, mouth, jaw movements; bone marrow suppression	Narcotics, fluconazole, erythromycin, ciprofloxacin, clarithromycin, propoxyphene
Fluphenazine Prolixin® Permitil®	Typical antipsychotic/schizophrenia	Dry mouth	Meperidine
Quetiapine Seroquel®	Atypical antipsychotic/schizophrenia, BPD, MDD	Hypersalivation, dry mouth, tongue sticking out	Fluconazole, itraconazole, ketoconazole, erythromycin, dexamethasone
Clozapine Clozaril® Fazaclo®	Atypical antipsychotic/schizophrenia	Bone marrow suppression, hypersalivation, dry mouth	Erythromycin

BPD, bipolar disease; ED, eating disorder; GAD, generalized anxiety disorder; MDD, major depression; NSAIDs, nonsteroidal anti-inflammatory drugs; OCD, obsessive–compulsive disorder; PTSD, posttraumatic stress disorder; SNRI, serotonin–norepinephrine reuptake inhibitor; SSRI, selective serotonin reuptake inhibitor.

supplementation, and may necessitate hospitalization for individuals who have life-threatening complications, including electrolyte abnormalities and cardiac arrhythmias.

III. Dental Management

Evaluation

Evaluation of the patient includes a thorough medical, behavioral, and social history, and determination of competency with regard to capacity to give informed consent for treatment. Level of control of the psychiatric illness and past successes with care and possible need for anxiety management or sedation should be determined.

Dental Treatment Modifications

Anxiety Disorders

GAD

Anxiety management must be tailored to individual patient needs.[58] Iatrosedative interview (dentist speaking in soothing tones and inviting patient to discuss fears) may decrease anxiety. During the patient interview, the dentist should look for verbal and nonverbal signs of anxiety and respond to those signs, while sitting eye to eye with the patient, speaking in a soothing tone of voice, and assuring the patient that he or she is in a safe environment. Nonverbal gestures, such as smiling, and explaining the next procedure/events (tell–show–do) are important. The patient should understand and not feel threatened by the treatment, but rather feel

---

Key questions to ask the patient (caregiver) with a psychiatric disorder

- What type of mental health disorder do you have?
- Are you under active psychiatric care? Is your condition under control? What types of behaviors/symptoms do you have when the condition is not under control?
- Are there certain things that we can do in the office to make you more comfortable?

Key questions to ask the physician for the patient with a psychiatric disorder

- If severe oral adverse side effects are noted from the psychiatric medications, are there alternative medications or dose/schedule/timing that might be possible to decrease the specific adverse effect?
- If an ED patient: What is the ED care plan?

Figure 15.3 Traumatic tongue biting and scalloped tongue border in a patient with panic disorder, a type of generalized anxiety disorder.

a part of the team making the decisions. There are advanced behavioral techniques that may be useful such as desensitization.[59] For some individuals, anxiety and stress can lead to self-injurious behaviors such as bruxism; parafunctional habits; temporomandibular disorders; and cheek-, lip-, and tongue-biting trauma. See Fig. 15.3.

OCD

Awareness of the particular obsessions/compulsions is helpful.

Phobias

The object of the patient's phobia should be identified and avoided. If the patient's specific phobia cannot be avoided (i.e., fear of injections), consultation with medical/behavioral specialists is advised as the patient may need behavioral therapy prior to initiating dental treatment.

PTSD

Poor oral hygiene, rampant caries, gingivitis, and bruxism have all been reported as frequent findings in patients with PTSD. Complaints of orofacial pain, temporomandibular joint (TMJ) pain, and burning tongue have also been noted.[34] If a stressor is related to dental treatment, involvement of the psychiatrist may be needed.

Mood Disorders

BPD

Disregard for oral hygiene by depressed patients and cervical abrasion by overzealous tooth brushing of manic patients may occur. Anticaries agents and saliva substitutes may be useful along with oral hygiene instruction.

MDD

Patients undergoing treatment for MDD may be reluctant to report such treatment to dental providers. It is important that providers assure patients of confidentiality and the importance of disclosing all medications. Patients with MDD may be uncooperative or irritable and have complaints that are inconsistent with objective findings during dental treatment. Neglect of oral hygiene, increased smoking, and altered immune responses may contribute to a breakdown of the periodontal attachment seen in patients with MDD.[60]

Psychotic Disorders

Schizophrenia

Schizophrenics are at great risk for poor oral health. The xerostomia caused by the anticholinergic action of many of the antipsychotics can lead to the development of rampant dental caries and periodontal disease. Patients with tardive dyskinesia may experience uncontrolled jaw movement that makes the wearing of removable prostheses impossible.

EDs

AN and BN

Caries and periodontal problems should be treated as necessary and a topical home fluoride regimen used for caries prevention. Patients should be advised that brushing teeth immediately after vomiting may result in increased enamel erosion; rather, rinsing the mouth with a baking soda and water mouth rinse (1 teaspoon baking soda in 8 oz of water) will help neutralize mouth acids. Brushing should be delayed for 40 minutes after vomiting and a soft or ultrasoft brush with low abrasive toothpaste should be used. Mouth guards can be made to cover teeth for use during vomiting episodes.

Nutritional issues related to the oral cavity should be discussed, including avoiding acidic and cariogenic foods and drinks. Due to its high solubility in acid, glass ionomer restorative materials should not be used in patients with BN. Some patients with severe dental erosion may require complete prosthetic coverage of teeth. There is no actual contraindication to placing crowns on teeth while a patient is still engaged in purging behavior, although there may be some concern that continued exposure to high acid levels could result in erosion to root surfaces on these teeth.[61]

The undiagnosed (in the closet) patient with an ED may exhibit oral signs of vomiting and may have calloused knuckles on the index and middle fingers of the dominant hand used to induce vomiting. Addressing with the patient the topic of a suspected ED is difficult and needs to occur in a nonthreatening and nonjudgmental way, by sharing concrete findings from the oral exam of dental destruction indicating acid erosion. The ED patient may not be ready to disclose the secret condition and present excuses. Reluctant adolescents should be given a short fixed amount of time to disclose the ED to a parent prior to the dentist sharing that suspicion. Those ready to disclose may need support for discussion with a parent/family member and referral to their physician or an ED management program.

Figure 15.4 Early generalized lingual erosion of the maxillary teeth as a result of gastric acid contact in a patient with bulimia nervosa. Permission from S. Karger AG, Basel, Switzerland, to reprint image originally published in Roberts MW & Tylenda CA. Pediatrician 1989;16:178–84.

- dental enamel erosion (most often associated with BN) on palatal surface of maxillary anterior teeth (see Figs. 15.4 and 15.5);
- gingival inflammation;
- trauma to soft palate (secondary to induction of vomiting);
- increased caries rate;
- xerostomia;
- parotid gland hypertrophy.

Risks of Dental Care

Hemostasis

High serotonin uptake SSRI antidepressants, fluoxetine, paroxetine, and sertraline have been reported to occasionally cause increased bleeding time by interfering with platelet aggregation.

Oral Lesion Diagnosis and Management

EDs

There are a number of orofacial conditions associated with ED[38]:

Susceptibility to Infection

Schizophrenics taking clozapine may develop agranulocytosis, which can manifest as intraoral mucosal ulcerations and/or candidal infections.[45]

Figure 15.5 (a) Severe incisal edge fractures of the teeth due to lingual erosion and thinning of tooth structure. Permission from S. Karger AG, Basel, Switzerland, to reprint image originally published in Roberts MW & Tylenda CA. Pediatrician 1989;16:178–84. (b) Lingual image of a patient showing extensive erosion of enamel and exposure of dentin. Occlusal metal restorations can appear raised. Permission from JADA to reprint image originally published in Tylenda CA, Roberts MW, Elin RJ, Li S-H, Altemus M. Bulimia nervosa. Its effect on salivary chemistry. J Am Dent Assoc 1991;122(6):37–41.

Drug Actions/Interactions

Drug interactions should be carefully avoided as some antibiotics and analgesics often used in dentistry may adversely react with antipsychotics, mood stabilizers, and other antidepressants.[62] Medications used to treat psychiatric disorders often have oral side effects such as xerostomia, dysgeusia, stomatitis, glossitis, and even sialorrhea. Atypical antipsychotics can also cause orthostatic hypotension.

Patient's Ability to Tolerate Dental Care

Poorly controlled patients may become agitated, irritated, hostile, and uncooperative with treatment. Various levels of iatrosedation, anxiolysis, conscious sedation, or general anesthesia may be required based on the patient's oral health and behavioral circumstances.

Medical Emergencies

In all psychiatric disorders, acute episodes of agitation or irrational behavior that may pose a threat to the patient or others is a medical emergency that requires hospitalization and medications such as mood stabilizers, antipsychotics, and benzodiazepines.[45]

IV. Recommended Readings and Cited References

Section 1. Neurodevelopmental Disorders

Recommended Readings

Wasserman BS, ed. The Special Care Patient. WB Saunders, Philadelphia, 2009.

Cited References

1. American Association on Intellectual & Developmental Disabilities, (AAIDD). Definition of Intellectual Disability. Available at: http://www.aaidd.org/content_100.cfm?navID=21. Accessed October 31, 2011.
2. Desai SS. Down syndrome: a review of the literature. Oral Surg Oral Med Oral Pathol Oral Radiol Endod 1997;84(3):279–85.
3. Bax M, Goldstein M, Rosenbaum P, Leviton A, Paneth N, Dan B, et al. Proposed definition and classification of cerebral palsy, April 2005. Dev Med Child Neurol 2005;47(8):571–6.

4. American Psychiatric Association. Diagnostic and Statistical Manual of Mental Disorders (DSM-IV), 4th ed. 2000. American Psychiatric Association, Washington, DC.
5. Chakrabarti S, Fombonne E. Pervasive developmental disorders in preschool children. JAMA 2001;285:3093–9.
6. Friedlander AH, Yagiela JA, Paterno VI, Mahler ME. The pathophysiology, medical management, and dental implications of children and young adults having attention-deficit hyperactivity disorder. J Calif Dent Assoc 2003;31(9):669–78.
7. Friedlander AH, Yagiela JA, Mahler ME, Rubin R. The pathophysiology, medical management, and dental implications of adult attention-deficit/hyperactivity disorder. J Am Dent Assoc 2007;138(4):475–82.
8. National Center for Biotechnology Information (NCBI). Online Mendelian Inheritance in Man, Johns Hopkins University. (n.d.). Available at: http://www.ncbi.nlm.nih.gov/omim. Accessed November 9, 2011.
9. Jacobbson B, Hagberg G. Antenatal risk factors for cerebral palsy. Best Pract Res Clin Obstet Gynaecol 2004;18(3):425–36.
10. Odding E, Roebroeck ME, Stam HJ. The epidemiology of cerebral palsy: incidence, impairments and risk factors. Disabil Rehabil 2006;28(4):183–91.
11. Friedlander AH, Yagiela JA, Paterno VI, Mahler ME. The neuropathology, medical management and dental implications of autism. J Am Dent Assoc 2006;137(11):1517–27.
12. Currenti SA. Understanding the etiology of autism. Cell Mol Neurobiol 2010;30(2):161–71.
13. Reichenberg A, Gross R, Weiser M, Bresnahan M, Silverman J, Harlap S, et al. Advancing paternal age and autism. Arch Gen Psychiatry 2006;63(9):1026–32.
14. Institute of Medicine. Adverse Effects of Vaccines: Evidence and Causality. Consensus Report August 25, 2011. Available at: http://iom.edu/Reports/2011/Adverse-Effects-of-Vaccines-Evidence-and-Causality.aspx. Accessed November 1, 2011.
15. Boyle CA, Cordero JF. Birth defects and disabilities: a public health issue for the 21st century. Am J Public Health 2005;95(11):1884–6.
16. Friedlander AH, Yagiela JA, Paterna VI, Mahler ME. The pathophysiology, medical management and dental implication of Fragile X, Rett, and Prader-Will syndrome. J Calif Dent Assoc 2003;31(9):693–702.
17. Shin M, Besser LM, Kucik JE, Lu C, Siffel C, Correa A, et al. Prevalence of Down syndrome among children and adolescents in 10 regions of the United States. Pediatrics 2009;124(6):1565–71.
18. National Down Syndrome Society. Information Topics. 2011. Available at: http://www.ndss.org. Accessed October 3, 2011.
19. Jones MW, Morgan E, Shelton JE, Thorogood C. Cerebral palsy: introduction and diagnosis (part 1). J Pediatr Health Care 2007;21(3):146–52.
20. Center for Disease Control and Prevention. Autism and Developmental Disabilities Monitoring Network. Available at: http://www.cdc.gov/ncbddd/autism/data.html. Accessed November 1, 2011.
21. Centers for Disease Control and Prevention. State-based prevalence data of ADHD diagnosis. Available at: http://www.cdc.gov/ncbddd/adhd/data.html. Accessed October 10, 2011.
22. Pilcher ES. Dental care for the patient with Down syndrome. Downs Syndr Res Pract 1998;5(3):111–6. Available at: http://www.down-syndrome.org/reviews/84/reviews-84.pdf. Accessed January 1, 2012.
23. Rosenbaum P. Cerebral palsy: what parents and doctors want to know. Br Med J 2003;326(7396):970–4.
24. Filipek PA, Accardo PJ, Ashwal S, Baranek GT, Cook EH Jr., Dawson G, et al. Practice parameter: screening and diagnosis of autism: report of the Quality Standards Subcommittee of the American Academy of Neurology and Child Neurology Society. Neurology 2000;55(4):468–79.
25. Fombonne E. Epidemiological surveys of autism and other pervasive developmental disorders: an update. J Autism Dev Disord 2003;33(4):365–82.
26. Pope JE, Curzon ME. The dental status of cerebral palsied children. Pediatr Dent 1991;13(3):156–62.
27. Winter K, Baccaglini L, Tomar S. A review of malocclusion among individuals with mental and physical disabilities. Spec Care Dentist 2008;28(1):19–26.
28. Glassman P, Subar P. Planning dental treatment for people with special needs. Dent Clin North Am 2009;53(2):195–205.

29. Reuland-Bosma W, van Dijk J. Periodontal disease in Down's syndrome. J Clin Periodontol 1986;13(1):64–73.
30. Ram G, Chinen J. Infections and immunodeficiency in Down syndrome. Clin Exp Immunol 2011;164(1):9–16.
31. Green D, Flanagan D. Understanding the autistic dental patient. Gen Dent 2008;56(2):167–71.
32. Klein U, Nowak AJ. Characteristics of patients with autistic disorder (AD) presenting for dental treatment: a survey and chart review. Spec Care Dentist 1999;19(5):200–7.

Section 2. Psychiatric Disorders

Recommended Readings/Resources

Friedlander AH, Mahler ME. Major depressive disorder. Psychopathology, medical management and dental implications. J Am Dent Assoc 2001;132(6): 629–38.

National Eating Disorders Association. Available at: http://www.nationaleatingdisorders.org/

Cited References

33. Fenske JN, Schwenk TL. Obsessive compulsive disorder: diagnosis and management. Am Fam Physician 2009;80(3):239–45.
34. Friedlander AH, Friedlander IK, Marder SR. Post-traumatic stress disorder: psychopathology, medical management, and dental implications. Oral Surg Oral Med Oral Pathol Oral Radiol Endod 2004;97(1):5–11.
35. Yehuda R. Post-traumatic stress disorder. N Engl J Med 2002;346(2):108–14.
36. Mayo Clinic Health Information, Bipolar Disorder. Available at: http://www.mayoclinic.com/health/bipolar-disorder/DS00356. Accessed October 30, 2011.
37. National Institute of Mental Health (NIMH). Schizophrenia. National Institute of Health. 2009. Publication #09-3517, Bethesda, MD.
38. Hague AL. Eating disorders: screening in the dental office. J Am Dent Assoc 2010;141(6):675–8.
39. Angst J, Vollrath M. The natural history of anxiety disorders. Acta Psychiatr Scand 1991;84(5):446–52.
40. Fenske J, Schwenk T. Obsessive compulsive disorder: diagnosis and management. Am Fam Physician 2009;80(3):239–45.
41. Kendler KS, Myers J, Prescott CA. The etiology of phobias: an evaluation of the stress-diathesis model. Arch Gen Psychiatry 2002;59(3):242–8.
42. American Psychiatric Association. Practice Guideline for the Treatment of Patients with Bipolar Disorder, 2nd ed. 2002, pp. 525–612. American Psychiatric Association, Washington, DC.
43. Fattal O, Budur K, Vaughan AJ, Franco K. Review of the literature on major mental disorders in adult patients with mitochondrial diseases. Psychosomatics 2006;47(1):1–7.
44. Kiyohara C, Yoshimasu K. Molecular epidemiology of major depressive disorder. Environ Health Prev Med 2009;14(2):71–87.
45. Friedlander AH, Marder SR. The psychopathology, medical management and dental implications of schizophrenia. J Am Dent Assoc 2002; 133(5):603–10.
46. Blazer DG, Hughes D, George LK, et al. Generalized anxiety disorder. In: Psychiatric Disorders in America. Robins LN, Regier DA, eds. 1991, pp. 180–203. The Free Press, New York, NY.
47. Brawman-Mintzer O, Lydiard RB. Generalized anxiety disorder: issues in epidemiology. J Clin Psychiatry 1996;57(Suppl. 7):3–8.
48. Kessler RC, Berglund PA, Demler O, Jin R, Merikangas KR, Walters EE. Lifetime prevalence and age-of-onset distributions of DSM-IV disorders in the National Comorbidity Survey Replication. Arch Gen Psychiatry 2005;62(6):593–602.
49. Kessler RC, Demler O, Frank RG, Oflson M, Pincus HA, Walters EE, et al. Prevalence and treatment of mental disorders, 1990–2003. N Engl J Med 2005;352(24):2515–23.
50. Kessler RC, Chiu WT, Demler O, Merikangas KR, Walters EE. Prevalence, severity, and comorbidity of 12-month DSM-IV disorders in the National Morbidity Survey Replication. Arch Gen Psychiatry 2005;62(6):617–27.
51. National Comorbidity Survey Replication (NCS-R). 2005. Available at: http://www.hcp.med.harvard.edu/ncs/publications.php. Accessed October 30, 2011.
52. Hoek HW. Incidence, prevalence and mortality of anorexia nervosa and other eating disorders. Curr Opin Psychiatry 2006;19(4):389–94.
53. Roy-Byrne PP, Craske MG, Stein MB, Sullivan G, Bystritsky A, Katon W, et al. A randomized effectiveness trial of cognitive-behavioral therapy and

medication for primary care panic disorder. Arch Gen Psychiatry 2005;62(3):290–8.
54. Koran LM, Hanna GL, Hollander E, Nestadt G, Simpson HB; American Psychiatric Association. Practice guideline for the treatment of patients with obsessive-compulsive disorder. Am J Psychiatry 2007;7(Suppl.):5–53.
55. Mayo Clinic Health Information. Phobia Available at: http://www.mayoclinic.com/health/phobias/DS00272. Accessed October 30, 2011.
56. Cleveland Clinic Center for Continuing Education Disease Management Project (Cleveland Clinic). *Bipolar disorder*. Available at: http://www.clevelandclinicmeded.com/medicalpubs/diseasemanagement/psychiatry-psychology/bipolar-disorder. Accessed October 30, 2011.
57. Kapur S, Mieczkowski T, Mann JJ. Antidepressant medications and the relative risk of suicide attempt and suicide. JAMA 1992;268(24):3441–5.
58. Peltier B. Psychological treatment of fearful and phobic special needs patients. Spec Care Dentist 2009;29(1):51–7.
59. Kemp F. Alternatives: a review of non-pharmacologic approaches to increasing the cooperation of patients with special needs to inherently unpleasant dental procedures. Behav Anal Today 2005;6(2):88–108. Available at: http://www.baojournal.com/BAT%20Journal/VOL-6/BAT-6-2.pdf. Accessed January 1, 2012.
60. Moss ME, Beck JD, Kaplan BH, Offenbacher S, Weintraub JA, Koch GG, et al. Exploratory case-control analysis of psychosocial factors and adult periodontitis. J Periodontol 1996;67(10 Suppl.): 1060–9.
61. Milosevic A. Eating disorders and the dentist. Br Dent J 1999;186(3):109–13.
62. Friedlander AH, Friedlander IK, Marder SR. Bipolar I disorder: psychopathology, medical management and dental implications. J Am Dent Assoc 2002;133(9):1209–17.

Substance Use Disorders

Abdel R. Mohammad DDS, MS, MPH

I. Background

Substance use disorders (SUDs) are characterized by potential for addiction. In 2011, the American Society of Addiction Medicine (ASAM) defined addiction as follows:

> Addiction is a primary, chronic disease of brain reward, motivation, memory and related circuitry. Dysfunction in these circuits leads to characteristic biological, psychological, social and spiritual manifestations. This is reflected in an individual pathologically pursuing reward and/or relief by substance use and other behaviors.
>
> Addiction is characterized by:
> - Inability to consistently abstain
> - Impairment in behavioral control
> - Craving
> - Diminished recognition of significant problems with one's behaviors and interpersonal relationships
> - A dysfunctional emotional response

Like other chronic diseases, addiction often involves cycles of relapse and remission. Without treatment or engagement in recovery activities, addiction is progressive and can result in disability or premature death.[1]

Description of Disease

Alcohol Abuse and Alcoholism

American Medical Association (AMA) and the World Health Organization (WHO) view alcoholism as a discrete disease. In 1992, a panel of members from ASAM and the National Council on Alcoholism and Drug Dependence (NCADD) defined alcoholism as follows:

> Alcoholism is a primary chronic disease with genetic, psychosocial, and environmental factors influencing its development and manifestation. The disease is often progressive and fatal. It is characterized by impaired control over drinking,

The ADA Practical Guide to Patients with Medical Conditions, First Edition. Edited by Lauren L. Patton.
© 2012 American Dental Association. Published 2012 by John Wiley & Sons, Inc.

preoccupation with the drug (alcohol), use of alcohol despite adverse consequences, and distortions in thinking, most notably denial. Each of these symptoms may be continuous or periodic.[2]

Opioid Abuse and Dependence

Opiate drugs, derived from the opium "poppy" are central nervous system (CNS) depressants or "downers" and include morphine, heroin, meperidine, hydromorphone, methadone, and codeine. The number of emergency department visits and hospital admissions related to opiate/narcotic abuse has been increasing. This trend is in contrast to other substances of abuse, such as cocaine and marijuana that are CNS stimulants or "uppers."

Methamphetamine Abuse

Methamphetamine abuse has been identified as an increasing problem in the United States and has surpassed both cocaine and marijuana as the greatest drug threat in most states. It is a CNS stimulant drug, similar in structure to amphetamine, that is taken orally, intranasally (snorting the powder), by needle injection, or by smoking. Methamphetamine increases the release and blocks the reuptake of the brain chemical (or neurotransmitter) dopamine creating an intense euphoria.

Tobacco Dependence

Tobacco dependence is a chronic medical condition that often requires repeated intervention and multiple attempts to stop. All tobacco forms contain tobacco toxins and carcinogens. Cigarettes consist of ground processed tobacco rolled in a flame retardant paper; a filter is usually added.

The morbidity and mortality from chronic cigarette smoking is closely related to:

- total years of smoking,
- number of cigarettes per day,
- depth of inhalation,
- use of filtered versus nonfiltered cigarettes,
- use of mentholated cigarette brands.

Smokeless tobacco (ST) is consumed orally, and the principal types of ST consumed in the United States are chewing tobacco (cut tobacco leaves) and snuff (moist ground tobacco), held between the gum and cheek.

Pathogenesis/Etiology
Alcohol Abuse and Alcoholism

Alcohol dehydrogenase (ADH) serves to break down ingested alcohol that is toxic. Genes for slower metabolizing forms of ADH and alcohol consumption during adolescence both increase the risk of adult alcoholism. Alcohol interacts extensively with the dopaminergic reward neurocircuitry and corticolimbic structures in the developing adolescent brain and alcohol-mediated cognitive dysfunction promotes maladaptive behaviors that lead to addiction.[3]

Recommendations of the National Institute on Alcohol Abuse and Alcoholism (NIAAA) regarding safe (moderate use) amounts of alcohol consumption include:

- up to two drinks per day for men;
- one drink per day for women and the elderly.
    - (one drink equals one 12-oz bottle of beer or wine cooler, one 5-oz glass of wine, or 1.5 oz of 80-proof distilled spirits).

Moderate use of alcohol in this fashion causes few if any problems and can have distinct health benefits including lowered risks for some forms of cardiovascular disease and cerebrovascular accident, and possibly even a mild protective effect against certain forms of dementia.

People who should not drink at all include:

- women who are pregnant or trying to become pregnant (ingestion during pregnancy can cause fetal alcohol syndrome);
- people who plan to drive or engage in other activities that require alertness and skill (such as operating heavy machinery);
- people taking certain over-the-counter (OTC) medications and prescription medications;
- people with medical conditions that can be exacerbated by drinking;
- recovering alcoholics;
- those <21 years old.

Opioid Abuse and Dependence

Some opiate abusers began their use with prescribed opiates to control pain, while others began their experience from social contacts. Opiate drugs compete with endogenously manufactured opiates at various receptor sites in the brain by attaching to opiate receptors on T lymphocytes and leukocytes.

Methamphetamine Abuse

Methamphetamines are widely used psychostimulant drugs that act on monoamine transporters. They have medicinal properties that are or may be useful in treating a variety of medical conditions but may also be abused. Alterations of intracellular messenger pathways, transcription factors, and immediate early genes within the brain reward system are essential to the development of methamphetamine addiction, with genetic risk factors and changes in gene expression less well understood. The abuse of methamphetamine has been related to neurotoxicity in human long-term abusers, increased risk of stroke, and Parkinson's disease.[4]

Tobacco Dependence

Tobacco products, whether pyrolytic or nonpyrolytic (see Table 16.1), should be considered contaminated nicotine delivery devices. Nicotine dependence is a SUD. Inhalation is not necessary for nicotine to be absorbed into the bloodstream. The pharmacological objective of any tobacco form is the delivery of nicotine to the user's brain. Tobacco initiation and progression to nicotine addiction is influenced by sociocultural, psychological, physiological, and genetic factors. Chronic tobacco use is characterized by psychological (habituation, behavioral) and pharmacological (addiction, chemical dependency) factors.

Table 16.1. Tobacco Products Consumed in the United States

Pyrolytic (Combustion)	Nonpyrolytic (Unburned)
1. Cigarettes (95% of U.S. tobacco consumed)	1. Smokeless (spit) (topical) tobacco
2. Cigars	2. Chewing tobacco
3. Pipes	3. Moist snuff
	4. Dry snuff (powdered)

A major barrier for most smokers who try to quit is the neurobiology of tobacco dependence, which is fed by the most efficient delivery device of nicotine that exists, the cigarette. Cigarette smoking delivers high concentrations of nicotine to the CNS within seconds of the first puff. The primary target for nicotine in the CNS is the cx4/32 nicotinic acetylcholine receptor. When this receptor is activated by nicotine binding, it results in the release of dopamine in the brain's reward center and provides the positive reinforcement observed with cigarette smoking.

Epidemiology

Alcohol Abuse and Alcoholism

The prevalence of risky use is 30%; problem drinking varies; harmful use/alcohol abuse

5%; and alcohol dependence/alcoholism 4%. Alcohol use accounts for 85,000 deaths per year and more than $185 billion of health-care spending in the United States.[5]

Opioid Abuse and Dependence

It is estimated that 5–23% of prescription opioid doses dispensed are used nonmedically (without a prescription for the high they cause), through sharing or diverting pills to help a friend or family member with symptoms of physical distress or pain. These unintended users are unlikely to receive information about individualized dosing, possible contraindications, drug interactions, side effects, allergies, or other warnings.[6]

Hydrocodone is the most commonly abused prescription narcotic. Although sometimes viewed as a "white collar" addiction, hydrocodone abuse has increased among all ethnic, age, and socioeconomic groups. Of particular concern is the prevalence of illicit use of hydrocodone among school-age children. In 2010, 4.8% (12 million) of the U.S. population age 12 and older reported using prescription painkillers nonmedically.[7]

Heroin is an abused illegal opiate drug synthesized from morphine and is associated with serious health conditions, including fatal overdose, spontaneous abortion, collapsed veins, pulmonary complications, and in users who inject the drug, infectious diseases.[8]

Methamphetamine Abuse

The 2008 U.S. National Survey on Drug Use and Health: National Findings report stated that the number of past month methamphetamine users aged ≥12 years decreased significantly to 314,000 in 2008.[9] Recent decreases are believed to have resulted from the U.S. government's *Combat Methamphetamine Epidemic Act of 2005*, which limited the amount of the precursor drugs—pseudoephedrine and ephedrine—that could be sold OTC and required secure storage of these drugs in pharmacies.

Tobacco Dependence

In 2010, an estimated 19.3% (45.3 million) of U.S. adults were current cigarette smokers, 78.2% smoke daily. Smoking prevalence is higher among men (21.8%) than women (17.3%).[10]

Tobacco use is responsible for approximately one death every 1.5 minutes (443,000 tobacco-related deaths annually). The average smoker begins at age 13 and becomes a daily smoker by age 14. Approximately 20% of all dental patients are tobacco users. Another 20% of all dental patients are young people who should be encouraged not to begin use of tobacco products.

In 2010, approximately 8.1 million (3.2%) of U.S. adults 12 years of age or older were current (within the past month) ST users, 13.3 million Americans (5.4% of the U.S. population aged 12 years or older) smoked cigars, and 2.0 million (0.8% of that same population) smoked pipes. Studies show that over 80% of tobacco users want to stop; however, because of the addictive properties of nicotine in tobacco products, many need professional intervention.

Coordination of Care between Dentist and Physician

Dentists have the responsibility to ask relevant questions about a patient's medical history and the opportunity to look for subtle clues that may lead to a diagnosis of substance abuse, and eventually to life-changing treatment. They should be vigilant in identifying the patient with active disease, so as to provide the appropriate referral to physicians and substance use support personnel.

Dental team members can assist patients and physicians by:

- screening for alcohol/drug/tobacco use and abuse;
- providing alcohol/drug/tobacco prevention information;
- providing brief interventions—directing patients with abuse problems to health-care providers for assessment and treatment;
- supporting dependent patients during their recovery and minimizing relapse in recovering patients.

The patient's primary care physician should be consulted initially when an alcohol, drug, or SUD is known or suspected. Some patients—those who have received professional treatment for SUDs—may have an ongoing relationship with an addictionist (i.e., a physician with advanced education and certification in treating addictive disorders). Given the breadth of potential medical problems associated with SUDs, including the prevalence of infectious diseases in the drug-using population, the physician can provide information of great value to the dentist.

In these medically complex patients, the dentist should review the accuracy of patient-provided information about current medications and overall health status. These patients may be poor medical historians because they do not understand what they have been told about their health status or because they deny the severity of it. The physician may be able to provide critical historical information. The physician should also be able to provide critical information to the dentist about hepatic status, clotting times, experience with pain management, the potential for unpredictable metabolism of medications, and drugs to be avoided. This is the appropriate time to discuss the use of sedatives, oral anxiolytics, anesthetics, and postoperative pain medication as well as relapse prevention strategies. Physicians may have very specific requests or contracts with their recovering patients (particularly those with a history of abusing prescription medications).

This may include that the patient ask each provider to consult with their physician, that the physician be aware of every prescription received from any provider, and that essential prescriptions be written or dispensed in such a way as to minimize abuse potential (i.e., several small prescriptions rather than one larger amount, or that the patient's sponsor dispense the medication).

II. Medical Management

Screening, Brief Intervention, Referral, and Treatment (SBIRT)[11]

SBIRT is a comprehensive, integrated, public health approach to the delivery of early intervention and treatment services for persons with SUDs, as well as those who are at risk of developing these disorders:

- *Screening* quickly assesses the severity of substance use and identifies the appropriate level of treatment.
- *Brief intervention* focuses on increasing insight and awareness regarding SUDs and motivation toward behavioral change.
- *Referral to treatment* provides those identified as needing more extensive treatment with access to specialty care.

A key aspect of SBIRT is the integration and coordination of screening and treatment components into a system of services. This system links a community's specialized treatment programs with a network of early intervention and referral activities that are conducted in medical and social service settings.

Identification

Alcohol, Opioid, and Methamphetamine Abuse

Primary care physicians should screen by history for substance use at every health maintenance exam or initial pregnancy visit. Several validated screening tools include Alcohol Use Disorders Identification Test (AUDIT), fast alcohol screening tool (FAST), TWEAK (for pregnant women), Michigan Alcohol Screening Test (MAST, MAST-Geriatric [MAST-G]), Paddington Alcohol Test (PAT), rapid alcohol problem screen (RAPS-4), CAGE Survey, and Substance Abuse Subtle Screening Inventory (SASSI).[12]

Health professionals should maintain a high index of suspicion for substance use in persons with:

- a family or personal history of an SUD;
- recent stressful life events and lack of a social support mechanism;
- chronic pain or illness (including a pattern of drug seeking), trauma, mental illness;
- at-risk substance use, which is defined as any illicit drugs; >3 drinks/day or >7 drinks/week in women; >4 drinks/day or >14 drinks/week in men; or >1 drink/day if age >65.
- physical and cognitive disabilities including alcohol use before age 15 and a medical condition associated with substance use.

Tobacco Dependence

Every health-care provider, including the dental team, should identify the smoking patient, advise him or her to quit, assess readiness to make an attempt, assist with the quit attempt (setting a quit date, motivational literature, pharmacotherapy), and arrange for follow-up. Even without full assist and arrange actions, using a practical "assisted referral" approach for assessing tobacco use, providing tailored advice and brief counseling, and encouraging smokers to talk by telephone with a specially trained tobacco counselor, the health team can contribute to increased abstinence rates and patient satisfaction among smoking patients.[13]

Medical History

Alcohol, Opioid, and Methamphetamine Abuse

A diagnosis of either substance dependence or abuse is made when symptoms indicate a maladaptive pattern of substance use resulting in clinically significant impairment or distress. Patients may directly report use or recovery

---

Substance use disorders assessment

A comprehensive psychiatric evaluation including:

1. a detailed history of the patient's past and present substance use and the effects of substance use on the patient's cognitive, psychological, behavioral, and physiological functioning;
2. a general medical and psychiatric history and examination;
3. a history of psychiatric treatments and outcomes;
4. a family and social history;
5. screening of blood, breath, or urine for substance used;
6. other laboratory tests to help confirm the presence or absence of conditions that frequently co-occur with substance use disorders;
7. with the patient's permission, contacting a significant other for additional information.

Modified from the National Guideline Clearinghouse of the Agency for Healthcare Research and Quality, http://www.guideline.gov/content.aspx?id=9316&search=substance+use+disorders, accessed 11/12/2011.

status on the health history or manifest signs that raise suspicion of undiagnosed and untreated dependence.

Tobacco Dependence

There are several forms in which tobacco can be used: cigarettes (traditional, herbal omni), cigars, pipes, smokeless, and lozenges. Smoking can result in systemic and upper aerodigestive tract diseases and increase the risk of several forms of cancer including lung cancer, heart disease, and a number of nonmalignant oral conditions and diseases.

Physical Examination and Laboratory Testing

Alcohol, Opioid, and Methamphetamine Abuse

Although the medical consequences of alcohol abuse are visible in almost every organ system of the body, to a large extent, the same is true for other drugs of abuse. A pathological condition in any organ system may affect the patient's oral health and subsequent dental treatment.

Analysis of body fluids, hair, or breath can document the presence or absence of a substance (or its metabolites) in the body, but it does not reveal anything about the cardinal symptoms of compulsion, loss of control, tolerance, or withdrawal. Medical test results such as liver function test patterns and altered platelet counts can be strongly indicative of alcoholism, but often do not appear until late-stage illness. The absence of abnormal test results does not indicate the absence of addictive illness. Currently, there is no definitive laboratory procedure for diagnosing alcohol dependence or identifying a genetic susceptibility for this or any of the other addictive illnesses.

Tobacco Dependence

Signs of chronic tobacco use:

- tobacco smell on clothes, hair, and skin;
- premature wrinkling of the skin and yellowing of the fingers and nails;
- presence of tobacco-related cancers and other diseases such as osteoporosis, emphysema, chronic obstructive pulmonary disease, and cardiovascular diseases;
- reduced taste and smell acuity that may result in dietary changes including increased dietary use of salt, sugar, and spices.

Biomarkers of tobacco control:

- Cotinine, the major metabolite of nicotine, has a half-life of 18–20 hours and can be used to quantify an individual's exposure to nicotine.
- Anabasine, present in trace amounts in tobacco smoke, may help distinguish abstinent tobacco users who are using nicotine replacement therapy (NRT) from those who are continuing to use tobacco.

Medical Treatment

Alcohol, Opioid, and Methamphetamine Abuse

A variety of approaches may be useful for the management of patients with SUDs involving integrated psychiatric, pharmacological, and psychosocial treatments.

Pharmacotherapy for Alcoholism[14]

Three oral medications are currently approved to treat alcohol dependence:

- *Disulfiram* (Antabuse®) discourages drinking by making the person taking it feel sick after drinking alcohol.
- *Naltrexone* (Depade®, ReVia®) acts in the brain to reduce the craving for alcohol after someone has stopped drinking.
- *Acamprosate* (Campral®) works by reducing symptoms that follow lengthy abstinence, such as anxiety and insomnia.

Substance use disorders management approaches

Psychiatric management has the following specific objectives:
- Motivating the patient to change.
- Establishing and maintaining a therapeutic alliance with the patient.
- Assessing the patient's safety and clinical status.
- Managing the patient's intoxication and withdrawal states.
- Developing and facilitating the patient's adherence to a treatment plan.
- Preventing the patient's relapse.
- Educating the patient about substance use disorders.
- Reducing the morbidity and sequelae of substance use disorders.

Modified from the National Guideline Clearinghouse of the Agency for Healthcare Research and Quality, http://www.guideline.gov/content.aspx?id=9316&search=substance+use+disorders, accessed 11/12/2011.

Substance use disorders management approaches—specific treatments

a. *Pharmacological treatments*
1. Medications to treat intoxication and withdrawal states
2. Medications to decrease the reinforcing effects of abused substances
3. Agonist maintenance therapies
4. Antagonist therapies
5. Abstinence-promoting and relapse prevention therapies
6. Medications to treat co-occurring psychiatric conditions

b. *Psychosocial treatments*
1. Cognitive–behavioral therapies (e.g., relapse prevention, social skills training)
2. Motivational enhancement therapy
3. Behavioral therapies (e.g., community reinforcement, contingency management)
4. 12-step facilitation
5. Psychodynamic therapy/interpersonal therapy
6. Self-help manuals
7. Behavioral self-control
8. Brief interventions
9. Case management
10. Group, marital, and family therapies

Modified from the National Guideline Clearinghouse of the Agency for Healthcare Research and Quality, http://www.guideline.gov/content.aspx?id=9316&search=substance+use+disorders, accessed 11/12/2011.

In addition, an injectable, long-acting form of naltrexone (Vivitrol®) is available.

Other types of drugs are available to help manage the symptoms of withdrawal (such as tremor, nausea, and diaphoresis) that may occur after someone with alcohol dependence stops drinking.

Pharmacotherapy for Opiate Abuse and Dependence[15]

Several treatment options are available for patients dependent on opiates:

- *Methadone*—Methadone is similar to morphine and is used in addiction detoxification and opioid maintenance therapy (OMT) programs to reduce the withdrawal symptoms for patients addicted to heroin or narcotics. (Methadone can also be prescribed in a physician's office, but only if it is being used to treat pain.)
- *Buprenorphine* sublingual tablets (Suboxone® and Subutex®)—Buprenorphine is a Schedule II narcotic but is a partial agonist with a long half-life, features that reduce its abuse potential. Suboxone also contains the narcotic antagonist naloxone, which is not absorbed when taken sublingually but discourages diversion for intravenous abuse. Buprenorphine can be used for both OMT and detoxification. In detoxification, it can be tapered comfortably on a symptom-based schedule.
- *Naloxone* (Narcan®)—An opioid antagonist used for the complete or partial reversal of opioid depression.

Tobacco Dependence

The national quit line program was developed in collaboration with and is sponsored by the states and the U.S. Department of Health and Human Services (USDHHS). 1-800-QUIT-NOW provides free cessation assistance and resource information to all U.S. tobacco users.

Counseling and pharmacotherapy are proven effective strategies to help smokers quit smoking. There are seven first-line medications that can be used individually or in combination. These include five nicotine replacement medications (nicotine gum, nicotine vapor inhaler, nicotine lozenges) and two non-nicotine medications (bupropion and varenicline). Short-acting NRT is best used for the acute management of nicotine withdrawal symptoms and cravings in combination with longer-acting medications such as nicotine patches, bupropion, or varenicline.

Pharmacotherapy for Tobacco Dependence[16]

1. *Nicotine Replacement Therapy (NRT)*
   NRT can be divided into two groups:
   - Short-acting NRT
     - *Nicotine gum*, available as an OTC product, in both 2- and 4-mg doses, can be used as monotherapy or in combination with other NRT or bupropion. Patients should be instructed in its proper use to "chew and park" and to avoid acidic beverages that lower the nicotine absorption.
     - *Nicotine lozenges* are available as an OTC product. Nicotine lozenges are available in 2- and 4-mg doses, with the latter indicated for use in "high"-dependence smokers (i.e., time to first cigarette of the day of less than 30 minutes after awaking). The method of delivery (i.e., transbuccal) is similar to that of nicotine gum, and can be used alone or in combination with other NRT or bupropion.
     - *Nicotine nasal spray* delivers nicotine directly to the nasal mucosa and has been observed to be effective for achieving smoking abstinence as monotherapy. This device delivers nicotine more rapidly than other therapeutic nicotine replacement delivery systems

and reduces withdrawal symptoms more quickly than nicotine gum.
- ○ *Nicotine vapor inhaler* has also been shown to be effective as monotherapy for increasing smoking abstinence. The device delivers nicotine in vapor form that is absorbed across the oral mucosa.
- Longer acting
  - ○ *Nicotine patches* deliver a steady dose of nicotine for 24 hours after a single application. The once-daily dosing enhances compliance. Nicotine patches are available without a prescription in doses of 7, 14, and 21 mg. The smoking rate can be used to determine the initial nicotine patch dose at a dose of approximately 1 mg of nicotine for each cigarette smoked per day (CPD). Thus, <10 CPD warrant a 7- to 14-mg dose, 10–20 CPD warrant a 14–21 mg per day dose, 21–40 CPD warrant a 21–42 mg per day dose, and >40 CPD warrant a dose of 42 mg per day or more. Adequacy of the initial dose is determined by assessing the patient's withdrawal symptoms and relief from cravings.

2. *Non-Nicotine Medications*
   - *Sustained-release bupropion* is a monocyclic antidepressant that inhibits the reuptake of both norepinephrine and dopamine and has an antagonist effect on nicotine acetylcholine receptors. Sustained-release bupropion (bupropion SR) has been shown to be effective and exhibits a significant dose–response effect.
   - *Varenicline* is a partial nicotine agonist/antagonist that selectively binds to the $c\alpha$ 4/32 nicotinic acetylcholine receptor. Varenicline both blocks nicotine from binding to the receptor (antagonist effect) and partially stimulates (agonist effect) receptor-medicated activity, leading to the release of dopamine, which reduces cravings and nicotine withdrawal symptoms. Varenicline is initiated at a dose of 0.5 mg once daily for 3 days followed by 0.5 mg twice daily for 4 days. The target quit date is day 8, when the maintenance dose of 1 mg twice daily begins. The length of treatment should be at least 12 weeks and can be extended for an additional 12 weeks.

All patients being treated with either bupropion or varenicline should be observed for neuropsychiatric symptoms that are a possible side effect.

Combination Pharmacotherapy

The 2008 USDHHS Public Health Service (PHS) Guideline[17] states that certain combinations of first-line medications have been shown to be more effective than monotherapy, with long-term (greater than 14 weeks) nicotine patch therapy combined with nicotine gum or nicotine nasal spray, nicotine patch therapy, plus nicotine vapor inhaler, and nicotine patch therapy plus bupropion SR cited as examples. No pharmacotherapy to date has been shown to be effective in treating ST users.

III. Dental Management

Evaluation

The health history should include questions about the use of tobacco, alcohol, and chemical substances. Substance users often use multiple substances discussed in this chapter. For example, there is a high prevalence of comorbidity with alcohol and nicotine dependence. With any dental patient, the assessment of their physical and behavioral presentation is important and may raise one's level of suspicion as the health history and oral examination progress. However, many who have SUDs in the early stages will not appear or behave differently than might be expected.

> **Signs of possible substance use disorder**
>
> - Obvious signs of intoxication: alcohol on the patient's breath, slurred speech
> - Odor of marijuana or tobacco smoke on clothing or hair
> - Extremely red eyes, swollen or puffy facial features, facial flushing
> - Fidgeting, rapid speech, difficulty sitting still
> - Spider angiomas on the face, needle tracks on hands or arms
> - Disruptive behavioral or emotional presentations suggestive of being "high"
> - A long-term patient of record who becomes less and less reliable in terms of keeping appointments, treatment compliance, and even basic oral hygiene
> - Adolescent wearing a T-shirt with alcohol- or drug-related art, or cannabis-leaf jewelry

As with any other component of the health history, questions about substance use should be asked matter-of-factly and professionally. Adolescents may be more receptive to questioning that begins indirectly—for example, "What kind of drugs are available to the kids you hang out with?" Adolescents may need realistic assurances about the privacy of information that they disclose. Dentists must be familiar with their state laws regarding disclosure of information to parents or guardians. For example, is there a legal obligation to inform parents?

Alcohol Abuse and Alcoholism

All adolescent and adult patients should be asked about the type, quantity, frequency, pattern of use, consequences of use, and family history of alcohol or drug use and/or dependence. In particular, dental professionals should be alert for alcohol-induced nutritional deficiencies resulting in such oral changes as angular chelitis, glossitis, and gingivitis. Signs of depression or other mood changes should be noted and appropriate referrals should be made.[18]

Opioid Abuse and Dependence

A key behavioral sign of opioid abuse and dependence is drug-seeking behaviors. Even when patients receive opiate medication through a health-care professional for the relief of pain, there is still a risk for those patients to become dependent. Those who abuse opiates are more prone to acquire oral fungal and viral infections, advanced periodontal disease, xerostomia, caries, and lost teeth.

Methamphetamine Abuse

Patients are often vague about their substance use. Additional questioning may be required to accurately assess the true quantity used. Date and time of last methamphetamine or cocaine use is critical information if you will be administering anesthetics. The patient may have signs of methamphetamine use, which include cutaneous lesions on the arms, an ill-defined febrile illness, cachexia, mood swings, violent outbursts, paranoia, poor coping skills, xerostomia, and rampant caries.

Tobacco Dependence

The oral health-care team should use the health history to identify every smoker, advise them to quit, assess their readiness to make an attempt, assist with the quit attempt (setting a quit date, motivational literature, pharmacotherapy), and arrange for follow-up.

The first step in treating tobacco use is to identify the tobacco users. Patients want and

Key questions to ask the patient who uses alcohol

*Exploring alcohol use patterns is easier in the context of related oral diseases.
1. Can you help me understand how often, how much, and for how long you have consumed alcohol?
2. Are you receiving any professional treatment for the use?

AUDIT-C—3-item alcohol screen to identify persons who are hazardous drinkers or active alcohol use disorders.
1. How often do you have a drink containing alcohol?
   Never = 0; monthly or less = 1; 2–4 times/month = 2; 2–3 times/week = 3; 4+ times/week = 5
2. How many standard drinks containing alcohol do you have on a typical day?
   1–2 drinks = 0; 3–4 drinks = 1; 5–6 drinks = 2; 7–9 drinks = 3; 10 or more drinks = 4
3. How often do you have 6 or more drinks on one occasion?
   Never = 0; Less than monthly = 1; Monthly = 2; Weekly = 3; Daily or almost daily = 5

SCORING: Men: score of 4 or more is positive; women: 3 or more is positive, unless all points are from question 1.
The higher the score, the more likely the drinking is affecting patient safety.
Reference: http://www.thenationalcouncil.org/galleries/business-practice%20files/tool_auditc.pdf, accessed November 12, 2011

Key questions to ask the physician of the patient who uses alcohol (see Chapter 6 for questions related to alcoholic liver disease)

Is the patient under your care or the care of an addictionist for his or her alcohol use disorder?
What medical problems has the patient developed related to the alcohol use?
Is the patient on Antabuse?
Should alcohol-containing mouth rinses be avoided for this patient?
Does the patient have hepatic damage?

Key questions to ask the patient with an opioid or methamphetamine use disorder

1. Can you help me understand how often, how much, and for how long you have consumed these drugs?
2. Are you receiving any professional treatment for the use?
3. Do you have a pain medicine contract with your physician? Do you have a sponsor/family member who will help dispense your pain medicine?

> **? Key questions to ask the physician of the patient with an opioid or methamphetamine use disorder**
>
> Is the patient under your care or the care of an addictionist for his or her substance use disorder?
> Do you have a narcotic prescription contract with this patient? Are all narcotics to be prescribed by a single provider? Is that you? What analgesics do you consider appropriate for this patient for varying levels of pain?
> Will the patient's dental pain be able to be controlled by the standard narcotic regimen?
> Do you feel sedatives and anxiolytics may be safely used for this patient?

> **? Key questions to ask the patient who uses tobacco**
>
> 1. Can you help me understand what kind of tobacco, how often, how much, and for how long you have consumed tobacco?
> 2. Have you tried to quit before? If so what assistance did you receive? Was this successful for a short time?
> 3. Are you currently receiving any professional treatment for the tobacco use?
> 4. Are you ready to quit? Do you have a quit date? What barriers to you have to quitting?

expect their health-care provider to ask and advise them about their tobacco use. Showing patients oral lesions related to their tobacco use is a powerful motivator for initiating a quit attempt. The PHS guideline[17] states that dentists can implement interventions, as brief as 3 minutes, and be effective in increasing cessation rates. Brief interventions are effective with all populations including older smokers, pregnant women, adolescent tobacco users, and racial and ethnic minorities.

The five A's of intervention are recommended by the National Cancer Institute and Public Health Service Guidelines: ASK the patient about tobacco use. ADVISE the patient to quit—strong, clear message. ASSESS the willingness of the patient to make an attempt to quit. ASSIST the patient who is willing to set a "quit date," likely with the use of pharmaco-therapy. ARRANGE for follow-up contact to prevent relapse; contact the patient 1–2 days prior to their quit date, 2 weeks after the quit date, and then follow-up as needed. See Appendix.

Dental Treatment Modifications

A general approach to deal with the dental care of addicts involves relief of pain as the prime concern. Once emergency care is completed, emphasis is redirected to improved oral hygiene and dietary advice to address the poor nutritional status and the high frequency of carbohydrate intake, which is strongly conducive to the predisposition of caries. Some patients who are addicted to opiates may want to retain carious teeth in order to try and seek a prescription for opiates.

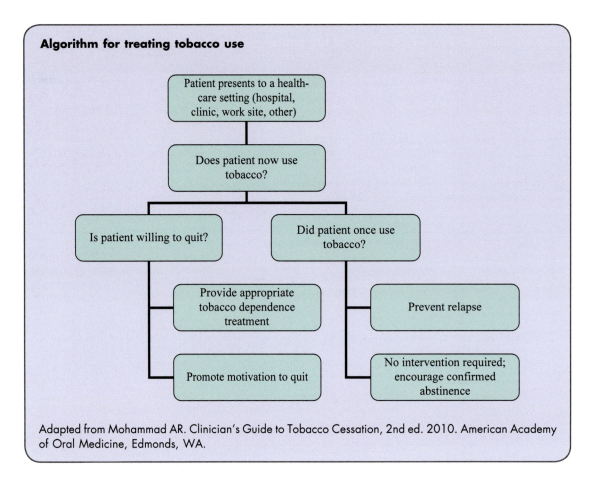

Adapted from Mohammad AR. Clinician's Guide to Tobacco Cessation, 2nd ed. 2010. American Academy of Oral Medicine, Edmonds, WA.

Pain Management

There is significant individual variation in the experience of acute pain in dental patients, and patients with SUDs may need more medication than might have been anticipated (due to increased levels of tolerance for analgesics). Inadequately managed pain, with its attendant anxiety and cravings, is a known risk factor for relapse, and is to be avoided.[19] Premedication with a nonsteroidal anti-inflammatory drug (NSAID) such as ibuprofen, 600–800 mg, 1–2 hours before the procedure, has been demonstrated to lower postoperative pain and to result in a decreased need for opiates. The administration of a long-acting anesthetic (such as bupivacaine) immediately following the procedure may also be of benefit in pain control. Whenever possible, non-narcotic analgesics should be recommended. As with all postoperative patients, the dentist will want to recommend the usual nonpharmaceutical strategies for pain management as appropriate—rest, relaxation, and ice. Patients should be cautioned against the use of nonprescribed psychoactive substances in the immediate postoperative period.

The undertreatment of pain in patients on OMT remains a serious problem. In cases of acute pain associated with surgery, trauma, or invasive dental treatment, physicians and dentists often and incorrectly assume that the maintenance dose of methadone or buprenorphine will also relieve any pain. The daily dose of OMT does not provide adequate analgesia for acute pain. Maintenance patients develop

ADA Statement on Provision of Dental Treatment for Patients with Substance Use Disorders. (2005:329)

- Dentists are urged to be aware of each patient's substance use history, and to take this into consideration when planning treatment and prescribing medications.
- Dentists are encouraged to be knowledgeable about substance use disorders—both active and in remission—in order to safely prescribe controlled substances and other medications to patients with these disorders.
- Dentists should draw upon their professional judgment in advising patients who are heavy drinkers to cut back, or the users of illegal drugs to stop.
- Dentists may want to be familiar with their community's treatment resources for patients with substance use disorders and be able to make referrals when indicated.
- Dentists are encouraged to seek consultation with the patient's physician when the patient has a history of alcoholism or other substance use disorder.
- Dentists are urged to be current in their knowledge of pharmacology, including content related to drugs of abuse; recognition of contraindications to the delivery of epinephrine-containing local anesthetics; safe prescribing practices for patients with substance use disorders—both active and in remission—and management of patient emergencies that may result from unforeseen drug interactions.
- Dentists are obliged to protect patient confidentiality of substance abuse treatment information, in accordance with applicable state and federal law.

Adapted from Statement on provision of dental treatment for patients with substance use disorders (2005:329). Chicago: American Dental Association; 2007:209 in Fung EYK and Giannini PJ. Implications of Drug Dependence on Dental Patient Management, General Dentistry, May/June 2010, page 236.

American Dental Association Statement on the Use of Opioids in the Treatment of Dental Pain (2005;328)

- The ADA encourages continuing education about the appropriate use of opioid pain medications in order to promote both responsible prescribing practices and limit instances of abuse and diversion.
- Dentists who prescribe opioids for treatment of dental pain are encouraged to be mindful of and have respect for their inherent abuse potential.
- Dentists who prescribe opioids for treatment of dental pain are also encouraged to periodically review their compliance with Drug Enforcement Administration recommendations and regulations.
- Dentists are encouraged to recognize their responsibility for ensuring that prescription pain medications are available to the patients who need them, for preventing these drugs from becoming a source of harm or abuse and for understanding the special issues in pain management for patients already opiate dependent.
- Dentists who are practicing in good faith and who use professional judgment regarding the prescription of opioids for the treatment of pain should not be held responsible for the willful and deceptive behavior of patients who successfully obtain opioids for nondental purposes.
- Appropriate education in addictive disease and pain management should be provided as part of the core curriculum at all dental schools.

Adapted from the American Dental Association. Current Policies Adopted. 1954–2009. Chicago: ADA; http://www.ada.org/sections/about/pdfs/doc_policies.pdf; page 227; accessed November 12, 2011.

> **Considerations to make when prescribing opioids to dental patients***
>
> - Be familiar with and consider evidence-based recommendations for the treatment of acute pain, including guidelines or suggestions for prescribing to patients with or without suspected substance abuse problems.
> - If available, use prescription monitoring programs to verify drug-use history.
> - Do not prescribe controlled drugs to patients you do not know, especially when the office is closed and there are few options available for seeing the patient.
> - Be suspicious of patients who ask for specific drugs or report that their medication was "lost," "stolen," or "dropped into the sink."
> - Discuss with your patients and determine whether they actually need an opioid for their pain and how likely they are to use the quantity you prescribe; if they do not need it, do not write it or write for smaller quantities with a limited number of refills if needed.
> - Secure (that is, lock up) all prescription pads when not in use.
> - Write out the quantity of doses on the prescription and indicate "No Refills" unless you are sure that the patient will require a specific number of refills.
> - Consider if you have received a referral from another dentist that the patient may already have been prescribed an analgesic (whether nonsteroidal anti-inflammatory drugs or opioids).
> - Advise all patients that if they do not destroy their remaining doses, they should properly secure any remaining medication.
> - For patients who acknowledge a substance use disorder, if opioids must be prescribed, ask if a responsible family member will safeguard and dispense the medication when needed to manage pain.
> - Discuss the patient's substance use history with his or her primary care physician or with another practitioner when referring the patient for specialized dental surgery.
>
> * American Dental Association.

full tolerance to the analgesic effects of the maintenance dose of methadone. During OMT, cross-tolerance develops to all opiate agonist drugs, accounting for the "blockade" effect. Patients on methadone therapy should be maintained on their current replacement therapy and, if needed, should receive additional opiate analgesics for pain, often at higher doses than usually given and at shorter dispensing intervals.[20]

Craniofacial Trauma

Chemical use, misuse, and abuse are often a causal factor in injuries producing craniofacial trauma. An accurate drug/alcohol use history is important to help predict the potential for acute withdrawal symptoms that can seriously complicate and compromise the treatment of maxillofacial injuries. Seizures are not uncommon during alcohol withdrawal and usually begin 24–48 hours after the last drink. Severe alcohol withdrawal is uncommon, but delirium tremens is life-threatening and should be prevented with careful medical management. Much craniofacial trauma is related to substance abuse by the perpetrator, and not to the victim. Trauma resulting from interpersonal violence presents a different set of challenges to the treating health-care professionals.

Oral Lesion Diagnosis and Management

Alcohol, Opioid, and Methamphetamine Abuse

The overall oral health of a patient with an SUD is generally related to the stage of the disease or disorder. The incidence of dental caries and subsequent tooth loss is far more pronounced in patients with SUDs. Neglect of oral hygiene associated with all substance use contributes to extensive dental caries. Nutritional deficiencies can result in glossitis and loss of tongue papillae along with angular and labial cheilitis, which may be complicated by concomitant candidal infections. Dry mouth and dry lips are common in patients who use alcohol, smoke tobacco, or smoke cocaine or methamphetamine:

Alcohol
- Oropharyngeal cancer
- Mucosal and gingival inflammation and discoloration[5]
- Parotid gland enlargement and increased flow with diminished buffering capacity
- Gingival bleeding
- Periodontitis

Methamphetamine
- Rampant dental caries (meth mouth) (see Figs. 16.1 and 16.2)
- Gingival inflammation
- Periodontitis
- Xerostomia
- Bruxism and tooth wear

Opioids
- Xerostomia
- Acute necrotizing ulcerative gingivitis
- Increased decay rate
- Periodontitis

Other substances of abuse, such as the addictive stimulant drug cocaine that can be snorted,

Meth mouth
- A distinctive rampant dental caries pattern can often be seen on the buccal smooth surfaces of teeth and the interproximal surfaces of the anterior teeth associated with methamphetamine use.
- Probably caused by a combination of drug-induced psychological and physiological changes resulting in:
  - xerostomia (dry mouth);
  - extended periods of poor oral hygiene;
  - frequent consumption of high calorie, carbonated beverages (e.g., Mountain Dew);
  - grinding and clenching;
  - acidic nature of the drug may be a contributing factor.

Figure 16.1 Methamphetamine mouth, front view.

Figure 16.2 Methamphetamine mouth, side view.

Figure 16.3 Cocaine dehiscence with gingival pallor.

Figure 16.4 Cocaine burn (cocaine pseudomembrane).

dissolved in water and injected, or processed into a rock crystal and smoked "crack" cocaine creating a 5- to 30-minute high, can result in similar oral lesions. Additionally, there may be an unusual pattern of burns present on the oral mucosa from smoking crack pipes. See Figs. 16.3 and 16.4.

Tobacco Dependence

Oral signs of tobacco use are numerous:

- Halitosis
- Tooth loss
- Tobacco stains on teeth, restorations, and dentures
- Periodontitis
- Gingival recession in areas of habitual ST use
- Aphthous ulceration
- Hairy tongue
- Median rhomboid glossitis
- Others below:

Figure 16.5 Leukoplakia lower lip and floor of mouth in edentulous chronic snuff user.

Leukoplakia

Leukoplakia is a white patch, which may be smooth or wrinkled with a pumice stone appearance. See Fig. 16.5. Leukoplakia occurs more frequently in smokers than in nonsmokers, and ST users may exhibit a mucosal lesion in the area where tobacco is held. Erythroplakia (speckled erythroplakia) is less common but has a higher risk of malignancy.

Chronic Hyperplastic Candidiasis

Chronic hyperplastic candidiasis exhibits a red or white plaque, which may be flat or slightly elevated. See Fig. 16.6. It is difficult to differentiate from leukoplakia, angular cheiltis, or denture stomatitis. This lesion is a combination of candidiasis and leukoplakia. This lesion should be biopsied to confirm the diagnosis.

Nicotine Stomatitis or Palatinus

Nicotine stomatitis is diffuse palatal keratosis with chronic inflammation of the palatal minor salivary glands. See Fig. 16.7. The color of the palate ranges from reddish to a diffuse grayish-white. The lesion is often seen in chronic moderate to heavy pipe and cigar smokers.

Figure 16.6 Chronic hyperplastic candidiasis in a smoker.

Figure 16.7 Nicotine palatinus.

Snuff Dipper's Lesion

This is considered a form of leukoplakia but varies in degree. The lesion initially is not thickened and shows no color changes, but later wrinkles, and may develop into deep furrows (pouch). See Figs. 16.8–16.10. The lesion will regress and may disappear when tobacco use is discontinued.

Smoker's Melanosis

Melanin pigmentation occurs in the attached gingiva of 5–10% of smokers. See Fig. 16.11. Frequency and extent may be dose–response related. No clinically significant risk is known.

Figure 16.8 Tobacco pouch with periodontal abrasion.

Figure 16.9 Smokeless tobacco pouch on lower lip.

Figure 16.10 Smokeless tobacco keratosis of buccal mucosa.

Figure 16.11 Smokers melanosis of buccal mucosa.

Figure 16.12 Squamous cell carcinoma of the edentulous right alveolar ridge.

Oral Squamous Cell Carcinoma

The incidence of oral cancer among smokers varies from 2 to 18 times that of nonsmokers. The greatest risk is among tobacco users who regularly use alcohol; both account for approximately 75% of all oral and pharyngeal cancers.[21] See Fig. 16.12. Refer also to Chapter 13.

 Risks of Dental Care

Denial and minimization of substance abuse is common. The dentist must stress to the patient that accurate information regarding their alcohol and/or drug use is imperative to avoid potential adverse drug interactions and assure safe provision of dental care.

Hemostasis

In SUD patients with liver damage that may alter coagulation mechanisms, it would be prudent to obtain laboratory studies—or to consult with the patient's physician—to assess their coagulation status prior to oral surgical procedures.

Cigarette smoke causes damage to vascular endothelium resulting in atherosclerosis, coronary artery vaso-occlusive factors, increased platelet aggregation, increased vasomotor reactivity (coronary artery vasospasm), increased prothrombotic state, increased fibrinogen levels, increased carbon monoxide, increased plasma viscosity, elevated total cholesterol, and decreased high-density lipoprotein.

Susceptibility to Infection

Susceptibility to infection is no greater among patients with SUDs unless they have generalized malnutrition.

Drug Actions/Interactions

Alcohol-containing mouthwashes or elixirs should be avoided in patients recovering from alcoholism (alcohol dependence), as even small amounts could precipitate a relapse. Such preparations should *never* be prescribed to patients taking disulfiram (Antabuse®) as they may trigger an adverse reaction. Patients on disulfiram also should not be given amoxicillin/clavulanic acid, metronidazole, cefuroxime, diazepam, midazolam, or alprazolam. Adverse interactions between alcohol and medications in dentistry are shown in Table 16.2.

In patients maintained on methadone, it is very important to avoid using mixed opiate agonist–antagonists such as pentazocine, butorphanol, and nalbuphine for pain relief, as these will precipitate acute withdrawal. Since naltrexone (ReVia®)—used as an adjunctive treatment of heroin or other opioid dependence—is an opioid antagonist, opioid analgesics will

Table 16.2. Adverse Interactions between Alcohol and Medications Used in Dentistry

Medication	Drug Interaction with Alcohol	Dentist's Guidance
Analgesics		
Aspirin	Excessive bleeding may occur because of aspirin-induced prolongation of bleeding time.	Counsel patient to discontinue alcohol use during analgesic therapy.
Ibuprofen	Increased risk of gastric mucosal ulceration; renal toxicity has been reported in association with binge drinking.	Counsel patient to discontinue alcohol use during analgesic therapy.
Antibiotics		
Cephalosporins Metronidazole Augmentin	A disulfiram effect may occur, permitting the accumulation of acetaldehyde, leading to facial flushing, headache, palpitations, and nausea.	Counsel patient to discontinue alcohol use during antibiotic therapy. Do not prescribe to active alcohol user.
Erythromycin	Decreased absorption of erythromycin with a resultant decrease in effectiveness.	Counsel patient to discontinue alcohol use during erythromycin therapy.
Tetracycline	Increased absorption and increased plasma concentration in normal subjects after acute ingestion of ethanol; diminished effectiveness in chronic alcoholism because of induction of metabolizing enzymes.	Counsel patient to discontinue alcohol use during tetracycline therapy.
Antifungals		
Ketoconazole	May increase risk of liver toxicity.	Counsel patient to discontinue alcohol during use of ketoconazole treatment.
Barbiturates		
Pentobarbital Secobarbital	Concurrent use may increase CNS depressant effects; diminished effectiveness in people with chronic alcoholism because of cellular tolerance to CNS depression, increased metabolism, or both.	Advise patients to never drink alcohol when taking barbiturates.
Benzodiazopines		
Diazepam Lorazepam	Concurrent use may increase CNS depressant effects; diminished effectiveness in people with chronic alcoholism because of cellular tolerance to CNS depression, increased metabolism, or both.	Initially decrease the usual dose of medication and observe for CNS depression; counsel patient to discontinue alcohol use during treatment.
Other medications		
Chloral hydrate	Concurrent use may significantly increase CNS depressant effects.	Initially decrease the usual dose of medication and observe for CNS depression; counsel patient to discontinue alcohol use during treatment.
Opioids	Sedative side effects are markedly increased.	Initially decrease the dose of medication and observe for CNS depression; counsel patient to discontinue alcohol use during treatment.

CNS, central nervous system.
Adapted from Friedlander et al.[14]

Table 16.3. Tobacco Cessation Therapies and Drug Actions/Interactions

Pharmacotherapy	Method of Delivery	Precautions/ Contraindications	Adverse Effects	Dosage	Duration	Availability	Cost per Day
First line							
Sustained release Bupropion Hydrochloride Zyban® (non-nicotine)	Tablet by mouth	History of seizure History of eating disorders	Insomnia Dry mouth	150 mg every morning for 3 days then 150 mg twice daily (begin treatment 1–2 weeks prequit)	7–12 weeks maintenance Up to 6 months	Prescription only	$3.33
Nicotine gum Nicorette® (polarcrilex)	Transmucosal	Do not use tobacco	Mouth soreness Dyspepsia	1–24 cigarettes/d: 2 mg gum (up to 24 pieces/d) ≥25 cigarettes/d: 4 mg gum (up to 24 pieces/d)	Up to 12 weeks	OTC only	$6.25 for ten 2-mg pieces $6.87 for ten 4-mg pieces
Nicotine inhaler	Oral cavity		Local irritation of mouth and throat	6–16 cartridges/d	Up to 6 months	Prescription only	$10.94 for 10 cartridges
Nicotine nasal spray	Nasal cavity		Nasal irritation	8–40 doses/d	3–6 months	Prescription only	$5.40 for 12 doses
Nicotine patch	Transdermal	Do not use tobacco	Local skin reaction Insomnia	21 mg/24 h 14 mg/24 h 7 mg/24 h 15 mg/16 h	4 weeks Then 2 weeks Then 2 weeks	Prescription and OTC	$4.22 $4.51
Second line							
Clonidine		Rebound hypertension	Dry mouth Drowsiness Dizziness Sedation	0.15–0.75 mg/d	3–10 weeks	Prescription only (oral formulation and patch)	$0.24 for 0.2 mg $3.50
Nortriptyline		Risk of arrhythmias	Sedation Dry mouth	75–100 mg/d	12 weeks	Prescription only	$0.74 for 75 mg

d, day; mg, milligrams; h, hour; OTC, over the counter.

not be effective in patients who take this medication.

Drug actions and interactions of tobacco cessation support products are shown in Table 16.3.

Patient's Ability to Tolerate Dental Care

Impaired Wound Healing

Alcohol: Alcohol interferes with proper formation of collagen, in a dose-related manner, so alcohol-dependent patients may have a prolonged postoperative healing time.

Tobacco: Impaired healing and poorer clinical results to both nonsurgical and surgical periodontal therapy and implant placement are problems that smokers experience. Impaired wound healing may be due to vasoconstriction and increased platelet aggregation (decreased blood flow). Increased levels of carboxyhemoglobin, decreased oxygen transport, changes in vascular endothelium, and elevated level of tumor necrosis factor-alpha (TNF-a) in gingival crevicular fluid are seen in smokers.

Minimizing Substance Use-Related Stress and Vasoconstrictor Interactions

Methamphetamine (and Cocaine)
Patients who are high on methamphetamine should not receive any dental treatment for at least 6 hours after the last administration of the drug. Due to the sympathomimetic effects of methamphetamine, the risk for significant myocardial ischemia and cardiac dysrhythmias is a significant concern.

Local anesthetics with vasoconstrictor (epinephrine or levonordefrin) should not be used within 24 hours of having used either meth or cocaine because of the risk of a hypertensive crisis, cerebral vascular accident, or a myocardial infarction. The biological half-lives of methamphetamine and cocaine in particular are fairly short, but the 24-hour rule provides a margin of safety. Local anesthetic without vasoconstrictor is safe at any time.

Supporting Dental Patients in Recovery and Minimizing the Risk of Relapse

Substance use dependence is a relapsing disease, as are many other chronic illnesses. Relapse (resumption of substance use, whether it is a return to the drug of choice or the initiation of another psychoactive substance) is to be taken very seriously. Dental patients in recovery will disclose their drug/alcohol use history, discuss any pain management issues, and trust the dentist not to prescribe medications or mouth rinses that will expose them to a drug of abuse or trigger cravings.

To minimize the risk of relapse, the dentist should avoid the use of psychoactive drugs, narcotics, sedatives, anxiolytics, and alcohol-containing medications in patients who are recovering from SUDs. If a potentially mood-altering drug is required, the patient's primary care physician or treatment professional should be consulted. If approved for use, the drug should be prescribed only in the amount needed without refills. Designating a family member to fill and dispense the drug can also minimize relapse. Advising a patient in recovery to intensify his or her recovery program (e.g., going to additional meetings or increased sponsor contact) is appropriate while undergoing any surgical dental procedures.

Medical Emergencies

Methamphetamine Overdose

In a patient experiencing methamphetamine toxicity, immediate medical attention should be sought:

- Tachypnea precedes respiratory depression so the patient should receive 100% supplemental oxygen.
- Ventricular dysrhythmias may also develop, so blood pressure and heart rate should be monitored.
- The patient may exhibit an acute paranoid psychosis and may become violent.

Special Considerations
Opioid Drug-Seeking Behaviors

Most dentists will encounter a drug-seeking patient at some point in their career. Dentists have a professional responsibility to prescribe controlled substances appropriately, guarding against abuse while ensuring that patients have medication available when they need it. Dentists also have a personal responsibility to protect their practice from becoming an easy target for drug diversion. They must become aware of the potential situations where drug diversion can occur and safeguards that can be enacted to prevent this diversion.

Typical Scenarios for Drug-Seeking Patients:
- Purpose of the first dental visit is an emergency, or for pain relief, at the end of the day on the last workday of the week.
- Gives some reason why the patient cannot come in to the office.
- Health history lists allergies to analgesics or the patient claims ineffectiveness of some specific analgesic (especially non-narcotic analgesics), and the patient can "only" take some other specific narcotic—like oxycontin or dilaudid.
- Shows interest in what narcotics are kept in the office.
- Is unwilling to schedule a follow-up visit to have the painful dental condition treated and only wishes pain medication.
- Claims to have "lost" a prescription or to have "forgotten" medications and to need a prescription from a local dentist.
- Assertively pressures or attempts to manipulate the dentist—"I'd heard you were a good dentist, I don't understand why you won't help me."
- Story is very complex and presentation so obnoxious that a dentist is tempted to prescribe a medication to get the patient to "go away."
- May take extreme measures, including breaking or extracting one of their own teeth, in order to obtain drugs.

The U.S. Drug Enforcement Agency (DEA) offers practitioners a list of directives for dealing with suspected drug abusers.[22]

IV. Appendix

Tobacco Cessation: The Five A's Brief Intervention[23]

1. **ASK**—Systematically identify all tobacco users at every visit.

    Expand the database of the patient's vital signs to include the use of any form of tobacco.

    Vital Signs

    Blood Pressure: Pulse: Weight:
    _____   _____   _____
    Temperature: Respiratory Rate:
    _____   _____

    Tobacco Use: Current Former Never
    (Circle one)
    Type of Tobacco _____

    Alternatives to expanding the vital signs are to:
    - Place tobacco-use status stickers on all patient charts.
    - Indicate tobacco-use status using electronic medical records or computer reminder systems.

2. **ADVISE**—Strongly urge all tobacco users to quit.

    Advice should be:
    - Clear—"I think it is important for you to quit smoking now, and I can help you." "Cutting down while you are ill is not enough."
    - Strong—"As your clinician, I need you to know that quitting smoking is the most important thing you can do to protect your health now and in the future. The clinic staff and I will help you."
    - Personalized—Link tobacco use to current health/illness, and/or its social economic costs, motivation level/readiness to quit,

and/or the impact of tobacco use on children and others in the household.
3. **ASSESS**—Determine willingness to make a quit attempt.
Assess patient's willingness to quit:
- If the patient is willing to make a quit attempt at this time, provide assistance.
- If the patient will participate in an intensive treatment, deliver such a treatment or refer to an intensive intervention.
4. **ASSIST**—Aid the patient in quitting
Preparations for quitting:
- **Set a quit date**; ideally, the quit date should be within 2 weeks.
    Encourage patient to:
    a. Tell family, friends, and coworkers about quitting, and request understanding and support.
    b. Anticipate challenges (nicotine withdrawal) to a planned quit attempt, particularly during the critical first few weeks.
- Remove tobacco products from your environment. Prior to quitting, avoid smoking in places where you spend a lot of time (e.g., work, home, car).
- Avoid situational cues, such as alcohol consumption or socializing with active smokers, which may facilitate unplanned relapse.
- **Provide motivational literature.**
- Consider pharmacotherapy.
5. **ARRANGE**—Set a follow-up appointment to prevent relapse
- Contact patient 1–2 days prior to quit date.
- Contact 2 weeks after quit date.
- Follow up as needed.

V. Recommended Readings and Cited References

Recommended Readings

Mecklenberg RE, Christen AG, Gerber B, Gift MC. How to help your patients stop using tobacco: a National Cancer Institute manual for the oral health team 1990. US DHHS Public Health Service, National Institutes of Health, National Cancer Institute. NIH Publication No. 91-3191, 1991.

Mohammad AR. Clinician's Guide to Tobacco Cessation, 2nd ed. 2010. American Academy of Oral Medicine, Edmonds, WA.

National Cancer Institute. Tobacco and the clinician: interventions for medical and dental practice. Monogr Natl Cancer Inst 5, 1-22. NIH Publication No. 94-3693, 1994.

Rees TD Oral effects of drug abuse. Crit Rev Oral Biol Med 1992;3(3):163–84.

Cited References

1. ASAM Board of Directors, April 19, 2011. ASAM Website. Available at: http://www.asam.org/advocacy/find-a-policy-statement/view-policy-statement/public-policy-statements/2011/12/15/the-definition-of-addiction. Accessed March 14, 2012.
2. Morse RM, Flavin DK. The definition of alcoholism. The Joint Committee of the National Council on Alcoholism and Drug Dependence and the American Society of Addiction Medicine to Study the Definition and Criteria for the Diagnosis of Alcoholism. JAMA 1992;268(8):1012–14.
3. Nixon K, McClain JA. Adolescence as a critical window for developing an alcohol use disorder: current findings in neuroscience. Curr Opin Psychiatry 2010;23(3):227–32.
4. Büttner A. Review: the neuropathology of drug abuse. Neuropathol Appl Neurobiol 2011;37(2):118–34.
5. Saitz R. Clinical practice. Unhealthy alcohol use. N Engl J Med 2005;352(6):596–607.
6. Denisco RC, Kenna GA, O'Neil MG, Kulich RJ, Moore PA, Kane WT, et al. Prevention of prescription opioid abuse: role of the dentist. J Am Dent Assoc 2011;142(7):800–10.
7. Centers for Disease Control and Prevention. Vital signs: overdoses of prescription opioid pain relievers—United States, 1999–2008. MMWR 2011;60(43):1487–92.
8. National Institute on Drug Abuse. 2010. NIDA InfoFacts: heroin. Available at: http://www.nida.nih.gov/infofacts/heroin.html. Accessed November 13, 2011.
9. National Institute on Drug Abuse. 2010. NIDA InfoFacts: methamphetamine. Available at: http://drugabuse.gov/infofacts/methamphetamine.html. Accessed November 13, 2011.

10. Centers for Disease Control and Prevention. Vital signs: current cigarette smoking among adults aged ≥18 years—United States, 2005–2010. MMWR 2011;60(35):1207–12.
11. Clay RA. 2009. Screening, Brief Intervention, Referral, and Treatment (SBIRT). Available at: http://www.samhsa.gov/samhsanewsletter/Volume_17_number_6/SBIRT.aspx. Accessed November 13, 2011.
12. Jones LA. Systematic review of alcohol screening tools for use in the emergency department. Emerg Med J 2011;28(3):182–91.
13. Little SJ, Hollis JF, Fellows JL, Snyder JJ, Dickerson JF. Implementing a tobacco assisted referral program in dental practices. J Public Health Dent 2009;69(3):149–55.
14. Friedlander AH, Marder MD, Pisegna MD, Yagiela JA. Alcohol abuse and dependence—psychopathology, medical management and dental implications. J Am Dent Assoc 2003;134(6):731–40.
15. Dodrill CL, Helmer DA, Kosten TR. Prescription pain medication dependence. Am J Psychiatry 2011;168(5):466–71.
16. Hughes JR, Goldstein MG, Hurt RD, Shiffman S. Recent advances in the pharmacotherapy of smoking. JAMA 1999;28(1):72–6.
17. Fiore MC, Jaen CR, Baker TB, Bailey WC, Benowitz WC, Burry SJ, et al. Clinical Practice Guideline. Treating Tobacco Use and Dependence: 2008 Update. Rockville, MD: U.S. Department of Health and Human Services, Public Health Service, May 2008. Available at: http://www.surgeongeneral.gov/tobacco/treating_tobacco_use08.pdf. Accessed November 13, 2011.
18. Friedlander AH, Norman DC. Geriatric alcoholism: pathophysiology and dental implications. J Am Dent Assoc 2006;137(3):330–8.
19. Lindroth JE, Herren MC, Falace DA. The management of acute dental pain in the recovering alcoholic. Oral Surg Oral Med Oral Pathol Oral Radiol Endod 2003;95(4):432–6.
20. Peng PW, Tumber PS, Gourlay D. Review article: perioperative pain management of patients on methadone therapy. Can J Anaesth 2005;52(5):513–23.
21. Anantharaman D, Marron M, Lagiou P, Samoli E, Ahrens W, Pohlabeln H, et al. Population attributable risk of tobacco and alcohol for upper aerodigestive tract cancer. Oral Oncol 2011;47(8):725–31.
22. Drug Enforcement Agency. 1999; 1(1). Don't be scammed by a drug abuser. Available at: http://www.deadiversion.usdoj.gov/pubs/brochures/drugabuser.htm. Accessed November 13, 2011.
23. Fiore MC, Bailey WC, Cohen SJ, Dorfman SF, Goldstein MG, Gritz E, et al. Treating tobacco use and dependence. Quick Reference Guide for Clinicians. Rockville, MD: U.S. Department of Health and Human Services. Public Health Service. October 2000.

17

Developmental Defects of the Craniofacial Complex and Orthopedic Disorders

J. Timothy Wright DDS, MS
Michael Milano DMD
Luiz Andre Pimenta DDS, MS, PHD

I. Background

Dentists are confronted with diagnostic and treatment challenges for patients with hereditary conditions and unique environmental exposures. Developmental and hereditary disorders vary in their prevalence, morbidity, and need for unique oral health-care management approaches. Providing optimal oral health care is predicated on having a basic understanding of the patient's underlying systemic and craniofacial condition, their current and future risk for developing oral pathology, and having the skills to manage their oral health needs. Depending on complexity, this can involve a team of oral and medical health-care providers. This chapter reviews some of the more common hereditary conditions affecting the skin, teeth, and bones, and presents dental management approaches.

Description of Disease/Condition

Hereditary Conditions Affecting the Teeth

Thousands of genes are expressed during tooth formation, so it is not surprising that there are many diverse hereditary conditions known to affect teeth. The defects can manifest as changes in the number, shape, size, and/or composition of the teeth. These conditions are genetically and clinically diverse in their presentations and can occur as part of a syndrome or can be isolated to the teeth. Two of the better known hereditary conditions affecting the composition and structure of teeth are amelogenesis imperfecta (AI) and dentinogenesis imperfecta (DGI). These conditions can be challenging to diagnose and manage depending on the specific subtype and its manifestations.

The ADA Practical Guide to Patients with Medical Conditions, First Edition. Edited by Lauren L. Patton.
© 2012 American Dental Association. Published 2012 by John Wiley & Sons, Inc.

Amelogenesis Imperfecta (AI)

- Most commonly classified into three main categories based on the nature of the enamel defect.[1]
- Hypoplastic: thin enamel (see Fig. 17.1).
- Hypomineralized: hypocalcified or hypomaturation.

Dentinogenesis Imperfecta (DGI)

DGI and dentin dysplasia type II (DD-II) are the most common hereditary dentin disorders and have an autosomal dominant inheritance. DGI can occur in association with osteogenesis imperfecta (OI) (type DGI-I) or as an isolated defect of teeth (type DGI-II) (see Fig. 17.2).

Figure 17.1 Hypomaturation amelogenesis imperfecta in a young female.

Figure 17.2 Blue-gray coloration, enamel fracturing, and severe attrition associated with DGI-II.

Hereditary Conditions Affecting the Skin

Many hereditary conditions affect the development of the skin and/or the ectoderm and its appendages. Affected individuals can have increased fragility of the skin or have a lack of development of ectodermally derived appendages and thus can have altered tooth formation.

Ectodermal Dysplasias (EDs)

- Characterized by abnormal development of ectodermally derived tissues, such as skin, hair, nails, sweat glands, and dentition (see Fig. 17.3).
- The current definition of an ED is any condition having two or more affected tissues that are of ectodermal origin.

Epidermolysis Bullosa (EB)

- Represents a spectrum of conditions having blistering and mechanical fragility of the skin as their hallmark feature (see Fig. 17.4).
- Given the developmental and structural complexity of the skin, it is not surprising that there is tremendous genetic heterogene-

Figure 17.3 Conical-shaped incisors and hypodontia in an X-linked hypohidrotic ectodermal dysplasia (HED) affected 4-year-old male.

ity and marked phenotypic variation in the EB disorders.

Orofacial Clefts (OFCs)

OFCs are congenital malformations characterized by incomplete formation of structures involving the nasal and oral cavities: lip, alveolus, hard and soft palate. OFC may also vary in size, from a defect of the soft palate only to a complete cleft that extends through the bone of the hard palate. Because the lips and the palate develop separately, it is possible for a child to be born with a cleft lip (CL) only, cleft palate

> **Facial clefting variations**
> - Cleft lip (cheiloschisis, CL)
> - Cleft palate (palatoschisis, CP)
> - Cleft lip and palate (cheilopalatoschisis, CLP)
> - Submucous cleft palate (SCP)

(CP) only, or the combination of both cleft lip and palate (CLP) (see Fig. 17.5).

Defects of the Limbs and Skeleton

Amputation or "removal of a limb or other appendage of the body," may be related to a surgical procedure or a vascular disturbance. Congenital "amputations" or developmental limb abnormalities are the result of growth inhibition during intrauterine development and are very diverse in their etiology.

Spinal Cord Injuries: Spinal cord injuries can be due to flexion, extension, or compression injuries to the spine. The location of the trauma has a direct impact on the individual's functional deficit. Table 17.1 indicates the relationship between the level of the injury and the resulting functional deficit.

Figure 17.4 Blistering of the skin and oral mucosa in a patient with recessive dystrophic epidermolysis bullosa.

Figure 17.5 Frontal view of a newborn with unilateral complete cleft lip and palate (a); occlusal view of the cleft palate (b). (courtesy of Dr. Pedro Santiago—Director of Orthodontics and Craniofacial Orthodontist, Duke Cleft/Craniofacial Team)

Table 17.1. Clinical Features Related to Level of Spinal Cord Injury

Level of Spinal Cord Damage	Associated Clinical Features
C1 to C4	Death secondary to respiratory paralysis
C4 to C5	Quadriplegia
C5 to C6	Arms paralyzed except for abduction and flexion
C6 to C7	Paralysis of hands and wrists but not arms
T11 to T12	Paralysis of legs above and below the knee
T12 to L1	Paralysis of the leg below the knee
S3 to S5	Loss of bladder and bowel control

C, cervical; T, thoracic; L, lumbar; S, sacral.

Scoliosis: Scoliosis is a lateral curvature of the spine, often with some rotation of the vertebrae. It ranges from mild to severe, and the degree of curvature can worsen over time. There are many diverse etiologies of scoliosis with a high percentage of cases in children being idiopathic.[2]

Spina Bifida: Neural tube defects are birth defects of the brain and spinal cord that are diverse in their etiology and clinical manifestations. The most common neural tube defect is spina bifida (myelomeningocele) where the fetal spinal column fails to close completely during the first month of fetal life.

Physical manifestations of scoliosis
- Lumbar area fatigue following extended standing or sitting
- Muscular backaches
- One hip more prominent than the other
- One shoulder higher than the other

Pathogenesis/Etiology

Hereditary Conditions Affecting the Teeth

AI

There are seven genes known to cause AI, with several more likely to be identified in the near future and multiple phenotypes associated with allelic mutations in several of these genes. Collectively, the allelic and nonallelic AI-associated gene mutations result in many different AI types at the clinical and molecular levels. These genes all code for proteins that are important in enamel formation and mineralization.

Hereditary Dentin Disorders

- OI
  - Associated with variable bone fragility that ranges from very mild to lethal at birth.
  - Caused by mutations in the genes that code for type I collagen and other genes involved in bone development.
- DGI in association with OI (type DGI-I)
  - Associated with a marked decrease in dentin mineralization.
- DGI as an isolated defect of teeth (type DGI-II)
  - Caused by mutations in the dentin sialophosphoprotein, a gene that codes for proteins that are critical for normal dentin mineralization.
  - Associated with a marked decreased in dentin mineralization.

Hereditary Conditions Affecting the Skin

EDs

There are many genes (over 50) known to cause ED, and many more will be discovered in the near future. Inheritance patterns include autosomal dominant, autosomal recessive, as well as the most frequently reported type, X-linked. If the mutated gene is critical for early oral epithelium events during tooth formation, such as invagination and proliferation of the oral epithelium, the result is likely to be missing teeth or hypodontia.

EB

The most recent classification of EB identifies four major EB groupings (Table 17.2) and over 30 EB subtypes.[3] The four major EB groups include intraepidermal EB (simplex), junctional EB, dermolytic EB (dystrophic), and mixed EB (Kindler syndrome).

EB is caused by mutations in at least 14 genes.[4] The causative genes for many of the EB subtypes code for proteins that are important in cell integrity, cell-to-cell adhesion and attaching the dermis and epidermis. Depending on the specific EB type, genetic mutation and thus missing or abnormal protein, there can be significant morbidity involving the soft and hard tissues of the craniofacial complex.

For example, Type VII collagen is critical for maintaining the integrity of the oral mucosa and skin. Consequently, individuals with Type VII collagen mutations (*dystrophic EB*) often have severely affected oral soft tissues that blister with minimal manipulation and frequently heal with scarring. Type VII collagen is not essential for normal tooth bud development so individuals with dystrophic EB typically have a normally developed dentition.

In contrast, laminin 332 is highly expressed during tooth development so individuals with mutations that affect laminin 332 function (*junctional EB*) have defects in the enamel of their teeth with generalized enamel hypoplasia. Individuals with recessive dystrophic and junctional EB are at increased risk for developing dental caries due to alterations in the soft tissue that make eating difficult and prolonged and home care difficult. The enamel defects in junctional EB produce additional risk for the development of dental caries.[5]

OFCs

OFC is a defect of formation of the frontonasal process that gives rise to the nose, superior lip, maxilla, and primary palate, or is a defect of the fusion of the frontonasal process with the two maxillary processes. The pathogenesis of CL and CP is complex; the most widely accepted model is multifactorial inheritance, with interaction of genetic and environmental factors.[6] Craniofacial defects such as CL and CP can occur as an isolated condition, or may be one component of an inherited disease or syndrome.

Defects of the Limbs and Skeleton

Amputation: Dysvascular amputations associated with diabetes account for the majority of amputations, more commonly affecting the lower extremities.[7] This type of amputation has increased over the past several decades as the prevalence of diabetes has risen. Limb defects in newborns are highly variable in their etiology and manifestations of affecting digits and long bones.[8] Vascular defects account for a high percentage of congenital limb defects.

Spinal Cord Injuries: The etiology of spinal cord injuries is diverse with trauma (automobile accidents, falls, and injury in sports activities or military service) being the most prevalent causes. Nontraumatic causes include arthritis, cancer, infections, or disk degeneration of the spine.

Scoliosis: Scoliosis can be divided into various categories based on etiology (congenital, paralytic, or idiopathic) or degree of curvature (functional or structural).[9]

Spina Bifida: This spinal defect is most commonly located in the lumbar, lower thoracic,

Table 17.2. Epidermolysis Bullosa Phenotypes and Treatment

Condition	Clinical Phenotype	Oral Manifestations	Treatment
Simplex	Severity varies but in most cases blistering is confined to hands and feet. There are severe simplex subtypes (i.e., dowling mera).	Slight increase in oral fragility. Teeth are normal and caries risk normal.	Typically, treatment is the same as for unaffected people. Appropriate oral disease prevention, sealants, bonding.
Junctional	Severity of blistering varies but can have extensive lesions on face and in perioral region. Can have significant scarring. Digits typically not fused.	Most will have increased fragility of intraoral soft tissues. All have enamel hypoplasia. Can have some microstomia due to perioral lesions.	Aggressive prevention and optimal use of fluorides/sealants can help control caries risk. Injections should be deep and slow to reduce risk of blister formation. No soft tissue shear force.
Dominant dystrophic	Tissue separation occurs in the dermis. Can have severe skin involvement with moderate–severe increase in tissue fragility. Lesions often heal with scarring. Oral opening relatively normal.	Mucosal fragility is increased and can develop lesions with minor soft-tissue manipulation. Teeth are typically normal. Caries risk is slightly increased.	Be cautious with soft tissue manipulation as can cause blisters and ulcerations. Optimize oral disease prevention. Typically treated in outpatient setting similar to unaffected patients.
Recessive dystrophic	Tissue separation in the dermis with typical severe skin involvement with marked tissue fragility. Can have severe scarring with digit fusion. Can have esophageal strictures, alopecia, and other manifestations.	Microstomia, vestibular obliteration, ankyloglossia, and loss of lingual papillae are all typical. Severe dental caries is common. Often develop periodontal disease if teeth retained. Mucosa is very fragile and oral ulcers are almost always present.	Aggressive prevention using optimal fluoride exposure (e.g., water, varnish, dentifrice, rinse). Restorative treatment: *primary–mixed dentition*: stainless steel crowns in posterior, resin, or resin-faced crowns in anterior; *permanent dentition*: stainless steel/cast/ceramic crowns in posterior teeth and resin or ceramic esthetic crowns in anterior.
Kindler syndrome	Skin blistering at birth, photosensitivity, and atrophy of skin, skin fragility.	Fragile oral mucosa, gingivitis and predilection to developing periodontitis, normal dentition.	Monitor periodontal status, periodontal maintenance therapy as needed, and rigorous caries prevention program.

or sacral regions and can involve up to six vertebral segments. Spina bifida has a multifactorial etiology with both environmental and genetic components. Maternal supplementation with folic acid during early pregnancy has helped reduce the frequency of this common developmental defect.[10]

Epidemiology

Hereditary Conditions Affecting the Teeth

AI

The AI conditions occur from about 1/700 to 1/15,000 depending on the population. It is believed that the prevalence in the United States is about 1:6000-8000.[11]

Hereditary Dentin Disorders

The prevalence of DGI-I is not known, although it is thought to occur in 30–50% of people with OI. DGI-III occurs in 1/8000 people in the United States.[11] The incidence of DGI-I is 1/100,000.[12]

Hereditary Conditions Affecting the Skin

EDs

The hypohidrotic or ED types associated with diminished sweat gland formation are the most common.

EB

The EB conditions are all rare with the milder forms (simplex) being more common than the severe forms.

OFCs

OFCs are among the most common and treatable birth defects in the United States.

Average prevalence of cleft lip and palate and number of births affected by these defects each year United States, 1999–2001

	Prevalence*	Annual Number of Cases
Cleft palate only	6.39	2567
Cleft lip with or without cleft palate	10.48	4209

* Prevalence per 10,000 live births.
Source: The Centers for Diseases Control and Prevention (CDC) National Birth Defects Prevention Network (NBDPN). 1999 to 2001 cleft lip and palate data collected from 11 states (Alabama, Arkansas, California, Georgia, Hawaii, Iowa, Massachusetts, North Carolina, Oklahoma, Texas, and Utah), adjusted for race-specific distribution of US live births.

Nonsyndromic OFC is the most common congenital malformation affecting on average of about 1/500–750 live newborns annually worldwide.[13] CL with or without CP is the second most common condition in the United States, with an adjusted prevalence of 10.63/10,000 live births or 1/940 live births.[14] The incidence of CL, with or without CP, varies among different ethnic populations and is presumed to be higher in developing countries. African-Americans have a lower prevalence rate compared with Caucasians.[14] Risk factors that have been identified with CP include maternal behavior (including alcohol and tobacco use); nutrition, and multiple environmental exposures.[15]

Defects of the Limbs and Skeleton

Amputation: The prevalence of dysvascular amputations increases with the diabetic population age.[7] Limb defects in newborns have a prevalence of about 0.8/1000 births.[8]

Spinal Cord Injuries: Overall males are more often afflicted than females. The prevalence is about 50/100,000 with cervical injury being the most common.[16]

Scoliosis: The U.S. adult prevalence of scoliosis is estimated at 8.3%, with women having twice the prevalence (10.7%) compared with men (5.6%).[17]

Spina Bifida: While it is reported that the worldwide incidence of all neural tube defects is thought to range from 1.0 to 10.0/1000 live births, spina bifida is one of the most common birth defects in the United States with a reported prevalence rate of 3.0–7.8/10,000 live births.[18]

Coordination of Care between Dentist and Physician

Treatment of patients with OFC or other craniofacial anomalies is widely regarded as a multi-interdisciplinary enterprise from prenatal and family counseling through adulthood. Patients with other hereditary conditions of skin and bone may require consultation between dentist and physician to safely provide care to allow maintenance of the dentition. Referral to a physician for genetic testing may benefit patients with suspected hereditary conditions of the teeth and skin that may be first recognized in the dental office based on tooth appearance.

Treatment of OFC patients may involve craniofacial or cleft teams and centers, sometimes working in coordination with private practitioners. These centers provide a coordinated, multidisciplinary approach generally including experienced and qualified physicians and health-care professionals from different specialties, such as surgical (plastic and maxillofacial surgeons), ear, nose, and throat specialists; pediatric and general dentists; orthodontists; prosthodontists; speech therapists; psychologists; social workers; and allied health disciplines. Teams have become the standard in assessment and treatment of children with craniofacial anomalies like OFC.[19] The role of dentistry in treating individuals with cleft and craniofacial anomalies is to provide comprehensive preventative and therapeutic oral health care.

II. Medical Management

Identification/Medical History/ Physical Examination/ Laboratory Testing

Hereditary Conditions Affecting the Teeth

AI

Genetic diagnosis is commercially available for several of the genes known to cause AI, thereby helping to confirm the diagnosis.

Hereditary Dentin Disorders

Several different tests are used to diagnose OI including evaluation of collagen formation by skin fibroblasts and gene sequencing. DGI-II is diagnosed clinically and can now be confirmed by gene sequencing.

Hereditary Conditions Affecting the Skin

EB

Most individuals are diagnosed by their dermatologist using skin biopsies or in consultation with medical geneticists in the natal or neonatal period. Genetic testing can now be used to confirm most EB types.

EDs

Diagnosis is based on initial recognition of the predominant clinical features, which may be first noted in the medical or dental office.

OFCs

Molecular testing is available to confirm the diagnosis of many specific ED types.

Prenatal diagnosis can be performed at 13–14 weeks of gestation, when the soft tissues of the fetal face will be clearly visualized sonographically. Ideally, coronal view and axial planes are optimal for visualization of the fetal lip and palate in ultrasound images.[20] Three-dimensional ultrasound[21] and magnetic resonance imaging[22] can also provide a clear image of the malformation and may enhance detection of isolated CP. Prenatal diagnosis of CLP is a reality today, and in cases of labial clefts detected during the prenatal period, parent's psychological aspects can be discussed before the birth of the child. Not only technical preparation regarding the birth, but also a moral and social preparation of the family and friends for the reception of a different child can be arranged, so the child with a malformation is accepted earlier.[23] In CP, the inability to separate the naso-oropharyngeal cavities results in feeding difficulties, speech unintelligibility, and maxillary growth abnormalities.[24]

Defects of the Limbs and Skeleton

Spinal Cord Injuries: The symptoms of the injury can include loss of limb function, bladder control, and even impaired respiration, depending on the height and extent of the injury.

Scoliosis: Scoliosis can be divided based on age of onset. Age of onset is related to future complications and the types of medical interventions that might be implicated for long-term management. Scoliosis can be found in association with a large number of medical conditions or syndromes.

Spina Bifida: Spina bifida can be diagnosed prenatally via amniocentesis. It is divided into two main forms: myelomeningocele and oculta (no external lesion):

- *Myelomeningocele (or open form)* is the most common and the more severe form.[10] In this form, there is not only incomplete fusion of the spine but also a protrusion of the spinal cord through this defective area.
  - This spinal defect can result in varying degrees of paralysis of the legs, anesthesia of the skin below the lesion, and can impact bladder and rectal function.[25]
  - Hydrocephalus occurs in over 80% of the cases of myelomeningocele.[25]
- *Spina bifida oculta* is often asymptomatic since even though the vertebrae may not be

---

Characteristics of early versus late onset scoliosis

Early Onset	Late Onset
• Presents before 5 years of age	• Presents after 5 years of age
• Uncommon	• Most common type
• Often resolves spontaneously	• Requires some form of intervention for resolution
• Can distort the chest resulting in interference with pulmonary function	• Results in deformity only

Conditions seen in association with scoliosis

- Cerebral palsy
- Duchene muscular dystrophy
- Spina bifida
- Rett syndrome
- Kabuki syndrome
- Goldenhar syndrome
- Neonatal Marfan syndrome
- Pseudo-achondroplasia
- VATER Association

> **Secondary conditions often associated with spina bifida**
>
> - Bladder and bowel incontinence
> - Mobility issues
> - Self-esteem issues
> - Pressure ulcers
> - Latex allergies
> - Respiratory problems

fully formed, there is no displacement of the spinal cord or the meninges.[10] The oculta form often is not diagnosed during the prenatal period and the impact it has on an individual is far less devastating than the open form.

Medical Treatment

Hereditary Conditions Affecting the Teeth

DGI-I patients will frequently be under treatment for OI. Management of individuals with OI will depend on the specific types and severity of the condition. Severely affected individuals must be handled with extreme caution due to their bone fragility to avoid causing iatrogenic fractures. Most individuals severely affected with OI are being treated with intravenous (IV) bisphosphonates.[26]

Hereditary Conditions Affecting the Skin

EDs

ED treatment is focused on the different abnormalities of ectodermal derivatives that are affected. For example, wigs for severe alopecia, topical emollients for dry skin and scalp care, hydration and air-conditioning for those lacking sweating capacity to thermoregulate, artificial tears and saline nasal spray, and antibiotics for infections in those with immune deficiencies.

EB

EB treatments focus on wound care with promise for newer therapies such as stem-cell transplants and administration of allogeneic fibroblasts or recombinant protein.[4] Treatment of EB acquisita may involve conventional immunosuppressive therapy, anti-inflammatory agents, biologics, extracorporeal photochemotherapy, and plasmapheresis.[27]

OFCs

Multidisciplinary management of OFC patients occurs in stages as the patient ages. Typically five to seven surgeries are required sequentially, extending into adolescence.

Newborn

- Feeding instructions, counseling, diagnosis by a geneticist, and a pediatric consultation.
- Hearing tests and assessment of the cleft.
- In case of wide clefts, lip taping can start immediately.[28]
- Surgical repair by 18 months in a normally developing infant.[29]
  - Surgical repair too early risks possible interference with normal craniofacial growth.
  - Surgical repair too late risks velopharyngeal insufficiency and speech delay.[30]
- Consideration of presurgical infant orthopedics (i.e., nasal alveolar molding or NAM) when appropriate. The conventional NAM protocol involves an orthodontic appliance covering the palate, worn from age 2 weeks to 6 months to assist alignment and approximation of the alveolar segments, repositioning deformed nasal cartilages, effective retraction of the protruded premaxilla, and lengthening of the deficient columella. This facilitates later surgical soft-tissue repair under minimal tension, with optimal condi-

Figure 17.6 Frontal view of a newborn with unilateral complete cleft lip and cleft palate (a); NAM appliance in place (b); child after NAM procedure with the cleft width reduced (c); postsurgery (d). *Courtesy of Dr. Pedro Santiago—Director of Orthodontics and Craniofacial Orthodontist, Duke Cleft/Craniofacial Team.*

tions for minimal scar formation and increased nose symmetry, thus reducing total number of surgeries and improving outcome[31] (see Fig. 17.6). During the NAM procedure, the family also meets with the counseling and feeding team. Lip surgery is usually performed between 3 and 6 months postnatally depending on the cleft severity. Palatal closure is performed at 12–14 months, prior to speech development.

Toddlers and Preschool Children

OFC toddlers and children often experience issues with feeding, swallowing, esthetics, and also poor oral health.[32,33]

School-Aged Children

Between age 9 and 12 years, secondary alveolar bone grafts are required to repair the CLP bony deficiency in the tooth-bearing alveolar region of the palate to provide adequate periodontal and bony support in which the canine can erupt.[34] Other surgical procedures are also used to improve velopharyngeal function, to improve speech development during this time period. If surgery is delayed, a prosthetic device can be fabricated to help with speech.

Adolescents

Adolescents have to deal with natural developmental changes and special concerns of integrating their facial differences into an already changing body image; establishing heterosexual relationships despite possible dissatisfaction with facial appearance; relating to medical staff as young adults rather than children; and coping with surgeries that may alter their facial appearance, but probably will not eliminate facial scarring.

Adults

Adult patients may have unrepaired OFCs or incompletely surgically corrected large clefts with residual oronasal fistulas and bone discontinuity defects in the alveolus, even though the primary cleft soft tissue defect may have been repaired. The severity of residual deformities of the repaired CL and nose may contribute to functional (mainly speech) and esthetic concerns.

Common sequelae of past cleft repair surgeries include:

- anterior and posterior crossbites;
- midface hypoplasia;
- anteroposterior, vertical, and transverse maxillary deficiency;
- residual lip and nasal deformities;
- speech problems.

Defects of the Limbs and Skeleton

Scoliosis: Medical treatment modalities for scoliosis fall into three main categories:
- Physiotherapy
  - Used in conjunction with orthosis to help control the negative effects associated with prolonged corset use.[35]
- Orthosis (orthopedic appliance or device used to support, align, prevent, or correct deformities or enhance movement)[9]
  - The use of casts, braces, or corsets has been a standard part of the treatment of scoliosis for decades. Although various types of braces exist, some can have a significant effect on dentofacial growth. For example, the Milwaukee brace can have a significant adverse impact on both maxillary and mandibular growth including flared incisors, alveolar bone resorption, and growth inhibition of the temporomandibular joint.[36]
  - It has been recognized that wearing a cast or brace can have a negative impact on a child or teenagers' self-image that must be weighed against continued spinal curvature that can eventually result in respiratory deterioration.
- Surgery
  - The final treatment modality is surgical intervention. Spinal fusion via the insertion of rods is considered if the curvature progresses. These fusions have been demonstrated to remain stable for decades.

Spina Bifida: The open spina bifida defect is surgically closed in utero or after birth, but closure surgery does not correct the lumbar and sacral area defect and restore normal function to the affected part of the spinal cord. Accompanying hydrocephalus is often treated by placing a ventriculoperitoneal (VP) shunt. Early placement of a VP shunt (which diverts cerebral spinal fluid) can aid in the functional recovery of a pediatric spina bifida patient.

III. Dental Management

Evaluation

Medical history can inform the dentist as to disorder-specific concerns and possible modifications that would support maintenance of oral health.

Key questions to ask the patient

With a hereditary condition affecting the teeth or skin
- If DGI-I patient with osteogenesis imperfecta: Are you receiving or have you ever received intravenous bisphosphonates?
- With mucosal fragility of EB: How have dental care procedures been most successful for you in the past?

With an orofacial cleft
- Is your care being coordinated by a Craniofacial Team? Who is the team contact person?
- Has your speech therapist recommended a prosthesis or speech aid appliance?

With defects of the limbs and skeleton
- If missing lower extremity: May we help you transfer to the dental chair or do you think this will not be possible?
- If missing upper extremity/digits: How has your brushing and flossing been going? Let's suggest some additional techniques.
- Scoliosis with brace: How long are you planned for wearing your brace?
- Spina bifida: Are you allergic to latex?

Key questions to ask the physician

For the patient with a hereditary condition affecting the teeth or skin
- If DGI-I: Is the patient on IV bisphosphonate therapy?

For the patient with an orofacial cleft
- From the Cleft Team coordinator: Who are the Cleft Team providers and what is the team's care plan for the patient? Where is the patient in planning surgeries for cleft repair? What general dental care needs are anticipated that I can help with for the patient?
- Does the patient require a speech aide appliance?

For the patient with a defect of the limbs and skeleton
- If the patient has a VP shunt: Do you recommend antibiotics prior to dental procedures?

Dental Treatment Modifications

Hereditary Conditions Affecting the Teeth

AI

Preventive and restorative treatment of the dentition in cases of AI will depend on the AI type and the severity of these manifestations (see Table 17.3). There is an increased prevalence of Class III and open-bite malocclusions that may require orthodontic and/or orthognathic surgery to correct. There can be strong self-image and quality of life issues associated with AI, and these should be considered when developing timing and approaches for treatment.

Hereditary Dentin Disorders

Dental treatment for DGI-I and DGI-II is essentially the same with treatment being largely focused on maintaining teeth if there is enamel loss and associated attrition and dealing with esthetics due to tooth discoloration and attrition (see Table 17.3).

Table 17.3. Amelogenesis Imperfecta and Dentinogenesis Imperfecta Phenotypes and Treatment

Condition	Clinical Phenotype	Radiographic Phenotype	Treatment
Amelogenesis imperfecta: hypoplastic	Color is normal to yellow with stains in pits. Enamel—thin, pitted, or grooved. Sensitivity usually not severe.	Enamel—thin, pitted, or not radiographically visible. Contrast to dentin often is normal.	Sealants, bonding, consider crowns if severe enamel hypoplasia and dental sensitivity.
Amelogenesis imperfecta: hypomineralized	Color varies: orange to yellow-brown. Enamel fracturing is common. Sensitivity—often severe. Calculus formation—often extensive.	Enamel—contrast to dentin may be minimal. Crown morphology in unerupted teeth appears normal. Often have cervical remnants or wings of enamel retained at cervical area.	*Primary—mixed dentition*: stainless steel crowns in posterior, resin, or resin-faced crowns in anterior. *Permanent dentition*: stainless steel/cast/ceramic crowns in posterior teeth and resin or ceramic esthetic crowns in anterior.
Dentinogenesis imperfecta	Color is blue-gray to yellow-brown. Enamel typically normal but can be hypoplasia and it frequently fractures leading to severe attrition. Crowns can be normal to small.	Dentin has reduced radiographic contrast. Can have marked cervical constriction, short pointed roots, pulp chamber obliteration.	If no enamel loss and wear then treatment is focused on esthetics. If enamel fracturing then: *primary—mixed dentition*: stainless steel crowns in posterior, resin, or resin-faced crowns in anterior; *permanent dentition*: stainless steel/cast/ceramic crowns in posterior teeth and resin or ceramic esthetic crowns in anterior.

Hereditary Conditions Affecting the Skin

EDs

Dental treatment for ED patients varies markedly depending on the clinical manifestations (see Table 17.4). Some ED conditions are associated with clefting and limb anomalies that can markedly influence the types and timing of oral health care that may be necessary. Affected individuals often will be missing or have malformed primary and permanent teeth requiring long-term treatment with short-term and long-term goals. Treatment goals are to optimize function and esthetics and thereby allow for the individuals optimal psychosocial development.

EB

Dental treatment of individuals with EB depends on the types of soft- and hard-tissue manifestations present. With extensive caries and severe soft-tissue involvement, such as in recessive dystrophic EB that has extreme tissue fragility, restorative and surgical care may be best provided with the use of general anesthesia. Special

Table 17.4. Ectodermal Dysplasia (ED) Phenotypes and Treatments

ED Type	Clinical Phenotype	Radiographic Phenotype	Treatment
Hypohidrotic	Sparse fine hair, missing teeth, lack of normal sweating, can have hyperthermia, and unexplained fevers	Multiple missing teeth, conical-shaped incisors, taurodont molars	*Infant*: age 1 year dental visit—diagnosis and anticipatory guidance. *Childhood*: bonding of conical-shaped teeth, prosthesis placement. *Adolescent-adult*: consider definite treatment of hypodontia with prostheses/implants.
Ectrodactyly-ectodermal dysplasia-clefting syndrome	Sparse hair, missing/malformed teeth, split hand/foot, cleft lip/palate	Hypodontia, malformed teeth, microdontia	*Infant*: age 1 year dental visit—diagnosis and anticipatory guidance, cleft management initiated, and continued through adolescence as needed. *Childhood*: bonding, crowns, extraction microdont/malformed teeth as needed, prosthesis placement. *Adolescent-adult*: consider definite treatment of hypodontia with prostheses/implants.
Focal dermal hypoplasia	Abnormal eye development, facial asymmetry, sparse hair, enamel hypoplasia, missing/malformed teeth, can include cleft lip/palate	Hypodontia, enamel hypoplasia, dental malformations such as talon cusps, malposition of the teeth	*Infant*: age 1 year dental visit—diagnosis and anticipatory guidance. *Childhood*: bonding/stainless steel crowns as needed on malformed teeth, prosthesis placement. *Adolescent-adult*: consider definite treatment of hypodontia with prostheses/implants.

protocols to protect the skin and reduce soft-tissue trauma have been developed and must be used to safely and effectively manage these patients. Individuals with extensive caries and/or generalized enamel hypoplasia will often be best treated using stainless steel crowns in the primary and young permanent dentitions.

OFCs

Newborn

During this time, a pediatric dentist should provide parental information and support; develop a strategy for caries prevention, growth, and development monitoring.

Toddlers and Preschool Children

During this period, it is important to inform parents and/or guardians of the importance of establishing a dental home when the first primary tooth erupts in the mouth or within the first year of age.[37]

- Preventative strategies: oral hygiene instructions, diet counseling and application of fluoride varnish.
- Evaluate water source (well or city water) for fluoride exposure.
- Fluoridated toothpaste should be used with amount limited to a grain of rice-sized smear, for caries prevention without increasing risk of dental fluorosis.[38]
- Frequency of sugar-based food intake should be limited to reduce the risk of dental caries. Until 6 years of age, sweet milk (such as chocolate milk), sodas, and juices should be limited to no more than 4 oz per day, at main meals, with their teeth cleaned afterward.

School-Aged Children

- Continued anticipatory guidance and preventative care.
- Surgical and restorative care as needed. Children with clefts are at a significant risk for caries of the primary incisors.[39]
- Despite the presence of clefts, the teeth adjacent to the cleft generally present good periodontal bone support during the stage of mixed dentition.[40]
- After surgery, canines in the cleft area will present normal root development in most cases with spontaneous eruption through autogenous bone grafting. Oftentimes, canines erupt more slowly through the bone graft and, in some cases, can require surgical and orthodontic intervention (exposure and bonding) to complete eruption.
- Buccal and mesiodistal orthodontic movement as well as rotational movements of maxillary anterior teeth before alveolar bone grafting should be avoided or carefully conducted in these patients.[41]
- Speech appliances can be fabricated to help with speech for children at least 5 years of age. These appliances are placed in the mouth like an orthodontic retainer. Parents should closely supervise the use of these appliances. There are two basic types of speech appliances for children:
  - *Speech Bulb:* For patients with short palate, the speech bulb can partially close off the space between the soft palate and the throat[42] (see Fig. 17.7).
  - *Palatal Lift:* In cases of inadequate muscle function, despite appropriate palatal length, a palatal lift appliance serves to lift the soft palate to a position that makes palatal closure possible.

Adolescents/Adults

- Most receive orthodontic treatment for alignment of their teeth, correction of the occlusion, and in preparation for orthognathic surgery (corrective jaw surgery) at skeletal maturity, if necessary.
- In patients with bilateral CLP, the premaxilla projects itself up and forward in various degrees because it is separated from the maxillary processes, which can be collapsed. The teeth adjacent to the cleft can present a

Figure 17.7 V-shaped cleft of the hard and soft palate (a); speech appliance with an acrylic velar section (b); appliance in place, note the speech bulb as an obturator (c); frontal view of the appliance, like an orthodontic retainer (d).

deficiency in the alveolar bone thickness and height, restricting the possibilities of orthodontic treatment.

- Orthognathic surgery is used to treat patients with CLP who have a large skeletal Class III malocclusion with variable degree of anteroposterior, vertical, and transverse maxillary growth deficiency. End-stage reconstruction should be considered at skeletal maturity, which is usually age 15 years for females and 16–18 years for males.[43] If surgery is performed prior to completion of facial growth, the adverse effect on maxillary growth, and the continued growth of the mandible will likely result in recurrence of the facial deformity and malocclusion. For esthetic and psychosocial reasons, surgery can be done at an earlier age with the understanding that it may need to be repeated after the growth is complete.
- Prevention and management of dental caries and gingival inflammation remain important.
- In some cases, esthetic modifications of anterior teeth with resin composite direct restorations are needed (see Fig. 17.8).
- If implant-supported prosthetic rehabilitation is planned, the patient will usually require a regraft of the cleft area. Complexity of the implant procedures in cleft spaces suggests referral to a specialist for implant placement and final oral rehabilitation.

Figure 17.8 A 15-year-old patient with unilateral left cleft lip and palate finishing orthodontic treatment, missing tooth #10 (a); lingual view of anterior teeth, teeth #8 and #9, with caries on mesial surfaces (b); tooth preparation and gingival cord packed prior to resin composite restoration (c); final aspect of resin composite restorations with canine transformation on tooth #11 (d).

Prosthetic Considerations in Oral–Facial Cleft Patients

Removable prostheses may be needed for speech appliances, for oronasal fistula closure, and when clefts were not surgically closed. Adult patients who did not receive proper treatment for CP are challenging for clinicians in terms of prosthetic habilitation. When patients become edentulous, prosthetic reconstruction becomes even more challenging.[44]

Adult patients who did not receive proper treatment for OFC often have several disorders:

- immature and collapsed maxillary arch,
- dysphagia,
- hypernasal speech,
- compromised chewing ability,
- palate with scar tissue,
- resorbed alveolar ridges,
- loss of vestibular depth,
- oronasal fistulas.

Management of the cleft after grafting involves either eruption of the canine in substitution for the missing tooth or tooth replacement using prosthetic means. Prosthetic methods include removable prosthesis, a fixed dental prosthesis, or a single-tooth dental implant. A variety of prosthetic appliances can be used to manage cleft patients and are listed in Table 17.5. Using

Table 17.5. Removable Prosthetic Appliances for Managing Oral–Facial Clefts

Appliance	Indication	Description
Palatal and palatopharyngeal obturator	Residual oronasal communication or fistula or palatopharyngeal insufficiency	Palatal obturator covers the fistula; palatopharyngeal obturator provides velopharyngeal closure; both appliances help reduce hypernasality and improve speech
Palatal lift appliance	Velopharyngeal incompetence where soft palate has appropriate length but inadequate innervation	Designed to elevate the soft palate and provide mechanical impedance of air from entering the nasal cavity
Tooth born fixed dental prostheses	Replace missing and/or malformed teeth	Constructed to replace missing teeth and can be conventional or resin bonded
Endosseous implant-based prostheses	Replace single or multiple missing or malformed teeth	May be single or multiple implants used depending on the number of teeth involved and relationship to cleft

Figure 17.9 A 65-year-old patient with unrepaired cleft palate and root caries on several teeth. (a); frontal view of the metal frame for a removable partial prosthesis (b); velar extension of the metal frame for a palatal obturator (c); final aspect of upper partial removable prosthesis with the palatal bulb (obturator) (d); adaptation of the acrylic bulb with the soft palate (e); final aspect of the full mouth rehabilitation with upper and lower partial removable prostheses (f).

appropriately designed appliances in conjunction with optimal, orthodontic, periodontal, surgical repairs, and bone-grafting patients with craniofacial and oral clefts can be treated effectively to provide excellent esthetics and function (see Fig. 17.9).

Defects of the Limbs and Skeleton

Amputations: Number and degree of limb involvement dictates the specific changes necessary in delivering oral health care.

Modifications include the following:
- Providing adequate handicapped access to the dental office.
- Proper positioning during dental care.
- Establishing home care routines that are compatible with the individual's limb involvement.
- If the patient must remain in the wheelchair, the dental team will need to modify how they deliver care based on the individual circumstances.
- For patients lacking lower extremities, transfer from the wheelchair to the dental chair should be performed with caution. Steps for a wheelchair transfer are outlined in Table 17.6 and shown in Fig. 14.6.
- For patients lacking upper extremities, modifications will center on manual dexterity and ability to participate in home care. If one arm remains functional, practice may result in the patient acquiring enough skill to achieve acceptable home care. See Fig. 18.3 for toothbrush modifications that may be useful for patients with missing digits.
- When a prosthetic arm has been placed, modifications on an individualized basis are needed. Children adapt better when prosthetics are placed early so they become part of the patient's development.

Spinal Cord Injuries: Because of the variation in functional limitation, modifications for dental treatment are equally variable. Table 17.7 indicates some common problems associated with spinal cord injuries that may need to be addressed by the dental team.

Scoliosis: Modifications for the delivery of dental treatment should focus on the following:
- Awareness of associated medical conditions or syndromes, which may require modifications.
- Periodic need to change positions in order to find the most comfortable position in the dental chair (especially with casts or braces). Finding the best position may be further complicated if any level of respiratory compromise has occurred.

Table 17.6. Steps for a Wheelchair to Dental Chair Transfer

1. Determine how much assistance the patient will require.
2. Move (or remove) any parts of the dental chair that might interfere with the transfer. Examples include the arm rest and foot controls.
3. Place the dental chair and wheelchair at approximately the same height. Move the wheelchair next to the dental chair and lock it in place.
4. Remove the wheelchair's arm and foot rests.
5. Perform the two-person transfer as illustrated in Fig. 14.6.
6. Position the patient in the dental chair and allow the patient to find a comfortable position (assist the patient as much as needed during this process).

Table 17.7. Modifications in Patients with Spinal Cord Injuries

Complication	Modification
Postural hypotension	Dental treatment in the supine position.
Paraplegia	See Table 17.6 and Fig. 14.6 for wheelchair transfers.
Quadriplegia	Assistance with home care required. Use general anesthesia with caution due to the risk of respiratory infections.
Possible use of long-term steroid therapy	Consult with physician regarding dosage modification prior to treatment.

- Monitoring of facial growth and development among brace wearers and if abnormal, consultation with the orthopedist and treatment or referral to an orthodontist.

Spina Bifida: There are multiple issues that will require modifications:
- Latex hypersensitivity (reported in up to 65% of children with spina bifida), related to the increased frequency of exposure to latex products secondary to medical procedures, including surgical management.[25,45] The possibility of latex hypersensitivity necessitates that no latex products be used at any time during the patient's treatment.
- Some degree of paralysis is likely. The patient may need assistance with mobility (the use of braces or a wheelchair).
- Additional medical conditions may require modifications ranging from using extra care when transferring to the dental chair, the patient who is catheterized and has a urinary collection device in place, to the use of antibiotic prophylaxis in those patients with a VP shunt. Antibiotic prophylaxis is typically not recommended for patients with VP shunts for hydrocephalus when undergoing dental procedures; however, the neurosurgeon may elect to have antibiotics given in patients with frequently infected shunts.[46]

Oral Manifestations

Hereditary Conditions Affecting the Teeth

Hereditary Dentin Disorders

- In *DGI* and *DD-II*, primary teeth range from yellow-brown to blue-gray and can be quite dark.
  - Underlying affected dentin shines through the translucent enamel giving the teeth an "opalescent" appearance.
  - The poorly mineralized dentin provides inadequate support for the rigid enamel layer.
  - If the enamel fractures and exposes underlying dentin, the dentin tends to be brown in appearance and then undergoes rapid attrition due to the low mineral content of the dentin.
- The permanent teeth in DGI-I (with OI) and DD-II are typically markedly less affected compared with the primary teeth, while DGI-II (without OI) permanent teeth can be severely affected similar to the primary teeth.

Hereditary Conditions Affecting Skin

EDs

The oral manifestations can be the first notable clinical manifestations:

- abnormalities in the number of teeth present,
- conical-shaped incisors,
- a lack of normal tooth development in infants.

EB

Soft tissue manifestations can include:

- microstomia,
- ankyloglossia,
- vestibular obliteration,
- increased risk for developing squamous cell carcinoma.

OFCs

- Alveolar clefts are frequently associated with missing teeth.[47]
- Dental anomalies, such as variations in tooth number and position, and reduced tooth dimensions, predominantly localized in the area of the cleft defect are common.[48] Children with OFC have a higher prevalence

of enamel discoloration compared with unaffected children.[49]

⚠️ Risks of Dental Care

Hemostasis

None.

Susceptibility to Infection

EB: Patients on immunosuppressants may require physician consultation regarding need for antibiotic premedication.

Spina Bifida: Patients with a VP shunt may require physician consultation regarding need for antibiotic premedication.

Drug Actions/Interactions

DGI-I Patients with OI: Although no cases of bone osteonecrosis have been reported in bisphosphonate-treated OI patients, there may be an increased risk for this potential complication from surgical procedures.

Patient's Ability to Tolerate Dental Care

DGI-I Patients with OI: Care is required in handling patients with bone fragility.

EB: There are significant risks of oral mucosal trauma.

Scoliosis: Patients may require positioning supports in the dental chair.

IV. Recommended Readings and Cited References

Recommended Reading

American Cleft Palate-Craniofacial Association Educational Resources. Available at: http://www.acpa-cpf.org/education/educational_resources/professional_enhancement_resources/slp_other_resources/.

Cited References

1. Wright JT, Torain M, Long K, Seow K, Crawford P, Aldred MJ, et al. Amelogenesis imperfecta: genotype-phenotype studies in 71 families. Cells Tissues Organs 2011;194(2–4):279–83.
2. Wang WJ, Yeung HY, Chu WC, Tang NL, Lee KM, Qiu Y, et al. Top theories for the etiopathogenesis of adolescent idiopathic scoliosis. J Pediatr Orthop 2011;31(1 Suppl.):S14–27.
3. Intong LR, Murrell DF. Inherited epidermolysis bullosa: new diagnostic criteria and classification. Clin Dermatol 2012;30(1):70–7.
4. Fine JD. Inherited epidermolysis bullosa: recent basic and clinical advances. Curr Opin Pediatr 2010;22(4):453–8.
5. Wright JT, Fine JD, Johnson L. Dental caries risk in hereditary epidermolysis bullosa. Pediatr Dent 1994;16(6):427–32.
6. Mangold E, Ludwig KU, Nothen MM. Breakthroughs in the genetics of orofacial clefting. Trends Mol Med 2011;17(12):725–33.
7. Dillingham TR, Pezzin LE, MacKenzie EJ. Limb amputation and limb deficiency: epidemiology and recent trends in the United States. South Med J 2002;95(8):875–83.
8. Gold NB, Westgate MN, Holmes LB. Anatomic and etiological classification of congenital limb deficiencies. Am J Med Genet A 2011;155A(6):1225–35.
9. Larson AN, Fletcher ND, Daniel C, Richards BS. Lumbar curve is stable after selective thoracic fusion for adolescent idiopathic scoliosis: a 20-year follow-up. Spine (Phila Pa 1976) 2011.
10. Venkataramana NK. Spinal dysraphism. J Pediatr Neurosci 2011;6(Suppl. 1):S31–40.
11. Witkop CJ Jr. Amelogenesis imperfecta, dentinogenesis imperfecta and dentin dysplasia revisited: problems in classification. J Oral Pathol 1988;17(9–10):547–53.
12. Barron MJ, McDonnell ST, MacKie I, Dixon MJ. Hereditary dentine disorders: dentinogenesis imperfecta and dentine dysplasia. Orphanet J Rare Dis 2008;3:31. doi:10.1186/1750-1172-3-31.
13. Walker SJ, Ball RH, Babcook CJ, Feldkamp MM. Prevalence of aneuploidy and additional ana-

tomic abnormalities in fetuses and neonates with cleft lip with or without cleft palate: a population-based study in Utah. J Ultrasound Med 2001; 20(11):1175–80, quiz 81-2.
14. Parker SE, Mai CT, Canfield MA, Rickard R, Wang Y, Meyer RE, et al. Updated National Birth Prevalence estimates for selected birth defects in the United States, 2004–2006. Birth Defects Res A Clin Mol Teratol 2010;88(12):1008–16.
15. Jia ZL, Shi B, Chen CH, Shi JY, Wu J, Xu X. Maternal malnutrition, environmental exposure during pregnancy and the risk of non-syndromic orofacial clefts. Oral Dis 2011;17(6):584–9.
16. Knutsdottir S, Thorisdottir H, Sigvaldason K, Jonsson H Jr., Bjornsson A, Ingvarsson P. Epidemiology of traumatic spinal cord injuries in Iceland from 1975 to 2009. Spinal Cord 2011.
17. Carter OD, Haynes SG. Prevalence rates for scoliosis in US adults: results from the first National Health and Nutrition Examination Survey. Int J Epidemiol 1987;16(4):537–44.
18. Liptak GS, El Samra A. Optimizing health care for children with spina bifida. Dev Disabil Res Rev 2010;16(1):66–75.
19. Grosse SD, Schechter MS, Kulkarni R, Lloyd-Puryear MA, Strickland B, Trevathan E. Models of comprehensive multidisciplinary care for individuals in the United States with genetic disorders. Pediatrics 2009;123(1):407–12.
20. Sommerlad M, Patel N, Vijayalakshmi B, Morris P, Hall P, Ahmad T, et al. Detection of lip, alveolar ridge and hard palate abnormalities using two-dimensional ultrasound enhanced with the three-dimensional reverse-face view. UltrasoundObstet Gynecol 2010;36(5):596–600.
21. Platt LD, Devore GR, Pretorius DH. Improving cleft palate/cleft lip antenatal diagnosis by 3-dimensional sonography: the "flipped face" view. J Ultrasound Med 2006;25(11):1423–30.
22. Mailath-Pokorny M, Worda C, Krampl-Bettelheim E, Watzinger F, Brugger PC, Prayer D. What does magnetic resonance imaging add to the prenatal ultrasound diagnosis of facial clefts? Ultrasound Obstet Gynecol 2010;36(4): 445–51.
23. Descamps MJ, Golding SJ, Sibley J, McIntyre A, Alvey C, Goodacre T. MRI for definitive in utero diagnosis of cleft palate: a useful adjunct to antenatal care? Cleft Palate Craniofac J 2010;47(6): 578–85.
24. Liau JY, Sadove AM, van Aalst JA. An evidence-based approach to cleft palate repair. Plast Reconstr Surg 2010;126(6):2216–21.
25. Northrup H, Volcik KA. Spina bifida and other neural tube defects. Curr Probl Pediatr 2000; 30(10):313–32.
26. Borromeo GL, Tsao CE, Darby IB, Ebeling PR. A review of the clinical implications of bisphosphonates in dentistry. Aust Dent J 2011;56(1):2–9.
27. Gürcan HM, Ahmed AR. Current concepts in the treatment of epidermolysis bullosa acquisita. Expert Opin Pharmacother 2011;12(8):1259–68.
28. Cassell CH, Daniels J, Meyer RE. Timeliness of primary cleft lip/palate surgery. Cleft Palate Craniofac J 2009;46(6):588–97.
29. Parameters for evaluation and treatment of patients with cleft lip/palate or other craniofacial anomalies. American Cleft Palate-Craniofacial Association. March, 1993. Cleft Palate Craniofac J 1993;30(Suppl.):S1–16.
30. Sullivan SR, Marrinan EM, LaBrie RA, Rogers GF, Mulliken JB. Palatoplasty outcomes in nonsyndromic patients with cleft palate: a 29-year assessment of one surgeon's experience. J Craniofac Surg 2009;20(Suppl. 1):612–6.
31. Ezzat CF, Chavarria C, Teichgraeber JF, Chen JW, Stratmann RG, Gateno J, et al. Presurgical nasoalveolar molding therapy for the treatment of unilateral cleft lip and palate: a preliminary study. Cleft Palate Craniofac J 2007;44(1):8–12.
32. Parapanisiou V, Gizani S, Makou M, Papagiannoulis L. Oral health status and behaviour of Greek patients with cleft lip and palate. Eur Arch Paediatr Dent 2009;10(2):85–9.
33. Miller CK. Feeding issues and interventions in infants and children with clefts and craniofacial syndromes. Semin Speech Lang 2011;32(2): 115–26.
34. Russell KA, McLeod CE. Canine eruption in patients with complete cleft lip and palate. Cleft Palate Craniofac J 2008;45(1):73–80.
35. Kotwicki T, Durmala J, Czaprowski D, Glowacki M, Kolban M, Snela S, et al. Conservative management of idiopathic scoliosis—guidelines based on SOSORT 2006 consensus. Ortop Traumatol Rehabil 2009;11(5):379–95.
36. Persky SL, Johnston LE. An evaluation of dentofacial changes accompanying scoliosis therapy with a modified Milwaukee brace. Am J Orthod 1974;65(4):364–71.

37. American Academy of Pediatric Dentistry reference manual 2010–2011. Pediatr Dent 2010;32(6 Reference Manual):1–334.
38. Richards D. Risk-benefit of fluoride toothpaste. Evid Based Dent 2010;11(1):2.
39. Johnsen DC, Dixon M. Dental caries of primary incisors in children with cleft lip and palate. Cleft Palate J 1984;21(2):104–9.
40. Lilja J. Alveolar bone grafting. Indian J Plast Surg 2009;42(Suppl.):S110–5.
41. Garib DG, Yatabe MS, Ozawa TO, Da Silva Filho OG. Alveolar bone morphology in patients with bilateral complete cleft lip and palate in the mixed dentition: CBCT evaluation. Cleft Palate Craniofac J 2012;49(2):208–14.
42. Dosumu OO, Ogunrinde TJ, Ogundipe OT. Prosthetic management of soft palate cleft—a case report. Afr J Med Med Sci 2006;35(3):391–3.
43. David DJ, Smith I, Nugent M, Richards C, Anderson PJ. From birth to maturity: a group of patients who have completed their protocol management. Part III. Bilateral cleft lip-cleft palate. Plast Reconstr Surg 2011;128(2):475–84.
44. Guven O, Gurbuz A, Baltali E, Yilmaz B, Hatipoglu M. Surgical and prosthetic rehabilitation of edentulous adult cleft palate patients by dental implants. J Craniofac Surg 2010;21(5):1538–41.
45. Agarwal S, Gawkrodger DJ. Latex allergy: a health care problem of epidemic proportions. Eur J Dermatol 2002;12(4):311–5.
46. Acs G, Cozzi E. Antibiotic prophylaxis for patients with hydrocephalus shunts: a survey of pediatric dentistry and neurosurgery program directors. Pediatr Dent 1992;14(4):246–50.
47. Aizenbud D, Camasuvi S, Peled M, Brin I. Congenitally missing teeth in the Israeli cleft population. Cleft Palate Craniofac J 2005;42(3):314–7.
48. Ribeiro LL, Das Neves LT, Costa B, Gomide MR. Dental development of permanent lateral incisor in complete unilateral cleft lip and palate. Cleft Palate Craniofac J 2002;39(2):193–6.
49. Lucas VS, Gupta R, Ololade O, Gelbier M, Roberts GJ. Dental health indices and caries associated microflora in children with unilateral cleft lip and palate. Cleft Palate Craniofac J 2000;37(5):447–52.

Geriatric Health and Functional Issues

Janet A. Yellowitz DMD, MPH

I. Background

Aging is a natural consequence of life and involves anatomical, biochemical, and physiological alterations in every system. These changes present with a high degree of heterogeneity, which challenge health-care providers to differentiate signs of normal aging from disease. Common age-related changes and age-related disorders of vision, hearing, mobility, and cognition will be discussed in this chapter. These health concerns often cause disability and vulnerability, and impact one's quality of life. Age-related visual and hearing impairments decrease one's ability to complete their activities of daily living (ADLs) and communicate with others, and can lead to isolation and depression.[1]

Description of Disease/Condition

Age-Related Visual Changes

The most common causes of vision impairment that lead to blindness are age-related macular degeneration (AMD), glaucoma, cataract, and diabetic retinopathy.

Presbyopia is the loss of visual acuity due to a progressive change in the optic compartment. Presbyopia presents with difficulties in the ability to focus at close range, read small print, see well in dim lighting, and differentiate colors. It is not a disease. Most with presbyopia do not become completely blind, but experience partial/moderate loss of vision and may need to develop new skills to remain self-reliant.

Cataract is a clouding or opacity of the lens of the eye that can range from a small, localized area to a diffuse loss of transparency. Most are related to aging. By age 80, >50% of Americans have a cataract or have had cataract surgery. The most common symptoms include cloudy or blurry vision, colors seem faded, glare from headlights and sunlight, poor night vision, double vision, or multiple images in one eye. See Fig. 18.1.

AMD is due to the abnormal vascularization under the retina, which causes progressive damage to the macula, the central part of the retina that allows fine details to be visible.[2]

The ADA Practical Guide to Patients with Medical Conditions, First Edition. Edited by Lauren L. Patton.
© 2012 American Dental Association. Published 2012 by John Wiley & Sons, Inc.

Figure 18.1 (a) Normal vision. (b) The same scene as viewed by a person with cataract. From the National Eye Institute, NIH, USDHHS. *Facts about Cataract.* September 2009. Adapted from *Don't Lose Sight of Cataract* (NIH Publication No. 94-3463) and *Cataract: What You Should Know* (NIH Publication No. 03-201). Available at: http://www.nei.nih.gov/health/cataract/cataract_facts.asp.

AMD leads to loss of central vision, which is needed for reading, driving, recognizing faces, and remaining independent. Peripheral vision is usually retained.

- Two forms:
  - Dry (atrophic) AMD accounting for 90% of cases.
  - Wet (neovascular/exudate) AMD is a more severe form, causing acute pain.

Glaucoma comprises a group of disorders characterized by optic nerve damage and visual field loss. It is chronic, progressive, and degenerative, usually occurs insidiously and is asymptomatic in early stages. Vision loss is caused by a progressive loss of optic nerve fibers. If not treated, it can cause irreversible blindness.[3] Those with glaucoma may have elevated intraocular pressure.[4]

- Two main types:
  - Open-angle (chronic) glaucoma—90% of cases
    - Characterized by a clinical triad:
      (1) elevated intraocular pressure;
      (2) development of optic nerve atrophy; and
      (3) loss of peripheral field of vision.[3]
  - Angle-closure (acute) glaucoma—10% of all cases
    - Causes a quick, severe, and painful rise in intraocular pressure.
    - Treatment must occur quickly as there is an increased risk of involvement of the second eye.

Diabetic retinopathy is a vascular complication of diabetes caused by poor blood glucose control. Diabetic retinopathy-related eye changes include micro-aneurysms, hemorrhages, hard and soft exudates, proliferation of newly formed vessels, retinal detachment, and the development of secondary glaucoma.[5] Early treatment can prevent blindness.

Age-Related Hearing Loss

Age-related hearing loss or presbycusis is a progressive sensorineural hearing loss that may involve both peripheral reduction in hearing threshold sensitivity and impairment of central processing. It is usually symmetric, though may have significant variation between ears. Age-related hearing loss often goes undetected and untreated, and has caused some with hearing loss to be wrongly labeled as "confused," "nonresponsive," or "uncooperative."

Hearing-impaired older adults may withdraw from social situations to avoid frustration and embarrassment, increasing their risk of social isolation, depression, and declining physical functioning—ultimately decreasing their quality of life.[6]

Mobility Limitations

Osteoarthritis (OA) or *degenerative joint disease* is a progressive pathological change of the hyaline cartilage and underlying bone of a joint, and is the most common type of arthritis. Joints most commonly affected are knees, hips, hands (Heberden's nodes are a visible sign, see Fig. 18.2), and spine. It is not caused simply by wear and tear. Presence of OA in weight-bearing joints has the greatest clinical impact. Disease onset is gradual and usually begins after the age of 40.

Cognitive Impairment/Dementias

The Role of Cognition in Older Adults

As people age, they are at an increased risk of having cognitive and memory problems, or cognitive aging. The cognitive functions most affected by age are attention and memory; however, age-related changes are not uniform across all cognitive domains[7] or across individuals. There is enormous variability in cognitive decline seen in older adults. Memory loss is not inevitable as people have lived to extreme old age without severe memory loss.[8]

The lack of cognitive health can have profound implications for a person's health and well being. Limitations in one's ability to manage medications, medical conditions, or to live safely are of particular concern when a person is experiencing a cognitive impairment. Poor cognitive health leads to increased vulnerability to disease, injury, malnutrition, crime, abuse, and eventually a loss of independence.

Cognitive declines range from mild cognitive impairment (MCI) to Alzheimer's disease (AD) and other dementias. Studies of brain abnormalities have recognized that AD, Lewy body disease, Huntington's disease, frontotemporal dementia, amyotrophic lateral sclerosis, Parkinson's disease, and Creutzfeldt–Jakob disease have similar clinical symptoms, including memory loss, movement problems, and sleep–wake disorders. Memory impairment can also be the result of cerebrovascular disease, hydrocephalus, hypothyroidism, vitamin B_{12} deficiency, central nervous system infection, a cognitive disorder related to human immunodeficiency virus infection, adverse effects of prescribed medications, substance abuse, and cancer.[9] See also Chapter 14 "Neurological Disorders."

Cognitive impairments adversely affect the person with the disease and their family, caregivers, and friends. Obtaining an early diagnosis of a cognitive impairment can make a significant difference in the lives of patients and their families; however, it is relatively rare that a cognitive disorder is diagnosed early in the course of the disease.[10]

Mild Cognitive Impairment (MCI)

MCI is a syndrome of having a cognitive decline greater than expected for an individual's age and education level that does not interfere notably with ADLs. MCI does not meet the criteria for dementia. MCI criteria include a

Figure 18.2 Heberden's nodes in osteoarthritic hand.

cognitive impairment, essentially normal functional activities, abnormal memory function for age and education (1–2 standard deviations), and absence of dementia.[11]

MCI is a risk state for AD, with the rate of conversion ranging from 10% to 15% per year, due to differences in assessment procedures, sample composition, and definition of cases. Early identification of MCI can lead to secondary prevention by controlling risk factors.[12]

There are two primary types of MCI:

1. *Amnestic MCI:* Presents with significant memory loss.
   - Has a high risk of progression to dementia particularly that of an Alzheimer's type;[13] averages 12% per year.
   - Neuropathology is typical of AD.
2. *Non-Amnestic MCI:* Memory is not impaired.
   - May be associated with cerebrovascular disease, frontotemporal dementias, or have no specific pathology.
   - Does not progress to AD.

Dementia

Dementia is a syndrome characterized by progressive deterioration in multiple cognitive domains, severe enough to interfere with daily functioning. Dementia is the umbrella term used to describe cognitive impairment.

- It affects one's memory, understanding and use of words, ability to identify objects, and ability to comprehend and act on messages.
- It is a principal cause of disability and institutionalization of older adults.
- Later stage present with total dependence on others.

Alzheimer's Disease (AD)

AD is a progressive, degenerative, neurological disorder that manifests by loss of intellectual functions, including memory, language, visuospatial skills, behavioral changes, problem-solving ability, and abstract reasoning.[14]

Early-onset AD, a rare disease inherited in an autosomal dominant pattern, occurs between 30 and 50 years of age. Late-onset AD typically affects those ≥65 years. AD is the most common type (60–80%) of dementia in the United States.

- Clinical hallmarks are progressive impairment in memory, judgment, decision making, orientation to physical surroundings, and language.

Disease onset is insidious; manifestations evolve over a period of years from mildly impaired to severe cognitive loss. Progression of the disease is inevitable and may include plateaus of 1–2 years.[9] Table 18.1 describes the seven stages of Alzheimer's.

Pathogenesis/Etiology

Age-Related Visual Changes

Age-related eye changes include the following:

- Retina: Colors appear less bright with contrast between colors less noticeable. Blue, black, and green colors appear faded and difficult to differentiate.
- Decreased visual field, around 1–3 degrees per decade of life; individuals 70–80 years have lost between 20 and 30 degrees of peripheral vision.
- Pupil gets smaller and pupil dilation decreases with age, resulting in less light reaching the retina.
- Ocular muscles weaken, with pupil and decreased elasticity of lens causing a delay in dark adaptation from bright areas, and may contribute to night vision problems.[15]
- Cornea and pupil are less responsive, resulting in the need for more light to see clearly.
- Lens yellows and becomes less clear, so light is scattered, which reduces color vision and contrast sensitivity.
- Lens hardens, which leads to decreased ability to accommodate.

Table 18.1. Seven Stages of Alzheimer's

Stage 1: *No impairment (normal function)*
The person does not experience any memory problems. An interview with a medical professional does not show any evidence of symptoms of dementia.

Stage 2: *Very mild cognitive decline (may be normal age-related changes or earliest signs of Alzheimer's disease)*
The person may feel as if he or she is having memory lapses—forgetting familiar words or the location of everyday objects. But no symptoms of dementia can be detected during a medical examination or by friends, family, or coworkers.

Stage 3: *Mild cognitive decline (early-stage Alzheimer's can be diagnosed in some, but not all, individuals with these symptoms)*
Friends, family, or coworkers begin to notice difficulties. During a detailed medical interview, doctors may be able to detect problems in memory or concentration. Common stage 3 difficulties include:
- Noticeable problems coming up with the right word or name
- Trouble remembering names when introduced to new people
- Having noticeably greater difficulty performing tasks in social or work settings
- Forgetting material that one has just read
- Losing or misplacing a valuable object
- Increasing trouble with planning or organizing

Stage 4: *Moderate cognitive decline (mild or early-stage Alzheimer's disease)*
At this point, a careful medical interview should be able to detect clear-cut symptoms in several areas:
- Forgetfulness of recent events
- Impaired ability to perform challenging mental arithmetic—for example, counting backward from 100 by 7's
- Greater difficulty performing complex tasks, such as planning dinner for guests, paying bills, or managing finances
- Forgetfulness about one's own personal history
- Becoming moody or withdrawn, especially in socially or mentally challenging situations

Stage 5: *Moderately severe cognitive decline (moderate or mid-stage Alzheimer's disease)*
Gaps in memory and thinking are noticeable, and individuals begin to need help with day-to-day activities. At this stage, those with Alzheimer's may:
- Be unable to recall their own address or telephone number or the high school or college from which they graduated
- Become confused about where they are or what day it is
- Have trouble with less challenging mental arithmetic; such as counting backward from 40 by subtracting 4's or from 20 by 2's
- Need help choosing proper clothing for the season or the occasion
- Still remember significant details about themselves and their family
- Still require no assistance with eating or using the toilet

(Continued)

Table 18.1. (Continued)

Stage 6:	*Severe cognitive decline (moderately severe or mid-stage Alzheimer's disease)* Memory continues to worsen, personality changes may take place, and individuals need extensive help with daily activities. At this stage, individuals may: • Lose awareness of recent experiences as well as of their surroundings • Remember their own name but have difficulty with their personal history • Distinguish familiar and unfamiliar faces but have trouble remembering the name of a spouse or caregiver • Need help dressing properly and may, without supervision, make mistakes such as putting pajamas over daytime clothes or shoes on the wrong feet • Experience major changes in sleep patterns—sleeping during the day and becoming restless at night • Need help handling details of toileting (e.g., flushing the toilet, wiping or disposing of tissue properly) • Have increasingly frequent trouble controlling their bladder or bowels • Experience major personality and behavioral changes, including suspiciousness and delusions (such as believing that their caregiver is an impostor) or compulsive, repetitive behavior like hand-wringing or tissue shredding • Tend to wander or become lost
Stage 7:	*Very severe cognitive decline (severe or late-stage Alzheimer's disease)* In the final stage of this disease, individuals lose the ability to respond to their environment, to carry on a conversation and, eventually, to control movement. They may still say words or phrases. At this stage, individuals need help with much of their daily personal care, including eating or using the toilet. They may also lose the ability to smile, to sit without support, and to hold their heads up. Reflexes become abnormal. Muscles grow rigid. Swallowing impaired.

It is difficult to place a person with Alzheimer's in a specific stage as stages may overlap.
Permission granted: "Alzheimer's Association 2011. All rights reserved."

  ○ Those ≥80 years need three to six times more light for comfortable reading than those in their twenties.

Cataract is an age-related condition.

AMD: Etiology is unknown.

- *Dry AMD:* Light-sensitive cells in macula break down causing distorted and blurred central vision with blind spots in advanced cases.
  ○ May precipitate the development of wet AMD.
- *Wet AMD:* A result of abnormal blood vessels growing under the retina and leaking blood and fluid and damaging the macula.

Glaucoma

- *Open Angle:* Unknown etiology.
- *Angle Closure:* Occurs when the aqueous humor fluid is blocked.

Diabetic retinopathy: Vision loss occurs through retinal detachment, vitreous hemorrhage, neovascular glaucoma, and macular edema or capillary nonperfusion.[5]

Age-Related Hearing Loss

- Results from peripheral cochlear defects and a defect in central auditory processing, but etiology is unknown. May be due to degenerative structural changes in the inner ear, genetic factors, or exposure to loud noises over a long period of time.
- Usually occurs slowly, affecting hearing of high tones (1000–8000 Hz range); thus, male voices are easier to hear than female voices.

Mobility Limitations

OA: Unknown etiology; classified as idiopathic and secondary (traumatic, congenital, or due to other causes).

Cognitive Impairment/ Dementias

MCI: Unknown etiology; likely multifactorial.

Dementia: Unknown etiology.

AD: Unknown etiology.

Epidemiology

Age-Related Visual Changes

- Occurs after age 40, considered almost universal for those ≥65 years.
- *Prevalence:* When asked "Do you have trouble seeing, even when wearing glasses or contact lenses?"; 25.6% of persons ≥65 years reported having trouble seeing.[16]
- Prevalence increases as age increases: 14.3% of those 65–74 years, 18.6% of 75–84 years, and 28.4% of people ≥85 years.[1]
- *Gender:* Compared with males ≥65 years (14.9%), females ≥65 years (19.4%) were more likely visually impaired.
- *Ethnicity:* Non-Hispanic blacks and Mexican-American older adults have a higher prevalence of vision impairment than non-Hispanic whites.[1]

Cataract

- *Prevalence:* 20.5 million (17.2%) Americans >40 years had a cataract in 2000; expected to rise to 30.1 million in 2020.[17] Prevalence increases with age: 2.5% of people aged 40–49 years, 20% of 60- to 69-year-olds, and 68% ≥80-year-olds.[17]
- *Risk factors:* Aging; secondary to diabetes mellitus, smoking, metabolic or nutritional disorders, medications, ultraviolet radiation, inflammation, and radiation.[18]
- *Gender:* Females had a higher prevalence among blacks and whites; white males had a higher prevalence than black males.[16]

AMD

- *Prevalence:* 1.75 million adults ≥40 years have AMD. Prevalence increases from 10% of those 66–74 years to 30% in those 75–85 years of age. It is expected to increase to 3 million adults in 2020.[2]
- *Race:* More prevalent among whites than blacks.[19]
- *Risk factors:* Advancing age, family history, hypertension, tobacco use, and high dietary fat.[20]

Glaucoma

- Prevalence increases with age; 1.57 million whites and 398,000 blacks ≥40 years had glaucoma in 2000; will likely increase to 3 million in 2020.[3]
- *Risk factors:*
  - Open-angle glaucoma: Family history, increasing age, high degree of myopia, hypertension, and diabetes.
  - Angle-closure glaucoma: More common in women, elderly, Asians, and those with a history of glaucoma or hyperopia.[3]
- *Race/ethnicity:* Blacks are three times more likely to have it than whites.

Diabetic Retinopathy

- *Prevalence:* 28.5% among persons with diabetes ≥40 years.

- Prevalence increases with amount of time a person has diabetes. Of those with diabetes, there is no significant difference in prevalence between age 40 and 65 years. Without regard for diabetes status, prevalence is higher for those ≥65 years.[21]
- *Gender*: Of those with diabetes, retinopathy is more prevalent among males than females.
- *Risk factors*: Being male, higher levels of HbA1c, longer diabetes duration, use of insulin, and higher systolic blood pressure.[21]

Age-Related Hearing Loss

- *Prevalence*: Around 20% of the U.S. population ≥65 years; 34.8% of persons ≥65 years reported having hearing loss.[16]
- *Prevalence increases as age increases*: 36% of adults aged 65–74 years; 43.7% of 75- to 84-year-olds; 66.7% of ≥85-year-olds.[16]
- Around 70% of older adults with hearing loss in at least one ear could potentially benefit from using a hearing aid, but do not use one.[16]
- *Gender*: 41.5% of males and 29.6% of females ≥65 years had trouble hearing.[16]
- *Risk factors*: Family history, repeated exposure to loud noises, trauma, certain medications, and smoking.

Mobility Limitations
OA

- *Prevalence*: 14% of adults ≥25 years, 34% of ≥65-year-olds; affects almost all adults to some degree by age 80.
- *Gender*: Before age 55, occurs equally in both genders; after age 55, it is more common in women.
- *Risk factors*: Primarily aging and may include mechanical and molecular changes in the joint; single or repeated injury, abnormal motion, metabolic disorders, joint infection, and obesity.

Cognitive Impairment/Dementias
MCI

- *Prevalence*: Ranges from 3% to 19% in adults ≥65 years old.[12]
- *Prevalence increases with age*: 10% in adults 70–79 years old to 25% in 80- to 89-year-olds.[23]
- *Risk factors*: Older age, diabetes, stroke, obesity, and the presence of the ApoE4 gene variant (linked to AD).

Dementia

- *Prevalence*: Around 1.5% for those aged 60–69 years to 40% for ≥90-year-olds. Rate almost doubles every 5 years.[22]
- *Risk factors*: Old age and genetic susceptibility.
- Other risk factors include: Midlife hypertension, obesity, diabetes mellitus, heart disease, cerebrovascular disease, hyperlipidemia, excessive alcohol consumption, cigarette smoking, dietary/nutritional factors, and inflammation.[9]

AD

- *Prevalence*: 5.3 million in the United States.
  - Around 13% of adults ≥65 years old; 16 million are expected to have AD by 2050.[25]
  - As age increases, prevalence increases: 30–50% of those age ≥85 years are diagnosed with AD. Formal studies of prevalence vary greatly.
- *Risk factors*: Family history.[23] Early-onset dementia has a very strong genetic association. For late-onset AD, first-degree relatives have approximately twice the expected lifetime risk.[9]
- *Gender*: Women are more affected 2:1 compared with men.

Coordination of Care between Dentist and Physician

Alert physician to ongoing oral health concerns for individuals with cognitive impairments.

II. Medical Management

Identification/Medical History/ Physical Examination/ Laboratory Testing

Age-Related Visual Changes

Age-related visual changes include the loss of ability to see fine details, focus at close range, see well in dim light, and to differentiate colors. Adults need annual eye examinations to identify and address age-related changes and disease.

Cataract symptoms include blurred or hazy vision, reduced intensity of colors, increased sensitivity to glare, and increased difficulty seeing at night.

AMD leads to the loss of central vision.

Glaucoma has no discernable symptoms until the optic nerve is damaged and peripheral vision is lost.

Age-Related Hearing Loss

In *age-related hearing loss*, a self-report of hearing difficulty or a need for hearing aids may be made. Examination by an audiologist is recommended when early signs are detected.

Mobility Limitations

OA

- Symptoms include pain, joint stiffness, swelling, and loss of function.
- Radiological findings include joint space narrowing, osteophytes, and/or bony sclerosis.
- Early diagnosis and treatment is recommended to reduce symptoms.

Cognitive Impairment/ Dementias

AD

Clinical presentation:

- Cognitive changes of AD tend to follow a somewhat characteristic pattern, beginning with memory impairment and spreading to language and visuospatial deficits. The cardinal feature is a progressive loss of memory of recent events/experiences.
- An inability to retain recently acquired information is typically an initial symptom. Memory for remote events is spared until later in the disease process.[9] Other changes include a decline in the ability to learn new information, perform routine tasks, and remain oriented in time and space. Difficulty with language, abstract reasoning, and executive function or decision making occurs as the disease progresses. Changes in mood and affect are common, as is the loss of communication skills, becoming incontinent, being disinhibited, unable to care for themselves, having speech and swallowing difficulties, and being at an increased risk for aspiration pneumonia (See Table 18.2.).[9]
- Prognosis: Disease can last 2–20 years.

Medical Treatment
Age-Related Visual Changes

Presbyopia may be corrected with glasses or contact lenses; there is no cure.

Cataracts

Surgery is readily available, effective, safe, and covered by Medicare. Over 90% of patients undergoing cataract surgery experience visual improvement and improved quality of life if there is no ocular comorbidity. There is no treatment to prevent or slow the progression of cataracts.

Table 18.2. Ten Signs of Alzheimer's

1. Memory loss that disrupts daily life
One of the most common signs of Alzheimer's is memory loss, especially forgetting recently learned information. Others include forgetting important dates or events; asking for the same information over and over; relying on memory aides (e.g., reminder notes or electronic devices) or family members for things they used to handle on their own. *What's a typical age-related change? Sometimes forgetting names or appointments, but remembering them later.*

2. Challenges in planning or solving problems
Some people may experience changes in their ability to develop and follow a plan or work with numbers. They may have trouble following a familiar recipe or keeping track of monthly bills. They may have difficulty concentrating and take much longer to do things than they did before. *What's a typical age-related change? Making occasional errors when balancing a checkbook.*

3. Difficulty completing familiar tasks at home, at work, or at leisure
People with Alzheimer's often find it hard to complete daily tasks. Sometimes, people may have trouble driving to a familiar location, managing a budget at work or remembering the rules of a favorite game. *What's a typical age-related change? Occasionally needing help to use the settings on a microwave or to record a television show.*

4. Confusion with time or place
People with Alzheimer's can lose track of dates, seasons, and the passage of time. They may have trouble understanding something if it is not happening immediately. Sometimes they may forget where they are or how they got there. *What's a typical age-related change? Getting confused about the day of the week but figuring it out later.*

5. Trouble understanding visual images and spatial relationships
For some people, having vision problems is a sign of Alzheimer's. They may have difficulty reading, judging distance, and determining color or contrast. In terms of perception, they may pass a mirror and think someone else is in the room. They may not realize they are the person in the mirror. *What's a typical age-related change? Vision changes related to cataracts.*

6. New problems with words in speaking or writing
People with Alzheimer's may have trouble following or joining a conversation. They may stop in the middle of a conversation and have no idea how to continue or they may repeat themselves. They may struggle with vocabulary, have problems finding the right word, or call things by the wrong name (e.g., calling a "watch" a "hand-clock"). *What's a typical age-related change? Sometimes having trouble finding the right word.*

7. Misplacing things and losing the ability to retrace steps
A person with Alzheimer's disease may put things in unusual places. They may lose things and be unable to go back over their steps to find them again. Sometimes, they may accuse others of stealing. This may occur more frequently over time. *What's a typical age-related change? Misplacing things from time to time, such as a pair of glasses or the remote control.*

8. Decreased or poor judgment
People with Alzheimer's may experience changes in judgment or decision making. For example, they may use poor judgment when dealing with money, giving large amounts to telemarketers. They may pay less attention to grooming or keeping themselves clean. *What's a typical age-related change? Making a bad decision once in a while.*

Table 18.2. *(Continued)*

9. Withdrawal from work or social activities
A person with Alzheimer's may start to remove themselves from hobbies, social activities, work projects, or sports. They may have trouble keeping up with a favorite sports team or remembering how to complete a favorite hobby. They may also avoid being social because of the changes they have experienced. *What's a typical age-related change? Sometimes feeling weary of work, family, and social obligations.*

10. Changes in mood and personality
The mood and personalities of people with Alzheimer's can change. They can become confused, suspicious, depressed, fearful, or anxious. They may be easily upset at home, at work, with friends, or in places where they are out of their comfort zone. *What's a typical age-related change? Developing very specific ways of doing things and becoming irritable when a routine is disrupted.*

Permission granted: Alzheimer's Association 2011. All rights reserved.

AMD

There is no cure for AMD:

a. Dry AMD can be treated in early stages to delay progression. Treatment for advanced stages is not available.
b. Wet AMD can be treated with medications, laser surgery, photodynamic therapy, and/or injections.

Glaucoma

Treatment is available to decrease eye pressure and to slow the progression of vision loss:

- Commonly used treatments include eyedrops (ocular hypotensive agents), laser, and surgery, which help to drain the fluid from the eye.[25]
- Eye drops are classified by their active ingredients: Prostaglandin analogs, beta-blockers, alpha agonists, carbonic anhydrase inhibitors and their combinations. Eyedrops can have systemic effects, although rare.

Diabetic Retinopathy

Maintaining intensive blood glucose control reduces the development and progression of retinopathy in both types 1 and 2 diabetes:

- Early recognition and treatment can prevent blindness. Surgical options are available for treatment.

Age-Related Hearing Loss

This is typically managed with hearing aids and generally not amenable to medical or surgical intervention. Primary goal is to maintain or improve daily function and to prevent social impairment.

Mobility Limitations

OA

There is no cure for OA. Management focuses on relieving symptoms and improving function.

- Treatment includes patient education, physical therapy, weight control, exercise, orthotics, and bracing; modification of ADLs and medications.
- Exercise can sometimes stop or reverse OA of the hip and knee.
- Analgesics are most frequently prescribed to reduce symptoms. Nonsteroidal anti-inflammatory drugs (NSAIDs) are used to decrease pain and swelling. Acetaminophen

is the preferred NSAID used for initial treatment, due to its effectiveness and safety.

Pharmacological therapies include the following:

- *Topical:* Capsaisin, topical NSAID preparations.
- *Systemic:* Acetaminophen, nonselective NSAIDs, COX-2-specific inhibitors, tramadol, narcotic analgesics.
- *Intra-articular:* Corticosteroid injection for short-term relief, hyaluronic acid derivatives.

Cognitive Impairment/Dementias

MCI: No U.S. Food and Drug Administration (FDA)-approved medications.
Dementia: There is no cure for dementia. Several medications are in use to reduce symptoms and modify behavior.
AD: Several medications are prescribed for AD; however, there are conflicting reports about their therapeutic value. See Table 18.3. Cholinesterase inhibitors (donepezil, rivastigmine, and galantamine) and N-methyl-D-aspartate receptor antagonist memantine are the only treatments for AD that have been FDA approved.[9] Studies have found significant but clinically marginal benefits for the use of cholinesterase inhibitor, with no significant difference in effects reported on cognitive performance among these medications.[26] Adverse effects of these medications include nausea, vomiting, diarrhea, dizziness, and weight loss.

III. Dental Management

Evaluation

Age-Related Visual Changes

Inability to complete health history forms may indicate visual impairment. Visual impairment also contributes to falls in the elderly, which may result in dental–facial trauma.

Age-Related Hearing Loss

Those with suspected hearing impairment need to be referred for evaluation and management and to reduce the risk for disease progression.

Table 18.3. Medications for Memory Loss

Brand Name	Generic Name	Approved for	Side Effects
Cholinesterase inhibitors			
Aricept®	Donepezil	All stages	Nausea, vomiting, loss of appetite, increased frequency of bowel movements
Exelon®	Rivastigmine	Mild to moderate	Nausea, vomiting, loss of appetite, increased frequency of bowel movements
Razadyne®	Glantamine	Mild to moderate	Nausea, vomiting, loss of appetite, increased frequency of bowel movements
Cognex®	Tacrine	Mild to moderate	Nausea, vomiting, possible liver damage (rarely prescribed due to more serious side effects)
Glutamate activity regulator			
Namenda®	Memantine	Moderate–severe	Headache, constipation, confusion, dizziness

- Assess degree of hearing impairment when taking a complete medical history. Individualize approach.

Cognitive Impairment/Dementias

Oral health professionals can have difficulty identifying individuals with cognitive changes due to their relatively isolated and brief patient encounters (see Table 18.3).

What to Ask Patient/Family Member

It is a good office policy to have all patients provide written permission to allow the dentist to talk with their physician, family member, and/or caregiver on an as-needed basis regarding their health care. This becomes important for older adults, when attempting to identify a cognitive change. Due to an increased level of suspiciousness, many individuals in the early stages of cognitive impairment(s) are less likely to provide authorization to talk with family members and or health-care providers:

- Whenever suspicious of a change in cognition, refer patient to health-care provider (preferably geriatrician or geriatric psychiatrist/psychologist) for comprehensive evaluation.
- Be aware that cognitively impaired persons tend to be poor/unreliable historians. As such, it is imperative to obtain supportive documentation from a family member, caregiver, or health-care provider.
- Update medication protocol at every visit.
- Stay informed of new medications used to treat AD. Web-based medical data sources can be helpful, that is, Epocrates® (available at http://www.epocrates.com)

Key questions to ask the patient with visual impairment

- Will wearing your glasses/corrective lenses help improve your daily mouth care? Do you wear them when brushing your teeth and/or dentures?
- Do you need to wear glasses/corrective lenses to read the health history form, appointment cards, instructions, and so on?
- Do you have your glasses/corrective lenses with you (in order to demonstrate or reveal an intraoral finding)?
- Do you have sufficient lighting available to evaluate your oral care technique?

Key questions to ask the patient with glaucoma

- Ask patient to include list of eye drops, ointments, and over-the-counter preparations in their medication list.

> **Key questions to ask the patient with age-related hearing loss**
>
> - Ask how best to communicate with them—lip reading, hearing aid, note writing, or combination.
> - Periodically confirm that you are understood throughout the appointment.

> **Key questions to ask the patient with mobility limitations**
>
> - What limitations do you have that affect your ability to provide good daily oral care?
> - What strategies do you use with food utensils? Can these be modified for your toothbrush, floss holder, denture brush, and/or to dispense toothpaste?

and Pepid™ (available at http://www.pepidonline.com).

Dental Treatment Modifications

Age-Related Visual Changes

- Ensure patient can clearly see demonstrations, written materials including appointment cards and instructions (see special considerations below).

Age-Related Hearing Loss

- Lip readers: Face patient while speaking, speak clearly and naturally; make sure your mouth is visible (remove mask). It is preferable to be at the same level as the individual.
- Gain patients' attention with a light touch or signal before beginning to speak. Be sure the patient is looking at you when you are speaking. Avoid technical terms. Use written instructions and facial expressions.
- Inform patient before starting to use dental equipment or when equipment is changed resulting in an altered experience, for example, vibrations from a slow speed handpiece.
- Hearing aids: Eliminate or minimize background noise (music, intercom) during conversation. Avoid sudden noises and putting your hands close to the hearing aid.
- Patient may want to adjust or turn off the aid during treatment.
- Written and illustrated materials and websites can be used to help explain dental information, procedures, and postoperative instructions.

Mobility Limitations

- Arthritis in the hand, finger(s), elbow, shoulder, and/or neck can affect one's ability to provide good daily oral health care.

Figure 18.3 Adaptations to make toothbrushes easier to grip. (a) Velcro® strap modified to hold brush. (b) Wide elastic or rubber band to hold brush. Make sure the band is not too tight. (c) Large toothbrush grips modified by cutting a slit in a tennis ball and sliding the handle into the ball or attaching a bicycle grip to a toothbrush. From the Dental Care Every Day: A Caregiver's Guide. NIH Publication No. 11-5191. Available at: http://www.nidcr.nih.gov/OralHealth/Topics/DevelopmentalDisabilities/DentalCareEveryDay.htm.

- Modified manual toothbrush handles or electric toothbrushes (wide handle) can help to accommodate for lost mobility.
- Interdental cleaners/brushes can assist when flossing is not possible.
- Increase frequency of oral prophylaxes and examinations to ensure optimal oral hygiene maintenance.

The following over-the-counter materials can be used to modify toothbrushes/denture brushes and floss holders: plaster, Velcro® (Velcro USA, Manchester, NH), nonslip mats/shelf liner, polyethylene pipe insulation tubing, modeling clay, tennis ball, bicycle handle, and aluminum foil. See Fig. 18.3.

Cognitive Impairment/ Dementias

Oral Disease Burden

- Individuals with dementias, like AD, are at increased risk for caries, periodontal disease, and oral infections due to self-care deficits; chronic disease burden; difficulty complying with medications, daily oral care, and appointments; dependence on caregivers; behavioral changes; swallowing difficulty; lack of understanding; and resistance to care.
- As a health-care provider, the relationship to the individual with cognitive impairments will change as the disease changes their cognition, mood, and behavior.
- Individuals with cognitive impairments may not be able to report symptoms of oral disease, but may display behavioral change when experiencing infection or pain.
- Many people with AD report brushing their teeth twice a day; however, this comment is most likely based on their long-term, not short-term memory.

Patient Management

- Following a diagnosis or when a cognitive decline appears likely, anticipate future oral

decline. Initiate aggressive preventive measures to include:
- increased frequency of preventive services;
- individualized schedules are needed;
- daily use of topical fluorides, chemotherapeutic rinses, fluoride varnish, and salivary substitutes.
* Chemotherapeutic rinses: Use a dip-and-brush approach when individual is unable to "swish and spit."
* Prosthesis(es): If not present, place patient's name on prosthesis.

Caregiver Education

Discuss the following with the caregiver (if available):

* Oral health concerns regarding the individual with disease and caregiver.
  - Ensure self-care of caregiver, as this is often neglected when serving as a full-time caregiver.
* Need for frequent visits to ensure oral and general health maintenance.
  - Encourage self-care as long as possible as some maintain some oral care skills when prompted.
  - Discuss current and/or future need for assistance with daily care, strategies to supervise and assist with daily care, methods to evaluate oral cleanliness, strategies for cooperation, and need for assistance from others.
* Dentate: Encourage frequent daily brushing and flossing (two or more times a day).
  - Modify toothbrush; consider electric or battery-operated toothbrush, if needed.
  - Encourage frequent brushing.
  - Follow same oral care routine(s) when possible.
  - Prosthetic devices: Daily cleaning strategies. Remove, inspect, and clean before bed. Return in the morning.

As the disease progresses, more supervision and professional care will be needed.

Risks of Dental Care

Hemostasis

With cognitive impairment or dementia affecting the patient's ability to follow instructions, it is highly recommended to ensure surgical hemostasis (sutures, local hemostatics, socket preservation techniques) prior to dismissal from dental practice. Patients with painful mobility limitations on aspirin or NSAIDs might have increased bleeding tendencies.

Susceptibility to Infection

Discuss concerns with family member/caregiver/power of attorney as individual is at increased risk for infection when daily oral care is neglected. Dental treatment poses no increased risk of infection.

Drug Actions/Interactions

With the exception of tacrine enhancing gastrointestinal ulcer bleeding potential in combination with NSAIDs, the other current medications used to treat AD do not have interactions with drugs used in dentistry. None of the medications for AD have oral side effects.

Patient's Ability to Tolerate Dental Care

The level of cooperation in a dental practice from patients with AD is quite variable and unpredictable. In general, utilizing good communication skills enhances cooperation; however, often times, behavior can become challenging and impede successful delivery of services. Some patients may benefit from short-term anti-anxiolytic medications (e.g., lorazepam), though results can be variable.

Special Considerations

Dental Office Modifications to Support Patients with Age-Related Vision Deficits

Having the following available can assist visually impaired older adults in the dental office:

1. Large print magazines in the waiting room
2. Nonprescription reading glasses (different strengths)
3. Ensure good lighting throughout the office
   a. Add spot/task lighting in areas used for completing forms
4. Large print on prescription bottles
5. Install blinds or shades to reduce glare
6. Use contrasting colors on door handles, towel racks, and stair markers

When to Be Suspicious That Your Patient Has a Cognitive Problem

Any of the following indicates a concern, especially when the behavior has changed:

1. Arrives for office visit on wrong day or time, or misses appointments
2. Calls office frequently for reassurance/reminders
3. Has trouble completing health history form
4. Has difficulty following instructions
5. Has repetitive speech
6. Has decreased ability to provide daily oral care
7. Presents signs of poor grooming or hygiene
8. Defers to others to answer questions

IV. Recommended Readings and Cited References

Recommended Readings

Figueiro MG. *Lighting the way: a key to independence*, 2001. Rensselaer Polytechnic Institute. From the Lighting Research Center, AARP Andrus Foundation. Available at: http://www.lrc.rpi.edu/programs/lightHealth/AARP/pdf/AARPbook3.pdf. Accessed November 27, 2011.

To learn about support groups, services, research centers, research studies, and publications about Alzheimer's disease, contact the following resources:

Alzheimer's Disease Education and Referral (ADEAR) Center
1-800-438-4380 (toll-free)
http://www.nia.nih.gov/alzheimers

Alzheimer's Association
1-800-272-3900 (toll-free)
1-866-403-3073 (TDD/toll-free)
http://www.alz.org

Cited References

1. Desai M, Pratt LA, Lentzner H, Robinson KN. Trends in vision and hearing among older Americans. Aging Trends 2001;2:1–8.
2. Maylahn C, Gohdes DM, Balamurugan A, Larsen BA. *Webcite: Eye Digest*. Available at: http://www.webcitation.org/63MvNQy6m. Accessed March 17, 2012.
3. Lee DA, Higginbotham EJ. Glaucoma and its treatment: a review. Am J Health Syst Pharm 2005;62(7):691–9.
4. Kwon YH, Fingert JH, Kuehn MH, Alward WL. Primary open-angle glaucoma. N Engl J Med 2009;360(11):1113–24.
5. Fong DS, Aiello L, Gardner TW, King GL, Blankenship G, Cavallerano JD, et al. Retinopathy in diabetes. Diabetes Care 2004;27(Suppl. 1):S84–7.
6. Dalton DS, Cruickshanks KJ, Klein BE, Klein R, Wiley TL, Nondahl DM. The impact of hearing loss on quality of life in older adults. Gerontologist 2003;43(5):661–8.
7. Glisky EL. Chapter 1. Changes in cognitive function in human aging. In: Brain Aging: Models, Methods and Mechanisms. Riddle DR, ed. 2007. CRC Press, Boca Raton, FL. Available at: http://www.ncbi.nlm.nih.gov/books/NBK3885/. Accessed November 28, 2011.

8. Bennett DA. Mild cognitive impairment. Clin Geriatr Med 2004;20(1):15–25.
9. Mayeux R. Clinical practice: early Alzheimer's disease. N Engl J Med 2010;362(23):2194–201.
10. Lawhorne L, Ogle KS. Approaches to the office care of the older adult and the specter of dementia. Prim Care 2005;32(3):599–618.
11. Petersen RC. Mild cognitive impairment: transition between aging and Alzheimer's disease. Neurologia 2000;15(3):93–101.
12. Petersen RC, Roberts RO, Knopman DS, Boeve BF, Geda YE, Ivnik RJ, et al. Mild cognitive impairment: ten years later. Arch Neurol 2009;66(12):1447–55.
13. Gauthier S, Reisberg B, Zaudig M, Petersen RC, Ritchie K, Broich K, et al. Mild cognitive impairment. Lancet 2006;367(9518):1262–70.
14. Friedlander AH, Norman DC, Mahler ME, Norman KM, Yagiela JA. Alzheimer's disease: psychopathology, medical management and dental implications. J Am Dent Assoc 2006;137(9):1240–51.
15. Owsley C. Aging and vision. Vision Res 2011;51(13):1610–22.
16. Dillon CF, Gu Q, Hoffman H, Ko CW. Vision, hearing, balance and sensory impairment in Americans aged 70 years and over: United States, 1999–2006. NCHS Data Brief 2010;31:1–8.
17. US Department of Health and Human Services, National Institutes of Health. National Eye Institute. Statistics and Data. Available at: http://www.nei.nih.gov/eyedata/pbd_tables.asp. Accessed March 16, 2012.
18. Robman L, Taylor H. External factors in the development of cataract. Eye (Lond) 2005;19(10):1074–82.
19. Ehrlich R, Harris A, Kheradiya NS, Winston DM, Ciulla TA, Wirostko B. Age-related macular degeneration and the aging eye. Clin Interv Aging 2008;3(3):473–82.
20. De Jong PT. Age-related macular degeneration. N Engl J Med 2006;355(14):1474–85.
21. Zhang X, Saaddine JB, Chou CF, Cotch MF, Cheng YJ, Geiss LS, et al. Prevalence of diabetic retinopathy in the United States, 2005–2008. JAMA 2010;304(6):649–55.
22. Qiu C, De Ronchi D, Fratiglioni L. The epidemiology of the dementias: an update. Curr Opin Psychiatry 2007;20(4):380–85.
23. Ferri CP, Prince M, Brayne C, Brodaty H, Fratiglioni L, Ganguli M, et al. Global prevalence of dementia: a Delphi consensus study. Lancet 2005;366(9503):2112–7.
24. Mayeux R. Epidemiology of neurodegeneration. Annu Rev Neurosci 2003;26:81–104.
25. Novack GD, O'Donnell MJ, Molloy DW. New glaucoma medications in the geriatric population: efficacy and safety. J Am Geriatr Soc 2002;50(5):956–62.
26. Hansen RA, Gartlehner G, Webb AP, Morgan LC, Moore CG, Jonas DE. Efficacy and safety of donepezil, galantamine and rivastigmine for the treatment of Alzheimer's disease: a systematic review and meta-analysis. Clin Interv Aging 2008;3(2):211–25.

Women's Health

Linda C. Niessen DMD, MPH

I. Background

In the mid-1980s, the United States Public Health Service defined women's health as "diseases or conditions that are unique to, more prevalent or more serious in women, have distinct causes or manifest themselves differently in women, or have different outcomes or interventions."[1] This task force raised the awareness among the scientific community that women were not "smaller" men and indeed had unique health problems, including oral diseases that may require different approaches. Later in 2001, the Institute of Medicine's Report "Exploring the biological contributions to human health: Does sex matter?"[2] focused the scientific community on the need to understand the roles that sex and gender play in disease prevention and management.

This chapter addresses the unique oral health needs that women have throughout their lives. While hormonal fluctuations during puberty, menses, and menopause can affect oral health, certain diseases such as osteoporosis, burning mouth, breast cancer, and autoimmune disorders (discussed in Chapter 10), are more common in women than men and present unique challenges for dental practitioners in caring for their women patients.

Description of Disease/Condition

Puberty Onset and Menses

At puberty, girls experience an increase in estrogen and progesterone. Puberty in girls is occurring at earlier ages,[3] with childhood obesity thought to be contributing to this change. Health concerns of early puberty onset include:

- potential increases in breast and uterine cancer in adult women,
- poor self-esteem,
- eating disorders,
- depression,
- earlier cigarette and alcohol use,
- earlier sexual activity.

As the age of puberty has decreased, the age of menarche has also decreased. Menstruation should occur regularly throughout a woman's life unless she is pregnant or using contraceptives.

The ADA Practical Guide to Patients with Medical Conditions, First Edition. Edited by Lauren L. Patton.
© 2012 American Dental Association. Published 2012 by John Wiley & Sons, Inc.

Pregnancy

From the first day of the woman's last menstrual period to delivery, a full-term pregnancy is considered to be 40 weeks and is divided into three trimesters each lasting approximately 3 months. Pregnancy is increasing among older women due to technological advances. Major organogenesis occurs in the first 3 months. The facial features begin to form in the 2nd month and become recognizably human in the 3rd month. In the 3rd month, the palate closes, allowing the fetus to begin to swallow by the 4th month. By the 5th month, the mother may feel the baby kick or move and the fetal heartbeat is audible by stethoscope. While lungs are not completely formed, a baby born during the 6th month, weighing 1–1.5 lb, can often survive in a neonatal intensive care unit.

Menopause

Menopause is a normal physiological event that signals the cessation of menses. The average age of menopause is 51 years, with a range from 48 to 55 years. Perimenopause is the 3- to 5-year period before the last menstrual period occurs and signals the changes in hormone levels. Women who smoke, have never been pregnant, and live at high altitudes are more likely to have an earlier menopause.

Osteoporosis

Osteoporosis is a systemic skeletal disease characterized by low bone mass and microarchitectural deterioration of bone tissue. These changes increase bone fragility and susceptibility to fracture.

Breast Cancer

Breast cancer is the most common cancer occurring among women. The two most common forms of breast cancer are ductal and lobular, and each can be either invasive or *in situ*.

Interpersonal Violence against Women

Violence against women, also called "domestic violence" or "spousal abuse," has been redefined as "intimate partner violence" (IPV). This new term recognizes that intimate partner violence occurs between two people in a close relationship, whether married or dating, men and women, and in gay and lesbian couples.[4] IPV can include four types of behaviors:

- physical violence,
- sexual violence,
- threats of physical or sexual violence,
- emotional abuse.[5]

Pathogenesis/Etiology

Osteoporosis

Osteoporosis risk factors

Nonmodifiable risk factors	Modifiable risk factors
Being female	Diet low in calcium
Small frame women	Sedentary lifestyle
Advanced age	Anorexia nervosa or bulimia
Family history of osteoporosis	Smoking
Early menopause (before age 45)	Excessive alcohol intake
	Prolonged use of certain medications (glucocorticosteroids, anticonvulsants, excessive thyroid hormone, and certain cancer treatments)

Breast Cancer

- The most common genetic risk factors for breast cancer are mutations in BRCA1 and/or BRCA2, affecting only 5–10% of women with breast cancer.
- Breast cancer risk is also elevated by
  - having a family member (first-degree relative) with breast cancer, particularly if the family member was diagnosed at an early age;
  - exposure to high levels of radiation in early life;
  - prior treatment for Hodgkin's disease.[6]

Epidemiology

Pregnancy

- In the United States in 2009, a little over 6 million pregnancies resulted in
  - 4,130,665 live births,[7]
  - about 1.2 million induced abortions,
  - about 1 million fetal losses from miscarriage or stillbirth.
- The mean age at first birth was 25.5 years, and 41% of the births were to unmarried women.
- Approximately 500,000 babies (12.2% of the births) were preterm.[7] A preterm low birth weight (LBW) baby is defined as a baby born before 37 weeks and weighing less than 2500 g (5 lb, 8 oz). Prematurity is a major risk for newborn death, chronic health problems, and developmental disabilities.
- The LBW rate (<2500 g) was 8.16%.[7]
- Breastfeeding for newborns increased in the United States from 2000 to 2008.[8]
  - Early postpartum breastfeeding (0–3 months) has increased from 71% to 75% of mothers in 2000–2007.
  - Mothers who breastfeed their babies at 6 months increased from 34.2% to 43.8%, from 2000–2007.
  - Mothers who exclusively breastfed their babies for the first 3 months were estimated at 35.0% and for the first 6 months were 14.8% in 2008.

Oral, Transdermal, and Implanted Contraception Use

Of the 62 million women between ages 15 and 44 in 2008, 62% were using some form of contraception.[9] Of these women, 35.7% or over 13 million women are using some form of oral, transdermal, or implanted contraception. Many systemic and oral side effects have been observed in women using hormonal contraception.

Osteoporosis

Approximately 30% of all postmenopausal women have osteoporosis in the United States and Europe.[10] At least 40% of these women and 15–30% of men will sustain one or more fractures in their remaining lifetime. The most common fracture sites are hip, radius, and vertebral compression fractures.

Breast Cancer

Each year, around 200,000 women will be diagnosed with invasive breast cancer and about 40,000 women will die from breast cancer.[6] Another 50,000 women will be diagnosed with noninvasive breast cancer. It is second to lung cancer in the number of cancer deaths in women. Although breast cancer is most common in Caucasian women, African-American women are more likely to die of breast cancer. While men are also diagnosed with breast cancer, the female-to-male ratio remains 100:1. Age and being female are the greatest risk factors for breast cancer, with breast cancer occurring more frequently in women over age 70 years.

Interpersonal Violence against Women

It is estimated that from 1 to 3 million women are battered each year by their intimate partner.[11]

IPV occurs along a continuum from a single episode of violence to continual battering. It is a leading cause of injury to women ages 15–44 years.

Nearly 3 in 10 women and 1 in 10 men have experienced rape, physical violence, or stalking by an intimate partner.[12]

Risk factors that contribute to intimate partner violence include:

- being violent or aggressive in the past;
- seeing or being a victim of violence as a child;
- using drugs or alcohol, especially drinking heavily;
- not having a job or other life events that cause stress.

Coordination of Care between Dentist and Physician

Critical times for the dentist and physician to work together to maintain and improve the woman's health (and that of her child) are during pregnancy, when breast cancer occurs and requires management with chemotherapy or intravenous bisphosphonates, and when interpersonal violence is suspected. Dentists should consult with the pregnant patient's obstetrician or other physician whenever management questions exist.

II. Medical Management

Identification/Medical History/ Physical Examination

Pregnancy

First Trimester (0–12 Weeks): Early symptoms of pregnancy include missed menstrual period, swelling and tender breasts, nausea and vomiting worse in the morning, fatigue, hunger and food cravings, frequent urination, and sensitivity to smells that may worsen nausea.

Second Trimester (13–28 Weeks): The woman becomes noticeably pregnant with enlarged uterus, darkening skin, darkening and enlarging nipples, with a feeling of being flushed and warm. The appetite increases and when nausea fades, energy returns, and heart rate increases with increased blood volume.

Third Trimester (29–40 Weeks): The woman experiences a variety of symptoms and may feel hot, sweat easily, find it difficult to get comfortable, develop stretch marks and lower back aches, and require more rest. Constipation, hemorrhoids, frequent urination, and swollen ankles are common in the last month. Healthy weight gain is 25–35 lb during the pregnancy. The average healthy birth weight is 7.5 lb for the baby and another 3.5 lb for placenta and fluid.

A history of pregnancies is often described by terms gravida (# of pregnancies), parida (# of deliveries after 20 weeks), and abortus (# of pregnancy losses prior to 20 weeks regardless of cause: spontaneous, elective, therapeutic abortion, or ectopic pregnancy). The sum of parity and abortus equals gravidy.

Menopause

Many women experience a variety of symptoms as a result of the hormonal changes associated with the transition through menopause. As women experience menopause, they are starting to lose bone mass and their risks for cardiovascular disease (CVD) increase as their cholesterol levels rise after menopause.

Hot flashes are the most common symptom of menopause affecting over 75% of women. These feelings of warmth throughout the body can last for about 30 seconds. Women usually experience them for 2–3 years, although some women have reported having them for up to 5 years. Night sweats can also signal menopause.

Interpersonal Violence against Women

Physical violence can result in broken bones, internal bleeding, or trauma to soft tissue and organs and even death. Trauma inflicted to the head and neck region is common.

Laboratory Testing
Pregnancy

Pregnancy tests (urine or serum) assess presence of human chorionic gonadotropin (hCG) produced by the placenta. Home urine tests can detect pregnancy as early as the day of the missed menstrual period.

Prenatal tests commonly include tests that assess for birth defects that may occur in up to 3% of pregnancies:

- Alpha-fetoprotein (AFP), a substance produced by the fetal liver. Abnormally low levels can suggest Down syndrome; abnormally high levels can suggest a fetal neural tube defect to include brain and spinal cord.
- Triple marker test: usually AFP, hCG, and unconjugated estriol.
- Other prenatal tests: tests for sexually transmitted diseases and human immunodeficiency virus, gestational diabetes screening at 24–48 weeks, blood tests for anemia and blood type, screening for immunity to various infectious diseases.
- Amniocentesis can also be used in the prenatal diagnosis of chromosomal abnormalities and fetal infections.

Osteoporosis

- Dual-energy X-ray absorptiometry (DXA) remains the most common diagnostic test for measuring bone mineral density.

Medical Treatment
Pregnancy

During pregnancy women are advised to take 400 µg folic acid supplement to prevent spina bifida; use precautions with all medications; eat a balanced diet with frequent small meals; and avoid smoking, drinking alcohol, recreational drugs, large amounts of caffeine, and artificial sweeteners.

Menopause

Hormone replacement therapy (HRT) was once fairly widely used to replace the hormones that were decreasing with menopause. Findings from the Women's Health Initiative of increased risks for CVD, breast cancer, and stroke when taking HRT resulted in the development of new guidelines supporting the use of HRT for only a short-term basis to help alleviate the symptoms of menopause. Recent studies demonstrate that estrogens exacerbate CVD in older women with existing atherosclerosis but may be protective from CVD in younger healthier women without atherosclerosis or inflammation.[13] The decision to take hormone therapy during and after menopause is based on medical history, severity of the symptoms, and potential risks and benefits of hormone administration.

Osteoporosis

Current treatment recommendations include antiresorptive agents to reduce bone resorption (and subsequently increase bone formation), leading to an increase in bone mineral density to varying degrees.

Antiresorptive agents include:

- estrogen,
- selective estrogen receptor modulators,
- bisphosphonates,

- the human monoclonal antibody to receptor activator of NFκB ligand (RANKL).

Bisphosphonates inhibit osteoclastic activity and have been shown to decrease vertebral fractures. They bind to bone mineral and have a long skeletal retention. Patients with a diagnosis of osteoporosis are also advised to take vitamin D and calcium, to maintain a proper diet, and to start or continue a program of weight-bearing exercise.

Breast Cancer

Treatment for breast cancer is determined by the stage of the tumor at the time of diagnosis, the aggressiveness of the tumor, and age of the patient.

Treatment options for breast cancer include:

- radiation to kill any additional cells to reduce the risk of recurrence;
- surgery to remove the tumor;
- chemotherapy, hormonal therapies, or biological therapies to treat systemic disease, reduce the risk of recurrence, and increase survival;
- targeted therapies are being developed based on various genetic markers found in the tumor.

These new treatments have increased the survival of breast cancer patients, and it is estimated that there are now 2.5 million survivors of breast cancer.

In cases of advanced breast cancer, metastases may be found in the lungs, bone, and liver. The mandible is a possible site of metastasis (see Fig. 19.1). Bone metastases can cause pain, fractures, and other bone problems. Intravenous bisphosphonates, potent inhibitors of osteoclastic activity, are the current standard of care for preventing and treating skeletal-related events for patients with advanced breast cancer with bone metastases.[14]

Figure 19.1 Metastatic lesion of the mandible in a 55-year-old woman with breast cancer.

III. Dental Management

Evaluation

As with every patient, the dental evaluation of the woman begins with a thorough history. Focused key questions for the patient and physician related to the health condition are shown on the next pages.

Dental Treatment Modifications

Puberty and Menses

Microbial changes in oral flora have been reported during puberty, attributed to responses to the sex hormones, estrogen, and progesterone, by the oral flora. *Capnocytophaga* species increase in incidence and proportion, and *Prevotella intermedia* has the ability to substitute estrogen and progesterone for vitamin K, an essential growth factor. These organisms, along with increased blood flow to gingival tissues as a result of hormonal changes, have been implicated in the increased gingivitis and gingival bleeding observed during puberty when oral home care is poor.

Oral changes may occur during menses and vary considerably among women.

Dental Treatment Considerations

- Early oral hygiene education.
- Scaling and improved daily oral hygiene care for mild cases of gingivitis.

> **? Key questions to ask the patient**
>
> **Pregnancy**
> What trimester are you in?
> Have you had any signs or symptoms of a high-risk pregnancy, such as hypertension, previous miscarriages, recent cramping, or bleeding?
> Have you noticed any intraoral changes?
>
> **Menopause**
> Have you experienced any oral pain, burning, or oral dryness? *If so, the dental professional should characterize the nature and frequency of the pain, burning, or oral dryness.*
>
> **Osteoporosis**
> Do you have osteoporosis? If yes, are you taking any bisphosphonates or other antiresorptive (bone strengthening) medication to prevent bone fractures? If yes, which one and for how long?
> Have you had teeth extracted while you were taking these medications?
> Have you ever experienced exposed bone in your jaw?
>
> **Burning mouth**
> How long have you noticed this burning? When does it start? Does anything precipitate it? How long does it last? Does anything relieve it?
> Have you started taking any new medications recently? Have you changed your toothpaste recently?
>
> **Breast cancer**
> What type of malignancy do you have? Do you have bone metastases? Are you taking any bisphosphonates or other antiresorptive medications to prevent bone pain and fractures?
> Have you ever had exposed bone in your jaw?
>
> **Suspected victim of interpersonal violence**
> How did this injury occur? Did anyone do this to you? How are things at home?

- More aggressive care and more frequent recalls for severe cases of gingivitis until the condition improves or resolves.

Pregnancy

Pregnancy is a stressor to oral health. It is not uncommon to encounter a woman today who still believes that you "lose a tooth for each pregnancy." This misconception arose from the belief that the calcium needed for the developing fetal bones was available from the teeth. The calcium in the teeth is in a stable crystalline form and is not bioavailable. Blood calcium serves as the reservoir for calcium required for fetal development.

- *Dental Caries*
  - The relationship between caries and pregnancy is not clearly defined. The

> **Key Questions**
>
> ### Key questions to ask the physician
>
> **Pregnancy**
> When is the expected delivery date?
> Is this a high-risk pregnancy? Do you have any special concerns about the patient?
> If medication use is planned: What medication do you advise be used for pain control or for control of a dental abscess?
>
> **Osteoporosis**
> If on an antiresorptive therapy: Which medication is the patient using? How long has the patient been on this therapy? What are your plans for continuation of antiresorptive therapy?
>
> **Breast cancer**
> What type and stage of malignancy does the patient have? Does the patient have bone metastases? What is the cancer treatment plan? Will there be use of myelosuppressive chemotherapy? Is the planned chemotherapy regimen expected to produce mucositis? Will there be use of an intravenous bisphosphonate or other antiresorptive therapy?
>
> **Suspected victim of interpersonal violence**
> Given concerns for new maxillofacial injury, has the patient had similar past injuries that seem unusual in pattern or number? Have you explored potential interpersonal violence with the patient and if so what result? What else do you suggest to help this patient?

relationship of increased parity to increased dental caries may relate both to biological and sociodemographic factors.[15]
- If the pregnant woman is craving cariogenic foods, her risk for caries may increase.
- Based on clinical trials showing no difference in early childhood caries outcome in the offspring,[16] current practice does not recommend the use of prenatal fluoride for pregnant women.
- *Periodontal Diseases*
  - Gingivitis is the most common oral condition, occurring in 60–75% of pregnant women.
  - It can range from mild inflammation to severe gingival overgrowth; be generalized or localized; occur at any time during pregnancy. The increase in hormones exaggerates the gum tissue's response to bacterial plaque. The gingival tissue is usually red and swollen, and bleeds easily. It often occurs in the anterior part of the mouth.
  - A "pregnancy tumor" or pyogenic granuloma (see Fig. 19.2) can occur in up to 10% of pregnant women. Pregnancy granulomas may be excised prior to delivery if the tissue becomes difficult to clean and interferes with chewing and speaking, but may recur.
- *Periodontal Disease and Risk of Preterm/LBW Delivery*
  - Periodontal disease has been investigated as a potential risk factor for preterm birth (PTB) and LBW babies. The mechanism of action suggests that throughout pregnancy, cytokines and prostaglandins

Figure 19.2 Severe pyogenic granuloma "pregnancy tumor" in a pregnant woman. (Slide courtesy of Dr. Terry D. Rees, Professor, Texas A&M Health Science Center, Baylor College of Dentistry, Dallas, TX.)

increase until a critical threshold is reached that induces labor and delivery. The bacteria associated with periodontal infection can stimulate excessive production of the mediators, which then induce labor and delivery too early.
   ○ Early studies of epidemiological associations between PTB/LBW and periodontal infection[17] and periodontal treatment intervention in pregnant women to prevent PTB/LBW babies[18–20] stimulated interest. However, a recent meta-analysis, which pooled results of 10 randomized controlled trials of periodontal interventions for prevention of PTB and 8 randomized controlled trials of periodontal interventions for prevention of LBW babies, did not support the hypothesis that reduction of PTB or LBW occurs in women who are treated for periodontal disease during pregnancy.[21] Nonetheless, dental professionals should provide advice and counsel on the importance of good oral health and periodontal disease prevention to their woman patients who are pregnant or considering becoming pregnant.

Preventive Dental Program during Pregnancy

Treatment planning objectives for the patient should include eliminating areas of infection, particularly periodontal infection, maintaining good oral hygiene, nutritional counseling, and tobacco cessation if the woman uses tobacco products:

- *Caries Risk Assessment and Caries Prevention Education*
  ○ Should be conducted to identify the patient's potential risk for dental caries. The best predictor for future caries is present caries.[22] As a result of food cravings, cariogenic foods consumed may increase caries risk.
  ○ Patient education on caries and its risk may be particularly important for preventing early childhood caries in her offspring. Figure 19.3 illustrates a caries risk assessment form for patients >6 years old. The American Dental Association (ADA) also has an early childhood caries risk assessment form for children <6 years old. Both forms are downloadable from the ADA website (ada.org, search "caries risk assessment form") and can be easily incorporated into your practice.
  ○ Preventive measures should be implemented based on the patient's caries risk status and monitored regularly.
- *Periodontal Risk Assessment*
  ○ Gingival and periodontal assessment should be conducted.
  ○ Scaling and root planing may be performed when needed during the pregnancy to treat any periodontal infection.
- *Oral Hygiene Education*
  ○ Education in proper oral self-care techniques is a critical component of the preventive treatment plan. Good oral hygiene and plaque control are especially important during pregnancy since the increase

(a)

Caries Risk Assessment Form (Age > 6)

Patient Name: Score:
Birth Date: Date:
Age: Initials:

		Low Risk (0)	Moderate Risk (1)	High Risk (10)	Patient Risk
Contributing Conditions					
I.	**Fluoride Exposure** (through drinking water, supplements, professional applications, toothpaste)	Yes	No		
II.	**Sugary Foods or Drinks** (including juice, carbonated or non-carbonated soft drinks, energy drinks, medicinal syrups)	Primarily at mealtimes		Frequent or prolonged between meal exposures/day	
III.	**Caries Experience of Mother, Caregiver** and/or other **Siblings** (for patients ages 6–14)	No carious lesions in last 24 months	Carious lesions in last 7–23 months	Carious lesions in last 6 months	
IV.	**Dental Home**: established patient of record, receiving regular dental care in a dental office	Yes	No		
General Health Conditions					
I.	**Special Health Care Needs***	No	Yes (over age 14)	Yes (ages 6–14)	
II.	**Chemo/Radiation Therapy**	No		Yes	
III.	**Eating Disorders**	No	Yes		
IV.	**Medications that Reduce Salivary Flow**	No	Yes		
V.	**Drug/Alcohol Abuse**	No	Yes		
Clinical Conditions					
I.	**Cavitated or Non-Cavitated** (incipient) **Carious Lesions or Restorations** (visually or radiographically evident)	No new carious lesions or restorations in last 36 months	1 or 2 new carious lesions or restorations in last 36 months	3 or more carious lesions or restorations in last 36 months	
II.	**Teeth Missing Due to Caries** in past 36 months	No		Yes	
III.	**Visible Plaque**	No	Yes		
IV.	**Unusual Tooth Morphology** that compromises oral hygiene	No	Yes		
V.	**Interproximal Restorations** - 1 or more	No	Yes		
VI.	**Exposed Root Surfaces** Present	No	Yes		
VII.	**Restorations with Overhangs** and/or **Open Margins**; **Open Contacts** with Food Impaction	No	Yes		
VIII.	**Dental/Orthodontic Appliances** (fixed or removable)	No	Yes		
IX.	**Severe Dry Mouth (Xerostomia)**	No		Yes	
				TOTAL:	

Patient Instructions:

*Patients with developmental, physical, medical or mental disabilities that prevent or limit performance of adequate oral health care by themselves or caregivers. © American Dental Association, 2009, 2011. All rights reserved.

ADA American Dental Association®

Figure 19.3 ADA Caries Risk Assessment form for patients over age 6. (a) Page 1; (b) page 2. (*Continued*)

(b)

Indicate 0, 1 or 10 in the last column for each risk factor. If the risk factor was not determined or is not applicable, enter a 0 in the patient risk factor column. Total the factor values and record the score at the top of the page.

A score of 0 indicates a patient has a low risk for the development of caries. A single high risk factor, or score of 10, places the patient at high risk for development of caries. Scores between 1 and 10 place the patient at a moderate risk for the development of caries. Subsequent scores should decrease with reduction of risks and therapeutic intervention.

The clinical judgment of the dentist may justify a change of the patient's risk level (increased or decreased) based on review of this form and other pertinent information. For example, missing teeth may not be regarded as high risk for a follow up patient; or other risk factors not listed may be present.

The assessment cannot address every aspect of a patient's health, and should not be used as a replacement for the dentist's inquiry and judgment. Additional or more focused assessment may be appropriate for patients with specific health concerns. As with other forms, this assessment may be only a starting point for evaluating the patient's health status.

This is a tool provided for the use of ADA members. It is based on the opinion of experts who utilized the most up-to-date scientific information available. The ADA plans to periodically update this tool based on: 1) member feedback regarding its usefulness, and; 2) advances in science. ADA member-users are encouraged to share their opinions regarding this tool with the Council on Dental Practice.

Signatures:

Patient, Parent or Guardian _____ _____ _____

Student _____ _____

Faculty Advisor _____ ___ _____ _____

Figure 19.3 (*Continued*)

in hormones results in an exaggerated inflammatory response to local irritants.
- Potentially at risk from lack of preventive oral health care during pregnancy is maternal to child transmission of cariogenic bacteria (such as *Streptococcus mutans*), which has been demonstrated to occur through kissing.[23]
- Mothers and their children are also known to share oral health behaviors and attitudes; thus, dental visits during pregnancy provide the opportunity to educate the expectant mother on the importance of infant oral health, oral hygiene techniques for infants and young children, and the role of fluoride in dental caries prevention for children.

Elective Dental Treatment during Pregnancy

- Expert opinion recommends providing elective care during the 2nd trimester or early half of the 3rd trimester. This recommendation is based on the pregnant woman having passed the 1st trimester, when the fetus is most susceptible to environmental influences during organogenesis, and not yet having reached the mid-late 3rd trimester when the woman is often less comfortable reclined in the dental chair.

Emergency Dental Treatment during Pregnancy

- Emergency dental treatment can be provided as needed any time during the pregnancy. The control of pain and elimination of infection, which would cause stress for the mother and endanger the fetus, should be addressed with emergency dental care.
- Emergency dental treatment may require a consultation with the patient's obstetrician, should concern about the medications required or the effect of the emergency dental treatment on the fetus arise.

Dental Radiographs during Pregnancy

- Dental radiographs may be required during routine or emergency dental care. Untreated dental infections may pose a greater risk to the developing fetus than the exposure to the radiation needed to treat the infection.
- Although radiation exposure from dental radiographs is extremely low, every precaution should be taken to minimize any radiation exposure to the mother and the fetus, including use of lower radiation emitting digital radiography and protective abdominal and thyroid shielding.[24]
- Dental radiographs are not contraindicated for women trying to become pregnant or who are breastfeeding.

Oral, Transdermal, and Implanted Contraception Use

- Hormonal oral contraceptives mimic pregnancy by increasing estrogen and progesterone levels, which can increase the body's inflammatory response to local oral irritants.
- A preventive program for oral hygiene is important for the patient using hormonal contraception.
- Some studies have demonstrated a two- to threefold increased risk of dry socket and postoperative pain following 3rd molar removal among women on oral contraceptives, possibly related to the fibrinolytic effect of oral contraceptives interfering with blood clotting.[25]
- If extractions are needed for patients on oral contraceptives, consider scheduling on days 23–28 of the oral contraceptive cycle, when estrogen influence is lower.[26]

Osteoporosis

- It is not clear if osteoporosis affects the maxillary and mandibular alveolar bone and incidence of tooth loss. Similarly in those

who are edentulous and experience alveolar ridge resorption, it is not clear if this condition is more pronounced in adults who have osteoporosis.
- Dental management for patients taking oral antiresorptive agents includes proper infection control, conservative surgical procedures, appropriate use of oral antimicrobials, and effective antibiotic therapy when indicated.
- Patients must be informed that their antiresorptive medications place them at a low risk for developing antiresorptive agent-induced osteonecrosis of the jaw (ARONJ) and the dental team will minimize this risk, but this risk can never be eliminated during dental treatment.
- A preventive program that includes thorough daily oral hygiene care at home and regular dental care may be the best approach to lowering the risk of ARONJ.
- No validated diagnostic test is currently available to determine which patients are at risk for ARONJ.
- Discontinuing the bisphosphonate therapy may not eliminate the risk and may have a negative effect on the low bone mass therapy.
- The ADA Council on Scientific Affairs Expert Panel[27] recommends that the dentist treat the patient who has active dental or periodontal disease despite the risk of developing ARONJ, since the risk and consequences of leaving active dental disease outweigh the risk of developing ARONJ. However, prior to starting dental treatment, the dentist and patient should discuss the benefits, risks, and treatment options, and obtain the patient's consent for treatment in writing.

Breast Cancer

Modifications will depend on use of myelosuppressive chemotherapy for treatment and use of bisphosphonates or other antiresorptive drugs, for prevention and treatment of bone metastases. For management recommendations for patients receiving chemotherapy, see Chapter 13.

Interpersonal Violence against Women

- Head and neck injuries occur in 75% of victims of IPV and broken jaws, fractured alveolus, or avulsed, subluxated, or fractured teeth result in care-seeking behavior (see Fig. 19.4).
- Dental professionals should be vigilant in evaluating patients with suspected IPV. The dental evaluation begins with the medical and dental history. Like child abuse, IPV should be considered if the patient experiences head and neck trauma and cannot provide a history consistent with the pattern of injuries. Multiple injuries or old, repeated injuries, delay in seeking care for injuries, and signs of neglect such as rampant caries or severe periodontal disease should alert the dental professional. Patient behavioral responses such as vague answers, or an overly protective, intrusive, or controlling partner joining the patient in the operatory, should raise the dental professionals' index of suspicion about the presence of IPV. If IPV is suspected or diagnosed by the dental team, the team must follow all state reporting requirements.
- Dental professionals should conduct an assessment for IPV for all patients who have experienced trauma to the head and neck. A model for assisting dental professionals in caring for patients who may be victims of IPV, called AVDR (steps are ask, validate, document, refer), has been shown to be effective[28]:
  - "Ask" refers to including questions about IPV in your dental history. Ask the patient in a nonjudgmental way and in private, if the patient has been a victim of IPV. Often patients do not want to discuss this or are

Figure 19.4 Pre and immediate post composite wire splint for patient who was hit in the mouth and sustained dento-alveolar fracture of lower incisor segment.

not ready to discuss this with a health professional requiring some persistence in questioning. The goal in questioning is not necessarily to "identify" the case but rather to begin the process of labeling the behavior as abuse. Victims of IPV have reported that when their health professionals labeled this behavior as abuse, it helped the victims to begin to recognize it, and ultimately take the needed steps to end the relationship. You may begin with "HATAH"—how are things at home?

- "Validate" refers to validating with the patient that battering is not normal behavior and that everyone deserves to feel safe in their home. Victims of IPV have reported that validating messages such as "you don't deserve to be abused" help, even when the patient is not ready to make a change.
- "Document" refers to the importance of your oral examination and dental record. Record all injuries both in written form and if possible with an intraoral camera. Identify the date of occurrence of the injuries, nature and physical description in as much detail as possible. Include in your record the words of the patient used to describe the injuries. If the patient ends the relationship or the matter becomes a criminal proceeding, your dental record may become evidence in any legal case.
- "Refer" If a patient reports that she is an IPV victim, provide referrals for her to the necessary medical and social services professionals. As dental professionals, we cannot solve the problem but we can assist our patients in identifying the resources they need to solve the problem. Some health professionals now place "shoe" referral cards (cards small enough to fit in the victim's shoe) about safe houses and homeless shelters in their rest rooms or dressing areas to assist individuals in seeking help to end abusive relationships.

Oral Lesions and Management

Temporomandibular Disorders (TMDs)

Most frequently in women of childbearing years, TMDs include a range of clinical problems involving the masticatory musculature, the temporomandibular joints (TMJs) and associated structures, or both.[29] TMDs are often associated with displacement of the disk and with arthritic and inflammatory changes in the joint. A good medical history, clinical examination, and imaging studies are necessary to make the diagnosis. Imaging includes an initial panoramic radiographic study; cone beam computed tomography (CBCT) to understand the nature of the osseous structures; and magnetic resonance imaging (MRI) as the gold standard for imaging TMD structure and allowing visualization of the disk, muscles of mastication, inflammatory changes, and effusions.[30] Treatment for these conditions is based on the diagnosis and focuses on addressing the causes of the joint pathology that led to the clinical problems, first with nonsurgical methods then using more invasive techniques only if the nonsurgical treatments are ineffective.

Menopausal Oral Mucosal Symptoms

Oral symptoms reported anecdotally include pain or burning sensations in the oral cavity, altered taste perceptions, and oral dryness. Treatment requires diagnoses of the underlying causes of these symptoms and use of palliative treatments. If a woman complains of oral dryness, salivary flow should be assessed to rule out Sjögren's disease. (For more on Sjögren's disease, see Chapter 10.)

Burning Mouth

Burning mouth has been defined as a chronic idiopathic oral pain condition characterized by burning pain in the tongue or oral mucous membranes without clinical lesion or laboratory findings of systemic disease.[31,32] It occurs more commonly in women after age 50 and is often associated with xerostomia and taste alterations. It has been associated with depression and anxiety in some patients and increasing pain throughout the day that results in sleep disturbances.

The etiology of burning mouth is unclear, but it has been proposed to be an oral dysesthesia or painful neuropathy.[32]

Workup involves the following:

- Clinical exam to rule out other possible causes of pain.
- Salivary flow evaluation to rule out salivary gland dysfunction.
- Oral cytology to rule out an oral candida infection.
- For the patient wearing dentures, the dentist should evaluate the lingual border of the mandibular denture to insure it is not impinging on the lingual nerve, causing pain or burning in the tongue.
- Patients may be encouraged to try a new toothpaste to insure that the ingredients in the toothpaste (e.g., cinnamon aldehyde flavoring) is not the cause of the burning.
- Blood studies should include a complete blood count (CBC) and differential, fasting glucose, iron, ferritin, folic acid, B_{12}, and a thyroid profile.

The diagnosis of burning mouth syndrome is made if the burning persists after all systemic and local factors are ruled out or treated.

Treatment of burning mouth is varied with uncertain success and includes the use of cognitive behavioral therapy, low-dose benzodiazepines, topical capsaicin, alpha-lipoic acid (ALA), clonazapam, tricyclic antidepressants, or anticonvulsants such as gabapentin.[32] Table 19.1 provides examples of medications that can be used to treat burning mouth.

Table 19.1. Medical Management of Burning Mouth Syndrome

Medications	Examples of Agents	Dosage	Common Prescription
Tricyclic antidepressants	Amitryptyline (Elavil®)	10–150 mg/day	10 mg at bedtime; increase dosage by 10 mg q4–7 days until oral burning is relieved or side effects occur
Benzodiazepines	Clonazepine (Klonopin®)	0.25–2 mg/day	0.25 mg at bedtime, increase dosage by 0.25 mg q4–7 days until oral burning is relieved or side effects occur
Anticonvulsants	Gabapentin (Neurontin®)	300–1600 mg/day	100 mg at bedtime; increase dosage by 100 mg q4–7 days until oral burning is relieved or side effects occur; as dosage increases, medication is taken in three divided doses

Modified from Grushka et al.[31]

Risks of Dental Care

Hemostasis

Women's health issues discussed in this chapter raise no increased risk for altered hemostasis.

Susceptibility to Infection

Oral, Transdermal, and Implanted Contraception Use Drugs

- Women taking hormonal contraceptives have been noted to have a higher risk for a localized osteitis (dry socket) after tooth extractions.
- Anecdotal reports suggest that scheduling dental extractions during nonestrogen days (days 23–28) of the oral birth control pill can lower the risk for this condition.

Drug Actions/Interactions

Pregnancy

Drugs that are known to be innocuous or have no effect on the developing fetus should be used during pregnancy. To guide health professionals in selecting medications, the U.S. Food and Drug Administration (FDA) developed a classification system to rate fetal risk associated with prescription medications. Drugs with unknown effects on the fetus should be avoided or used only in consultation with the patient's obstetrician. Drugs classified as A or B are recommended for use in pregnant patients. Drugs in the C category are sometimes administered during pregnancy. If these drugs are selected for use, consultation with the patient's obstetrician may be advisable prior to prescribing. Drugs in category D and X should be avoided during pregnancy.

Most of the drugs commonly used in dental practice can be used when caring for the pregnant patient. Table 19.2 provides a list of drugs used during dental practice and the FDA classification. Local anesthetics cross the placenta and enter the fetal circulation. Toxicological assessment of lidocaine administration in pregnant rats gave no indication of fetal toxicity.[33] Retrospective studies of pregnant women receiving local anesthesia during the 1st trimester of pregnancy have found no evidence of

> **FDA pregnancy classification categories**
>
> Five category system used by the FDA to classify systemically absorbed drugs based on their potential or known teratogenic effects.
>
> **A.** Adequate well-controlled studies in pregnant women have failed to demonstrate a risk to the fetus in the first trimester (and there is no evidence of a risk in later trimesters). The possibility of fetal harm appears remote.
> **B.** Animal-reproduction studies have failed to demonstrate a risk to the fetus and there are no adequate and well-controlled studies in pregnant women. OR Animal-reproduction studies have shown an adverse effect (other than decrease in fertility), but adequate and well-controlled studies in pregnant women have failed to demonstrate a risk to the fetus during the first trimester (and there is no evidence of a risk in later trimesters).
> **C.** Animal reproduction studies have shown an adverse effect on the fetus and there are no adequate and well-controlled studies in humans, and the benefits from the use of the drug in pregnant women may be acceptable despite its potential risks. OR There are no animal reproduction studies and no adequate and well-controlled studies in humans.
> **D.** There is positive evidence of human fetal risk based on adverse reaction data from investigational or marketing experience or studies in humans, but the potential benefits from the use of the drug in pregnant women may be acceptable despite its potential risks.
> **X.** If studies in animals or humans have demonstrated fetal abnormalities or there is positive evidence of fetal risk based on adverse reaction reports from investigational or marketing experience, or both, and the risk of the use of the drug in a pregnant woman clearly outweighs any possible benefit (e.g., safer drugs or other forms of therapy are available).
>
> These 1975 FDA categories are available at: http://www.accessdata.fda.gov/scripts/cdrh/cfdocs/cfcfr/cfrsearch.cfm?fr=201.57. Accessed January 23, 2012.
> There is an FDA proposal of a **New Pregnancy and Lactation Labeling Rule** under consideration that would give health-care providers better information for making prescribing decisions and for counseling women who are pregnant, breastfeeding, or of childbearing age. A summary for the proposed rule is available at: http://www.fda.gov/Drugs/DevelopmentApprovalProcess/DevelopmentResources/Labeling/ucm093310.htm.

fetal toxicity.[34] Since organogenesis occurs during the 1st trimester, routine dental care is recommended during the 2nd and 3rd trimester of pregnancy.

Breastfeeding

Many drugs used in dental practice can enter the breast milk of the nursing mother. Table 19.2 lists the drugs commonly used in dental practice and guidelines for their use with breastfeeding mothers. In addition, Appendix C in the ADA/PDR Guide to Dental Therapeutics provides a list of agents that are known to affect the fetus or nursing infant.[34]

Oral, Transdermal, and Implanted Contraception Use Drugs

The role of antibiotics in interfering with the effectiveness of oral contraceptives is controversial and a recent large case-crossover study has failed to demonstrate risk of breakthrough pregnancy.[35] The suggested biological

Table 19.2. Dental Drug Administration during Pregnancy and Breastfeeding

Drug	FDA Category	During Pregnancy	During Breastfeeding
Local anesthetics[a]			
Lidocaine	B	Yes	Yes
Mepivacaine	C	Use with caution; consult physician	Yes
Prilocaine	B	Yes	Yes
Bupivacaine	C	Use with caution; consult physician	Yes
Etidocaine	B	Yes	Yes
Procaine	C	Use with caution; consult physician	Yes
Analgesics			
Aspirin	C/D 3rd trimester	Caution; avoid in 3rd trimester	Avoid
Acetaminophen	B	Yes	Yes
Ibuprofen	B/D 3rd trimester	Caution; avoid in 3rd trimester	Yes
Codeine[b]	C	Use with caution; consult physician	Yes
Hydrocodone[b]	B	Use with caution; consult physician	Yes
Oxycodone[b]	B	Use with caution; consult physician	Yes
Propoxyphene	C	Use with caution; consult physician	Yes
Antibiotics			
Penicillins	B	Yes	Yes
Erythromycin	B	Yes; avoid estolate form	Yes
Clindamycin	B	Yes	Yes
Cephalosporins	B	Yes	Yes
Tetracycline	D	Avoid	Avoid
Metronidazole	B	Avoid; controversial	Avoid
Sedative hypnotics			
Benzodiazepines	D	Avoid	Avoid
Barbiturates	D	Avoid	Avoid
Nitrous oxide	Not assigned	Avoid in 1st trimester; otherwise, use with caution; consult physician	Yes

[a] Can use vasoconstrictors if necessary.
[b] Avoid prolonged use.
Source: American Dental Association. Women's Oral Health Issues. American Dental Association. Chicago, November 2006.

mechanism is that broad-spectrum antibiotics (e.g., ampicillin) might disrupt the intestinal bacterial flora, thus altering hormone levels by interfering with the enterohepatic recirculation of hormone metabolite. Should a dentist prescribe antibiotics to a woman taking oral contraceptives, the patient should be advised of the potential interaction between these medications resulting in decreased efficacy of the oral contraceptives for the hormonal cycle in which the antibiotics are taken, generally the subsequent 4 weeks.

Dentists who need to prescribe antibiotics for the woman on oral contraceptives should follow the ADA Council on Scientific Affairs[36] recommendations. These include "1) advise the patient to maintain compliance with oral contraceptives when using the antibiotics; 2) advise the patient of the potential risk for the antibiotics' reduction of the effectiveness of the oral contraceptive; 3) recommend that the patient discuss with her physician the use of an additional nonhormonal means of contraception."

Osteoporosis

Osteonecrosis of the jaw (ONJ) has been reported in patients taking bisphosphonates and other oral antiresorptive agents (see Table 19.3), leading the name of this necrotic bone sequelae to be changed from "bisphosphonate-associated osteonecrosis of the jaws" (BRONJ) to ARONJ. New recommendations from the ADA's Council on Scientific Affairs have been published on managing patients who are taking antiresorptive therapy for the prevention of osteoporosis.[27] The authors note that the risk of developing ARONJ in patients who do not have cancer appears to be low, at 0.00038–0.10%. ARONJ can occur spontaneously but is more commonly associated with specific medical or dental procedures that cause bone trauma, such as tooth extractions. The risk for ARONJ increases for patients over age 65, with periodontitis, taking bisphosphonates for more than 2 years, smoking, wearing a denture, and with diabetes. The dentist must be informed if a patient is taking an antiresorptive agent and must inform the patient of the ARONJ risk for certain dental procedures if the patient is taking these medications. See Table 19.4 for ARONJ prevention strategies.

Breast Cancer

Dental professionals should be alert to any patient with a malignancy who is receiving antiresorptive therapy or myelosuppressive and cytotoxic chemotherapy. Mucositis is a common side effect of chemotherapy agents used to treat breast cancer. For patients receiving bisphosphonates for bone metastases, such as those with metastatic breast cancer, the nitrogen-containing bisphosphonates typically delivered intravenously have been shown to have a greater risk of causing ARONJ, with cumulative incidence of 0.8–12% of patients (see Fig. 19.5). Patients receiving once monthly intravenous bisphosphonates may fail to report this medication use on the health history if they interpret the question as asking about oral medications. A specific query should be made about current or past use of bisphosphonate medications. The American Society of Clinical Oncology advised that all patients should receive a dental examination and appropriate preventive dentistry before bone-modifying agent therapy and maintain optimal oral health.[14]

A staging scheme, as shown in Table 19.5, has been proposed for ARONJ with management strategies suggested based on stage, as described in guidelines by the American Association of Oral and Maxillofacial Surgeons.[37]

Patient's Ability to Tolerate Dental Care

Pregnancy

- Increased treatment disruptions from increased need to urinate that accompanies the fetus placing pressure on the bladder.
- During the latter part of the 3rd trimester, the patient may have difficulty sitting in a reclining or semisupine position due to compression on the superior vena cava by the gravid uterus. This compression can cause maternal hypotension, decreased cardiac output, and eventual loss of consciousness. Turning the patient on her left side will relieve this pressure (see Fig. 19.6).

Table 19.3. Bisphosphonates and other Antiresorptive Agents

Drug	Dosing Interval	Indication
Parenteral drugs		
Pamidronate (Aredia®)	Monthly	Metastatic bone disease, multiple myeloma, hypercalcemia, Paget's disease of the bone
Zolendronic acid (Zometa®)	Monthly	Metastatic bone disease, multiple myeloma, hypercalcemia
Denosumab (Xgeva®)	Monthly	Metastatic bone disease, multiple myeloma, hypercalcemia
Zolendronic acid (Reclast®; Aclasta®[a])	Every 12 months' treatment; every 24 months' prevention	Osteoporosis, Paget's disease of the bone
Ibandronate (Boniva®)	Every 3 months	Osteoporosis
Denosumab (Prolia®)	Every 6 months	Osteoporosis
Clodronate (Bonefos[a])	Daily	Paget's disease of the bone, hypercalcemia from metastatic disease, multiple myeloma and parathyroid carcinoma
Oral drugs		
Alendronate (Fosamax®)	Daily or weekly	Osteoporosis, Paget's disease of the bone
Risedronate (Actonel®; Atelvia®)	Actonel®: daily, weekly, two consecutive days per month or monthly. Atelvia®: weekly	Osteoporosis, also Paget's disease of the bone for Actonel
Ibandronate (Boniva®)	Monthly	Osteoporosis
Etidronate (Didronel®)	Daily	Paget's disease of the bone, treat or prevent hypertrophic ossification after hip replacement, osteoporosis
Tilurdronate (Skelid®)	Daily	Paget's disease of the bone, osteoporosis
Clodronate (Bonefos[a])	Daily	Osteoporosis, hypercalcemia and osteolytic metastatic disease, reduce occurrence of bone metastases in primary breast cancer

[a] Not commercially available in the United States.

Table 19.4. Prevention Strategies for Patients Receiving Antiresorptive Therapy for Prevention and Treatment of Osteoporosis

Duration of Therapy	Oral Health Management Considerations
Before start	• Establish lifetime oral health awareness. • Remove unsalvageable teeth and perform invasive dentoalveolar procedures (more important for cancer patients receiving antiresorptive therapy). • Assess caries and periodontal risk, patient dental compliance and motivation to establish treatment plan in consultation with physician.
<2 years	• Continue as above. • ARONJ risk is very low. • Serum C-terminal telopeptide level testing is not recommended as it has no predictive reliability for ARONJ. • Chlorhexidine rinses are advised whenever periosteal or medullary bone exposure is anticipated or observed. • Dentoalveolar procedures involving periosteal penetration or intramedullary bone exposure (extractions, apicoectomies, periodontal surgery, implants or biopsies) carry minimal risk. • If multiple surgical needs, a trial segmental/sextant approach may help assess the patient's risk and reduce the risk of developing multifocal ARONJ.
≥2 years	• Continue as above. • Advise patient and physician who prescribe antiresorptive agents that the risk of ARONJ increases with extended drug use.
Any length of therapy	• Good oral health and routine dental care are always recommended. • The dentist should discuss antiresorptive therapy with the patient's physician as it relates to the patient's oral health with any decision to discontinue antiresorptive therapy based primarily on risk of fracture, not on risk of ARONJ. • No oral or maxillofacial surgery is strictly contraindicated, but plans that minimize periosteal and/or intrabony exposure and disruption are preferred. • All extractions or dentoalveolar surgery based on medical or dental emergencies are appropriate.

ARONJ, antiresorptive agent-induced osteonecrosis of the jaw.
Adapted from Hellstein et al.[27]

Figure 19.5 Osteonecrosis of the right mandible in an edentulous area in a 45-year-old woman with metastatic breast cancer on intravenous zolendronic acid for the prior 2 years.

Table 19.5. American Association of Oral and Maxillofacial Surgeons Recommendations for Management of Bisphosphonate Osteonecrosis of the Jaw

Bisphosphonate Osteonecrois of the Jaw Stage[a]	Treatment Strategies[b]
At risk: No apparent necrotic bone in asymptomatic patients who have been treated with intravenous or oral bisphosphonates.	No treatment indicated; patient education
Stage 0: No clinical evidence of necrotic bone, but nonspecific symptoms or clinical and radiographic findings: *Symptoms* • Odontalgia not explained by an odontogenic cause • Dull, aching bone pain in the body of the mandible, which may radiate to the temporomandibular joint region • Sinus pain, which may be associated with inflammation and thickening of the maxillary sinus wall • Altered neurosensory function *Clinical findings* • Loosening of teeth not explained by chronic periodontal disease • Periapical/periodontal fistula that is not associated with pulpal necrosis due to caries *Radiographic findings* • Alveolar bone loss or resorption not attributable to chronic periodontal disease • Changes to trabecular pattern—dense woven bone and persistence of unremodeled bone in extraction sockets • Thickening/obscuring of periodontal ligament (thickening of the lamina dura and decreased size of the periodontal ligament space) • Inferior alveolar canal narrowing	Systemic management, including antibiotics and pain medication

Table 19.5. (Continued)

Bisphosphonate Osteonecrois of the Jaw Stage[a]	Treatment Strategies[b]
Stage 1: Exposed and necrotic bone in patients who are asymptomatic and have no evidence of infection.	Antibacterial mouth rinse; clinical follow-up on a quarterly basis; patient education and review of indications for continued bisphosphonate therapy
Stage 2: Exposed and necrotic bone in patients with pain and clinical evidence of infection.	Symptomatic treatment with oral antibiotics; oral antibacterial mouth rinse; pain control; superficial debridement to relieve soft tissue irritation
Stage 3: Exposed and necrotic bone in patients with pain, infection, and one or more of the following: • Exposed necrotic bone extending beyond the region of alveolar bone, that is inferior border and ramus in the mandible, maxillary sinus, and zygoma in the maxilla • Pathological fracture • Extraoral fistula • Oral antral/oral nasal communication • Osteolysis extending to the inferior border of the mandible or sinus floor	Antibacterial mouth rinse; antibiotic therapy and pain control; surgical debridement/resection for longer-term palliation of infection and pain

[a] Exposed bone in the maxillofacial region without resolution in 8–12 weeks in person treated with bisphosphonate, but not radiation therapy.
[b] Regardless of stage, mobile segments of bony sequestrum should be removed without exposing uninvolved bone. Symptomatic teeth in exposed bone should be extracted. If systemic conditions permit, modification or cessation of bisphosphonates should be done only in consultation with the treating physician and patient. There is limited benefit unless discontinuation exceeds 6 months. Adapted from Ruggiero et al.[37]

Figure 19.6 Pregnant patient comfort during dental treatment. (a) Pregnant patient in 2nd trimester. Left lateral decubitus position. Using a support under the right hip and buttocks to create a 15-degree elevation can help to prevent supine hypotensive syndrome where decreased blood pressure and cardiac output result from gravid uterus compression on inferior vena cava. (b) Rolled to the left. Recovery position from supine hypotensive syndrome.

IV. Recommended Readings and Cited References

Recommended Readings

American Dental Association Council on Scientific Affairs. Dental management of patients receiving oral bisphosphonate therapy: expert panel recommendations. J Am Dent Assoc 2006;137(8): 1144–50.

American Dental Association Council on Scientific Affairs. Professionally applied topical fluorides. Evidence based clinical recommendations. J Am Dent Assoc 2006;137(8):1151–9.

Giglio JA, Lanni SM, Laskin DM, Giglio NW. Oral health care for the pregnant patient. J Can Dent Assoc 2009;75(1):43–8.

Lyons MF. Current practice in the management of temporomandibular disorders. Dent Update 2008; 35(5):314–6, 318.

Cited References

1. U.S. Public Health Service. Report of the public health service task force on women's health issues. Public Health Rep 1985;100:73–106.
2. Wizemann TM, Pardue ML, eds. Exploring the Biological Contributions to Human Health. Does Sex Matter? 2001. National Academy Press, Washington, DC. Available at: http://www.nap.edu/openbook.php?isbn=0309072816. Accessed January 22, 2012.
3. Biro FM, Galvez MP, Greenspan LC, Succop PA, Vangeepuram N, Pinney SM, et al. Pubertal assessment method and baseline characteristics in a mixed longitudinal study of girls. Pediatrics 2010;126(3):e583–e590.
4. Centers for Disease Control and Prevention. 2006. *Understanding intimate partner violence*. Available at: http://www.cdc.gov. Accessed January 12, 2012.
5. Gunter J. Intimate partner violence. Obstet Gynecol Clin North Am 2007;34(3):368–88.
6. American Cancer Society. 2011. *Breast cancer: facts and figures 2011–2012*. Atlanta, GA. 36 pp. Available at: http://www.cancer.org/Research/CancerFactsFigures/BreastCancerFactsFigures/breast-cancer-facts-and-figures-2011-2012. Accessed January 22, 2012.
7. Martin JA, Hamilton BE, Ventura SJ, Osterman MJ, Kirmeyer S, Matthews TJ, et al. Births: final data for 2009. Natl Vital Stat Rep 2011;60(1):1–104. Available at: http://www.cdc.gov/nchs/data/nvsr/nvsr60/nvsr60_01.pdf. Accessed January 22, 2012.
8. Centers for Disease Control and Prevention. 2011. *Breastfeeding among US children born 2000–2008, CDC national immunization survey*. Available at: http://www.cdc.gov/breastfeeding/data/NIS_data/index.htm. Accessed December 31, 2011.
9. The Alan Guttmacher Institute. *Facts on contraceptive use in the United States*. New York. June, 2010. Available at: http://www.guttmacher.org. Accessed December 31, 2011.
10. International Osteoporosis Foundation. 2011. *Facts and statistics about osteoporosis and its impact*. Available at: http://www.iofbonehealth.org. Accessed December 31, 2011.
11. Department of Justice. Bureau of Justice Statistics. Intimate Partner Violence. 2000. U.S. Department of Justice, Washington DC.
12. Black MC, Basile KC, Breiding MJ, Smith SG, Walters ML, Merrick MT, et al. *The National Intimate Partner and Sexual Violence Survey*. 2010 Summary Report. Atlanta, GA: National Center for Injury Prevention and Control. Centers for Disease Control and Prevention, 2011. Available at: http://www.cdc.gov/ViolencePrevention/pdf/NISVS_Report2010-a.pdf. Accessed January 22, 2012.
13. American College of Obstetricians and Gynecologists Committee on Gynecologic Practice. ACOG Committee Opinion No. 420, November 2008: hormone therapy and heart disease. Obstet Gynecol 2008;112(5):1189–92.
14. Van Poznak CH, Temin S, Yee GC, Janjan NA, Barlow WE, Biermann JS, et al. American Society of Clinical Oncology executive summary of the clinical practice guideline update on the role of bone-modifying agents in metastatic breast cancer. J Clin Oncol 2011;29(9):1221–7.
15. Russell SL, Ickovics JR, Yaffee RA. Parity & untreated dental caries in US women. J Dent Res 2010;89(10):1091–6.
16. Leverett D. Appropriate uses of systemic fluoride: considerations for the 90s. J Public Health Dent 1991;51(1):42–7.
17. Offenbacher S, Katz V, Fertik G, Collins J, Boyd D, Maynor G, et al. Periodontal infection as a

possible risk factor for preterm low birth weight. J Periodontol 1996;67(10 Suppl.):1103–13.
18. Jeffcoat MK, Hauth JC, Geurs NC, Reddy MS, Cliver SP, Hodgkins PM, et al. Periodontal disease and preterm birth: results of a pilot intervention study. J Periodontol 2003;74(8):1214–8.
19. Lopez N, Smith PC, Gutierrez J. Higher risk of preterm birth and low birth weight in women with periodontal disease. J Dent Res 2002;81(1):58–63.
20. Davenport ES, Williams CE, Sterne JA, Murad S, Sivapathasundram V, Curtis MA. Maternal periodontal disease and preterm low birthweight: case-control study. J Dent Res 2002;81(5):313–8.
21. Uppal A, Uppal S, Pinto A, Dutta M, Shirvatsa S, Dandolu V, et al. The effectiveness of periodontal disease treatment during pregnancy in reducing the risk of experiencing preterm birth and low birth weight. J Am Dent Assoc 2010;141(12):1423–34.
22. Fontana M, Zero DT. Assessing patients' caries risk. J Am Dent Assoc 2006;137(9):1231–39.
23. Dye BA, Vargas CM, Lee JJ, Magder L, Tinanoff N. Assessing the relationship between children's oral health status and that of their mothers. J Am Dent Assoc 2011;142(2):173–83.
24. Brent RL. Commentary on JAMA article by Hujoel et al. Health Phys 2005;88(4):379–81.
25. Garcia AG, Grana PM, Sampedro FG, Diago MP, Rey JM. Does oral contraceptive use affect the incidence of complications after extraction of a mandibular third molar? Br Dent J 2003;194(8):453–5.
26. Catellani JE, Harvey S, Erickson SH, Cherkin D. Effect of oral contraceptive cycle on dry socket (localized alveolar osteitis). J Am Dent Assoc 1980;101(5):777–80.
27. Hellstein JW, Adler RA, Edwards B, Jacobsen PL, Kalmar JR, Koka S, et al. Managing the care of patients receiving antiresorptive therapy for prevention and treatment of osteoporosis. J Am Dent Assoc 2011;142(11):1243–51.
28. Love C, Gerbert B, Caspers N, Bronstone A, Perry D, Bird W. Dentists' attitudes and behaviors regarding domestic violence: the need for an effective response. J Am Dent Assoc 2001;132:85–93.
29. Dym H, Israel H. Diagnosis and treatment of temporomandibular disorders. Dent Clin North Am 2012;56(1):149–61.
30. Wiese M, Wenzel A, Hintze H, Petersson A, Knutsson K, Bakke M, et al. Influence of cross-section temporomandibular joint tomography on diagnosis and management decisions of patients with temporomandibular joint disorders. J Orofac Pain 2011;25(3):223–31.
31. Grushka M, Epstein JB, Gorsky M. Burning mouth syndrome. Am Fam Physician 2002;65(4):615–20.
32. Patton LL, Siegel MA, Benoliel R, De Laat A. Management of burning mouth syndrome: systematic review and management recommendations. Oral Surg Oral Med Oral Pathol Oral Radiol Endod 2007;103(Suppl.):S39.e1–13.
33. Ramazzotto LJ, Curro FA, Paterson JA, Tanner P, Coleman M. Toxicological assessment of lidocaine in the pregnant rat. J Dent Res 1985;64(10):1214–7.
34. Ciancio SG, ed. ADA/PDR Guide to Dental Therapeutics, 5th ed. 2009. American Dental Association, Chicago, IL.
35. Toh S, Mitchell AA, Anderka M, De Jong-Van Den Berg LT, Hernández-Díaz S; National Birth Defects Prevention Study. Antibiotics and oral contraceptive failure—a case-crossover study. Contraception 2011;83(5):418–25.
36. ADA Council on Scientific Affairs. Antibiotic interference with oral contraceptives. J Am Dent Assoc 2002;133:880.
37. Ruggiero SL, Dodson TB, Assael LA, Landesberg R, Marx RE, Mehrotra B, et al. American association of oral and maxillofacial surgeons position paper on bisphosphonate-related osteonecrosis of the jaw—2009 update. Aust Endod J 2009;35(3):119–30.

Medical Emergencies

Lauren L. Patton DDS

I. General Principals of Emergency Medical Care

Medical emergencies are best prevented. Regardless of prevention approaches, emergencies occur in dental practice, and preparation

> **Keys to prevention of medical emergencies in the dental office**
>
> **"Never treat a stranger."**
> - Obtain written and interview dialog health history or updates at each visit.
> - Obtain vital signs at initial and recall exams and prior to use of local anesthetic or surgical procedures, or more frequently as health history dictates.
> - Make needed treatment modifications, including use of stress and anxiety management protocols.
> - Recognize early signs of patient distress and address the cause to prevent escalation, including terminating dental treatment if needed.

enhances the dental team's ability to recognize patient distress and react immediately to the emergency. Obtaining adequate perioperative pain, fear, and anxiety control plays an important role in preventing escalation of the stress response into an emergency situation.

Preparation includes dentist and staff training and maintaining in the office basic airway rescue and monitoring equipment and basic emergency medications.

The likelihood of a competent and timely initial emergency response in the dental office is enhanced by the dental team receiving annual medical emergency education updates. Team participation in mock medical emergency drills in the office, were members actually rehearse the roles they would play in responding to potential emergency scenarios, can create a safer dental office environment.[1-3] Emergency response scenarios that are routinely practiced by the dental team in a nonemergency situation, will come more naturally, without the initial panic typically generated by the emergency, should the emergency situation arise

The ADA Practical Guide to Patients with Medical Conditions, First Edition. Edited by Lauren L. Patton.
© 2012 American Dental Association. Published 2012 by John Wiley & Sons, Inc.

with a real patient where response times and professional decision making can matter between life and death or morbidity.

> **Keys to preparation for managing medical emergencies**
>
> - Learn to identify signs of patient distress related to the most common medical emergencies in the dental office.
> - Maintain current basic life support (BLS) certification for all office staff.
> - Attend continuing education courses in emergency medicine.
> - Conduct periodic office "mock" emergency drills.
> - Post the telephone number of the emergency medical response service (e.g., 911) near each telephone.
> - Maintain an updated emergency drug kit and automated external defibrillator equipment, where required by state law, and have staff demonstrate the knowledge to properly use all items.

Figure 20.1 Portable oxygen cylinder with regulator and nasal cannula and nonrebreathing mask in plastic attached of handle of cart.

> **Basic medical emergency equipment for the dental office**
>
> - Portable oxygen cylinder (E size) with regulator (see Fig. 20.1)
> - Supplemental oxygen delivery devices (nasal cannula, non-rebreathing mask with oxygen reservoir, nasal hood)
> - Bag/valve/mask device with oxygen reservoir (see Fig. 20.2)
> - Oropharyngeal airway (adult sizes 7, 8, 9 cm)
> - Magill forceps
> - Automated external defibrillator
> - Stethoscope
> - Sphygmomanometer with adult small, medium, and large cuff sizes
> - Wall clock with second hand

Figure 20.2 Bag/valve/mask.

> **Oxygen delivery systems**
>
> - Positive pressure/demand valve:
>   - Full mask permitting 100% O_2 delivery
> - Bag/valve/mask device:
>   - Full mask permitting delivery of 21% O_2 ambient air, or enriched O_2 if attached to an E cylinder (25–90% O_2)
> - Pocket mask:
>   - Face mask that permits mouth-to-mask ventilation, providing 16% O_2 (exhaled air)

As shown in Table 20.1, surveys of dentists indicate that vasovagal syncope, affecting most dentists, is the most commonly reported

Table 20.1. Frequency of Occurrence of Medical Emergencies in Dental Practices, Based on Dentist Surveys

Order	United States (Malamed[4])		United States (Fast et al.[5])		Germany (Müller et al.[6])		Britain (Girdler and Smith[7])	
	Survey of Dentists, n = 2704 Relative Prevalence of Episodes Reported in a 10-Year Period		Survey of Dentists, n = 1605 Relative Prevalence of Episodes Reported in a 10-Year Period		Survey of Dentists, n = 620 Yearly Prevalence		Survey of Dentists, n = 302 Yearly Prevalence	
	Emergency	% Episodes Reported	Emergency	% Episodes Reported	Emergency	% Dentists Affected	Emergency	% Dentists Affected
1	Vasovagal syncope	30.1	Vasovagal syncope	67.0	Vasovagal syncope	57.7	Vasovagal syncope	62.9
2	Mild allergic reaction	18.7	Angina	11.4	Seizures	6.8	Angina	11.9
3	Postural hypotension	17.9	Asthma	6.0	Hypertensive crisis	6.6	Epileptic fit	9.9
4	Hyperventilation	9.6	Seizures	5.7	Asthma	3.9	Hypoglycemia	9.6
5	Hypoglycemia	5.1	Epinephrine reaction	5.4	Hypoglycemia	3.5	Asthma	4.6
6	Angina	4.6	Cardiac arrest	1.1	Acute coronary syndrome	3.5	Choking	4.5
7	Seizures	4.6	Hypoglycemia	1.1	Anaphylaxis	1.1	Anaphylaxis	0.9
8	Asthma	2.8	Anaphylactic reaction	0.8	Airway obstruction	0.8	Hypertensive crisis	0.9
9	Local anesthetic overdose	1.5	Diabetic coma	0.6	Stroke	0.6	Myocardial infarction	0.7
10	Myocardial infarction	1.4	Myocardial infarction	0.6	Cardiac arrest	0.3	Cardiac arrest	0.3
11	Anaphylactic reaction	1.2	Acute pulmonary edema (heart failure)	0.2	Other emergencies	2.9	Unspecified collapse	2.3
12	Cardiac arrest	1.1						
13	Acute pulmonary edema	0.8						

427

emergency episode in dental offices.[4-7] Other common emergencies include angina/acute coronary syndrome, mild allergic reactions, seizures, postural hypotension, asthma, hypoglycemia, hyperventilation, hypertensive crisis/epinephrine reaction, choking/airway obstruction, myocardial infarction, local anesthetic overdose, anaphylaxis, and cardiac arrest.[4-7]

When the emergency medical service (EMS) first responders are called to the office, the dental team should be prepared to quickly and efficiently relay information about the patient, the emergency situation, and the efforts made to manage the condition.

> **Information the dental staff should give to emergency medical service (EMS) and first responders**
>
> - **Presumed diagnosis** (e.g., "possible myocardial infarction")
> - **Patient information** (e.g., "Mr. Smith is a 63-year-old male with a history of angina, currently experiencing chest pain not relieved by sublingual nitroglycerin. He is conscious, with blood pressure of 161/93 and heart rate of 88 beats per minute.")
> - **Current patient supportive care** (e.g., "The patient is supine and has received three sequential sublingual nitroglycerine tablets, followed by 325 mg chewed aspirin. The patient is receiving 4 L of oxygen by face mask.")
> - **Location of office where emergency responders need to report** (e.g., "Dr. Sweet's dental office on the ground floor suite 100 at 495 East Avenue at the corner of East Avenue and Northern Boulevard.")
> - **Phone number from which the call is being made** (The dental staff caller should stay on the line with EMS until they have arrived at the office. Giving the phone number allows EMS responders to contact the office should the line be inadvertently disconnected.)

II. Emergency Drugs and Use

Emergency drugs that the dentist knows how to use should be readily available.[1] While there is no universal agreement as to which drugs should be included in the basic kit, most agree upon inclusion of a positive pressure oxygen delivery system, 1:1000 injectable epinephrine, injectable histamine-blocker-diphenhydramine, nitroglycerine sublingual tablet or spray, bronchodialator-albuterol, aspirin, glucose-sugar packet, and aromatic ammonia as shown in Table 20.2.[1,2] Emergency kits should be routinely maintained with replacement of soon to expire medications. Dentists should consult their state laws and liability insurance carrier to ascertain if there is a mandated list of emergency drugs and equipment that they must have available at the office.[2] Increasingly, states are requiring dental offices to have an automated external defibrillator (AED) on-site and have staff trained in its use.

Depending on the dentist's level of training in management of medical emergencies, types of procedures and techniques, levels of sedation offered, and special needs of the dental office, additional emergency drugs such as naloxone, flumazenil, midazolam, morphine, nitrous oxide, hydrocortisone, ephedrine, atropine, and glucagon may be warranted.[1,8]

III. Common Emergencies, Recognition, and Initial Management

The basic components of position (P), airway (A), breathing (B), circulation (C), and definitive treatment (D) (differential diagnosis, drugs, defibrillation) applies to each medical emergency.[9] However, the American Heart Association's Healthcare Provider guidelines

Table 20.2. Basic Emergency Drugs for the Dental Office

Drug	Indication	Action	Administration
Epinephrine	Bronchospasm (severe allergic reaction, severe asthma)	α- and β-adrenergic receptor agonist (bronchodilator)	1:1000 solution, subcutaneously, intramuscularly, or sublingually; dose 0.3 mg adults, 0.15 mg children
Diphenhydramine	Mild allergic reaction	Antihistamine	50 mg intramuscularly; 25–50 mg orally every 3–4 hours
Nitroglycerine	Angina	Vasodilator	Sublingual spray: 0.4 mg per metered dose, one spray every 5 minutes up to three times; sublingual tablet: one every 5 minutes up to three doses
Albuterol	Bronchospasm (mild asthma)	Selective β2-adrenergic receptor agonist	Inhaler: two to three inhalations every 1–2 minutes, up to three times
Aspirin	Myocardial infarction	Antiplatelet	One full-strength 325 mg tablet (not enteric coated) chewed and swallowed
Glucose (orange juice, sugar packet, glucagon)	Hypoglycemia (insulin shock)	Antihypoglycemic	If the patient is conscious, ingest
Aromatic ammonia (see Fig. 20.3)	Syncope	Respiratory stimulant	Inhalant crushed and held 4–6 inches under the nose

Figure 20.3 Crushable ammonia inhalant (close-up, see insert) affixed to each operatory overhead light for ease of access. Tape holding stimulant is marked with expiration date. Aromatic ammonia spirit crushed and held 4 inches from the nose, acts as a respiratory stimulant for syncope treatment by causing peripheral irritation of the sensory receptors in the nasal mucous membranes. Avoid use in patients with known respiratory disease.

for cardiopulmonary resuscitation (CPR) changed in 2010 for the unresponsive adult victim with no breathing or no normal breathing (i.e., only gasping) to C-A-B: compressions (C), airway (A), and breathing (B).[10] For healthcare providers, the 2010 CPR changes are deletion of the initial sequence of opening the airway, look/listen/feel while crouching over the patient, and giving a subsequent two breaths in the nonresponsive nonbreathing patient prior to pulse assessment and starting compressions.[10] The new emphasis is on immediate activation of EMS, simultaneous check for unresponsiveness and lack of adequate breathing, and lack of pulse (within 10 seconds), chest compressions started early and delivered at a rate of at least a 100/minute, with use of the AED when available. The airway is opened and two breaths are given after each set of 30 chest compressions at a depth of at least 2 inches.[10]

Typically, the position is supine for the unconscious patient, Trendelenburg (see Fig. 20.4) for the patient with syncope, and whatever position is most comfortable for the conscious distressed patient. Airway, breathing, and circulation should be supported first, followed by consideration of drug therapy.

Conditions of unconsciousness, respiratory difficulty, and chest pain that create emergency management needs in dental practices are discussed below.

Unconsciousness

Vasovagal Syncope

Cause: Decreased cerebral blood flow due to fear, anxiety, stress, and/or pain.

Prevention: Identify patients at risk; adequate sedation; administer oxygen; place patient in supine position for injection.

Signs and Symptoms:
  Early: Diaphoresis/complaints of warmth, tachycardia, nausea, pale appearance.
  Late: Hypotension, bradycardia, hyperpnea, pupillary dilation, visual disturbances, dizziness, loss of consciousness.

Management: Place patient in Trendelenburg (head down position) (pregnant patient in the left lateral position). Establish airway and administer oxygen; monitor vital signs; reassure and support patients, cold towels to head; aromatic ammonia, if available. If delayed recovery (>5 minutes unconsciousness or >20 minutes until complete recovery), consider other causes and need for medical assessment; must be accompanied if sent home.

Figure 20.4 Dental chair in sitting position (left panel) and Trendelenburg (right panel) where the patient's feet are 15–30 degrees higher than the head.

Hypoglycemia (Insulin Shock)

Cause: Blood glucose <70 mg/dL (normal before meal blood glucose range 70–130 mg/dL).

Prevention: Assure insulin-using diabetics have eaten a meal (more than having had morning coffee or tea) prior to the dental appointment. Have patient bring own home glucose monitor and check blood sugar level prior to treatment.

Signs and Symptoms:
  Early: Nervousness, shakiness, nausea, weakness, hunger, headache, tachycardia.
  Late: Increasingly bizarre behavior, diminished cerebral function, seizure activity, unconsciousness.

Management: Administer oxygen, check glucose level, administer glucose as needed.
  Glucose administration:
    Responsive patient: Give 15–20 g of carbohydrates or three to four chewable glucose tablets; after 15 minutes, recheck vitals and glucose levels and treat again if warranted. Give ½ cup regular (not diet) soda; give 15 mL (tbs) sugar dissolved in water (target glucose >70 mg/dL).
    Unresponsive patient: Start IV or IM 1 ampule 50% dextrose (D50) or glucagon injection: if >44 lb (20 kg) = 1 mg; if <44 lb (20 kg) = 0.5 mg. May inject glucagon into muscle or subcutaneous tissue in upper arm or thigh. Place patient on side, monitor vital signs and neurological status.

Hyperglycemia (Diabetic Ketoacidosis)

Cause: Excess blood glucose (usually >300 mg/dL) due to not enough insulin (normal before meal blood glucose range 70–130 mg/dL).

Prevention: Adequate insulin management, prevention of acute dental infection in diabetics. Have patient bring own home glucose monitor and check blood sugar level prior to treatment.

Signs and Symptoms:
  Early: Increased thirst and urination, high blood glucose level.
  Late: Shortness of breath, fruity breath odor, nausea and vomiting, decreased consciousness.

Management: Prevention is key. Patient may require insulin adjustment or initiation.

Convulsions/Seizures

Cause: Epilepsy, hypoglycemia, hypoxia following syncope, intracranial pathology, local anesthetic overdose. Predisposing factors include anticonvulsant medication noncompliance, fatigue and/or stress, flickering lights.

Prevention: Appropriate management of hypoglycemia and syncope. Avoidance of local anesthetic overdose. For epileptics: careful seizure history and medication use history. Consider sedation with nitrous oxide/oxygen or benzodiazepines.

Signs and Symptoms: Preseizure aura: for example, visual and auditory premonitions, taste and smell changes.

Management: Administer oxygen, protect head and neck from injury, supportive airway measures. In prolonged seizures (>5 minutes; status epilepticus), activate EMS and consider parenteral administration of a benzodiazepine.

Respiratory Difficulty

Hyperventilation

Cause: Ventilation in excess of that required to maintain a normal PaO_2 and $PaCO_2$.

Prevention: Manage anxiety.

Signs and Symptoms: Anxiety, hypertension, tachycardia, elevated respiratory rate, muscle pain, cramps, tingling and numbness of extremities, dizziness, chest pain.

Management: Suspend or terminate procedure, position patient sitting upright, monitor vital signs, do not give oxygen, have patient rebreathe exhaled air (e.g., into a brown paper bag, full face mask, hands cupped over face), reassure patient.

Asthmatic Attack

Cause: Bronchospasm, inflammation, and increased mucus production resulting in reduced airflow.

Prevention: In severe asthmatic, preprocedure use of bronchodilator may be beneficial. Avoid known triggers of asthmatic attacks.

Signs and Symptoms:
  Early: Wheezing, coughing, rapid breathing, chest pain or pressure, pale, sweaty face.
  Late: Cyanotic lips, "silent chest" where lungs tighten to the point of lack of airflow stopping the wheezing sound.

Management: Terminate procedure and assist patient with best positioning, typically sitting. Administer albuterol (Proventil® HFA) bronchodilator in metered-dose inhaler (MDI) with supplemental oxygen as needed.
  Proventil administration: Sitting upright, breathe out fully, place mouthpiece between teeth and seal lips around it, press down on inhaler to release mist of drug and breathe in slowly; hold breath for about 10 seconds.
Monitor vital signs and reassure patient. If no improvement, consider additional inhaler treatment or activating EMS.

Anaphylaxis/Life-Threatening Allergic Reaction

Cause: Medications (aspirin, ibuprofen, penicillin, biological modifiers like cetuximab, infliximab, and omalizumab), latex, radio-contrast dye, foods, insect venom, and exercise.

Prevention: Avoid contact with allergens to which patient is allergic or has demonstrated a past anaphylactic response.

Signs and Symptoms:
  Skin reaction: Urticaria (hives), angioedema.
  Respiratory reaction: Rhinitis, laryngeal edema, bronchospasm.
  Cardiovascular reaction: Circulatory collapse, dysrhythmias, cardiac arrest.

Management: Activate EMS. Administer parenteral epinephrine, albuterol MDI and oxygen. Prepare for CPR and use of an AED.
  Epinephrine administration: Epinephrine 0.3–0.5 mL IM injectable (1:000 concentration).
    Adult: 0.3 mL of 1:1000 Epi = 0.3 mg.
    Child: 0.3 mL of 1:2000 Epi = 0.15 mg.
  Alternative: EpiPen® Auto-Injector (see Fig. 20.5); only effective for 10–15 minutes, typically until EMS responds.
    Adult: EpiPen Auto-Injector; dose: 0.3 mg (0.3 mL, 1:1000); for patient >66 lb; >30 kg.
    Child: EpiPen Auto-Injector; dose: 0.15 mg (0.3 mL, 1:2000); for patient 33–66 lb; 15–30 kg.
    EpiPen Auto-Injector Administration: Pull off safety release cap; firmly push tip against outer thigh until a "click" is heard; hold on outer thigh for 10 seconds to deliver drug.

Note: Non-life-threatening allergic reaction can be treated with Benadryl® (diphenhydramine) 50 mg for adults or 1 mg/kg for children.

Aspiration or Swallowing a Foreign Object

Cause: Patient in reclined position and object falls in posterior oropharynx. Object is typically a tooth or root during extraction or crown/bridge during try-in and cementation.

Figure 20.5 (a) EpiPen Auto-Injector (yellow label) and trainer (blue label). (b) Diagram of how to administer.

Prevention: Use of a gauze throat screen, throat pack, or rubber dam during procedures.
Signs and Symptoms:
  Aspiration: Choking, coughing, high-pitched wheezing, cyanosis, absence of air entry, asymmetrical chest movement.
  Swallowed object: None early; the majority pass safely through the gastrointestinal tract and are passed in the feces. Patients may develop vague sensation of something being stuck in the center of the chest or epigastric region. Drooling, gagging, vomiting, retching, inability to swallow fluids, neck and throat pain, and abdominal distension may result. Gastrointestinal perforation is rare.
Management: Determine if foreign object was swallowed or aspirated. Remain with patient and monitor signs and symptoms, observing for respiratory distress. Aspiration is life threatening. Activate EMS and provide oxygen. If there is complete airway obstruction, provide Heimlich maneuver and prepare for CPR. Chest radiograph, computed tomography (CT) scans, endoscopy, and other test may be needed to identify location of object.

Chest Pain

Angina

Cause: Chest pain caused by transient myocardial ischemia without necrosis of the heart muscle signifying significant coronary artery disease. Myocardial oxygen demand is greater than oxygen delivery.
Prevention: Avoid precipitating episodes that produce increase in myocardial oxygen requirement, such as physical exertion, stress, hot humid environment, or cold weather. Administer oxygen, sedation with nitrous oxide/oxygen, obtain good local anesthesia.
Signs and Symptoms: Dull, usually substernal pain, described as tightness, pressing, or burning. Pain may radiate to left shoulder

and arm and be relieved by rest or nitroglycerin. Usually accompanied by elevated blood pressure and tachycardia.

Management: Stop treatment and place the patient in the most comfortable position, administer oxygen, monitor vital signs, use nitroglycerin sublingual spray or tablet. If no relief after third spray or tablet, activate EMS as patient needs medical assessment to rule out myocardial infarction. If no history of prior chest pain episodes, activate EMS immediately.

Nitroglycerine administration: One spray lingually or sublingually or one tablet (0.3–0.4 mg) sublingually. Repeat every 5 minutes as needed, up to three times. Do not use for systolic BP <90 mmHg. If no relief after 3rd dose, patient needs medical assessment to rule out myocardial infarction (MI). (Note: Nitroglycerine spray bottle should be primed before first use. Do not shake. Point away from you and depress nozzle once, a "click" should be heard indicating it is ready to spray onto or under the tongue.)

Myocardial Infarction

Cause: Usually coronary occlusion due to atherosclerotic clot leads to inadequate blood supply to the heart muscle, leading to muscle necrosis, electrical instability, and finally death.

Prevention: Diet, physical activity, body weight maintenance, smoking cessation, cholesterol control, hypertension control.

Signs and Symptoms: Severe chest pain or discomfort unrelieved by nitroglycerin, weakness/dizziness, nausea, vomiting, diaphoresis, palpitations, premature ventricular contractions.

Management: Activate EMS. Administer oxygen at 4 L/min, nitroglycerin, and crushed non-enteric coated aspirin placed sublingually. (Aspirin is contraindicated in aspirin allergy, active bleeding or bleeding disorder, patients on warfarin.) Prepare for CPR and use of an AED.

IV. Recommended Readings and Cited References

Recommended Readings

Malamed SF. Medical Emergencies in the Dental Office, 6th ed. 2007. Elsevier Health Sciences, Philadelphia, PA.

Niwa H, Hirota Y, Shibutani T, Matsuura H. Systemic emergencies and their management in dentistry: complications independent of underlying disease. Anesth Prog 1996;43(1):29–35.

Cited References

1. Rosenberg M. Preparing for medical emergencies: the essential drugs and equipment for the dental office. J Am Dent Assoc 2010;141(Suppl. 1):14S–9S.
2. ADA Council on Scientific Affairs. Office emergencies and emergency kits. J Am Dent Assoc 2002;133(3):364–5.
3. Haas DA. Preparing the dental office staff members for emergencies: developing a basic action plan. J Am Dent Assoc 2010;141(Suppl. 1):8S–13S.
4. Malamed SF. Managing medical emergencies. J Am Dent Assoc 1993;124(8):40–53.
5. Fast TB, Martin MD, Ellis TM. Emergency preparedness: a survey of dental practitioners. J Am Dent Assoc 1986;112(4):499–501.
6. Müller MP, Hänsel M, Stehr SN, Weber S, Koch T. A state-wide survey of medical emergency management in dental practices: incidence of emergencies and training experience. Emerg Med J 2008;25(5):296–300.
7. Girdler NM, Smith DG. Prevalence of emergency events in British dental practice and emergency management skills of British dentists. Resuscitation 1999;41(2):159–67.
8. Haas DA. Management of medical emergencies in the dental office: conditions in each country,

the extent of treatment by the dentist. Anesth Prog 2006;53:20–6.
9. Reed KL. Basic management of medical emergencies: recognizing a patient's distress. J Am Dent Assoc 2010;141(Suppl. 1):20S–4S.
10. Hazinski MF, ed. Highlights of the 2010 American Heart Association Guidelines for CPR and ECC. 2010. American Heart Association, Dallas, TX. Available at: http://www.heart.org/idc/groups/heart-public/@wcm/@ecc/documents/downloadable/ucm_317350.pdf. Accessed December 30, 2011.

Index

Note: Page numbers in *italics* indicate figures; those in **boldface**, tables.

ablative radioactive iodine therapy (I^{131}), 88
absence seizures, 283
acamprosate (Campral), 337
acquired immune deficiency syndrome (AIDS), 149
  coordination with physician of patient with, 219
  definition of, 217, **219**
  dental management
    evaluation, 223
    questions for patient with, 223
    treatment modifications, 223–224
  epidemiology of, 218
  medical management
    identification, 220
    laboratory testing, 220–222, *222*
    medical history, 220
    physical examination, 220
    treatment, 222–223
  pathogenesis/etiology, 217
acquired immunodeficiency syndrome (AIDS)
  antiretroviral drugs for, **233–236**
  dental management
    coinfections of, 224–225
    oral lesions, 225, **225–226**, 227–231, *227–231*
    questions for physician of patient with, 224
  risks associated with, 231–232, **233–236**, 236
activated partial thromboplastin time (aPTT), 178, **179**, 180
activities of daily living (ADLs), in geriatric health, 381
acute coronary syndrome (ACS), 27
acute lymphocytic leukemia (ALL), 143
  HSCT for, 158, *159*
  laboratory testing, **152**
  pathogenesis/etiology of, 145
acute myeloid leukemia (AML), 144
  HSCT for, 158, *159*
  laboratory testing, **152**
  pathogenesis/etiology of, 145
acute myocardial infarction (AMI), 26
acute necrotizing ulcerative gingivitis (ANUG), 229
acute renal failure (ARF), 95
addiction, defined, 331. *See also* substance abuse disorders
adenomatous polyposis coli (APC) gene, 131
adjuvant therapy, 270

The ADA Practical Guide to Patients with Medical Conditions, First Edition. Edited by Lauren L. Patton.
© 2012 American Dental Association. Published 2012 by John Wiley & Sons, Inc.

adolescents
  dental management of OFCs in, 367–368
  with hypertension, **35**
  OFCs in, 372–373
adrenal cortex, 79
adrenal failure, signs and symptoms of, 84
adrenal insufficiency (AI)
  classification of, 358, *358*
  coordination with physician of patient with, 79–80
  dental management
    adrenal crisis, 83–84
    evaluation, 81
    oral lesions, 81–82, *82*
    questions for patient with, 81
    questions for physician of patient with, 82
    risks associated with, 82–84
  epidemiology, 79, 363
  medical management, 80–81, 364
  oral hyperpigmentation associated with, 82, *82*
  pathogenesis/etiology, 79, 360
  and steroid supplementation, 83
Advisory Opinion, on patients with bloodborne pathogens, 239
African Americans, head and neck cancer in, 260
age-related macular degeneration (AMD), 381–382
  dry *vs.* wet, 386
  epidemiology, 387
  forms of, 382
  pathogenesis/etiology, 386
  treatment for, 390
aging, nature of, 381. *See also* geriatric health
AIDS-defining conditions, 218
albumin, in CKD, **100**
albuterol, in dental office, **429**
alcohol
  and dental management, 187
  drug interactions with, **19**
  and head and neck cancers, 258
  impact on wound healing, 353
alcohol abuse and alcoholism, 331–332
  defined, 331
  dental management

    evaluation, 341
    questions for patient with, 342
    questions for physician of patient with, 342
  epidemiology, 333–334
  medical management
    identification, 335–336
    medical history in, 336–337
    treatment, 337–340
  oral lesions associated with, 346, 347, *347*
  pathogenesis/etiology, 332–333
  pharmacotherapy for, 337–339
  physical exam/laboratory testing, 337
alcoholic cirrhosis, purpura due to, *12*
alcoholic liver disease (ALD), 115
  epidemiology, 118
  medical management
    medical history/physical exam, 119, *119*
    treatment, 121
  pathogenesis/etiology, 117
allergic reactions
  classification of, 244
  life-threatening, 432
allergies
  dental, *244*
  drug, 17
alpha-adrenergic blockers, in patient with CVD, **31**
alveolar clefts, 376–377
Alzheimer's disease (AD), 383
  characteristics of, 384
  diagnosis of, 389
  epidemiology, 388
  pathogenesis/etiology, 384
  signs of, **390–391**
  stages of, **385–386**
  treatment for, 392, **392**
amelogenesis imperfecta (AI), 357, 370, **370**
American Academy of Orthopedic Surgeons (AAOS), 208
American Association of Oral and Maxillofacial Surgeons, **420**
American Cancer Society Cancer Facts & Figures, 132
American College of Rheumatology, SLE criteria of, 194

American Dental Association (ADA)
    on opioid use, 345
    principles of ethic and code of professional conduct of, 239
    on provision of dental treatment for patients with SUDs, 345
American Diabetes Association, diagnostic criteria of, 71, **72**
American Heart Association (AHA)
    antibiotic premedication guidelines of, **37**
    on antibiotic prophylaxis, 232
    Healthcare Provider guidelines of, 428, 430
American Joint Committee for Cancer (AJCC), TNM classification system of, 265–266
American Medical Association (AMA), 331
American Society of Addiction Medicine (ASAM), 331
American Society of Anesthesiologists (ASA)
    baseline health and stress status of, 17
    physical status classification system of, 34
    Physical Status Score of, 5, **6**
amifostine, 270
amitriptyline, side effects associated with, **321**
ammonia inhalant, crushable, *429*
amputation, congenital, 359
    dental management for patient with, 375–376, **376**
    epidemiology, 363
    pathogenesis/etiology, 361
amyotrophic lateral sclerosis (ALS), 282
    dental management, 296
    epidemiology of, **284**
    medical management, 292
    pathogenesis/etiology of, 286
    symptoms of, 291
    tolerance to dental care in, 302
analgesics
    in hepatic disease, 124
    interaction with alcohol of, **351**
anaphylaxis/life-threatening allergic reaction, 432
anemia
    in CKD, 99
    classification of, 144
    dental management, 164
        evaluation, 160, 161
        oral lesions, 165–166, *166*, *167*
        questions for patient with, 161
        questions for physician of patient with, 161
    drug actions/interactions in, 169
    epidemiology, 149, 150
    medical management
        identification, 151, **153–154**
        laboratory testing, 151, **153–154**
        treatment, **153–154**, 158
    pathogenesis/etiology, 146–149, *147*, *148*
    susceptibility to infection in, 169
anemia, aplastic, 12
anemia, pernicious, 148
anesthetics
    allergy to, 17
    in patient with COPD, 64
angina, as medical emergency, 433–434
angina pectoris (AP)
    CCS guidelines for, 34, 36
    classification of, 25–26
    defined, 25
angioedema
    forms of, 244
    with systemic drugs, **20**
angiotensin-converting enzyme (ACE) inhibitors, in patient with CVD, **31**
angiotensin II receptor blocker, in patient with CVD, **31**
angular chelitis, treatment of, **225**
anorexia nervosa (AN), 315
    dental management, 324
    epidemiology of, 317–318
    identification of, 319
    medical management, 320, 323
    pathogenesis/etiology, 316
antagonists, drug interactions with, **19**
anti-arrhythmics, for patient with CVD, **32**
antibiotic coverage, for susceptibility to infection, 14
antibiotic prophylaxis, 21
    for bacteremia in patients with joint replacements, 208–209
    for HD patients, 108–109
    for HIV-infected patients, 232
    for kidney transplant patients, 109
    for patients with CVD, **37**, **38**

antibiotics
    in COPD, 55
    in hepatic disease, 124
    interaction with alcohol of, **351**
anticholinergics, in PD, **288**
anticoagulants
    in older adults, 16
    for patient with CVD, **32**
anticonvulsants, side effects associated with, 321
antidepressants, side effects associated with, 321–322
antiepileptics, drug interactions with, **19**
antifibrinolytics, postoperative, 22
antifungals, interaction with alcohol of, **351**
anti-inflammatory drugs, in dental practice, **18–19**
antimicrobial drugs, in dental practice, **18**
antiplatelet agents, 175
antiplatelet therapy, 13
antipsychotics, side effects associated with, 321
antiresorptive agents
    examples of, 403–404
    for preventing osteoporosis, 417, **418**
antiresorptive therapy
    for prevention of osteoporosis, 417
    prevention strategies during, **419**
antiretroviral drugs, for HIV-infected patients, 233–236
antiretroviral therapy (ART), during pregnancy of HIV-infected mothers, 218
anxiety, dental, 21
anxiety disorders, 314–315
    dental management, 323–324, *324*
    diagnosis of, 318
    epidemiology of, 317
    medical management, 320
    pathogenesis/etiology, 316
anxiolytics, in hepatic disease, 124
anxiolytic therapy, for asthma patients, 64
aphthous stomatitis, medical management of, 250–251, *251*
aphthous ulcerations, 139
    in HIV-infected patients, 230, *231*
    treatment for, **226**

aplastic anemia (AA), 144
    epidemiology, 150
    hemostasis in, 168
    HSCT for, 158, *159*
    laboratory testing, **154**
    pathogenesis/etiology, 149
apnea, 44. *See also* obstructive sleep apnea
apnea-hypopnea index (AHI), 44
arrhythmias, cardiac, 28, 36
arthritis, dental management of patient with, 393, *395*. *See also* rheumatoid arthritis
aspiration, of foreign object, 432–433
aspirin
    in dental office, **429**
    and platelet disorders, 175
aspirin therapy, and dental extractions, 12–13
asthma, 43
    classification of, **50**
    dental management
        oral lesions, 62, *62*
        treatment modifications, 59, 60
    drug interactions in patient with, 63
    management of asthma attack in, 64–65
    medical management
        epidemiology, 47
        medical history/physical examination, 48–49, **49**
        pathogenesis/etiology, 44–45
        treatment, **54**, 54–56
    medications for, 54, **54**
    questions for patient with, 56
    questions for physician of patient with, 57
    tolerance to dental care of patient with, 63–64
asthmatic attack, 64–65, 432
atonic seizures, 283
attention deficit hyperactivity disorder (ADHD), 306
    diagnosis of, 308–309
    epidemiology, 307–308
    pathogenesis/etiology, 307
    treatment for, 309, **311**
autistic spectrum disorder (ASD), 306
    diagnosis of, 308
    epidemiology, 307

pathogenesis/etiology, 306–307
tolerance to dental care in, 314
treatment for, 309, **310**
autoimmune diseases. *See* connective tissue and autoimmune diseases
automated external defibrillator (AED), 39, 428
AVDR assessment, of violence against women, 411

bacilli Calmette-Guerin (BCG) vaccine, 52
bacterial infections, in HIV-infected patients, 231
barbiturates, interaction with alcohol of, **351**
Barrett's esophagus, 128, 129129
basophils, in differential WBC count, **157**
Behçet's disease (BD), 251, 252
Bence-Jones proteins, 158
benzodiazepines, interaction with alcohol of, **351**
beta-adrenergic blockers, in patient with CVD, **31**
beta-blockers, drug interactions with, **19**
betel quid, and head and neck cancers, 259
Bethesda inhibitor assay (BIA), 175
biopsy, in head and neck cancer, 265
biphosphonates, for preventing osteoporosis, 417, **418**
bipolar disorder (BPD)
    characteristics of, 315
    dental management of, 324
    epidemiology of, 317
    identification of, 318
    medical management of, 320
    pathogenesis/etiology, 316
bisphosphonate-related osteonecrosis of jaw (BRONJ), 163, 164, *170*, 417, **420–421**
black hairy tongue, 140, *141*
bladder cancer, 110
bleeding. *See also* hematological disease; hemostasis
    local control of, 14
    in risk assessment, **8**
bleeding disorders, 173, **174**. *See also* hemostasis
    coagulation disorders, **174**, 174–175

coordination with physician of patient with, 176–177
dental management
    evaluation, 181
    oral lesions, 186, *186*
    questions for patient with, 182
    questions for physician of patient with, 182
    risks associated with, 186–187, *187*
    treatment modifications, 181, 183–184, *183–185*, 186
epidemiology, 176
medical management
    identification, 177, **177**
    laboratory testing, 178–180, **179**
    medical historyidentification, 177–178
    physical examination, 178
    treatment, 180–181
oral signs of, 176, *176*
pathogenesis/etiology, 173
platelet disorders, 173–174, **174**
screening test results for, **179**
symptoms of, **177**
blistering disease, 247
blood exposures, occupational, 236, **237**, 238
blood pressure
    baseline, 21
blood product administration, 21
blood urea nitrogen (BUN), in CKD, **100**
blue bloaters, 51. *See also* bronchitis
bone loss, in untreated DM, 75, *76*, 77. *See also* osteoporosis
breast cancer, 400
    dental management of patient with, 411
    and drug interactions, 417, *420*
    epidemiology, 401
    menopause, 400
    pathogenesis/etiology, 401
    treatment for, 404, *404*
breastfeeding
    dental drugs during, **416**
    drug interactions in, 415, **416**
bridging therapy, 184, *185*
bronchitis
    in COPD, 46, 51
    signs and symptoms of, 51

bruising, 173. *See also* bleeding
bulimia nervosa (BN), 315
    dental management of, 324
    epidemiology of, 317–318
    erosion of teeth in, 325, *325*
    identification of, 319
    medical management of, 320, 323
    pathogenesis/etiology, 316
buprenorphine (Skuboxone, Subutex)
bupropion, sustained-release, 340
burn, cocaine, 348, *348*
burning mouth syndrome, 413, **414**
burning mouth/tongue, in risk assessment, **8**

cahexia, in risk assessment, **8**, **10**
calcifiedcarotid artery atheromas (CCAAs), 3–2
calcium, in CKD, **100**
calcium channel blockers, for patient with CVD, **32**
Canadian Cardiovascular Society (CCS), AP guidelines of, 34, 36
cancer. *See also* breast cancer
    colorectal, 128, 131, 132, 137
    gastric, 128–132, 136
    hepatocellular carcinoma, 115, 116, 118, 119, *119*, 121
    of hypopharynx, 268
    of larynx, 268
    lung, 44, 47, 56, 60–61
    of nasopharynx, 268
    of oropharynx, 268, 347
    pancreatic, 69, 70, 71, 72, 73, 76–76, 78
    prostate, 110–111
    of salivary glands, 268
    thyroid, 85–87, 88, 90, 91
candidiasis
    in immune-suppressed post-liver transplant patients, 123, *123*
    in kidney transplant patients, 110
    in tobacco dependence, 348, *349*
    in xerostomia, 75, *76*
candidiasis, oral
    in aplastic anemia, 165, *166*
    erythematous, 227, *227*
    in HIV-infected patients, 227, *227*–228

    with nebulized corticosteroids, 62
    pseudomembraneous, 227, *227*
    treatment of, **225**
cardiopulmonary resuscitation (CPR), 39, 430–431
cardiovascular diseases (CVDs), 25
    coordination with physician of patient with, 29
    dental management
        evaluation, 33
        questions for patients, 33
        questions for physicians of patients with, 34
        risks associated with, 37–39
        treatment modifications, 33–34, **35**, 36
    medical management, 29
        epidemiology of, 28–29
        identification, 29
        laboratory testing, 30–31
        medical history in, 29–30, *30*
        physical examination, 30
    medications for, **31–32**
    pathogenesis/etiology, 25–28, **26**, *26*, *28*
    risk factors for, 25, **26**
caregiver education, in cognitive impairment/dementia, 396
caries, dental
    and cancer therapy, 276, *276*
    during pregnancy, 405–407, *408–409*
    in risk assessment, **9**
    in SS, 210, *211*
caries, radiation, 276, *276*
Caries Risk Assessment Form, *408–409*
carotid artery calcification, in risk assessment, **11**
cataracts, 381, 386
    epidemiology, 387
    treatment, 389–391, **391**
CBCT tomography, in TMD, 413
CD4+ lymphocyte counts, 221
celiac disease (gluten-sensitive enteropathy), 128
    epidemiology, 132
    medical management, 136
    oral lesions in, 138
    pathogenesis/etiology, 130

Center for Disease Control and Prevention
    (CDC), infection control measures
    recommended by, 236
cerebral palsy (CP)
    definition for, 305
    diagnosis of, 308
    epidemiology, 307
    oral manifestations of, 309, 312
    pathogenesis/etiology, 306
    tolerance to dental care in, 314
    treatment for, 309
cerebrovascular accident (CVA), 281–282
    classic warning signs for, 291
    dental management, 296, **297**
    diagnosis of, 289
    epidemiology of, **284**
    medical management, 291
    pathogenesis/etiology of, 285–286
chair, dental, in Trendelenburg position, 430, *430*
chemiluminescence, for head and neck cancer, 262–263
chemo-osteonecrosis of jaw
    with systemic drugs, **20**
chemotherapy
    and dental management, 163–164, 271–272, 273
    for head and neck cancer, 270
chemotherapy agents, 270
chest pain, as medical emergency, 433–434
Child Health/Dental History Form, 4, *5*
children
    dental management of craniofacial anomalies in, 372, *373*
    dental management of OFCs in, 367
    prescribing drugs for, 16
Child-Tucotte-Pugh classification, 121
chloride, in CKD, **100**
chronic kidney disease (CKD). *See also* kidney disease
    classification of, **98**
    clinical features of, **98**
    laboratory changes in, **100**
    stage 4, 99
chronic lymphocytic leukemia (CLL), 143–144
    laboratory testing, **152**
    pathogenesis/etiology of, 145

chronic myeloid leukemia (CML), 144
    laboratory testing, **152**
    pathogenesis/etiology of, 145
chronic obstructive pulmonary disease (COPD), 43
    classification of severity of, 45, **45**
    dental management
        risks associated with, 63–65
        treatment modifications, 60
    medical management
        epidemiology, 47
        medical history/physical examination in, 49, 51
        pathogenesis/etiology, 45–46
        treatment, 54–55
    medications for, 54, **54**
    pulmonary functions in, **53**
    questions for patient with, 57
    questions for physician of patient with, 58
chronic renal failure (CRF), 95. *See also* dialysis
    epidemiology, 96
    medical management of, 96–97
    pathogenesis/etiology, 95
    treatment considerations in, 105, **106–107**
cigarette smokers, 257
cleft lip and palate (CLP), 359, *359*. *See also* orofacial clefts
    in adolescents, 372–373, *374*
    adult patient with unrepaired, 375, *375*
    medical management of, 366–368, *367*
    prevalence of, 363
    V-shaped cleft, 372, *373*
clonic seizures, 283
Clostridium. difficile, 130, 135
cluster of differentiation, 144
coagulation cascade, 173
coagulation disorders, **174**, 174–175, **177**
    acquired, 175
    dental management, 183
    drug-induced, **174**, 175–176, 181
    treatment, 180–181
cocaine
    oral lesions associated with, 347–348, *348*
    and tolerance to dental care, 353
cocaine burn, 348, *348*
cognition, in older adults, 383–384

cognitive impairment/dementia, 383
  in cognitive impairment/dementia, 396
    dental management
      questions for patient/family member, 394
      treatment modifications, 393, 395–396
    diagnosis of, 389
    epidemiology, 388
    indications of, 397
    pathogenesis/etiology, 387
    patient management in, 395–396
    treatment for, 392
Collis-curve, 293, 295, *295*
colorectal cancer, 129
  epidemiology, 132
  medical management, 137
  pathogenesis/etiology, 131
Combat Methamphetamine Epidemic Act (2005), 334
complete blood cell (CBC) count, and disease-related changes, **156**
computed tomography (CT), in head and neck cancer, 264
COMT inhibitors, in PD, **288**
concurrent chemoradiation for organ preservation, 270
condyle articular space destruction, in risk assessment, **11**
condyloma acuminatum, in HIV-infected patients, 228–229, *229*
congenital heart disease, 27–28, *28*
connective tissue and autoimmune diseases, 191
  coordination with physician of patient with, 193–194
  dental management
    evaluation, 203–205
    medical emergencies, 214
    oral lesions, 209–211, *210*, *211*
    risks associated with, 211–214
    treatment modifications, 205, **206**
  epidemiology, 193
  medical management
    identification, 194–197, *195*, *196*
    laboratory testing, 199–202, **201**
    medical history and physical exam, 197–199, *198*, *199*
    treatment, 202, **203**
    medications for, **213**
  multiple sclerosis, 281
  pathogenesis/etiology, 192–193
contact stomatitis, 243–244, *244*
  clinical features of, 243–244
  of maxilla, *244*
continuous ambulatory peritoneal dialysis (CAPD), 102
continuous cycling peritoneal dialysis (CCPD), 102
continuous renal replacement therapy (CRRT), 99, 102
contraception use
  antibiotics and, 415–417
  and dental management, 410
  epidemiology, 401
convulsions, 431
Cooley's anemia, 146
coronary artery bypass grafts (CABG), 30
coronary artery disease (CAD), 25, **26**
Correa pathway, 131
cortical bone density, in risk assessment, **11**
corticosteroid therapy
  and antibiotic prophylaxis, 82–83
  following ASCT, 160
  oral, 64
coumadin, dental management of patient on, 183–184, *184*, *185*
craniofacial anomalies. *See also* orofacial clefts
  coordination with physician of patient with, 364
  dental management
    evaluation, 368
    oral manifestations, 377–378
    risks associated with, 378
    treatment modifications, **370**, 370–375, **371**, *373–375*, **375**
  epidemiology, 363
  medical management
    diagnosis, 364–365
    treatment, 366–368, *367*
  questions for patient with, 369
  questions for physician of patient with, 369
craniofacial trauma, dental management of, 346
creatinine, in CKD, **100**

cretinism, 85
Crohn's disease (CD), 128
    cobblestone appearance of buccal mucosa in, 139, *140*
    medical management of, 135
    oral lesions in, 138–139
    pathogenesis/etiology, 129
Cushingoid facies, in risk assessment, **8**, **10**
Cushing's disease, 81
Cushing's syndrome (CS)
    and glucocorticoid replacement therapy, **80**
    pathogenesis/etiology of, 79
cyclosporine, following ASCT, 160
cystic fibrosis (CF), 43–44
    clubbing of fingers in, 48, *48*
    dental management
        oral lesions, 63
        treatment, 60
    medical management
        epidemiology, 47
        treatment, 55
    questions for patient with, 58
    questions for physician of patient with, 58
cytomegalovirus (CMV), in leukemic patient, 165

dabigatran (Pradaxa), 175–176, 186
DDAVP (desmopressin [1-deamino-8-D-arginine vasopressin]), 105, 180–181
degenerative joint disease, 383, *383*
dementia, 383. *See also* cognitive impairment
    characteristics of, 384
    epidemiology, 388
    treatment for, 392
dental care, ability to tolerate, 17, 19–21. *See also* tolerance
dental care providers, exposure to HIV of, 238
dental office
    emergency response in, 425
    equipment in, 425, 426, *426*
    prevention of medical emergencies in, 425
dental skeletal delay, and cancer therapy, 278
dentin dysplasia type II (DD-II), 358
dentinogenesis imperfecta (DGI), 357
    dental management, 370, *370*
    DGI-I, 366

epidemiology, 363
pathogenesis/etiology, 360
types of, 358, *358*
desmopressin (1-deamino-8-D-arginine vasopressin [DDAVP]), 180–181
diabetes mellitus (DM)
    classification of, 70
    coordination with physician of patient with, 71
    dental management
        evaluation, 73
        oral lesions, 75, *76*
        questions for patient with, 74
        questions for physician of patient with, 74
        risks associated with, 76, 78
        treatment modifications, 73, 75
    drug actions/interactions in, 78
    epidemiology, 70–71
    medical emergencies in, 78
    medical management, 71–72, **72**, **73**
    oral signs of undiagnosed/uncontrolled, *76*
    pathogenesis/etiology, 69–70
    prognosis for, 72
diabetic retinopathy. *See* retinopathy, diabetic
Diagnostic and Statistical Manual of Mental Disorders (DSM-IV), 315
dialysis
    CAPD, 102
    CCPD, 102
    hemodialysis, 99, *101*, 102, *102*, 105
    peritoneal, 99
diet, and head and neck cancers, 259–260
dietary supplements
    commonly used, **16**
    in older adults, 16
digital rectal exam, 133
diphenhydramine, in dental office, **429**
dipyridamole (Persantine, Aggrenox), platelet disorders caused by, 175
direct-acting peripheral vasodilators, for patient with CVD, **32**
discoloration, tooth
    in risk assessment, **9**
    with systemic drugs, **20**
disease-modifying antirheumatic drugs (DMARDs), 202

disseminated intravascular coagulation (DIC), **174**, 175
disulfram (Antabuse), 337
diuretics, for patient with CVD, **32**
dopamine, in PD, **288**
Down syndrome (DS), 305
  dental management in, 313
  diagnosis of, 308
  epidemiology, 307
  oral manifestations of, 309, 312, *313*
  orofacial features of, 309, *313*
  pathogenesis/etiology, 306
  tolerance to dental care in, 314
drooling
  in Parkinson's disease, 287, 298
  in risk assessment, **8**
drop seizures, 283
drug actions/interactions, 3
  of antiretroviral drugs, **233–236**
  in autoimmune and connective tissue diseases, 212
  in bleeding disorders, 187
  commonly used drugs, 14, **15**
  in dentistry, 17, **18–19**
  in DG-I patients with OI, 378
  in endocrine and metabolic disorders, 78
  in geriatric health, 396
  in GI disease, 140–141, *141*
  in glucocorticoid therapy, 83
  in head and neck cancer, 278
  in hematological disease, 169
  in hepatic disease, 124
  with herbal supplements, 14, **16**
  in HIV-infected patients, 232, **233–236**
  in kidney disease, 111
  in neurodevelopmental disorders, 314
  in neurological disease, 300
  in patients with SUDs, 350, **351**, **352**, 353
  in patient with CVD, 38
  in psychiatric disorders, **321–322**, 326
  in pulmonary diseases, 63
  in thyroid disease, 91
  with vitamins/minerals, 14, **16**
  in women's health, 414–415, **416**
drug-drug interactions, in older adults, 16
drug-induced bleeding disorders, dental management of, 183–184, *184*, 185, *185*

drugs. *See also* medications
  common interactions with dental, **18–19**
  emergency, 428, *429*, **429**
  oral consequences of systemic, 17, **20**
  in patient management, 17
  platelet disorders caused by, 175–176
  side effects of, **20**
drug-seeking patients, 354
dry mouth. *See also* xerostomia
  effects of, 199
  in Parkinson's disease, 298
  questionnaire for, 205
dysarthria, in MS, 299
dysgeusia, and cancer therapy, 275
dyspepsia, 127
  epidemiology, 131
  medical management of, 133
  pathogenesis/etiology, 129
dysphagia, in MS, 299
dysrhythmias, cardiac, 28, 36

eating disorders (EDs), 315
  dental management, 361
    oral lesions associated with, 325, *326*
    oral manifestations, 377
    treatment modifications, 324
  epidemiology, 317–318, 363
  identification of, 319
  medical management
    diagnosis, 364–365
    treatment, 320, 323, 366
  pathogenesis/etiology, 316, 360–361
  phenotypes for, **371**
eating disorders not otherwise specified (EDNOS), 315–316
ecchymoses
  dental management of, 186, *186*
  in risk assessment, **8**, 11, *12*
ectodermal dysplasias (EDs), 358, *359*
ejection fraction (EF), in CVDs, 30
electrocardiogram, 26
emergencies, medical
  in bleeding disorders, 187
  common, 428, 430–434, *433*
  in connective tissue diseases, 214
  drugs for, 426, 428, *429*, **429**
  equipment for, 425, *426*, 428

frequency in dental practice, 425, **427**
in patients with CVD, 39
preparation for managing, 426
prevention of, 426
in psychiatric disorders, 326
emergency medical care, principles of, 425–426, *426*, **427**
emergency medical service (EMS), 39, 302, 303, 428
in CVA, 291
information for, 428
emphysema
in COPD, 46, 49
signs and symptoms of, 51
enamel erosion, in risk assessment, **9**
endocarditis, infective, antibiotic premedication guidelines for, **37**, **38**
endocardium, infection and inflammation of, 28
endocrine and metabolic disorders
of adrenal gland, 79–84, **80**, *82*
of pancreas, 69–76, **72**, **73**, *76*, *77*, *78*
of thyroid, 84–92, **85**
endoscopy
for head and neck tumors, 263–264
nasal flexible, 263
end-stage cirrhosis, intraoral spontaneous bleeding in, 123
end-stage heart failure, dental management of patient with, 36
end-stage renal disease (ESRD)
dental management of patient with, 187
incident rate of, 96
progression to, 95–96
risk for bleeding in patients with, 111
entry inhibitors, **236**
enzyme-linked immunosorbent assay (ELISA), 221
eosinophils, in differential WBC count, **157**
epidermolysis bullosa acquisita (EBA), 246, 247–248
epidermolysis bullosa (EB), 247–248, 358–359, *359*
dental management, 361–372, **362**, 377
epidemiology, 363
medical management
diagnosis, 364
treatment, 366
pathogenesis/etiology, 361, **362**, 363
phenotypes, **362**
susceptibility to infection in, 378
tolerance to dental care of patient with, 378
epigastric pain syndrome, 127
epilepsy, 282
dental management, 297, **298**
diagnosis of, 293
epidemiology of, **284**
medical treatment of, 293, **294**
medications used in, **294**
pathogenesis/etiology of, 286
tolerance to dental care in, 302
epinephrine, in dental office, **429**
EpiPen Auto-Injector, 432, *433*
ε-aminocaproic acid (EACA), 181
Epstein-Barr virus (EBV)
and head and neck cancers, 259
and Hodgkin's disease, 149
equipment, for medical emergencies, 425, *426*, 428
erythema, linear gingival, treatment for, **226**, *229*, 229–230
erythema multiforme (EM)
medical management, 248
precipitating factors of, 248
with systemic drugs, **20**
ethics, and HIV-infected patients, 238, 239
exopthalmos, in Graves' disease, 85

facial musculature, in risk assessment, **8**
facial skeletal delay, and cancer therapy, 278
factor replacement therapy, 181
Factor VIII, deficiency of, 174–175
factor VIII concentrate, self-infusion of, 183, *183*
family history, 4–5. *See also* history, medical
fibromyalgia (FM), 191–192
dental management, 206–207
drug interactions in, 212, **213**
epidemiology, 193
medical management
identification, 195
laboratory testing, 201
medical history/physical exam, 198, *198*
treatment, 202
pathogenesis/etiology, 192
tolerance to dental care in, 214

fine needle aspiration (FNA), in head and
    neck cancer, 265
focal seizures, 283
folate-deficiency anemia, 145, 148–149
    epidemiology, 150
    laboratory testing, **154**
Food and Drug Administration (FDA)
    pregnancy classification categories, 415
forms
    ADA Health History, 4, *4*
    Child Health/Dental History Form, 4, *5*
fractures
    dento-alveolar, 411, *412*
    incisal edge, 325, *326*
fungal infections
    and cancer therapy, 275
    in leukemia, 165

gastric cancer, 128
    diffuse type of, 131
    epidemiology, 132
    intestinal type, 130
    medical management, 136
    pathogenesis/etiology, 130–131
gastroesophageal reflux disease (GERD), 127
    epidemiology, 131
    medical management, 134
    oral lesions in, 138, *139*
    pathogenesis/etiology, 129
gastrointestinal (GI) disease
    common disorders, 127–128
    coordination with physician of patient with, 132–133
    dental management
        evaluation, 137
        medical emergencies in, 141
        oral lesions, 138–139, *139*, *140*
        questions for patient with, 137
        questions for physician of patient with, 137
        risks associated with, 140–141
        treatment modifications, 138
    epidemiology, 131
    medical management
        diagnosis, 133
        treatment, 133, 137
    pathogenesis/etiology, 129–131

gender, and head and neck cancer, 260
generalized anxiety disorder (GAD), 314–315
    dental management, 323–324, *324*
    diagnosis of, 318
    epidemiology of, 317
    pathogenesis/etiology, 316
    treatment for, 320
geriatric health
    age-related hearing loss, 282–283
    cognitive impairment/dementias, 383–384, **385–386**
    coordination with patient's physician, 389
    dental management
        evaluation, 392, 394
        risks associated with, 396
        treatment modifications, 393, 394–396, *395*
    epidemiology, 387–388
    medical management
        identification of problems, 389
        treatment, 389–391, **391**
    mobility limitations, 383
    pathogenesis/etiology, 384, 386–387
    sensory limitations, 381–382, *382*
    suspicion of cognitive problems in, 397
gingival bleeding, in leukemia, 164–165
gingival erythema, in leukemic patient, 164, *164*
gingival inflammation/hyperplasia, in aplastic anemia, 165, *166*
gingival overgrowth
    dilantin-induced, 299, *299*
    in kidney transplant patients, 110, *110*
    in risk assessment, **8**
    with systemic drugs, **20**
gingivitis, necrotizing ulcerative, 229, *229*
Glasgow Coma Scale (GCS), 292
glaucoma, 382
    epidemiology, 387
    pathogenesis/etiology, 386
    questions for patient with, 393
    treatment for, 390
glomerular filtration rate (GFR), 96
glossitis, with systemic drugs, **20**
glucocorticoids, characteristics of, **80**
glucocorticoid therapy, 93
glucocortisol (cortisol), 79

glucose, in dental office, **429**
gluten-sensitive enteropathy (celiac disease), 128
glycated hemoglobin (HbA1c) test, 72
glycosylated hemoglobin (HbA1C), 21
goiter, diffuse toxic, 84
G6PD anemia, 144
   epidemiology, 149–150
   laboratory testing, **153**
   pathogenesis/etiology, 146
graft-*versus*-host disease (GVHD), 160, 244–245
   clinical features of, 244–245
   clinical similarity to autoimmunity of, 245
   complications of, 163
   oral findings in, 245
   oral lesions associated with, 168
   oral lichenoid lesions associated with, 253
   risk factors for, 245
   treatment of, 245
granuloma, pyogenic, during pregnancy, 406, *407*
Graves' disease, 84–85

hairy leukoplakia, oral, in HIV-infected patients, 228
hard tissue enlargements, in risk assessment, **8**
Hashimoto's thyroiditis, 85
HATAH assessment, of violence against women, 412
head and neck, anatomic glossary of, 258
head and neck cancer, 257
   coordination with physician of patient with, 261
   dental management
     evaluation, 271
     oral lesions, 274–278, *275–277*
     questions for patient with, 271
     questions for physician of patient with, 272
     risks associated with, 278
     treatment modifications, 271–274
   epidemiology, 260–261
   location of, 259
   lymphatic drainage patterns in, *264*
   medical management
     adjunctive screening tests, 261–263, **262**
     identification, 261, *262*
     laboratory testing, 264–266, *266*
     medical history/physical examination, 263–264, *264*
     treatment, 267, 267–270, *269*
   mortality associated with, 260–261
   pathogenesis/etiology, 257–260
   prognosis for, 266
   SCC, 257
   signs and symptoms of, 261
   staging of, 265–266, *266*
health history. *See also* history, medical
hearing loss, age-related, 382–383
   dental management
     evaluation, 392
     questions for patient with, 394
     treatment modifications, 394
   diagnosis of, 389
   epidemiology, 388
   pathogenesis/etiology, 387
   treatment for, 390
heart
   anatomy of, *26*
   healthy, *26*
heart failure (HF)
   dental management of patient with, 36
   pathophysiology of, 27
heart rate, baseline, 21
Heberden's nodes, 383, *383*
Helicobacter pylori infection, 129, 132, 134
hemarthrosis, 186
hematocrit (HCT), in CBC, **156**
hematological disease
   classification of, 143–145
   coordination with physician of patient with, 150–151
   dental management, 163
     evaluation, 160–162
     oral lesions in, 164–168, *164–168*
     risks associated with, 168–169, *170*
   epidemiology, 149–150, **150**
   medical management
     identification, 151
     laboratory testing, 151, **152–157**
     treatment, **152**, **153–154**, **155**, 158–160, *160*
   pathogenesis/etiology, 145–149, *147*, *148*

hematology, of HIV-positive patients, 222
hematomas, dental management of, 186, *186*
hematomas, in risk assessment, 11, *12*
hematopoetic stem cell transplant (HSCT), 158, *159*, 160, 163–164
hemodialysis (HD), 99, *101*, 102, *102*
　access shunts for, *102*
　dental management of patients in, 105
　equipment for, *102*
　hemostasis in patients on, 111
　at outpatient dialysis center, *101*
hemoglobin (Hb), in CBC, **156**
hemophilia, treatment of, 180, 181
hemophilia A, *12*, *13*, **174**
　dental management, 183
　epidemiology, 176
　tooth extraction in patient with, 186, *187*
hemophilia B, **174**, 176
hemorrhage, gingival, in risk assessment, 11, *13*
hemosiderin staining, in risk assessment, 11, *13*
hemostasis, 3. *See also* bleeding disorders
　and anticoagulant medications, 12
　in bleeding disorders, 186, *187*
　in connective tissue diseases, 211–212
　in CVD patient, 37
　in DM, 76
　in geriatric health, 396
　in GI disease, 140
　in head and neck cancer, 278
　in hematological disease, 168
　in hepatic disease, 123
　in HIV-infected patients, 231
　indications of risk for, *11*, 11–13, *12*
　in kidney disease, 111
　in neurological diseases, 299–300
　in pancreatic cancer, 76
　in patients with SUDs, 350
　phases of, 11, 173
　in psychiatric disorders, 325
　and pulmonary disease, 63
heparin
　coagulation disorders caused by, 175
　dental management of patient on, 183–184, *185*, 187

hepatic disease. *See also* viral hepatitis
　alcoholic liver disease, 115
　coordination with physician of patient with, 118
　dental management
　　evaluation, 122
　　oral lesions, 123, *123*
　　questions for patient with, 122
　　questions for physician of patient with, 122
　　risks associated with, 123–124
　　treatment modifications, 123
　epidemiology, **117**, 117–118
　hepatocellular carcinoma, 115
　medical management
　　identification, 118
　　laboratory testing, 119–120
　　medical history/physical examination, 118–119
　　treatment, 120–122
　pathogenesis/etiology, 115–117, **116**
　viral hepatitis, 115
hepatitis A virus (HAV) infection, 115, **116**
　epidemiology, **117**
　symptoms of, 118–119
　testing for, 119
　treatment for, 120
hepatitis B virus (HBV) infection, 115, **116**
　coinfection with HIV, 225
　diagnosis of, 116
　epidemiology, **117**
　symptoms of, 118–119
　testing for, 119–120
　transmission of, 125
　treatment for, 120–121
hepatitis C virus (HCV) infection, 115, **116**
　coinfection with HIV, 225
　diagnosis of, 116
　epidemiology, **117**
　symptoms of, 119
　testing for, 120
　transmission of, 125
　treatment for, 121
hepatitis D virus (HDV) infection, 115, **116**
　clinical expression of, 116
　testing for, 120
　treatment for, 121

hepatitis E virus (HEV) infection, 115, **116**
   testing for, 120
   treatment for, 121
hepatocellular carcinoma, 115
   annual incidence of, 116
   epidemiology, 118
   medical management of
      medical history/physical exam, 119, *119*
      treatment, 121
herbal supplements
   commonly used, **16**
   drug interactions with, 14
Herbst appliance, 65, *65*
hereditary conditions
   affecting skin, 358–359, *359*
   affecting teeth, 357–358
   defects of limbs and skeleton, 359–360, **360**
   orofacial clefts, 359, *359*
hereditary dentin disorders
   dental management, 377
   epidemiology, 363
   medical management, 364
   pathogenesis/etiology, 360
hereditary nonpolyposis colorectal cancer (HNPCC), 131
heroin, 334
herpes simplex virus (HSV) infection
   in HIV-infected patient, 230
   in leukemic patient, 165, *165*
   treatment for, **226**
herpes zoster (shingles), treatment for, **226**
herpetic lesions, in kidney transplant patients, 109, *109*
herpetiform aphthous ulcers, 251
hiatal hernias, 129
highly active antiretroviral therapy (HAART), 223, 227
histological tumor grading, in head and neck cancer, 265
history, medical, 3
   ADA Health History Forms, 4, *4*
   in AIDS, 220
   in bleeding disorders, 177–178
   Child Health/Dental History Form, 4, *5*
   in CVDs, 29–30, *30*
   family history in, 4–5

and privacy rules, 3
in SUDs, 336–337
HIV antibody tests, 220–221, *222*
HIV-infected patients
   antibiotic prophylaxis for, 232
   antiretroviral drugs for, **233–236**
   bacterial infections of, 231
   candidiasis in, *227*, 227–228
   drug actions/interactions in, 232, **233–236**
   with TB, 224
HIV viral load, 221–222
Hodgkin's lymphoma, 145
   epidemiology, 150
   HSCT for, 158, *159*
   laboratory testing, **155**
   pathogenesis/etiology, 149
hormone replacement therapy (HRT), 403
hormones, thyroid, 84, **84**
hospitalization, for patients on coumadin, 184
HSCT. *See* hematopoetic stem cell transplant
human immunodeficiency virus (HIV)
   definition of, 217, **219**
   detection of, 217
   occupational exposures to, 236, **237**, 238
   transmission and replication of, 217–218
human immunodeficiency virus (HIV) infection
   oral lesions associated with, 225, **225–226**, 227–231, *227–231*
   surveillance case definition for, **219**
human papilloma virus (HPV)
   and head and neck cancers, 258
   in HIV-infected patients, 228–229, *229*
   screening for, 263
hydrocodone, 334
hyperglycemia
   detection and management of, 78
   as medical emergency, 431
hyperpigmentation, in risk assessment, **8**
hypersensitivity reactions, classification of, 244
hypertension (HTN), 21, 27
   and dental treatment, 34, **35**
   outpatient dental care guidelines for patients with, **35**
   in patients with CKD, 99

hyperthyroid crisis, management of, 92
hyperthyroidism, 84, **85**
  coordination with physician of patient with, 87
  dental management
    evaluation, 88
    oral lesions, 90
    questions for patient with, 88, 89
    treatment modifications, 90
  diagnosis of, 87
  drug actions/interactions in, 91
  drugs used for, 88
  epidemiology, 86
  medical emergency in, 92
  pathogenesis/etiology of, 86
  susceptibility to infection in, 91
  treatment of, 87–88
hyperventilation, as medical emergency, 431–432
hypogeusia, and cancer therapy, 275
hypoglycemia
  as medical emergency, 431
  recognition and management of, 78
hypopharynx, cancer of, 268
hypopnea, 44
hyposalivation, clinical complications of, 210–211, *211*
hypothyroidism, 85, **85**
  congenital, 85
  coordination with physician of patient with, 87
  dental management
    evaluation, 88
    oral lesions, 90
    questions for patient with, 89
    questions for physician of patient with, 89
    treatment modifications, 90
  diagnosis of, 87
  drug actions/interactions in, 91
  epidemiology, 86
  medical emergencies in, 91–92
  medical management, 88
  pathogenesis/etiology of, 86
  susceptibility to infection in, 91

IGRAs, 52
image-guided radiotherapy (IGRT), 270

immune system, 243
  allergic reactions, 243–244, *244*
  graft-*versus*-host disease, 244–245
  vesiculobullous conditions, 245–248
immune thrombocytopenic purpura (ITP), **174**, 176
immunosuppressant therapy, following ASCT, 160
impaired fasting glucose (IFG), 70
impaired glucose tolerance (IGT), 70
implantable cardioverter-defibrillator (ICD), 30, *30*
implant brachytherapy, 270
induction chemotherapy, 270
infection
  distant-site, 14
  fungal, 165, 275
  late prosthetic joint infections (LPJIs), 208
  odontogenic, 151
  opportunistic, **9**, 218
  viral, 165, *165*, 275 (*see also* human immunodeficiency virus)
infection, susceptibility to, 3
  in autoimmune and connective tissue diseases, 212
  in COPD, 63
  for CVD patient, 37–38, **38**
  in DM, 76
  of DS patients, 314
  in gastric disease, 140
  in geriatric health, 396
  of HD patients, 108
  in head and neck cancer, 278
  in hematological disease, 169
  in hepatic disease, 124
  in HIV-infected patients, 231, 232
  in kidney disease, 111
  in neurological disease, 300
  of oral cavity, 14
  in pancreatic cancer, 76, 78
  in patients with SUDs, 350
  in psychiatric disorders, 325
  of RA patients, 198
  in thyroid diseases, 91
  in women's health, 414
infection control, for patients with HIV/AIDS, 236

Infectious Diseases Society of America (IDSA), 208
inflammatory bowel disease (IBD), 128
  dental management of, 138
  epidemiology, 132
  medical management of, 135
  oral lesions in, 138–139
  pathogenesis/etiology, 129
influenza vaccine, 55
Institute of Medicine (IOM), 399
insulins, standard, **73**
insulin shock, 431
insulin supplementation, in DM, 72
integrase inhibitor, **236**
intellectual disabilities (IDs)/mental retardation, 305
  coordination with physician of patient with, 308
  dental management in, 313
  diagnosis of, 308
  epidemiology, 307
  pathogenesis/etiology, 306
intensity modulated radiotherapy (IMRT), 270
International Classification for Diseases (ICD), 281
international normalized ratio (INR), 178, **179**, 180
International Workshop on Definition and Classification of Cerebral Palsy, 305
intimate partner violence (IPV), 400. *See also* violence against women
iron-deficiency anemia, 144
  epidemiology, 149
  laboratory testing, **153**
  pathogenesis/etiology of, 146
irritable bowel syndrome (IBS), 128
isoniazid (INH), 55
Ivy bleeding time, 178, **179**

jaundice, in risk assessment, **8**, 11, *13*
jaw. *See also* biphosphonate-associated osteonecrosis; temporomandibular disorders
  physical therapy for, 207
  total joint replacement for, 208–209

Joint National Committee on Prevention, Detection, Evaluation, and Treatment of High Blood Pressure (JNC 7), 27

Kaposi's sarcoma, in HIV-infected patients, 228, *228*
ketoacidosis, diabetic, 431
kidney, malignant neoplasms of, 110
kidney disease. *See also* chronic renal failure
  chronic, **98**, 99, **100**
  classification of, 95
  coordination with physician of patient with, 96
  dental management
    coordination with physician of patient with, 104
    evaluation, 103–104
    HD patients, 105, *108*, 108–109
    questions for patient with, 104
    questions for physician of patient with, 104
    risks associated with, 111–112
    treatment modifications, 104–105
  medical management
    laboratory testing, 97, 99, **100**
    medical history, 97
    physical examination, 97
    treatment, 99, **100**, *101*, *102*, 102–103, *103*
  medications adjusted for patients with, **106–107**
  NKF definition of
Kidney Disease Outcome Quality Initiative (K/DOQI), 99, **100**
kidney transplantation, 99
  dental management following, *109*, 109–110, *110*
  donors for, 103, **103**
  immunosuppressant medications in, **103**
  long-term care following, 110
Kindler syndrome, 361

laboratory testing. *See also specific disease or disorder*
  in bleeding disorders, 178–180, **179**
  in connective tissue and autoimmune diseases, 199–202, **201**
  in CVDs, 30–31

laboratory testing (continued)
  in DM, 71, **72**
  in hematological disease, 151, **152–157**
  in kidney disease, 97, 99, **100**
  in pulmonary diseases, 53, **53**
laryngoscopy, indirect, 263
larynx, cancer of, 268
latent TB infection (LTBI), 46, 51, 55
late prosthetic joint infections (LPJIs), 208
Lauren classification, 130
leukemia
  classification of, 143
  dental management, 163
    evaluation, 160, 161
    oral lesions, *164*, 164–165, *165*
    questions for patient with, 160
    questions for physician of patient with, 161
  epidemiology, 149, **150**
  gingival oozing in, 176, *176*
  hemostasis in, 168
  HSCT for, 158, *159*
  medical management
    identification, 151, **151**
    laboratory testing, 151, **152**
    treatment, **152**, 158
  pathogenesis/etiology of, 145
  susceptibility to infection in, 169
leukoplakia
  hairy, in HIV-infected patients, 228
  in tobacco dependence, 348, *348*
levothyroxine, drug interactions with, **19**
lichenoid reactions, with systemic drugs, **20**
lichen planus (LP)
  medical management, 253–254
  white reticular pattern of, *253*
linear gingival erythema, **226**, *229*, 229–230
lip, tumors of, 267
lipid regulators (statins), for patient with CVD, **32**
liver cirrhosis, jaundice of, *13*
liver disease. *See also* hepatitis
  bleeding disorders associated with, 175
  prescribing drugs in, 16
  spider angioma of, *13*
liver enzymes, 120

liver function tests, 180
liver transplantation, 121–122
lorazepam (Ativan), in patient with COPD, 64
loss of consciousness (LOC), in CVA, 303
Lou Gehrig's disease, 282. *See also* amyotrophic lateral sclerosis
low birth weight (LBW) babies, and periodontal disease, 401, 406–407
low-molecular-weight heparins (LMWHs)
  coagulation disorders caused by, 175
  dental management of patient on, 183–184, *185*
lung cancer
  dental management, 60–61
  description, 44
  epidemiology of, 48
  medical management, 56
  pathogenesis/etiology of, 47
lungs, function of, 43
lung transplantation, 44
  dental management
    posttransplant, 61–62
    pretransplant, 61–62
  epidemiology of, 48
  medical management, 56
lupus erythematosus-like lesions, with systemic drugs, **20**
lymphocytes, in differential WBC count, **157**
lymphoma, 145. *See also* non-Hodgkin's lymphoma
  dental management, 163
    evaluation, 160–162
    oral lesions, 166–167, *167*
    questions for patient with, 161
    questions for physician of patient with, 162
  epidemiology, 150
  hemostasis in, 168
  HSCT for, 158, *159*
  medical management
    identification, 151, **155**
    laboratory testing, 151, **155**
    treatment, **155**, 158
  pathogenesis/etiology, 149
  radiotherapy in, 169
  susceptibility to infection in, 169

macular degeneration, age-related, 381–382
magnetic resonance imaging (MRI)
   in head and neck cancer, 264–265
   in TMD, 413
major depressive disorder (MDD), 315
   dental management of, 324
      epidemiology of, 317
      identification of, 319
      medical management of, 320
      pathogenesis/etiology, 316
malar rash, in risk assessment, **8**, **10**
malignancy, oral, 160
malocclusion, from oral appliance, 66, *66*
mandible. *See also* biphosphonate-associated osteonecrosis of the jaw; temporomandibular disorders
   BRONJ in, *170*
   fibula reconstruction of, *269*
   metastatic lesion of, 404, *404*
   in MM, 168, *168*
   osteonecrosis of, 417, *420*
   plasmacytoma in, 167, *168*
   in risk assessment, **11**
mandibular advancement devices, 65, *65*
Mantoux skin test, 52, *52*, 224
marrow hyperplasia, in risk assessment, **11**
marrow hypoplasia, in risk assessment, **11**
maxillofacial defects, surgery for, 268–269, *269*
medical disease. *See also specific disease*
   dental radiographic signs of, 10, **11**
   dental signs of, **9**
   facial signs of, **8**
   indications of, 7
   oral signs of, **8–9**
medications
   adjusted for patients with kidney disease, **106–107**
   for burning mouth syndrome, **414**
   for connective tissue diseases, **213**
   for CVDs, **31–32**
   in epilepsy, **294**
   interaction with alcohol of, **351**
   for memory loss, **392**
   in multiple sclerosis, **290**
   in neurodevelopmental disorders, **310–311**
   in older adults, 16
   oral antidiabetic, **73**
   in Parkinson's disease, **288**
   for prevention of osteoporosis, 417, **418**
   in psychiatric disorders, **321–322**
   for systemic disease management, 17
   and tobacco cessation therapiess, **352**
megaloblastic anemia, 145
memory loss, 383
   causes of, 383
   medications for, **392**
menopause, 400
   diagnosis of, 402–403
   medical management of, 403
   oral mucosal symptoms of, 413
menstruation, 399, 404–405
mental retardation. *See* intellectual disabilities (IDs)/mental retardation
metabolic syndrome, 70
metered-dose inhalers (MDIs), 54
methadone, 339
methamphetamine abuse, 332
   dental management
      evaluation, 341
         questions for physician of patient with, 343
         tolerance to dental care, 353
   epidemiology, 334
   medical management
      identification, 335–336
      medical history in, 336–337
      treatment, 337–340
   oral lesions associated with, 346, 347, *347*
   pathogenesis/etiology, 333
   physical exam/laboratory testing, 337
methamphetamine overdose, 353
methicillin-resistant *Staphylococcus aureus* (MRSA), and hospitalized immunosuppressed patients, 110
meth mouth, 347, *347*
microstomia
   in PSS, 209, *210*
   in risk assessment, **8**, **10**
mikulicz aphthae, 251
mild cognitive impairment (MCI), 383–384
   epidemiology, 388
   treatment for, 392
   types of, 384

mineralocorticoid (aldosterone), 79
minerals, commonly used, **16**
mobility limitations
   dental management
      questions for patient with, 394
      treatment modifications, 394–395, *395*
   diagnosis of, 389
   epidemiology, 388
   pathogenesis/etiology, 387
   treatment for, 390
Model for End-Stage Liver Disease (MELD) score, 121–122
monoamine oxidase β inhibitor, in PD, **288**
monocytes, in differential WBC count, **157**
mood disorders, 315
   dental management, 324
   epidemiology of, 317
   identification of, 318
   medical management, 320
   pathogenesis/etiology, 316
Mouth. *See* burning mouth syndrome
mucocutaneous disorders
   Behçet's disease, 251–252, *252*
   erythema multiforme, 248–249, *249*
   lichen planus, 253–254, *254*
   Steven-Johnson syndrome, 249
   toxic epidermal necrolysis, 249
mucosa
   in aplastic anemia, 166, *166*
   hyperpigmentation of, 81–82, *82*
   in leukemic patient, 164, *164*
   in risk assessment, **8**, 11, *12*
mucosa, buccal
   cobblestone appearance of, 139, *140*
   oral candida of, 140, *140*
mucositis, caused by cancer therapy, 274–275, *275*
mucous membrane pemphigoid, 247, *247*
multi-infarct dementia (MID), 286
Multinational Association of Supportive Care in Cancer, 274
multiple myeloma (MM), 145
   dental management, 162, 163
      oral lesions, 167–168, *168*
      questions for patient with, 162
      questions for physician of patient with, 162

   drug actions/interactions in, 169, *170*
   epidemiology, 150
   laboratory investigation in, 158
   medical management
      identification, 151
      treatment, **155**, 158
   oral manifestations of, 151
   pathogenesis/etiology, 149
   susceptibility to infection in, 169
multiple sclerosis (MS), 281
   dental management in, 296
   epidemioloy of, **284**
   medical treatment for, 289
   medications used in, **290**
   pathogenesis/etiology of, 285
   patterns of disease in, *289*
   presenting symptoms of, 289
   tolerance to dental care in, 300
multispectral technology, for head and neck cancer, 263
Mycobacterium tuberculosis, 224
myelomeningocele, 360, 365
myocardial infarction (MI), 26
   dental management of patient with, 36
   as dental office emergency, 434
   with ST elevation (STEMI), 26
myoclonic seizures, 283
myxedema, 85

naltrexone (Depade), 337
narrow-emission tissue autofluorescence, in head and neck cancer, 263
nasal alveolar molding (NAM), 366–367, *367*
nasopharynx, cancer of, 268
National Institute on Alcohol Abuse and Alcoholism (NIAAA), 332
National Kidney Foundation (NKF)
   classification of chronic kidney disease of, **98**
   CRF definition of, 96–97
   D/DOQI of, 97
National Survey on Drug Use and Health, U.S., 334
necrotizing ulcerative gingivitis, 229, *229*
necrotizing ulcerative periodontitis, **226**, *229*, 229–230

neoadjuvant therapy, 270
nephroblastoma, 110
neural tube defects, 360
neurodevelopmental disorders, 305–307
   dental management
      evaluation, 309
      oral manifestations, 309, 312, *313*
      questions for patient with, 312
      questions for physician of patient with, 312
      risks associated with, 314–315
      treatment modifications, 312–314.*314*
   epidemiology, 307–308
   medical management
      diagnosis of, 308
      treatment, 309
   medications in, **310–311**
   pathogenesis/etiology, 306–307
neuroleptics, drug interactions with, **19**
neurological diseases and disorders
   classification of, 281
   coordination with physician of patient with, 287
   dental management
      evaluation, 293
      medical emergencies, 302
      oral lesions, 298–299, *299*
      questions for patient with, 294
      questions for physician of patient with, 295
      risks associated with, 299–300, **301**, 302, 1*201*
      treatment modifications, 293, *295*, 295–297, *297*, **298**
   epidemiology, 283, **284**
   medical management, 287–293, **288**, 289, **290**
   pathogenesis/etiology, 285–287
neutrophils, in differential WBC count, **157**
newborn
   dental management of craniofacial anomalies in, 372
   OFCs in, 366–367
New Pregnancy and Lactation Labeling Rule, of FDA, 415
nicotine dependence, 333
nicotine palatinus, 348, *349*
nicotine patches, 340

nicotine replacement therapy (NRT), 330–340
nicotine stomatitis, 348, *349*
Nikolsky's sign, 248
nitroglycerine
   administration of, 434
   in dental office, **429**
non-Hodgkin's lymphoma (NHL), 145
   epidemiology, 150
   laboratory testing, **155**
   oral lesions in, 166–167, *167*
   pathogenesis/etiology, 149
non-nucleoside reverse transcriptase inhibitors (NNRTIs), **235–236**
nonsteroidal anti-inflammatory drugs (NSAIDs), 45
   in dental management of SUDs, 344
   in GI disease, 141
   in hepatic disease, 124
   platelet disorders caused by, 175
   for RA, 202
nucleoside/nucleotide reverse transcriptase inhibitors (NRTIs), **233–236**
nutritional status, and cancer therapy, 278

obsessive-compulsive disorder (OCD), 315
   dental management, 324–325
   epidemiology, 317
   medical management
      diagnosis, 318
      treatment, 320
   pathogenesis/etiology, 316
obstructive sleep apnea (OSA), 44
   medical management
      epidemiology, 47
      medical history/physical exam, 53
      pathogenesis/etiology, 47
      treatment, 56
   oral appliance for, 65, *65*
   questions for patient with, 59
   questions for physician of patient with, 59
occupational blood exposures, management of, 236, **237**, 238
odor, oral, in risk assessment, **9**
older adults. *See also* geriactric health
   prescribing drugs for, 16
   role of cognition in, 383–384

Open Wide® Disposable Mouth Rest, 295, *295*
opiate drugs, 332
opiate maintenance therapy (OMT), 344
opioid abuse and dependence, 332
   dental management
      evaluation, 341
      questions for patient, 342
      questions for physician of patient, 343
   epidemiology, 334
   medical management
      identification, 335–336
      medical history in, 336–337
      pharmacotherapy, 339
      treatment, 337–340
   oral lesions associated with, 346, *348*
   pathogenesis/etiology, 333
   physical exam/laboratory testing, 337
opioid drug-seeking behaviors, 354
opioid maintenance therapy (OMT), 339
opioid use
   ADA on, 345
   for dental patients, 346
opportunistic infections
   in AIDS, 218
   in risk assessment, **9**
oral cavity, SCC of, 267, 267–268
oral contraceptives, and antibiotic therapy, 416. *See also* contraceptive use
oral disease. *See also specific disease*
   in geriatric health, 395
   systemic disease in, 7, **8–9**, 10, *10*, *11*
oral/jaw pain, in risk assessment, **9**
oral malodor, in risk assessment, **9**
oral squamous cell carcinoma, 350, *350*. *See also* squamous cell carcinoma
OraQuick ADVANCE® Rapid HIV-1/2 antibody test, 221, *222*
OraQuick HCV Antibody Test, 125
orofacial clefts (OFCs), 359, *359*
   dental management
      oral manifestations, 377
      treatment modifications, 372–375, *373–375*, **375**
   epidemiology, 363
   medical management
      diagnosis, 365
      treatment, 366–368, *367*
   pathogenesis/etiology, 361
   prosthetic considerations in, 374–375, **375**, *375*
   questions for patient with, 369
   questions for physician of patient with, 369
orofacial findings, in PSS, 207, **207**
orofacial granulomatosis (OFG), 244
oropharynx, cancer of, 268, 347
orthopedic disorders
   dental management, 378
   epidemiology, 363
   hereditary, 359–360, **360**
   medical management
      diagnosis, 365
      treatment, 368
   and oral health care, 375–377, **376**
   pathogenesis/etiology, 361
   questions for patient with, 369
   questions for physician of patient with, 369
OSAHS (obstructive sleep apnea/hypopnea syndrome), 44
osteoarthritis (OA), 383, *383*
   diagnosis of, 389
   epidemiology, 388
   treatment for, 390
osteogenesis imperfecta (OI), 358, 360
osteolysis, in MM, 158
osteonecrosis
   of mandible, 417, *420*
   in risk assessment, **9**
osteoporosis, 400
   dental management, 410–411
   and drug interactions, 417, **418**, **419**
   epidemiology, 401
   laboratory testing in, 403
   medications for prevention of, 417, **418**
   pathogenesis/etiology, 400
   treatment for, 403–404
osteoradionecrosis (ORN), and cancer therapy, 277, 277–278
outpatient dental procedures, for patients on coumadin, 184, *184*, *185*
overdose, methamphetamine, 353
oxygen, supplemental
   during dental treatment, 22
   in patient with COPD, 64

oxygen delivery systems, 426
oxygen therapy
   for asthma attack, 65
   in COPD, 55
   in medical emergency, 302

pacemaker, 30, *30*
pain management, 19, 22
   in hepatic disease, 124
   in SUDs, 344, 346
palatal lift, 372
pancreatic cancer, 69
   coordination with physician of patient with, 71
   dental management
      evaluation, 73
      oral lesions, 75–76
      questions for patient with, 74
      questions for physician of patient with, 75
   drug actions/interactions in, 78
   elective dental treatment during, 75
   medical management, 72
   pathogenesis/etiology, 70, 71
parathyroid hormone, in CKD, **100**
Parkinson's disease (PD), 281
   classical features of, 287
   compared with HD, 102–103
   dental management, 109, 296
   epidemioloy of, **284**
   medical management of, 287, 289
   medications used in, **288**
   pathogenesis/etiology of, 285
   tolerance to dental care in, 300
patient education
   for HIV-infected patients, 238
   for oral hygiene during pregnancy, 407, 410
   in RA, 205
patient instruction sheet, for transplant patients, 112
patient management, in cognitive impairment/dementia, 395–396
pemphigus vulgaris (PV), 246, *246*
peptic ulcer disease (PUD), 128
   dental management, 138
   epidemiology, 132
   medical management, 134

oral lesions in, 138
pathogenesis/etiology, 129
periodontal disease
   HIV-associated, 229, 229–230
   osteoporosis-related, 82
   during pregnancy, 406, 407, *407*
   and risk of preterm/LBW delivery, 406–407
   in untreated DM, 75, *76*
periodontitis
   in leukemia, 164–165
   necrotizing ulcerative, **226**, *229*, 229–230
peritoneal dialysis (PD), 99, 102
pernicious anemia, 148
petechiae
   in aplastic anemia, 166, *166*
   in bleeding disorders, 186
   in risk assessment, **8**, 11, *12*
petit malseizures, 283
phobias, 315
   dental management, 324–325
   diagnosis of, 318–319
   epidemiology of, 317
   medical management, 320
   pathogenesis/etiology, 316
phosphorus, in CKD, **100**
physical evaluation
physical evaluation, in risk assessment, 5, 7
physical examination, in CVD, 30. *See also specific disease*
Physical Status Score of, of ASA, 5, **6**
physicians, patient, communication with, 7, 34
pink puffers, 49. *See also* emphysema
platelet count, 178, **179**
platelet defects, drug-induceed, 186
platelet deficiencies, in patients with CKD, 99
platelet disorders, 173–174, **174**, **177**
   dental management of, 183
   drug-induced, **174**, 175–176
   treatment for, 180
platelet function analyzer 100 (PFA-100), **179**, 180
platelet inhibitors, for patient with CVD, **32**
Pneumocystis carinii pneumonia (PCP), 218
polyps, inflammatory, 130
positron emission technology (PET) scan, in head and neck cancer, 265

postexposure prophylaxis (PEP), for
    HIV-infected patients, 236, **237**, 238
postprandial distress syndrome, 127
posttraumatic stress disorder (PTSD), 315
    dental management, 324
    epidemiology, 317
    identification, 318
    medical management, 320
    pathogenesis/etiology, 316
potassium, in CKD, **100**
potassium channel opener, for patient with
    CVD, **32**
prediabetes, 70
pregnancy, 400
    dental management
        dental radiographs during, 410
        drugs during, **416**
        elective treatment, 410
        emergency treatment, 410
        positioning, 417, *421*
        preventive program during, 407, *408–409*,
            410
        questions for patient's physician, 406
        treatment modifications, 405–410, *407*,
            408–409
    diagnosis of, 402
    drug actions/interactions during, 414–415,
        416
    epidemiology, 401
    laboratory testing in, 403
    medical management of, 403
"pregnancy tumor," 406, *407*
presbycusis, 382–383
presbyopia. *See* age-related macular
    degeneration
preschool children
    dental management of craniofacial
        anomalies in, 372
    dental management of OFCs in, 367
preterm birth (PTB), and periodontal disease,
    401, 406–407
primary biliary cirrhosis (PBC), 191
    dental management
        oral lesions, 209, *210*
        treatment modifications, 205–206
    drug interactions in, 212, **213**

epidemiology, 193
hemostasis in, 212
medical management
    identification, 195
    laboratory testing, 201
    medical history/physical exam, 198
    treatment, 202
pathogenesis/etiology, 192
susceptibility to infection in, 212
tolerance to dental care in, 212
professional conduct, and HIV-infected
    patients, 238, 239
progressive systemic sclerosis (PSS), 192
    dental management
        oral lesions, 209, *210*
        treatment modifications, 207
    epidemiology, 193
    medical management
        identification, 195–196, *196*
        laboratory testing, 201
        medical history/physical exam, 198–199
        treatment, 202, **203**
    pathogenesis/etiology, 192
    tolerance to dental care in, 214
propranolol, drug interactions with, **19**
prostate cancer, 110–111
prosthetic appliances, for managing OFCs,
    374, **375**
prosthetic joints, dental treatment of patients
    with, 208
protease inhibitors, **234–235**
protein restriction, in renal insufficiency, 99
prothrombin time (PT), 178, **179**, 180
proton beam therapy (IMPT), 270
pseudomembranous colitis (PC), 128
    epidemiology, 132
    medical management of, 135
    pathogenesis/etiology, 130
pseudopolyps, 130
psychiatric disorders, 314–316
    coordination with physician of patient with,
        317
    dental management
        evaluation, 323
        medical emergencies, 326
        oral lesions, 325, *326*

questions for patient with, 323
questions for physician of patient with, 323
risks associated with, 325
treatment modifications, 323–325, *324*
drugs used in, **321–322**
epidemiology of, 317–318
medical management
diagnosis, 318–319
treatment, 319, **321–322**, 323
pathogenesis/etiology, 316–317
psychological stress, of dental treatment, 21
psychotic disorders, 315
dental management, 324–325
epidemiology of, 317
identification of, 319
medical management, 320
pathogenesis/etiology, 316
ptosis, in risk assessment, **8**
puberty, 399, 404
pulmonary disease, 43–44
coordination with physician of patient with, 48
dental management
evaluation, 56
medical emergencies, 64–65
oral lesions, 62–63
risks associated with, 63–65
treatment modifications, 59–62
epidemiology of, 47–48
laboratory testing in, 53, **53**
medical history in, 48–58, **49**, **50**, **53**
medical management
identification, 48, *48*
treatment, **54**, 54–56
pathogenesis/etiology of, 44–47
physical examination in, 48–58, **49**, **50**, **53**
purpura, in risk assessment, 11, *12*
pyoderma gangrenosum, 139
pyostomatitis vegetans, 139, *139*

quality of life, and age-related hearing loss, 383

radiation caries, 276, *276*
radiation therapy
dental management of, 163–164, 273–274, *274*
for head and neck cancer, 269–270

radiographic signs, of medical disease, 10, **11**
radiographs, dental, during pregnancy, 410
range of motion (ROM), in RA, 197
RANKL, 404
Raynaud's phenomenon, 194, *195*
records, patient's, confidentiality of, 239
red blood cells (RBCs)
in CBC, **156**
sickle-shaped, 146, *147*
renal cell carcinoma, 110
renal diseases, 95. *See also* kidney disease
renal impairment, prescribing drugs in, 16
renal transplant recipients, dental management of, 111–112. *See also* kidney transplantation
rescue inhaler, prophylactic use of, 64
respiratory difficulty, as medical emergency, 431–433, *433*
restrictive lung diseases, 44
dental management, 60
medical history/physical examination in, 51, **53**
medical management of, 55
pathogenesis/etiology of, 46
positioning of patient with, 64
pulmonary functions in, **53**
retinopathy, diabetic, 382, 386
epidemiology, 387–388
treatment for, 390
reverse transcriptase-initiated polymerase chain reaction (RT-PCR), 221
review of systems, in physical evaluation, 7
rheumatoid arthritis (RA), 191
autoantibodies associated with, **201**
dental management, 205
diagnosis criteria for, 196
drug interactions in, 212, **213**
epidemiology, 193
hemostasis in, 211–212
medical management
identification, 194–195, *195*
laboratory testing, 201
medical history and physical exam, 197–198
treatment, 202
pathogenesis/etiology, 192

rheumatoid arthritis (RA) (continued)
  progression of, **195**
  susceptibility to infection in, 212
  tolerance to dental care in, 212
risk assessment
  communication with patient's physician in, 7
  and dental management modifications, 21–22
  physical signs in, 5, 7
  Physical Status Score in, 5, **6**
  purposes of, 5
  systemic disease in, 7, **8–9**, 10, *10*, *11*
risks of dental care, four key, 3. *See also specific conditions*
rivaroxaban (Xarelto), 176, 186
rubber dams, in patient with COPD, 64

salivary glands
  cancer of, 268
  and cancer therapy, 275–276, *276*
saliva substitutes, 230
SBIRT (screening, brief intervention, referral, and treatment), in SUDs, 235
SCA. *See* sickle cell anemia
schizophrenia, 315
  dental management, 324–325
  epidemiology of, 317
  identification of, 319
  medical management, 320
  pathogenesis/etiology, 316
sclerodactyly, *196*
scleroderma, 192. *See also* progressive systemic sclerosis
  autoantibodies associated with diffuse, **201**
  in risk assessment, **10**
sclerosing syndromes, 191, 192
scoliosis, 360
  conditions associated with, 365
  dental management, **376**, 376–377
  early *vs.* late onset, 365
  medical management
    diagnosis, 365
    treatment, 368
  pathogenesis/etiology, 361
  physical manifestations of, 360

  prevalence of, 364
  tolerance to dental care in patient with, 378
screening
  for head and neck cancer, 261–263, **262**
  for hemostatic disorders, **179**
  for oral SCC, **262**
  for SUDs, 336
sedatives
  drug interactions with, **19**
  in hepatic disease, 124
seizure disorders, 282
  dental management, 297, **298**
  diagnosis of, 293
  medical treatment of, 293, **294**
  pathogenesis/etiology of, 286
  tolerance to dental care in, 302
seizures, 431
  absence, 283
  atonic, 283
  drop, 283
  generalized, 283
  myoclonic, 283
  partial, 282–283
  petit mal, 283
  tonic-clonic, 283
"shoe" referral cards, 412
Sicca symptoms, 199
sickle cell anemia (SCA), 144
  epidemiology, 150
  inheritance pattern for, *148*
  laboratory testing, **153**
  oral lesions in, 167
  pathogenesis/etiology of, 146, *147*, *148*
  stair step appearance of alveolar bone in, 166, *166*
sickle cell trait, 146
side effects, of systemic drugs, **20**
Sjögren's syndrome (SS), 191, 192
  autoantibodies associated with, **201**
  dental management
    evaluation, 203–205
    oral lesions, 210–211, *211*
    questions for patient with, 204
    questions for physician of patient with, 204
    treatment modifications, 207

epidemiology, 193
international classification criteria for, 200
medical management
  identification, 196–197
  laboratory testing, 201–202
  medical history/physical exam, 199
  treatment, 202, **203**
pathogenesis/etiology, 192–193
xerostomia in, 210, *211*
skin
  hereditary conditions affecting, 358–359, *359*
  in risk assessment, **8**, **10**
  in scleroderma, 195–196, 202
smokeless tobacco (ST), 332
smoker's melanosis, 349, *350*
snuff dipper's lesion, 349, *349*
sodium, in CKD, **100**
speech, and cancer therapy, 278
speech bulb, 372, *373*
spider angioma, in risk assessment, 12, *13*
spina bifida, 360
  dental management, 377
  medical management
    diagnosis, 365
    treatment, 368
  pathogenes/etiology, 361, 363
  prevalence of, 364
  secondary conditions associated with, 366
  susceptibility to infection in, 378
spina bifida oculta, 365
spinal cord injuries, 359–360, **360**
  clinical features related to, **360**
  dental management, 376, **376**
  medical management, 365
  pathogenesis/etiology, 361
  prevalence of, 364
squamous cell carcinoma (SCC)
  of head and neck, 257
  of lower lip, *260*
  oral, *267*, 267–268, 350, *350*
  screening for oral, **262**
stenosis, valvular, 27
steroid supplementation, 21
steroid therapy, 82–83
steroid use, in risk assessment, **10**
Steven-Johnson syndrome (SJS), 248, *249*

stomatitis
  aphthous, 250–251, *251*
  contact, 243–244, *244*
  nicotine, 348, *349*
  with systemic drugs, **20**
stress
  body's response to, 17
  of dental treatment, 3, 17–19
stress management
  during dental treatment, 22
  postoperative, 22
stress reduction, 21
stroke, 281–282. *See also* cerebrovascular accident
  dental management for patient with, **301**
  as medical emergency, 302–303
  tolerance to dental care in, 300, **301**, *301*, 302
Sturge-Weber syndrome, in risk assessment, **10**
substance use disorders (SUDs), 331–332
  coordination of care with physician of patient with, 334–335
  craniofacial trauma associated with, 346
  dental management
    evaluation, 340–343
    medical emergencies, 353
    oral lesions associated with, 346–350, *347–350*
    pain management, 344, 346
    risks associated with, 350–351, **351–352**, 353
    treatment modifications, 343–346
  epidemiology, 333–334
  management of
    pharmacological, 338
    psychiatric, 338
    psychosocial, 338
  medical management
    identification, 335–336
    medical history in, 336–337
    SBIRT, 235
    treatment, 337–340
  pathogenesis/etiology, 332–333, **333**
  physical exam/laboratory testing, 337
  signs of, 341
sulfasalazine, in GI disease, 141, *141*

Surgeon General, family health history
  initiative of, 5
surgery
  and anticoagulant therapy, 13–14
  for head and neck cancer, 268–269, *269*
Surveillance Epidemiology and End Results
  (SEER), for head and neck cancer, 260
Sutton's disease, 251
swallowing
  and cancer therapy, 278
  of foreign object, 432–433
swelling, soft tissue, in risk assessment, **9**
systemic diseases, stomatitis-like ulcers
  associated with, 250. *See also specific
  disease*
systemic lupus erythematosus (SLE), 191
  autoantibodies associated with, **201**
  dental management
    oral lesions, 209, *210*
    treatment modifications, 205
  drug interactions in, 212, **213**
  epidemiology, 193
  hemostasis in, 211
  laboratory testing in, 199, **201**
  medical management
    identification, 194, *195*
    medical history and physical exam, 197
    treatment, 202
  pathogenesis/etiology, 192
  in risk assessment, **10**
  susceptibility to infection in, 212
  tolerance to dental care in, 212

taste alteration, with systemic drugs, **20**
teeth
  early loss of, **9**
  hereditary conditions affecting, 357–358
telangiectasias, in risk assessment, **8**
temporomandibular disorders (TMDs), 413
  in FM, 206–207
  in patients with RA, 205
temporomandibular joint (TMJ) articular space
  destruction, in risk assessment, **11**
tender-point examination, in FM, 198, *198*
thalassemia, 144–145
  epidemiology, 150

  laboratory testing, **153**
  pathogenesis/etiology of, 146
theophylline, 55
thrombin time (TT), 178, **179**, 180
thrombocytopenia, **174**, 175
  gingival oozing, 176, *176*
  in risk assessment, **12**, **13**
  treatment, 180
thyroid cancer
  coordination with physician of patient with,
    87
  dental management
    evaluation, 90
    treatment modifications, 90, 91
  diagnosis of, 87
  epidemiology, 86–87
  histological types, 86
  medical management, 88
  susceptibility to infection in, 91
  types of, 85–86
thyroid crisis, signs of, 86
thyroid disease
  characteristics of, **85**
  dental management
    evaluation, 88
    medical emergencies, 91–92
    oral lesions, 90
    risks associated with, 91
    treatment modifications, 90
  epidemiology, 86–87
  etiology of, 84–85
  major, 84–85
  medical management
    diagnosis, 87
    treatment, 87–88
  pathogenesis/etiology, 86
thyroidectomy, 88
thyrotoxic crisis (thyroid storm), 88
tissue reflectance test, for head and neck
  cancer, 262–263
tobacco
  and head and neck cancer, 257–258, *260*
  impact on wound healing, 353
tobacco cessation
  and drug actions/interactions, **352**
  five A's brief intervention for, 354–355

tobacco control, biomarkers of, 337
tobacco dependence, 332
   dental management
      evaluation, 341, 343
      questions for patient with, 343
   epidemiology, 334
   medical management
      combination pharmacotherapy, 340
      identification, 336
      medical history, 337
      pharmacotherapy, 339–340
      treatment, 339–340
   oral lesions associated with, 348–350, *348–350*
   pathogenesis/etiology, 333.**333**
   physical exam/laboratory testing, 337
tobacco use, treating, 344f
toddlers
   dental management of craniofacial anomalies in, 372
   dental management of OFCs in, 367
tolerance to dental care, 17, 19–21
   in autoimmune and connective tissue diseases, 212–214
   of DGI-1 patients with OI, 378
   in DM, 78
   in endocrine and metabolic disorders, 93
   in geriatric health, 396
   in GI disease, 141
   in head and neck cancer, 278
   in hematological disease, 169
   in hepatic disease, 124–125
   in HIV-infected patients, 232, 236
   in neurodevelopmental disorders, 314
   in neurological disease, 300, **301**, *301*, 302
   in pancreatic cancer, 78
   in patients with SUDs, 353
   of patient with CVD, 38–39
   in pregnancy, 417, *421*
   in psychiatric disorders, 326
   in pulmonary diseases, 63
   in thyroid disease, 91
toluidine blue screening test, for head and neck cancer, 261–262
tongue, coated, with systemic drug use, **20**
tongue-retaining device, 65

tonic seizures, 283
toothbrushes
   adaptations for, 393, *395*
   modification of, 295
toxic epidermal necrolysis (TEN), 248, 249–250
transepithelial oral cytology, 262
transient ischemic attack (TIA)
   defined, 285
   as medical emergency, 302–303
transitional cell carcinoma, of kidney, 110
TRAP findings, in PD, 287, 296
trauma, in risk assessment, **8**
traumatic brain injury (TBI), 282
   classification of, 292
   dental management, 297
   epidemiology of, **284**
   medical management, 292–293
   pathogenesis/etiology of, 286
tricyclic antidepressants, drug interactions with, **19**
trigeminal neuralgia (TN), 287, 299
trismus
   and cancer therapy, 277
   in risk assessment, **9**
Trisomy 21. *See* Down syndrome
TSH suppression, 88
tuberculosis (TB), 44
   coinfection with HIV virus, 224
   dental management, 60, 61
   drug interactions in patient with, 63
   epidemiology of, 47
   Mantoux tuberculin skin test for, 52, **52**
   medical history/physical examination in, 51–53
   medical management of, 55
   pathogenesis/etiology of, 46
   questions for patient with, 58
   questions for physician of patient with, 59

ulcerations. *See also* aphthous ulcerations; stomatitis
   in Behçet's disease, *252*
   palliative management of oral, 165
   with systemic drugs, **20**

ulcerative colitis (UC), 128
　medical management of, 135
　oral lesions in, 138–139, *139*
　pathogenesis/etiology, 129
ultraviolet light, and head and neck cancers, 259
unconsciousness, as medical emergency, 430
uremia, dental management in, 187
uremic bleeding diathesis, treatment considerations in, 105
urinary tract, cancers of, 110
urinary tract diseases, 95

vaccination, HBV, 125
vaccination programs, for hepatitis disease, 117
valvular cardiomyopathy, dental management of patient with, 36
valvular heart disease, 27–28
varenicline, 340
varicella zoster virus infection, in HIV-infected patients, 230
vasovagal syncope, 426, **427**, 430
velopharyngeal function, 367
vesiculobullous diseases, 245–248
　epidermolysis bullosa (EB), 247–248
　mucous membrane pemphigoid, 247, *247*
　pemphigus group, 246, 247–248
violence against women, interpersonal, 400
　dental management, 411–413, *412*
　epidemiology, 401–402
　medical management, 403
viral hepatitis, 115
　epidemiology, **117**, 117–118
　medical management
　　laboratory testing, 119–120
　　medical history/physical examination, 118–119
　　treatment, 120–121
　pathogenesis/etiology, 115–117, **116**
viral infections
　and cancer therapy, 275
　in leukemic patient, 165, *165*
viruses, hepatitis, **116**
visual changes, age-related
　dental management
　　evaluation, 392
　　questions for patient with, 393
　　treatment modifications, 394
　dental office accommodations for, 397
　medical management
　　diagnosis of, 389
　　epidemiology, 387–388
　　treatment, 389–390
　pathogenesis/etiology, 384, 386
vital signs
　in physical evaluation, 7
　in physical examination, 30
vitamin B$_{12}$-deficiency anemia, 145, 148–149
　epidemiology, 150
　laboratory testing, **154**
vitamin K, coagulation disorders caused by, 175
vitamins, commonly used, **16**
von Willebrand disease (vWD), **174**
　dental management in, 183
　epidemiology, 176

warfarin (coumadin)
　coagulation disorders caused by, 175
　dental care of patients receiving, *185*
　epidemiology of anticoagulation disorders caused by, 176
warfarin therapy. *See also* anticoagulants
　laboratory testing in, 31
　management of dental patients on, 13
warts, oral, in HIV-infected patients, 228–229, *229*
wasting syndrome, in risk assessment, **10**
Western blot assay, 221
wheelchair
　positioning for providing oral hygiene for patient in, *313*
　transfer to dental chair from, 376, **376**
wheelchair transfer, two-person, *301*
white blood cell (CBC) count, and disease-related changes, **156**
Wickham's striae, 253
Wilms' tumor, 110
wire splint, for dento-alveolar fracture, 411, *412*
women's health
　breast cancer, 400

coordination with woman's physician, 402
defined, 399
dental management
  and contraception use, 410
  evaluation, 404
  oral lesions, 413, *414*
  questions for patient, 405
  risks associated with, 414–421, **416**, **418–421**
  treatment modifications, 404–412, *407–409*, *412*
epidemiology, 401–402
interpersonal violence, 400
medical management
  diagnoses, 402–403
  laboratory testing, 403
  treatment, 403–404
menopause, 400
osteoporosis, 400
pathogenesis/etiology, 400–401
pregnancy, 400
puberty onset and menses, 399
Women's Health Initiative (WHI), 403
World Health Organization (WHO), 331
wound healing, in risk assessment, **9**

xerostomia, 75. *See also* dry mouth
  and cancer therapy, 275–276, *276*
  in HIV-infected patients, 230–231
  in patients with RA, 205
  in SS, 210, *211*
  with systemic drugs, **20**
  in untreated DM, 75, *76*
x-rays, chest, in head and neck cancer, 264
x-rays, dental, in head and neck cancer, 264

zidovudine, for occupational blood exposure, 238